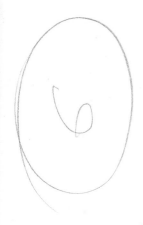

The Practice of Emergency Nursing

James H. Cosgriff, Jr., M.D., F.A.C.S.

Clinical Assistant Professor of Surgery, State University of New York at Buffalo

Chairman, New York State Emergency Medical Services Council

Member, Advisory Committee of the Emergency Department Nurses Association

Diann Laden Anderson, R.N., M.N.

Instructor, Department of Health Sciences, San Jose City College

Staff Nurse Emergency Department, Good Samaritan Hospital, San Jose, California

Chairman, Committee on Educational Standards, Emergency Department Nurses Association

J. B. Lippincott Company

Philadelphia

New York   Toronto

Distributed in Great Britain by Blackwell Scientific
Publications, London, Oxford, Edinburgh.

ISBN 0-397-54169-4

Printed in the United States of America

3   5   7   9   8   6   4   2

Library of Congress Cataloging in Publication Data

Main entry under title:

The Practice of emergency nursing.

   Includes bibliographies and index.
   1.   Emergency nursing.   I.   Cosgriff, James H.
II.   Anderson, Diann.   [DNLM: 1.   Emergencies—
Nursing texts.   2.   Hospital emergency service.
WY156 C834]
RT42.P7   610.73   75-20303
ISBN 0-397-54169-4

dedication

To
Mary Louise, Nancy, Maribeth and Jim

To
Carl, Kirsten and Eric

contributors

Carl T. Anderson, R.P.T., M.A.
Assistant Professor, Department of Occupational Therapy, San Jose State University, San Jose, California

John D. Bartels, M.D., F.A.C.O.G.
Associate Clinical Professor of Obstetrics and Gynecology, State University of New York at Buffalo
Attending Obstetrician and Gynecologist, Sisters of Charity Hospital, Buffalo, New York

Barbara Bates, M.D.
Professor of Medicine, School of Medicine and Dentistry, University of Rochester, Rochester, New York

Rita E. Caughill, R.N., M.S.
Associate Professor, School of Nursing, State University of New York at Buffalo

Gregory M. Chudzik, Pharm. D.
Assistant Professor of Pharmacy, State University of New York at Buffalo

James M. Cole, M.D.
Associate Clinical Professor of Surgery (Orthopedics), State University of New York at Buffalo
Chief, Department of Orthopedic Surgery, Buffalo General Hospital, Buffalo, New York

Jane C. Donahue, R.N., J.D.
Assistant Professor, School of Nursing, and Assistant Clinical Professor, School of Medicine, State University of New York at Buffalo

Karilyn R. Duarte, R.N., M.S.
Instructor, Department of Health Sciences, and Coordinator, Emergency Medical Technician Program, San Jose City College, San Jose, California

Donna Duell, R.N., M.S.N.
Assistant Professor, San Jose State University
CPR Instructor, American Heart Association, San Jose, California

Florence B. Dziekan, R.N.
Supervisor, Burn Treatment Center, Emergency Hospital, Buffalo, New York

Mildred K. Fincke, R.N., B.S.
Associate Director, Emergency/Ambulatory Services, and Project Director, Emergency/Ambulatory Nurse Practitioner Program, Allegheny General Hospital, Pittsburgh, Pennsylvania
President, Emergency Department Nurses Association (1975)

Mary Furth, M.D., M.P.H.
Associate Clinical Professor, School of Pharmacy, University of Maryland Coordinator, Adolescent Suicide Program, University of Maryland Hospital, Baltimore

Joseph P. Gambacorta, M.D.
Attending Surgeon (Urology), Sisters of Charity Hospital, St. Joseph's Intercommunity Hospital and Emergency Hospital, Buffalo, New York

Cathy Gray, R.N.
Emergency Department Nurse, Maricopa County General Hospital, Phoenix, Arizona

Harry W. Hale, Jr., M.D., F.A.C.S.
Chairman, Department of Surgery, Maricopa County General Hospital, Pheonix, Arizona
Member, Emergency Care Committee, Maricopa County Medical Society

Paul A. Kennedy, M.D., F.A.C.S.
Associate Clinical Professor of Surgery, Stanford University, Palo Alto, California
Attending Surgeon, Peninsula Hospital, Burlingame, California; Mills Memorial Hospital, San Mateo, California; and Chope Hospital, San Mateo, California

Betty N. Lawson, R.N., M.S.
Associate Professor, School of Nursing, State University of New York at Buffalo

Joan E. Lynaugh, R.N., M.S.N.
Assistant Professor, School of Nursing, University of Rochester, Rochester, New York
Nurse Clinician, Ambulatory Care, Strong Memorial Hospital, Rochester, New York

Gordon F. Madding, M.D., F.A.C.S.
Associate Clinical Professor of Surgery, Stanford University, Palo Alto, California
Attending Physician, Peninsula Hospital, Burlingame, California and Mills Memorial Hospital, San Mateo, California

Albert D. Menno, M.D., F.A.C.S.
Assistant Clinical Professor of Surgery, State University of New York at Buffalo
Attending Surgeon, Deaconess Hospital and E. J. Meyer Memorial Hospital, Buffalo, New York
Director, Dialysis and Transplant Unit, Deaconess Hospital, Buffalo, New York
Executive Director, Kidney Bank of Buffalo, New York

Thomas S. Morse, M.D., F.A.C.S.
Associate Professor of Surgery, College of Medicine, Ohio State University, Columbus, Ohio
Director, Surgical Outpatient Services, Children's Hospital, Columbus, Ohio
President, American Trauma Society

M. Kathleen Pendleton, R.N., M.S.
Associate Professor, Department of Nursing, San Jose State University, San Jose, California

R. Brian Pendleton, Ph.D.
Associate Professor, Department of Psychology, San Jose State University, San Jose, California

George Reading, M.D., F.A.C.S.
Associate Professor of Surgery, School of Medicine, State University of New York at Buffalo
Attending Plastic Surgeon, E. J. Meyer Memorial Hospital, Buffalo, New York

A. J. Rice, M.D.
Physician, Emergency Department, Kaweah Delta Hospital, Visalia, California

Mary C. Sand, R.N.
Head Nurse, Department of Urology, Sisters of Charity Hospital, Buffalo, New York

Arthur J. Schaefer, M.D., F.A.C.S.
Associate Clinical Professor, School of Medicine, State University of New York at Buffalo
Chief of Ophthalmology, Sisters of Charity Hospital and St. Joseph's Intercommunity Hospital, Buffalo, New York
Director, Ophthalmic Plastic and Reconstructive Surgery Clinic, E. J. Meyer Memorial Hospital and Deaconess Hospital, Buffalo, New York

Joseph C. Serio, M.D.
Chief of Otolaryngology, Sisters of Charity Hospital and Emergency Hospital, Buffalo, New York
Attending Physician, Veteran's Administration Hospital, Buffalo, New York

Sandra M. Stewart, M.D.
Assistant Medical Director, Ambulatory Services, Children's Hospital, Columbus, Ohio

James S. Williams, M.D., F.A.C.S.
Associate Clinical Professor, School of Medicine and Dentistry, University of Rochester, Rochester, New York
Surgical Consultant, Willard Psychiatric Center, Rochester, New York
Attending Physician, Strong Memorial Hospital and Rochester General Hospital, Rochester, New York
Director, American Trauma Society, New York State Chapter

William D. Ziter, D.M.D.
Associate Professor and Acting Chairman, Department of Oral Surgery, State University of New York at Buffalo
Attending Oral Surgeon, Buffalo General Hospital and E. J. Meyer Memorial Hospital, Buffalo, New York
Consulting Oral Surgeon, Roswell Park Memorial Institute and Veteran's Administration Hospital, Buffalo, New York

contents

preface

Emergency nursing is perhaps the most recently recognized specialty in the nursing profession, and it is unique in several other ways. In no other specialty is there such a close professional relationship between nurses and physicians as exists in the emergency department, where both function independently and interdependently. Many activities of patient management which have been traditionally within the practice of medicine may be the responsibility of the nurse, in whole or in part, in the emergency setting.

As the emergency department has evolved in the years following World War II, demands for broader services have arisen. The emergency nurse, of necessity, has broadened her knowledge and increased her level of competence, to enable her to expand and extend her role in patient care. Because the "typical" patient presenting to the emergency department has an undiagnosed problem, the nurse in this situation must develop skills in the observation and identification of clinical signs and symptoms which are life-threatening, carry a high measure of risk or are pertinent to arriving at a correct diagnosis. Beyond this, the nurse must, if required, be able to initiate and maintain life-support measures for any critically ill or injured patient.

It was with these concepts in mind that we authors developed this volume as a single, comprehensive, practical source of information, which will provide the emergency nurse with sound principles, on which she can develop a plan of nursing management for her patient.

The material contained in this volume includes a philosophy of emergency nursing which has been recognized and accepted by the Board of

Directors of the Emergency Department Nurses Association. Other aspects of concern to the emergency nurse include staffing and equipping a hospital emergency department, the role of the emergency department in a regionalized system of care, the legal aspects of emergency care and acquisition of donor organs for transplantation. The chapters devoted to clinical areas cover a broad range of subjects, from triage and assessment to specifics of wound management and care of a wide range of medical and surgical emergencies. Acute psychiatric problems are discussed in detail, but more importantly, this chapter stresses the importance of awareness on the part of the emergency nurse in detecting *any* deviation from normal behavior in a patient.

It is hoped this volume will enable the nurse to participate knowledgeably as a clinical specialist and as a colleague with the physician to provide quality emergency care. Because we believe this is most important, the majority of chapters in this text have been coauthored by a physician and a nurse, recognizing their goals to be similar and their roles symbiotic.

While we are keenly aware of the increasing numbers of men in the nursing profession and the mixture of male and female patients visiting the emergency department, a decision was made to take editorial license when reference is made to nurses and patients. Throughout the text, the emergency nurse is referred to in the female gender only, while patients are described in the male gender, except where the description applies only to a female patient.

This work has been conceived and written in response to an expressed need by *nurses* involved in giving emergency *nursing* care. In addition to emergency nurses, this includes industrial and/or school nurses who, more often than not, function independently. To date, no such book has met this need. It is hoped *The Practice of Emergency Nursing* will.

James H. Cosgriff, Jr.
Diann Anderson
July 1975

acknowledgments

It is difficult indeed to adequately express our appreciation to our many colleagues and friends who willingly gave us support, advice and guidance during the 3-year preparation of this volume. In particular, mention must be made of the following: Doctors Gaspare Alfano and John Curtin, each of whom read a portion of the manuscript and provided critical comments and helpful suggestions; Jane Lipp, M.D., who took time from the preparation of her own book to help us with ours; and to Maynard Schaus, who gave thoughtful direction during the earliest phase of the work. Special thanks are in order for Mrs. Anne Cohen, Medical Librarian at Sisters of Charity Hospital, for her help in obtaining reference volumes.

Rosanne Bratty, Maribeth Cosgriff, Nancy Cosgriff, Eleonore Barlog, Sandra Bogdanowicz and Linda Longoria spent many hours typing the manuscript and making textual corrections along the way. We are most grateful for their skill and untiring patience.

The teaching value of a volume such as this is greatly enhanced by well-conceived and factually correct illustrations. For these, we must acknowledge Dana Cadille, who prepared most of the illustrations initially, and Neil Hardy, who made most of the final drawings. Doctors Oscar Llugany and Humberto Revollo of the Department of Radiology of Sisters of Charity Hospital kindly made available the many fine x-rays which are presented throughout the text.

David T. Miller, Managing Editor of the Nursing Department of J. B. Lippincott, gave us not only the benefit of his years of experience in the field, but his personal support in this endeavor from the outset. We are personally grateful to him and to the J. B. Lippincott Company for their awareness of the need for a volume of this type and for sharing our interest in a high-quality publication.

It was a delightfully educational experience working with Gale Schricker, our copy editor. Her scrupulous reading of the manuscript and cogent suggestions added considerably to the readability of many difficult passages. She has "put it all together" in such a way that the seemingly endless proofreading was almost enjoyable. A special thanks is also due Lars Egede-Nissen for his availability and guidance when the inevitable problems arose.

Our warmest thanks go to our loving families, who shared in our daily joys and frustrations and who reluctantly, but good-naturedly, loaned us time to work on the manuscript.

Finally, we are deeply appreciative of our colleagues, our teachers, our students and our patients, who have taught us more than they will ever realize.

1

Introduction to
emergency nursing practice

DIANN ANDERSON

GENERAL CONSIDERATIONS

The typical image of the emergency nurse is of one who institutes grand and glorious life-saving activities in the busy emergency department of a large metropolitan hospital. What is not generally understood, however, is that such life-threatening emergencies comprise only about 5 percent of emergency department patient visits. Less well known to the general public are the more typical emergency department scenes: a nurse teaching first aid to lay persons or advanced training courses to emergency medical technicians and other nurses; a nurse helping a patient to understand his health problem and the ways he can cope with or control it; a nurse communicating information to a referral agency for provision of follow-up care for a previous patient.

From another point of view, emergency nursing is generally considered as that aspect of nursing care which is given in emergency department settings, although emergency nursing is practiced in many settings: schools, industries, mobile health units, community agencies and hospitals. Emergency nurses do not only initiate life-support measures; they also teach, counsel, comfort and refer. Thus, defining the practice of emergency nursing is a difficult, if not impossible, task, for emergency nursing is as varied as nursing practice itself.

If emergency nurses could be labeled at all, they might be called generalists in acute nursing care. Emergency nurses must possess an understanding of all kinds of health problems in all age groups, from the neonate to the very elderly person, and must understand the physical and emotional developmental tasks of each age group, especially as they relate to presenting health problems. Emergency nursing expertise must encompass the basic nursing specialty areas (obstetrics and gynecology, pediatrics, medical-surgical nursing, psychiatric–mental health nursing and community health nursing), to the extent that each one relates to acute care, and it must draw knowledge from subspecialty areas, such as rehabilitation, orthopedics and coronary care nursing, as well as many others.

Despite the encompassment of the above "definition" of emergency nursing practice, 2 commonalities are generally found in the patients cared for by emergency nurses: they have health problems which are (1) undiagnosed and (2) sufficiently acute to seek emergency care. These two characteristics, which serve to separate the emergency nurse from other nursing realms, mandate astute patient evaluation by the nurse.

Thus, assessment skills are as important in emergency nursing as life-support measures. Like technical skills, assessment skills require practice before perfected; unlike most technical skills, nursing assessment skills must be based on a wide foundation of knowledge, which serves to guide the nurse in collecting information, making observations and interpreting medical and nursing diagnoses to the patient and his family. This knowledge base is also needed as the nurse sorts and analyzes relevant information, communicates it to the patient's physician and develops her nursing care plan.

Because assessment, based on in-depth knowledge, is so important to emergency nursing practice, much of the content of subsequent chapters relates to the assessment of patients with selected complaints, signs and symptoms and to the knowledge base underlying it. While some of this information may initially seem more applicable to medical practice, it must be emphasized that effective nursing practice, especially in the newly expanding nursing roles, requires the acquisition of facts and concepts which are not found in traditional nursing knowledge.

Growing recognition of the breadth and depth of the knowledge and expertise needed to practice emergency nursing has raised it to the level of a nursing specialty. A national organization, the Emergency Department Nurses Association,* was formed in 1970 to meet the need of many emergency care nurses for an organization sensitive to their problems and goals. Its membership growth has been rapid; numerous local chapters have formed across the country.

Consistent with the activities of the American Nurses Association and other specialty organizations, the Emergency Department Nurses Association is refining criteria and developing educational programs and examinations for the certification of emergency nurses — the purpose being to recognize nursing excellence in this specialty and, ultimately, to improve the overall quality of health care given to the patient in the emergency department as well as at the scene of injury.

THE CHANGING SCOPE OF NURSING PRACTICE

The National Commission for the Study of Nursing and Nursing Education reported in 1970 that in the early years of the decade the nursing profession would be affected in 3 important areas:

> . . . striking changes in the levels of nursing; greater development of clinical specialization; and significant alterations in the reciprocal roles held by nurses and other health personnel, particularly the physician.[8, p. 69]

These changes apply to nursing practice in general and to emergency nursing practice in particular.

Levels of competence

Recognition of differences in emergency nurses' levels of competence has been a high-priority undertaking of the Emergency Department Nurses Association, which, as previously mentioned, is creating a core curriculum and certifying examinations to develop and recognize competence and excellence in emergency nursing practice. As one result of the Association's efforts, the certified "emergency nurse specialist" will represent a high level of competency in emergency nursing, by virtue of her in-depth knowledge and technical skill in this specialty area of nursing practice.

At another level, nurse-practitioner programs in emergency care are being planned and implemented, and nurse-practitioners †

---

* Headquarters office: The Emergency Department Nurses Association, P.O. Box 1566, East Lansing, Michigan 48823.

† While there is much variation in the educational programs which prepare nurses in this expanded role, generally nurse-practitioners share these commonalities: (1) they are registered professional nurses and graduates of basic nursing programs; (2) they have nursing and medical skills, notably history-taking and physical assessment skills; (3) they employ independent judgments within their

prepared in other specialties are now being employed in emergency care settings. It is already safe to state that much diversification in the nursing role is occurring and that competence at varying levels of practice in emergency care is emerging.

Clinical specialization

Programs to develop clinical specialization are also becoming evident in emergency nursing. One is the Trauma Nurse Specialist program in Illinois.[10] This intensive 4-week program prepares nurses to knowledgeably assess and care for injured patients. Other programs, ranging from one to 4 academic semesters, provide classroom and clinical experience to help the nurse more effectively assess and intervene in the care of patient problems common to the emergency setting.[1]

Reciprocal roles

As these changes in nursing education occur, so do changes in nursing practice. Nurses are increasingly finding that their roles are overlapping other roles, particularly the role of the physician. This overlapping is especially obvious in the emergency department, when nurse and physician work hand-in-hand to resuscitate a patient or when the nurse completes an initial assessment, including indicated laboratory tests and x-rays, before the physician is notified or sees the patient. While this sharing of responsibilities is discomforting to those who prefer to view nurse and physician functions in separate and well-defined spheres of medical and nursing practice, one can be more objective when these functions are seen in terms of patient care needs, as detailed in Figures 1–1, 1–2 and 1–3. (See pages 6–7.)

In the acute, episodic health care setting (such as the emergency department), the patient's problem is assessed by the most qualified available professional, and if im-

mediate intervention is needed, that, too, is initiated by the most qualified available professional. Providing quality care to the patient is more important than who does what; however, *quality care* implies competence in the provider of that care. Competence must be evaluated individually and must not be confined by traditional, often archaic modes or boundaries of practice. *Of particular importance is that adequate supervision and consultation be available whenever needed to insure that safe, quality care is given to the patient.*

In summary, changes in competence levels of nursing, development of clinical specialization and alterations in the reciprocity of roles are together changing the scope of nursing practice. These trends will invariably lead to increased confusion among nurses, other health care providers and consumers and will emphasize the need for nursing to articulate its beliefs and goals through a nursing philosophy.

A PHILOSOPHY OF EMERGENCY CARE NURSING

A philosophy takes time to articulate, for one must be introspective and analytical before being able to state with assurance, "This is what I believe and value." Although many nurses have not systematically described their own professional beliefs, they do possess them, and these beliefs are or should be a very important part of how nurses practice their profession. Bevis fittingly defines philosophy as:

> . . . the picture window through which the world is viewed. [It] . . . provides a point of view; it is a belief construct, a speculation about the nature and value of things.[3, p. 99]

Hence, the beliefs and values an individual holds about his or her own profession enable that individual to determine those professional activities which are important and the manner in which they are conducted. Stated another way, the professional philosophy one holds determines both one's practice of the profes-

---

own areas of competence; and (4) they participate in patient care directly or in consultation with the physician, while the final responsibility for medical care rests with the physician.

sion and one's goals for personal professional growth.

Just as the individual's philosophy is important, so, too, is the articulation of beliefs and values by the profession itself. Once the philosophy of nursing is defined, nurses can begin to make sense of it all; they can better identify who they are, what they are about and where they are going. With this self-knowledge, nursing can increase its influence over those activities which affect the profession and patient care. Bevis elaborates:

> It will be a foundation for a sense of identity, security, confidence and ultimately will enable a clear or a better identification of *purpose,* evolution of a *system* to achieve that purpose, and *creation* of new approaches to nursing problems.[3, p. 100]

Emergency nursing, as a clinical specialty within nursing, holds a philosophy which is consistent with the beliefs and values held by the profession. Important features of this shared philosophy are highlighted and developed here.

(1) *The central focus of emergency nursing practice is helping the patient to attain his highest possible level of general health.* This value is basic to nursing; in fact, it is the central focus of nursing practice, the reason for the profession's existence. It implies that nurses focus on:

> (1) motivating people to seek health; (2) identifying deviations from health; and (3) enhancing the coping mechanisms available for man's overcoming threats to health, his being restored to the highest possible level of health and function, and his adapting to circumstances that require alteration in life style and those over which he has no control.[12, p. 245]

In emergency nursing practice, patients are seen at all levels of wellness and with varying abilities to cope emotionally and physically with their health problems. The astute emergency nurse can identify and build upon the capabilities of individual patients and their families, as in the following examples.

An aware and concerned mother, who had little experience with childhood illnesses, brought her 1-year-old to the emergency department for the treatment of vomiting and diarrhea. The mother reported that the child had eaten nothing all day but a few french fries, which he loved. The child was diagnosed as having a viral gastroenteritis, and the mother was advised to limit his dietary intake until the medication took effect and the symptoms subsided. The nurse, recognizing the mother's need for dietary information and assessing her ability to comprehend it, explained the dietary plan. The nurse provided the mother with dietary instruction sheets, supplemented this information with her own knowledge and experience and responded to the mother's questions.

A young mother brought her feverish 10-month-old child to the emergency department for evaluation and treatment. The nurse observed that the baby and his sibling were unkempt and very dirty, as well as scantily clothed for the cold weather. During the interview, the nurse learned that the mother was unmarried, living alone and unaware of the basic health needs of children. The mother also indicated that she would welcome information and assistance concerning better care for her children. The nurse discussed her findings with the attending physician, who agreed that this family could benefit from a referral to a public health nurse. The emergency nurse recorded the relevant information she had collected about the family on the appropriate referral form and sent it to the public health nursing office in the family's residential area.

Emergency nurses care for those who are ill or injured, but they focus on assisting every patient to attain or maintain his best general level of health. This requires skills in assessment, decision making and patient teaching. Other skills used by emergency nurses derive from the areas of communication, leadership and problem solving and are particularly useful in team conferences and other activities which either directly or indirectly affect the quality of patient care.

(2) *Nursing's uniqueness lies in the synthesis of basic social and biological sciences into functions that promote health.* Almost every nursing act is an amalgamation of knowledge from many of the basic social and biological sciences: psychology, sociology,

bacteriology, chemistry, physics, anatomy and physiology. All of these sciences are used in unique ways within the practice of nursing, with little regard to individual levels of education and experience.

It is true that all professionals who provide health care do so through the application of some of the basic sciences, although their goals are different and separate from nursing goals. It is also generally agreed that medicine shares more commonalities with nursing than any other group of health care providers: both fields draw from a broad, eclectic knowledge base, both are concerned with total patient care and both rely on one another for the complete delivery of this care.[2] The roles of these 2 primary health professionals (nurses and doctors) are coordinate and complementary; yet, they are not the same. Wherein lies the difference? Schlotfeldt defines the difference in terms of primary intellectual concern—the central goal to which the professional's behavior is directed:

> The nurse's *primary* intellectual concern, and functions related thereto, is that of helping each person attain his highest possible level of general health; the physician's *primary* intellectual concern, and functions related thereto, is the diagnosis and treatment of illness.[11, p. 769]

The examples cited previously (concerning the mother who needed dietary information and the mother of the feverish child, who needed further evaluation, assistance and support) illustrate keen observation skills, coupled with concepts from the basic sciences which aid in planning nursing interventions which promote health. Another good example is the common and simple nursing act of elevating the head of the bed for an anxious, dyspneic patient with congestive heart failure. This action applies principles from anatomy, physiology, physics, chemistry and psychology.

In short, the nurse assesses the patient's deviation from health and his capabilities to cope with the problem; then the nurse plans for interventions to enable the patient to return to health or to a level of well-being, through the selective application of scientific knowledge known to alleviate the problem.

New trends in nurses' and physicians' roles are providing more complete and comprehensive care to the patient through an increased sharing of patient care activities between the 2 professions. It is expected that as new role relationships continue to evolve, those activities once unique to one profession will undoubtedly be more and more difficult to delineate. In her study of nurse-physician relationships in recent years, Bates notes this fact and that the role changes and merges can be represented schematically, as they are here, in Figures 1–1, 1–2 and 1–3.*

As may be seen in Figure 1–1, traditional nurse-physician roles involved some overlapping of activities, but it was minimal. Note also that a good share of the psychosocial needs of patients was left unmet.

The increased population growth and extended life expectancy of the 1960s placed greater work pressures on the physician, and he was often forced to limit his activities to the physical diseases and reduce his concern for the social and personal influences relating to the diseases. Figure 1–2 demonstrates how medicine retracted into the diagnostic and treatment role. Nursing moved to fill the gap created in the psychosocial area of patient care needs and ancillary nursing personnel increasingly tended to the physical and assistive needs of patients.

Finally, Figure 1–3 represents the efforts of both nursing and medicine to provide more complete and comprehensive health care to patients. The scope of their patient care activities has become broader than ever before, as is the overlapping of these activities. This trend is not universal; however, it does represent the influence of emerging roles in medicine and nursing on patient care.

* The concepts represented here by Figures 1–1, 1–2, and 1–3 were originally developed by Barbara Bates in *The New England Journal of Medicine* 283 (3):129–133 (July 16, 1970). The diagrams were not published, however, until Dr. Bates contributed them to The National Commission for the Study of Nursing and Nursing Education.[9]

Patient Care Needs

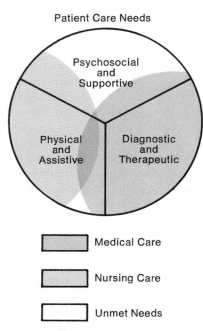

Medical Care

Nursing Care

Unmet Needs

Figure 1–1 Traditional breakdown of nurse and physician roles. As this diagram illustrates, there traditionally was little overlapping of nursing and medical roles, and much of patient care needs was left unmet. Source: National Commission for the Study of Nursing and Nursing Education, *From Abstract into Action,* p. 39. Copyright © 1973 by McGraw-Hill, Inc. Used with permission of McGraw-Hill Book Company.

These trends do not imply that either profession will lose its identity or total uniqueness. Rather, through close communication and collaboration, nursing and medicine will complement and support one another's roles, toward the enhancement of patient care.

(3) *Nursing functions are independent, interdependent and collaborative.* This statement affirms that nurses can and do function independently in patient care, including such activities as case finding, health counseling and teaching and providing care and comfort supportive to life or well-being. But, as nurses are prepared for new nursing roles, nursing activities will extend beyond the traditional boundaries of nursing practice. The Secre-

tary's Committee to Study Extended Roles for Nurses of the U.S. Department of Health, Education, and Welfare suggests that, one day, the following functions will be routine in acute care nursing:

(1) Securing and recording a health and developmental history and making a critical evaluation of such records as an adjunct to planning and carrying out a health care regimen in collaboration with medical and other health professionals.

(2) Performing basic physical and psychosocial assessments and translating the findings into appropriate nursing actions.

(3) Discriminating between normal and abnormal findings on physical and psycho-

Patient Care Needs

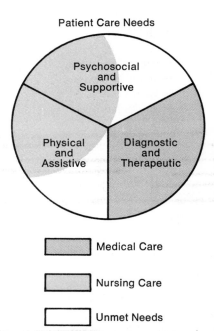

Medical Care

Nursing Care

Unmet Needs

Figure 1–2 Reoriented nurse and physician roles. The diagram illustrates that medicine has retreated into its strict domain, while nursing has adjusted its domain to include physical and psychological duties equally. However, a sizable portion of patient needs remains unmet. Source: National Commission for the Study of Nursing and Nursing Education, *From Abstract into Action,* p. 40. Copyright © 1973 by McGraw-Hill, Inc. Used with permission of McGraw-Hill Book Company.

Patient Care Needs

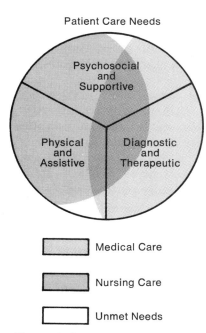

Medical Care

Nursing Care

Unmet Needs

Figure 1–3 Emergent nurse-physician roles. As medicine and nursing expand to include each of the 3 areas of patient care needs, entirely or in part, the total amount of patient care needs is almost completely covered.
Source: National Commission for the Study of Nursing and Nursing Education, *From Abstract into Action,* p. 41. Copyright © 1973 by McGraw-Hill, Inc. Used with permission of McGraw-Hill Book Company.

social assessments and reporting findings when appropriate.

(4) Making prospective decisions about treatment in collaboration with physicians. . . .

(5) Initiating actions and treatments within a protocol developed by medical and nursing personnel, such as making adjustments in medication, ordering and interpreting certain laboratory tests, and prescribing certain rehabilitative and restorative measures.[5, p. 10]

While these may become independent functions of the prepared nurse, in no way do the collaborative and interdependent components become less important. Patient problems and the knowledge and technology to treat them are so complex that the expertise of many health care providers is necessary. Communication, collaboration and teamwork now comprise an *essential* component in quality health care.

(4) *Nurses are responsible and accountable for their own actions.* Since nursing activities are independent, as well as interdependent and collaborative, nurses are becoming increasingly responsible and accountable for the care they give. Taking call and carrying a patient load are examples of increased responsibility for patient care which are operative in some nursing roles.

In addition, revisions and amendments to nursing practice acts and laws and legal decisions in malpractice suits in a number of states emphasize the fact that nurses can no longer rely on immunity from prosecution. Although in most states nurses function to a certain extent under the protective umbrella of the employing agency or supervising physician, as clinical expertise and expanded nursing roles are authorized and practiced, increased accountability for nursing actions will inevitably follow.[6] Hence, the practicing nurse must be competent in her specialty area, must seek learning experiences to supplement her knowledge and competence and must be cognizant of the legal limitations of practice.

Further, nurses must become more involved in the decisions and programs which affect their practice. Conversely, changes in agency policy, planning of educational offerings and other activities which affect nursing practice require input from nurses to insure success and relevancy.

(5) *Emergency nursing care is given both within and without hospital settings.* Lysaught stresses that "patient condition rather than location defines the care given."[7, p. 165] This applies especially to emergency nursing care. Emergencies arise in every imaginable location, and the possible variety of emergencies, singly and in combination, is infinite. Thus, concepts of emergency nursing practice apply to the care given in emergency situations, wherever they occur, in the community as well as in emergency departments of hospitals.

Nurses in all settings give emergency care in some form when necessary.

Emergency department nursing offers a wealth of learning experiences for developing competence in emergency nursing care, since applications can be made to any other patient care setting. In his discussion of episodic nursing practice, Lysaught affirms:

> (1) Nursing practice is broader than the traditional concerns of the hospital for treatment of grave illness, injury, or disease in the sense that nursing has long included elements of health maintenance, disease prevention, and nonacute patient care.
>
> (2) Acute, or episodic, nursing practice is not synonymous with hospital care even though this institution is the most common location for the provision of that care because of the concentration of personnel, resources, and equipment.[7, p. 165]

His point is that one of the key problems in health care is the system of *delivering* that care and bringing the needs and the resources into optimum balance.

Nurses can be directly involved in achieving this goal of optimal delivery of health care by supporting and contributing to activities that foster a closer relationship between the hospital and the community. Developing educational experiences is one such activity, for example, bringing an emergency medical technician into the emergency department to learn from demonstrations and practice of life-support skills. Nurses in some emergency departments accompany the trained ambulance attendant on special calls and initiate emergency care in the field. Nurses who staff poison control centers bring the resources of the center to the public and to other health service agencies. Other innovative educational experiences are being sought and developed to ultimately improve the delivery of emergency care in both hospital and community settings.

Communication is another mechanism for bringing health care needs and resources into better balance, and it is being utilized in a number of ways. One is participation on committees, at the hospital, community, state and national levels. Nurses must seek active membership and representation on these committees. Another is the use of liaison or coordinator nurses, who promote continuity of care between the hospital emergency department and the community nursing service agency. Technology has provided yet another avenue: sophisticated communication instrumentation, such as radio and telemetry equipment, can link the emergency department directly with the ambulance.

To summarize, emergency nursing is considered to be a specialty practice area within the nursing profession, but it is an area which is very broad in scope, as it encompasses acute patient care, wherever it is needed.

BIBLIOGRAPHY

(1) Anderson, D.: "Continuing Education and the Emergency Room Nurse," *Hospital Topics,* 52 (1974):9.

(2) Anderson, D., and Cosgriff, J.: "Partners in Practice," *Supervisor Nurse,* 5 (1974):8.

(3) Bevis, E.: *Curriculum Building in Nursing: A Process* (Saint Louis: C. V. Mosby Company, 1973).

(4) Cosgriff, J.: "Emergency Nursing," *Supervisor Nurse,* 5 (1974):30.

(5) "Extending the Scope of Nursing Practice: A Report of the Secretary's Committee to Study Extended Roles for Nurses" (Washington, D.C.: U.S. Department of Health, Education, and Welfare, 1972).

(6) Kelly, L.: "Nursing Practice Acts," *American Journal of Nursing,* 74 (1974):1310.

(7) Lysaught, J. (ed.): *Action in Nursing: Progress in Professional Purpose* (New York: McGraw-Hill Book Company, 1974).

(8) National Commission for the Study of Nursing and Nursing Education: *An Abstract for Action* (New York: McGraw-Hill Book Company, 1970).

(9) ———: *From Abstract into Action* (New

York: McGraw-Hill Book Company, 1973).

(10) Romano, T.: "Trauma Nurse Specialist," *American Journal of Nursing,* 73 (1973):1008.

(11) Schlotfeldt, R.: "Planning for Progress," *Nursing Outlook,* 21 (1973):766.

(12) ——: "This I Believe—Nursing is Health Care," *Nursing Outlook,* 20 (1972):245.

2

Functional requirements
of an emergency department

MILDRED K. FINCKE
JAMES H. COSGRIFF, JR.

How a hospital sees the roles and obligations of its emergency department in the community and how it attempts to meet those roles and obligations may well determine the quality of its service. There must be no haphazard management of emergency patients, and the service provided is dependent upon proper utilization of personnel, equipment and facilities.*

HOSPITAL POLICIES

Emergency department policies and procedures should be documented in a procedure manual, which is really a compendium of all the activities of this area of the hospital. It should be an all-inclusive volume, listing the objectives and goals of the department's particular services and establishing rules and regulations for staffing patterns and individual responsibilities. This manual must clearly reflect the attitudes and policies of the hospital's administrative, medical and nursing staffs with regard to the management of emergency patients; therefore, it is properly prepared by representatives of hospital administration, medical staff and emergency department personnel.

The manual should also serve as a resource for information on management of particular patient problems, including those pertaining to medical and social service needs and those dealing with law enforcement officers, the press and medical examiners. All personnel should be required to be familiar with its contents and adhere to its directives. Especially with respect to the use of part-time employees, this volume will help provide for patient management and appropriate follow-up of care consistent with the standards maintained by the hospital. No emergency department can afford to turn a patient away to another system or service or make a referral where inadequate follow-up may result.

Most hospitals make use of a system of committees to communicate the needs and policies of various hospital services. Two which relate closely to the emergency depart-

---

* Throughout this chapter, the reader might refer to the 3 tables in Appendix A, on pages 32–36, for a summary of the functional requirements of 4 levels of emergency departments.

ment are the emergency department and disaster committees. (The disaster committee is discussed later in this chapter, under "Disaster Planning.") The emergency department committee serves as a policy-making and advisory body to the director of the department; it is not responsible for the day-to-day operation of the department. The committee must not be awkwardly large, but it must be broadly representative of the hospital administration, medical staff and nursing service. Its purview may or may not include the outpatient department. In those hospitals in which it does, the group is frequently referred to as the ambulatory care or out-of-hospital services committee.

The committee should be responsible for making the department responsive to community needs yet adherent to hospital policy. This means that an ongoing review of department activities, equipment and service is required, accompanied by recommendations for appropriate changes as indicated. With the current emphasis on consumerism, many believe that responsible members of the community should be seated on the committee, to state the views of those they represent (the patients). This idea may have some merit, but, clearly, the dominant force of the group must derive from the physicians and nurses, those most knowledgeable of and intimately involved in maintaining quality patient care.

EMERGENCY DEPARTMENT STAFF

The capabilities of the emergency department in the daily routine of caring for patients depend largely on the staff. Continuous patient traffic flow, without delay in treatment or admission, is the responsibility of the personnel who work day-to-day in the emergency department, for it is they who know best how the department is geared to function.

There are many considerations involved in selecting the type of personnel for a hospital emergency department. What may be adequate, even recommended for one department may not be at all suitable for another.

The geographic location, the proximity of other area hospitals, the local population, the medical services offered and, in general, the particular hospital's concept of the function of its emergency department should determine staffing. The department itself and the quality of its services to all patients are only as efficient as the capabilities of those persons employed in the department.

Physicians and nurses

Physician coverage of emergency departments varies tremendously, from 24-hour physician coverage exclusively devoted to the emergency department; to doctors on dual assignment, both in the emergency department and the remainder of the hospital; to on-call, off-premises coverage. One recent study revealed that the vast majority of smaller hospitals provide the latter coverage.[19]

The level of training of the emergency department physician also varies greatly, from a new graduate (intern or resident) to a senior attending physician. Younger physicians are often found staffing university hospital emergency departments. Some difference of opinion exists regarding the propriety of staffing an emergency department with interns and resident physicians without adequate supervision. Staffing by attending physicians may assume a variety of methods, the Pontiac and Alexandria plans being 2 examples.*

The vast majority of emergency department nurses are registered nurses, but licensed practical/vocational nurses comprise a significant number. Their role in the emergency setting is considerably different from that of the traditional floor nurse. At varying times the emergency nurse must perform triage, assist patients, perform cardiopulmonary resuscitation, institute life-support measures, start intravenous solutions, draw blood samples, give comfort and solace to families, counsel patients and perform any number of other tasks.

* See Chapter 3, pp. 28–29, for more information on the Pontiac and Alexandria plans.

Recognizing the nature of the emergency nurse's broad range of responsibilities and the services she provides, physicians, nurses and nurse educators have become more aware of the need for special educational programs prepared specifically for the emergency department nurse. Such courses are being offered on an ever-widening basis, and more in-depth educational experiences are evolving to develop clinical specialists in emergency nursing.

The Emergency Department Nurses Association serves as a pool for knowledge and provides a reference point for solutions to the myriad problems arising in all phases of the emergency care system. It also provides a means for developing standards and improved methods of delivering efficient and effective emergency medical and nursing care and has had the encouragement and assistance of the American College of Surgeons, the American College of Orthopedic Surgeons and the American College of Emergency Physicians. This is as it should be, for in no other area of the health care system do nurses and physicians work so closely, in teams, through the 24 hours of every day.

Teaching and learning are invaluable experiences in the emergency unit, and these organizations have much to offer each other, for theirs is a common goal: the best care for each emergency patient. The training and knowledge of emergency nurses are supplemented by postgraduate courses, scientific assemblies, workshops and conferences presented by these organizations. As in all health care services, the providers must continually keep up with current improvements and innovations in technology and instrumentation. Independent study and continuing education courses must be available, to qualify workers in the emergency department. Emergency service is a dynamic field, and all organizations concerned with keeping up with the changes in this specialty will demand eligible, qualified and certified nurses as well as physicians.

Management of the emergency department is accomplished by the attending physician and his colleague, the clinical nursing supervisor. This is the beginning of setting the functions of the department. Without team participation in the management of the emergency department there may be mismanagement, and the inevitable victim of mismanagement is the patient. For example, ready assistance at the emergency entrance for the incoming patient by trained hospital emergency, security and/or ancillary personnel is very important. (In many instances, such broadly qualified assistance is a necessity for good patient management, as well as good public relations.)

Priority of care should be ascertained by triage, to determine not only the urgency of the patient's problem but to maintain a smooth patient flow pattern through the treatment areas. The triage officer is preferably a physician or nurse. In smaller departments with relatively light patient loads (less than 10,000 patient visits a year), a paraprofessional, such as a secretary, may be specially trained to function in this role. Also, there must be no delay in treating such patients in any emergency department. In the absence of a physician, the nurse must respond appropriately to initiate resuscitative and life-support measures.

Allied health care personnel

In addition to nursing and medical professionals, nurses' aides, emergency medical technicians, orderlies, clerks, secretaries, social workers, ombudsmen and voluntary workers provide further support to the emergency department. Spiritual support should also be available, at the request of the patient or his family.

The need for a social worker in the emergency department has been established. Unfortunately, this service is often only available during daytime hours and not in the evening, or on weekends, when the need is often greater. Many hospitals have become aware of this inadequacy and now provide a social service representative on an around-the-clock basis. Depending on volume and patient need, late evening and night coverage might be satisfactorily furnished by a person with an on-call service.

The respiratory (inhalation) therapist has assumed a unique role in certain aspects of emergency care. This individual is trained in a variety of skills, including endotracheal intubation, airway maintenance and use of mechanical ventilators, among others. The inhalation therapist is an important member of the cardiopulmonary resuscitation team and, in this regard, works closely with the emergency department staff.

Teamwork depends on all emergency personnel being oriented and trained in the policies and procedures of the department. This is an ongoing process, geared for change, since changes occur constantly in both concepts and methods. Newer techniques of patient care, management of specific problems and development of more advanced and sophisticated instrumentation demand that every effort be made by the emergency department to maintain pace with current trends.

All allied health professionals can play leading roles in the delivery of emergency health services, but the placement and training of these persons must fit into the specific hospital emergency department system. The roles and the values each can contribute should be assessed and evaluated to determine how the emergency department can operate to its fullest potential.

Staff, regardless of job classification, must be understanding of the importance of public relations and must be emotionally stable, able to make quick and accurate decisions and responsible for their actions. And all this must be coupled with compassion without personal involvement.

Today's emergency health workers are diverse and multidisciplinary, and they must have the ability to grow, as must all health professionals, as medical science progresses.

It is not enough to expect experience to be the only teacher. All health professionals must be trained and educated in the common goal of good emergency health care delivery.

EMERGENCY DEPARTMENT FACILITIES

Good design of or use of existing facilities is another factor affecting the quality of care given in the hospital emergency department. It is obvious that the emergency department should be located in an area of the hospital where it is most easily accessible. It should be on the ground floor and have entrances from both outside and within the hospital. Adequate walking access for ambulatory patients is needed, as well as sufficient parking areas for patients arriving by ambulance or automobile. The ambulance receiving area must be large enough to allow for entry and exit without delay. Overhead protection is advisable, to shield the patient in all types of weather conditions. A ramp permits easier access by patients with crutches or in wheelchairs. (See Figure 2–1.)

Interior emergency department design is an equally important aspect of providing efficient emergency care. A treatment room must be available at all times for the immediate care of the patient who is in an acute, life-threatening situation. Experience has shown that the main treatment area should be a large, open room which can be partitioned into cubicles by separating stretchers with curtains. In-wall oxygen, suction, etc., should be available near each stretcher. (See Figure 2–2.) Departments which are divided into a number of private, walled cubicles are not usually conducive to good emergency care, unless *each* is fully equipped and staffed. Ordinarily such luxury is not feasible. Staff must have ready access to each and every patient with a minimum of delay, and this the "open" unit allows.

A security room for the inebriated, unruly or unmanageable patient or for the acutely disturbed patient is essential to assure main-

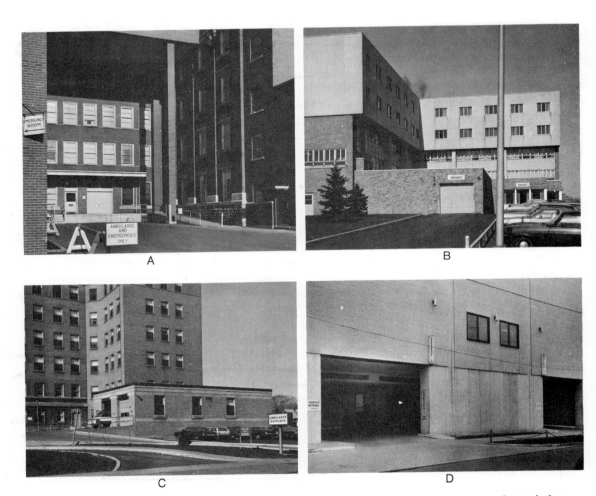

Figure 2–1 Emergency department entrances. A: Photo shows a large, open entrance for ambulances. Note the dock to unload patients, with an automatic overhead door. The ramp on the right may be used for wheelchair patients. This entrance allows at least 2 ambulances to load or unload patients at one time; it is protected by high-rise walls on 3 sides and a limited overhang. B: Photo shows a completely enclosed ambulance entrance immediately adjacent to the hospital emergency department. Readily accessible, it is protected from the weather, but limits access to one ambulance at a time. C: Photo shows a completely enclosed ambulance entrance immediately adjacent to the hospital emergency department, as in "B". But this entrance has room for 2 ambulances to load or unload patients at any one time. D: Photo shows an enclosed "in-and-out" ambulance entrance, immediately adjacent to the street. It is fully protected from the weather.

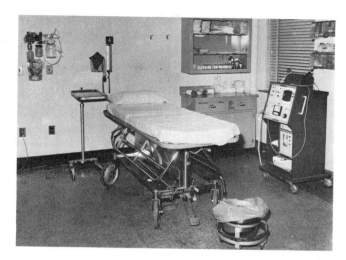

Figure 2–2 Example of an emergency department "open" treatment cubicle. Note the open area, storage cabinet, in-wall oxygen and suction, cardiac monitor-defibrillator unit. Privacy is assured by overhead curtain enclosures, not shown in the photograph.

tenance of the safety and dignity of the patient, the staff and other emergency patients. Such precautionary interior design as a minimum of furniture, soundproof walls and a door that locks only on the outside are recommended.

The waiting room ought to be large enough to provide uncrowded seating for relatives and friends of patients under care, thus discouraging any milling about the treatment area. A supply of reading material or a television may serve as diversionary measures. Public telephones are needed for use by relatives; booths are preferable, to allow for privacy. Special provisions may be required for the press or the police in instances when prominent citizens or public officials are under emergency care. These needs will vary from hospital to hospital and from incident to incident.

A secluded and quiet room is worthwhile, affording privacy to relatives and friends of patients who are critically ill or injured and in imminent danger of death. It also provides a setting for a physician, nurse or clergyman to keep the family informed of the patient's progress and provide comfort and solace when needed, including times when the physician must inform the family of the patient's death and request a postmortem examination or the donation of organs for transplantation.

Whether or not the hospital emergency department should have an observation area depends on the space available and on the need for such a service. If there is an observation area, there must also be a policy specifying the types of patients to be held there and the average length of stay allowed. It must not become a disposition area or misused by the staff to delay the admission of patients. The emergency nursing staff is responsible for the care of the patients in the observation area, and if such an area is separate and adjacent to the emergency department, nursing staff must be available to provide for patient needs separately from those of patients seen in the emergency department for treatment and discharge.

X-ray and laboratory services

Under ideal circumstances, x-ray services are available in the emergency department or immediately adjacent to it. In a busy department it is indeed inefficient and a waste of valuable time to maintain a shuttle service for patients between a ground floor emergency department and an x-ray department on the third or fifth floor or elsewhere. Naturally, this requirement must be flexible, for some hospitals do not treat enough patients to warrant this service; however, if the best interest of the patient were foremost in mind, there would be strong support for an x-ray service in *every* emergency department.

An emergency x-ray service should be staffed by qualified technicians capable of assuming the responsibility of managing acutely ill or injured patients while in their care. Radiological consultation should also be available to the emergency department at all times. Some services are staffed on an around-the-clock basis, others only during busy hours and on an on-call basis the remainder of the day.

Laboratory services, including hematology, chemistry and blood bank capabilities, should be available to emergency department patients as needed. Basic blood count and electrolyte determination services must be available to patients 24 hours a day. With improved technique, arterial blood gas determinations can be available at all times, consistent with the needs of emergency patients. The patient load of trauma or acute cases seen in any emergency service must be used as a guideline to which laboratory services must be provided and when and for what period of time.

Blood bank capability is needed at all times. In hospitals which do not have this service around the clock, it would behoove the emergency department staff to be familiar with the use of universal donor blood (Type O, Rh negative) and with plasma expanders or blood substitutes. Long delays for type-specific blood are unpardonable, especially when a life is in danger.

EQUIPMENT

Since emergency nurses and others are required to make quick and accurate medical decisions, equipment and supplies must be adequate and on the unit. No equipment in the emergency department should ever be borrowed or removed from the unit, for no one can foresee when or how quickly it may be needed. The lack of any necessary equipment could easily cost a patient his life and result in a legal entanglement for the hospital and the responsible medical and nursing staff. All personnel working in the emergency department must know the location of all equipment.

There should be a list of all supplies and equipment, and the quotas for each item should appear. This list should be all-inclusive, from wheelchairs, stretchers, gloves, soap, drugs, to tongue blades and safety pins.

All nursing and medical personnel must be trained to use every item of the intricate, sophisticated electrical and electronic monitoring equipment in the department. Since there are many varieties of cardiac monitoring and defibrillating equipment essential to the emergency department, this equipment should be chosen by the emergency physician in consultation with the emergency nurse supervisor. Joint selection of equipment will insure the best and most knowledgeable use of it by both physicians and nurses.

Individually wrapped suture sets and special trays must be kept sterilized and ready for immediate use. If the hospital has a materials management distribution plan which insures delivery of sterile equipment and maintenance of quotas at all times or if supplies of instruments and special trays are more than adequate, a sterilizer in the emergency department may not be necessary. But there can be no breakdown in the system and no chance ever taken that would leave the emergency department without needed sterile supplies readily available.

All emergency supplies must be clearly marked and strategically placed. Finally, equipment and supplies must be constantly checked, both for adequacy and readiness and for maintenance needs.

Equipment essential to the emergency department

CPR

Cardiac and pulmonary resuscitation equipment may be conveniently located in a "resuscitation cart," which is easily movable from one area of the emergency department to another.*

* See the section on "The Resuscitation Cart," which follows.

Airway

(1) Bag-valve mask combination.
(2) Oropharyngeal and nasopharyngeal airways, pediatric and adult sizes.
(3) Orotracheal (endotracheal) tubes, cuffed, pediatric and adult sizes. (Tubes less than 0.5 cm. in external diameter are not cuffed.)
(4) Laryngoscope with varying sized blades.
(5) Oxygen, wall and portable.
(6) Mechanical ventilator, volume type.
(7) Suction apparatus.

Cardiac

(1) Monitor-defibrillator unit with cardio-scope and direct-writing electrocardiograph.
(2) Portable monitor-defibrillator for accompanying patients being transferred to other units.
(3) Intravenous equipment, including needles, plastic catheters, scalp vein needles, calibrated I.V. drip chambers and blood infusion sets.
(4) Specific cardiac drugs. (See Chapter 14, "Cardiac Emergencies.")
(5) Chest tray and rib spreaders.

Special trays

(1) Tracheostomy trays with varying sizes of cuffed tracheostomy tubes.
(2) Venous cut-down trays.
(3) Thoracostomy trays with chest catheters and chest bottles.
(4) Suture trays, including trays which contain finer instruments for facial wounds or plastic closure (e.g., Adson toothed forceps, tenotomy scissors, skin hooks).
(5) Catheter trays (French and Foley catheters), with special catheters as needed. (See Chapter 23, "Genitourinary Emergencies.")
(6) Bleeder trays.
(7) Irrigation trays, including gastric lavage equipment, nasogastric tubes, Ewald tube.

(8) Emergency childbirth tray.
(9) Thoracentesis tray.
(10) Abdominal paracentesis and/or peritoneal lavage tray.
(11) Sengstaken-Blakemore tube tray.
(12) Cul-de-sac aspiration tray, vaginal packing.

General equipment

(1) Splints, including simple board type, plastic inflatable type, traction splints, spine boards (half-length and full-length). (See Chapters 24 and 25.)
(2) Sandbags.
(3) Cast material.
(4) Restraints, including those for children. (See Papoose boards, Figure 10–4.)
(5) Stretchers, such as those used in a recovery room.
(6) I.V. stands and portable I.V. equipment for stretchers.
(7) Portable floor lights.
(8) Portable x-ray equipment (especially if the fixed x-ray unit is not available in the emergency department).
(9) Special equipment (eye, ear, nose, throat, gynecology, urology). (See appropriate chapters.)
(10) Medications for emergency use.
(11) Intravenous solutions, including glucose, electrolytes, Ringer's lactate, plasma expanders, 50% glucose.
(12) Poison antidotes. (See Chapter 12.)

The resuscitation cart

When a cardiopulmonary emergency occurs in the emergency department, regardless of cause, prompt action on the part of the staff is required. A variety of special equipment, drugs and supplies may be needed on short notice to initiate and maintain the resuscitation effort. Considerable time can be saved by storing all the necessary gear in one or two units which are mobile and thus can be moved to any point in the department as circumstances require. Such a device is known by a

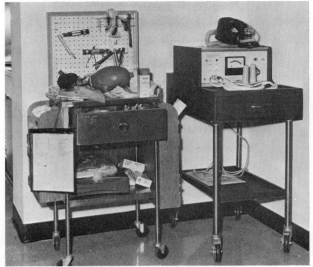

A

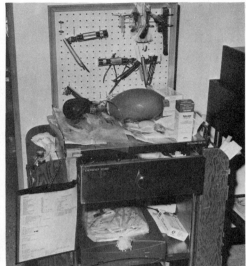

B

Figure 2–3 Emergency resuscitation carts. A: This cart has been modified to contain all drugs and equipment necessary for a cardiopulmonary emergency. It is used in conjunction with bag-valve-mask units and a cardiac defibrillator. This particular unit was used in a location where in-wall continuous monitoring equipment was available, hence the simple defibrillator unit alone was needed. B: Photo shows a close-up of the resuscitation cart in "A". Note the laryngoscope handles and varying sizes of blades on the pegboard, along with oropharyngeal airways. Sterile endotracheal tubes are individually packaged on top, with bag-valve-mask and individual-dose prefilled syringes. I.V. solutions are in the rack at left, and plastic veinways and central venous pressure catheters are in the rack on the right. The drawer contains individual ampules and prefilled syringes. All equipment is easily accessible. C: Photo shows another type of resuscitation cart, to be used with a monitor defibrillator. This cart has been modified from a standard tool chest. The disadvantage of this type of cart is that all the drawers cannot be opened at one time for ease of accessibility.

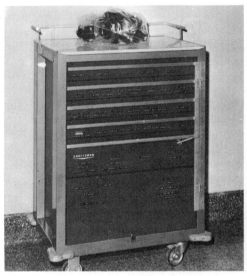

C

variety of names, such as "code cart," "emergency cart," "CPR cart," but perhaps is best termed a "resuscitation cart."

While a number of such carts have been designed and produced commercially, many hospitals have ingeniously modified standard storage chests for this purpose. (See Figure 2–3.) Some contain all necessary items, including cardiac monitoring equipment, on one cart, while others are used for airway equipment, drugs and supplies only, with the cardiac monitors being available on a separate movable device. Whatever contrivance is chosen, it should be of a type that is easily moved but of sufficient size to store all needed items in drawers or in compartments which permit full display of equipment and ease of accessibility for rapid retrieval.

COMMUNICATIONS

Communications equipment is a necessity in the emergency department, more so than in any other department of the hospital. Voice link to other in-hospital facilities, such as the laboratory, dietary department, x-ray department, operating room, pharmacy, admission office, lends immeasurable efficiency to the department. Many hospitals utilize a vacuum tube system to quickly send and receive small items, such as drugs and reports, among all areas of the hospital.

Interdepartmental services must be immediately accessible and available. If they are not, the efficiency of the emergency department suffers, and the patient can be seriously and adversely affected. For example, delays in obtaining an available operating room, in initiating x-ray and diagnostic laboratory studies or in obtaining the services of the blood bank can bring about problems which, in addition to influencing patient care, may give rise to medicolegal issues.

Extra-hospital communications include links with ambulances and the emergency departments in other hospitals. The hospital-ambulance radio link is recognized as an important factor in improving the prehospital phase of emergency care, as well in alerting the emergency department to the patient's condition and special needs, thus allowing for advance preparations by emergency department personnel.*

Telemetry of biomedical data (blood pressure, pulse, electrocardiogram, electroencephalogram) is common today from fixed points in communities. It is likely to be available wherever mobile shock, intensive or coronary care units are operating.

Hospital-to-hospital voice links are used in day-to-day emergency department activities, usually of an administrative nature, but are absolutely necessary in the event of disaster. Such links permit the development of regional emergency medical services systems with a minimum of duplication of expensive, sophisticated equipment and specialized medical services.

RECORDS

Emergency records, containing *factual* medical and legal information, must be made up for all who are treated in the emergency department. For patients who are examined, treated and released, only the emergency record is required, but it should be complete, with physician's history, physical examination, diagnosis, diagnostic procedures, treatment and disposition.

The emergency nurse should enter the time and her initials with the record of treatment and note whether written or verbal instructions for specific care were given to the patient. Patients being detained for observation or being admitted to the hospital from the emergency department should have full medical charts prepared for them, with therapeutic and diagnostic treatments noted and initialed and nursing notes recorded. Good nursing standards and practice begin with the emergency nurses's notes; they constitute a factual record of the case for following shifts of nurses, so that there is never any doubt as to diagnosis, treatment and management.

DISASTER PLANNING

Disaster planning involves all hospital departments and personnel and should be the responsibility of the emergency department or disaster committee. The coordinators for a disaster plan should be the senior surgeon of the medical staff and the emergency department physician. Committee members should include physicians, nurses and administrative personnel from key departments, such as administration, operating room, nursing services, outpatient, pharmacy, materials management, engineering and maintenance and public relations, in addition to representation of the major medical services.

---

* See Chapter 3 for discussion of a federally mandated emergency medical services radio frequency.

In a disaster, the emergency department should be the triage area, with the senior surgeon as the physician-in-charge. Areas for treating the urgent and nonurgent must be decided and defined and teams assigned for immediate staffing when needed. Ongoing orientation for all personnel and a written disaster plan, with a personnel and department disaster chart outline, should be placed on every unit of the hospital. When a disaster strikes is not the time for needed staff to ask, "Where do I go?" or "What can I do?"

A "disaster run" should be planned and implemented at least twice a year, in accordance with the policy outlined by the Joint Commission on Accreditation of Hospitals.[14] All personnel involved, including police and fire departments, should participate. Experience with these "runs" has proved to be valuable when an actual disaster occurs. While every contingency cannot be acted out, many deficiencies are often brought to light, and ways to effect improvements become readily apparent.

SUMMARY

As it is inclusive of many medical and nursing disciplines, emergency medicine is dependent on these disciplines for back-up support if optimal care is to be given. The practice of emergency medicine is best carried out by physicians and nurses with a special interest and expertise in this field of care, trained in emergency medicine and, therefore, best qualified to assess the medical problems presented and deal with them competently and expeditiously.

The roles of the emergency physician and the emergency nurse are essentially episodic and must include the capability to initiate resuscitative and life-support measures with a wide spectrum of mechanical and electronic devices. Extrahospital, interdepartmental and intradepartmental communications, input from medical staff and house physicians and proper use of facilities and equipment are all important and helpful in the delivery of emergency medicine.

Ultimately, decisions for the organization and function of the emergency department are within the province of the emergency department committee. Yet, day-to-day operations and decisions must be made by the emergency physician and the emergency nurse, with input from all emergency department personnel. Team effort is the key to a well-organized and -administered department and to attaining its primary objective of giving each emergency patient the highest level of care and of assuring prompt and adequate examination and treatment of each patient.

BIBLIOGRAPHY

(1) Cobb, L. A.; Conn, R. D., and Samson, W. E.: "Pre-Hospital Coronary Care: The Role of Rapid Response Mobile Intensive/Coronary Care System," *Circulation,* 44, supplement II (1971).

(2) *Communications Guidelines for Emergency Medical Services* (Washington, D.C.: U.S. Department of Transportation, DOT Publication No. [H.S.] 820–214, 1972).

(3) Cosgriff, J. H., Jr.: "Emergency Nursing," *Supervisor Nurse,* 5 (1974):30.

(4) Eckert, C. (ed.): *Emergency Room Care* (Boston: Little, Brown & Company, 1967).

(5) "Editorial Notes: The Potentials and Limitations of EMS," *Hospitals,* 47 (1973):57.

(6) *Emergency Medical Services Communications System* (Washington, D.C.: U.S. Department of Health, Education and Welfare, DHEW Publication No. [HSM] 73–2003, 1972).

(7) *Emergency Service: The Hospital Emergency Department in an Emergency Call System* (Chicago: American Hospital Association, 1972).

(8) Gibson, G.: "EMS: A Facet of Ambulatory Care," *Hospitals,* 47 (1973):59.

(9) Grace, W. J., and Chadbourne, J. A.: "The Mobile Coronary Care Unit," *Chest,* 55 (1969):452.

(10) Hannas, R. R., Jr.: "Staffing the Emergency Department," *Hospitals,* 47 (1973):83.

(11) Harvey, J. C.: "Categorization of Emergency Capabilities," *Hospitals,* 47 (1973):69.

(12) Holmes, R. H.: "Emergency Room Organization: A General Concept of EMS," in W. W. Oaks and Stanley Spitzer (eds.), *Twenty-third Hahnemann Symposium on Emergency Room Care* (New York: Grune & Stratton, 1970).

(13) Horty, J. F.: "Categorization: A Legal View," *Hospitals,* 47 (1973):75.

(14) Joint Commission on Accreditation of Hospitals: *Accreditation Manual for Hospitals* (Chicago: JCAH, 1970).

(15) Kesserman, J.: "Staffing the Emergency Room," in W. W. Oaks and Stanley Spitzer (eds.), *Twenty-third Hahnemann Symposium on Emergency Care* (New York: Grune & Stratton, 1970).

(16) *Nursing Clinics of North America,* 2 (1967):2.

(17) Riehl, C. L.: *Emergency Nursing* (New York: Charles A. Bennett Company, 1970).

(18) *Roles and Resources of Federal Agencies in Support of Comprehensive Emergency Medical Services* (Washington, D.C.: Committee on EMS, Division of Medical Service, Nation Academy of Science — National Research Council, 1972).

(19) Rossman, J.; Esselstyn, C. B., *et al.:* "Emergency Care in Northeastern New York Hospitals: Report of a Survey," *Journal of Trauma,* 13 (1973):994.

(20) Spencer, J. H.: *The Hospital Emergency Department* (Springfield, Ill.: Charles C Thomas, 1972).

(21) Strensky, C.: "Medical Social Worker," *Hospitals,* 44 (1970):58.

(22) Taubenhaus, L. J., and Simon, J.: "To Build a Better Emergency Practice," *Emergency Medicine,* 5 (March 1973): 38.

(23) Uhley, H. N.: "Electrocardiographic Telemetry from Ambulances: A Practical Approach to Mobile Coronary Care Units," *American Heart Journal,* 80 (1970):838.

(24) Warren, J. V.: *A Workshop: Mobile Coronary Care Unit* (Columbus: Ohio State University, College of Medicine, 1969).

3

Evolving roles and trends in emergency health care

JAMES H. COSGRIFF, JR.
DIANN ANDERSON

"Emergency health services" has been developed in recent years as a generic term to refer to all aspects of emergency health care, from time of incident to final rehabilitation and discharge of the patient. Formerly, hospital physicians and nurses regarded emergency care as that care given the acutely ill or injured, which only concerned the hospital emergency department. In recent years, especially with the advent of consumerism and the passage of the Highway Safety Act (1966) and the Partnership for Health Act (1966), many other agencies, including governments, have become involved. The term is thus broad enough to include any and every type of health care a patient may receive—that rendered by oneself or a friend, trained ambulance attendant, fireman, nurse, physician or social worker, to name but a few.

HISTORICAL PERSPECTIVE

Prior to World War II, the emergency room, or "accident room" as it was then called, primarily served the acutely ill and injured. It played an inconspicuous role in the day-to-day operation of the hospital and was thus usually located in an inconspicuous part of the building. The staff was frequently limited to a nurse who functioned quite independently. In smaller facilities, the emergency room was often covered by a "float" nurse, who was assigned to duties elsewhere in the hospital but opened up the emergency area when a patient was brought in by ambulance.

In the years following World War II and up to the present time, the emergency department played an increasingly prominent role in health care. Patient visits increased 380 percent during that time. Provision of services broadened, so that the emergency department today no longer exists primarily to serve the acutely ill and injured. Rather, it has taken on the functions of a community health center. Estimates of the percentage of patients seen in the emergency department with problems that are not *clinically* emergent vary between 60 and 80 percent. Further, many persons now use the emergency department as their primary source of medical care. Currently, one third of all outpatient visits and 25 percent of all hospital admissions are made in the emergency department. Nationally, the number of annual emergency department visits exceeds 60,000,000.

While this period of tremendous growth has placed an inestimable burden on hospitals, present trends indicate no diminution of use, rather an ever higher utilization of emergency department facilities.* The reasons for the staggering increase in utilization of the emergency department are many and include: (1) advances in medical technology, (2) population migration, (3) failure to establish a professional relationship with a physician, (4) decline in the actual number of family practitioners, (5) intervention of third-party fiscal intermediaries and (6) public and physician convenience. These factors could well serve as subject matter for an entire book and thus cannot be covered here. Study of these factors, however, would probably help those in the health professions to be more responsive to the demands placed on them.

This tremendous growth in use of the emergency department has reached a level of significant impact on the delivery of emergency care services. At this time, patient (consumer) demands or needs are straining the existing facilities and making apparent the need for change. This chapter will discuss the changes that are occurring within the emergency health services to adapt to the growing demands on them.

THE REGIONAL SYSTEM OF EMERGENCY HEALTH CARE

Of all the efforts to improve the delivery of emergency health care and make it available to all segments of the population, the most promising is the development of the "regional system." In such a system, the resources of the community or region are pooled and coordinated, so that a complete range of services suited to community need can be economically provided. Thus, a regional

* National Center for Health Statistics, *Physician Visits: Volume and Interval Since Last Visit: United States, 1969* (Washington, D.C.: U.S. Department of Health, Education and Welfare, 1973).

system should have a total capability for delivery of health care. The Emergency Medical Service Systems Act of 1973 (Public Law 93–154) has encouraged such an approach.

This plan is well suited to the changing patterns of American life. Population migration and development of satellite communities away from large cities have progressed at a rate which currently exceeds the capability of establishing new health centers. In many instances, the migration has followed no specific pattern, making health planning difficult or impossible. With improvement of methods of transportation and through regionalization, optimal use of existing resources, supplemented with additional needed services, can provide continuous care, from time of incident until final discharge of the patient.

The designation of a "region" will vary from one area of the country to another. One region may include an entire state, while another may include a number of counties within a state or a single large metropolitan area. Determining considerations must include local need, population density and geographic, industrial and environmental factors.

The major components of an emergency medical services system include: (1) *personnel,* trained to manage any potential patient, especially physicians, nurses, ambulance attendants and physician's assistants (all personnel must be totally familiar with the following 2 factors); (2) *facilities* appropriate to the needs of the region, including ambulances, first aid stations and hospital emergency departments supported by such ancillary services as blood bank, laboratories, radiology, poison control, heart-lung machine, coronary care and intensive care units, hyperbaric chamber and so on; (3) *equipment,* encompassing not only rescue and life-saving gear but also cardiac monitors, defibrillators, ventilators and, of the utmost importance, communications equipment. (See "Communications" at the end of this chapter.)

Development of a regional system

In establishing a regional emergency services system, 3 preliminary procedures must be carried out: (1) determination of existing services and capabilities, (2) assessment of local needs and (3) development of recommendations to effect the changes necessary to coordinate local needs and services. It should be kept in mind that regional planning does not necessarily imply a major alteration in existing facilities and services. It is better viewed as a coordination of the services available in a region and a development of a built-in system of patient referral based on medical indications.

Providing the forum for discussion of this enormous task usually falls to an emergency medical services committee or council.[3, 7] This committee should be broadly representative of all involved in emergency health care, including the consumer. It may either be an action-oriented group or serve in an advisory or consultative capacity to the local health commissioner. Above all, it must be nonpartisan and not subject to political pressures.

Because of their expertise, medical societies and nursing organizations must assume the leadership in developing regional systems. Health planners are generally uninformed in such matters, and successful development depends to a great extent on clinical experience. These organizations must also work closely with local health officials, hospital administrators, the hospital association and representatives of all available ambulance services to provide an overview of the regional capability and to make judgments and recommendations from a wide knowledge base.

The system that is developed must be able to handle day-to-day problems as well as a community disaster. To achieve the broadest possible capability, each regional system should be integrated with adjacent regional systems, with a mutual aid component built in. To be most effective and to achieve the highest level of cooperation, the planning initiative has to originate from the grass roots of the community rather than by state fiat. Of particular importance to the success of a regional system is the education of the consumer to act responsibly in terms of his own health care and to utilize the available services in an appropriate manner.

Categorization of hospital emergency services

Most general hospitals operate an emergency department, but the quality and scope of capability of the medical services available vary considerably. There is no valid reason why this should be otherwise. It is neither economically prudent, nor feasible, nor technically possible for every hospital to develop a full range of emergency services. At the same time, the patients with life-threatening conditions require the immediate availability of highly sophisticated equipment and medical skills if successful medical care is the goal.

In recognizing the variations in emergency services, a system of categorization of hospital emergency departments was first proposed in 1966 by The National Academy of Sciences — National Research Council.[2] Of the 4 categories proposed, Category I included those hospitals with minimal service, while Category IV designated those with the maximum capability. Subsequently, several leading physicians' organizations became interested in the concept, and a variety of categorization plans were developed, with some using 3 and others as many as 5 categories. In 1971, The American Medical Association convened a national conference to establish guidelines for categorization. A 4-level system was devised, reversing the categories proposed by the NAS-NRC committee. Thus, according to the AMA system, a Category I hospital provided the widest range of services and a hospital in Category IV the least. In addition, the rating system included consideration not only of a hospital's emergency department capability but of the complete range of services and staff available to receive and treat the emergency patient. (See the tables comprising Appendix A, at the end of this chapter.)

From a practical standpoint, implementation of the AMA categorization is limited, for it does not take into account those institutions which specialize in limited areas of care. In addition, and perhaps more important, it is unlikely that any hospital in the United States could meet the criteria of an AMA Category I facility. Among others, Boyd has adopted a 3-level system of categorization in Illinois.[5, 6]

Despite the advantages of categorization, its drawbacks must also be recognized, for it could force some hospitals to close their emergency facilities. Nevertheless, in a regional system approach to emergency care, there is a need to identify and properly utilize the special medical services and capabilities that are available in every emergency department. It should be expected, as an absolute minimum, that every hospital emergency department should qualify as an Advanced Life Support Station.* But whether strict and universal application of the principles of categorization will occur in the future is a moot question; the emergency nurse should be familiar with the concept in order to evaluate the services available within her own hospital and region.

Critical care units

Experience has demonstrated significant advantages to the critically ill or injured patient when special care units are available. The military, particularly during time of war, has applied the concept by designating various hospitals as centers for special care. Specific examples are centers for amputees, frostbite victims, those with spinal cord injury and burns, to name but a few. The principles

---

* In emergency cardiac care, there are stratified levels of care available (or that should be available). A "Basic Life Support Station" includes the capability to (1) recognize airway obstruction, respiratory arrest and cardiac arrest and (2) administer the appropriate application of cardiopulmonary resuscitation (CPR). An "Advanced Life Support Station" includes the capabilities of (1) a Basic Life Support Station and (2) the proper use of adjunctive equipment and intravenous lines, administration of drugs, control of cardiac arrhythmias, cardiac monitoring and postresuscitation care. It also requires the supervision of a physician.[29]

which evolved as a result of this practice have application in the overall management of patients who enter the emergency health care system.

In community hospitals, the development of critical care units devoted to the treatment of such patients as those with severe burns, acute myocardial infarction, spinal cord injury or multiple trauma or as the neonate in acute distress has resulted in a lower morbidity rate, shortened hospital stays and earlier returns to the home environment and productivity. In effect, the results have reaffirmed this approach to patient care. Such special units will become an integral part of any regional system of emergency care and undoubtedly will be expanded to include other clinical areas, for example, poison control, drug abuse, mental health, alcoholic detoxification and complicated, high-risk pregnancy.

The need for these clinical units within a particular region will depend, in part, on population size, incidence of population at risk and frequency of occurrence of specific disease entities. Indeed, in some areas of the country, one unit may serve patients from several adjacent regions. As critical care units evolve within a region, a patient referral mechanism must be developed, to maintain maximum utilization and high quality of care.

CHANGING ROLES OF EMERGENCY CARE PROVIDERS

Because of changes in community needs and in the delivery of emergency health care services, the roles of all health care providers are changing as well. Some confusion and controversy exist among those who give care regarding the capabilities and responsibilities inherent in each professional role. The need to develop a continuing dialogue, interdisciplinary collaboration, teamwork and evaluation of the care given among the groups is obvious. Furthermore, the newly expanded and/or extended roles of nurses and allied health workers must be developed and practiced with the support and cooperation of physicians and hospital administrators. This will probably require changes in the basic philosophies of all concerned.

For practical purposes, emergency health care may be considered as having 2 phases: the prehospital phase and the hospital phase. The prehospital phase is from the time of incident until the victim arrives at the hospital. The hospital phase takes place in the hospital setting. Both must be coordinated to provide a continuum of care. Examining the roles of the ambulance attendants, emergency nurses and physicians in both phases may be helpful in elucidating the independent yet interdependent aspects of each role within this continuum of care.

Ambulance attendants

The ambulance attendant is the medical services representative most likely to provide on-site emergency care. Depending on location and circumstances, this person may be referred to as an emergency medical technician (EMT), a rescue worker, a public service technician or the like. He or she may be an employee of a hospital-based or commercial ambulance company or a member of a volunteer fire and/or rescue company.

The level of formal training of ambulance attendants varies from none, to a standard or advanced first aid course, to completion of a standardized emergency medical technician training program or an extended educational experience which involved work in mobile coronary care/intensive care units. To provide a national standard, an 81-hour training program was established by the U.S. Department of Transportation after meetings with national medical organizations. Those who complete it successfully may be certified as an Emergency Medical Technician (EMT-I). Unfortunately, at the present time the vast majority (about 80 percent) of ambulance attendants in the country do not have this minimum standard of training.[13] It is important to be aware of these varied training experiences in order to properly assess the merits and/or deficiencies of the on-site emergency care service in a given community.

The capability of an ambulance crew will be determined for the most part by the amount of training each member has received. The EMT-I level attendant has knowledge and skills in all phases of first aid, plus emergency childbirth, artificial ventilation and closed chest cardiac massage. More advanced training, varying in time up to 480 hours, elevates an individual to the level of EMT-II, which includes management of certain cardiac arrhythmias, defibrillation, endotracheal intubation and initiation of intravenous lines with giving medication. In most areas of the country, the EMT-II has radio voice communication with a physician or specially trained nurse who prescribes the necessary treatment.

The significant role that *trained* ambulance attendants can play in the initial phase of emergency care must be recognized and accepted by physicians and nurses alike. There is need for more communication and cooperation among these 3 disciplines, including such experiences as having the EMT participate and assist in the early hospital care of the patients he transports to the emergency department. Such an exercise would allow for better understanding and better communications, but more importantly, it would give the EMT an opportunity to evaluate his treatment and at the same time sharpen his skills. Deficiencies in the prehospital phase of care (e.g., inadequate control of hemorrhage, lack of immobilization of suspected fractures, failure to properly dress wounds) should be noted and the EMT apprised of them. At the same time, proper care should be noted and the ambulance attendant encouraged to continue his good efforts. If at all possible, the emergency nurse or physician should accompany the attendant on an ambulance call.

Preferably, the patient's record of emergency assessment and treatment should be initiated by the EMT and made a permanent part of the patient's hospital record. In many instances, information gathered at the scene of the incident is valuable to emergency department personnel in the evaluation and further treatment of the patient.

Emergency nurses

The findings and recommendations of the National Commission for the Study of Nursing and Nursing Education [23, 24] have begun to have significant impact in all areas of nursing education and practice. Of the many worthy recommendations of the initial study now being implemented, one stressed the importance of a career plan to develop and reward increasing levels of competence within each functional specialty.[23]

Committees within the Emergency Department Nurses Association are working toward this goal by identifying knowledges and skills in emergency nursing which demonstrate competence and excellence in practice. A core curriculum, educational materials and a certifying examination for the "emergency nurse specialist" are being developed based on this data, so that nurses can obtain additional education and gain recognition for excellence in practice.

The "emergency nurse specialist" is one who, through education and practice, has attained a high level of competence in the delivery of emergency nursing care, particularly as it applies to the hospital emergency department setting. This nurse specialist is able to knowledgeably assess life-threatening situations and initiate appropriate interventions, independently if necessary.

The emergency nurse specialist is not to be confused with the nurse practitioner, who uses physical assessment skills mainly in assessing and treating common health problems of patients. Most nurse practitioners practice in ambulatory care settings, directing their attentions to promoting health, using the tools of health screening, supervision and teaching.[11] Physician consultation is usually available for medical advice when needed. While nurse practitioners generally have not practiced in emergency department settings, their service in the emergency department may be appropriate in some situations.

The "general" nature of emergency care and the broad scope of nursing practice itself allow for much innovation toward the ultimate improvement of nursing care in the emergency department. Some possibilities follow. (As with any new or innovative plan, bureaucratic details and obstacles must be addressed.)

(1) *Rotate nurses through other patient care settings* to enhance learning and communication as well as relieve the stress or routine of the emergency department. Such settings may include intensive and coronary care units, ambulances, outpatient clinics or community health services or agencies. This approach can be beneficial to both the nurse and employing agency when the focus is on patient care rather than on managerial functions. It is recognized that this particular activity may be difficult to implement, yet the outcome may be well worth the effort.

(2) *Utilize the services of a psychiatric-mental health nurse or a crisis team.* Staff, as well as patients, react to the stress that is prominent in any emergency department. A specially prepared nurse or group of providers comprising a "crisis team" can allay staff and/or patient anxiety and facilitate early intervention, referral and continuity for those needing further help.

(3) *Provide in-service programs on a regular and continuing basis.* Nurses and nursing personnel are both more competent and content when they feel they are "growing" with the job. In-service education is everyone's business and the responsibility of each team member. An in-service coordinator is helpful but need not be responsible solely to the emergency department. However, commitment and willingness to participate by each staff member *is* necessary. In-service programs should involve nurses, physicians and emergency department staff and ought to be

geared to broaden the knowledge base and sharpen the technical skills of all. Thought should be given to having emergency medical technicians participate in some teaching exercises. Both patients and staff reap benefits from a well-informed, challenged emergency care team.

(4) *Peer evaluation* is an excellent mechanism to appraise the quality of care if the emergency department staff is functioning as a closely knit team. Such an activity can point out the strengths and weaknesses of the department and can result in recommendations to effect needed change. Peer review must be carried out with an eye toward constructive criticism rather than as a punitive exercise.

Emergency physicians

As the demands on emergency departments have increased and changes in emergency care have developed, a new area of special practice has evolved within the medical profession — that of the emergency physician.

Among the personnel in the emergency department, the physician has the ultimate responsibility in the medical care of the patient. In general, he must have the versatility to deal with all types of emergencies which might threaten life, limb or psyche, in addition to assuming a leadership role in the work of the emergency team.

Physician staffing patterns vary with need. Most hospital emergency departments do not have physician coverage at all hours of the day, particularly those without university affiliation and those in suburban or rural areas. In hospitals with residency training programs, the emergency department is usually covered by house officers from the surgical and medical services under the supervision of attending physicians. Consultation with various specialty services may be available from either the resident or attending staff.

Hospitals without a resident staff and with limited coverage by attending physicians may use residents who "moonlight" on their time off from the hospitals where they are regularly employed. There are some drawbacks to this method of staffing, particularly if the resident is regularly employed in a specialty which is not ordinarily oriented to emergency care, such as pathology, dermatology, gastroenterology. These "moonlighting" residents are usually backed-up by an attending physician on call to the emergency department.

Approximately 80 percent of hospitals in the United States do not have house officers and thus must rely on the attending staff for coverage of the emergency department. With the marked increase in emergency department utilization subsequent to World War II and the Korean Conflict, the problem of staffing became acute. Various plans were devised for the attending medical staff to cover the emergency department. One method was to assign the staff on a rotation basis, with each member expected to cover a certain number of hours or days a month. This met with protests from senior staff members and those not usually involved in direct patient care. And, while physicians in many specialties are qualified and capable of providing emergency care, it is reasonable to state that some who practice in highly specialized fields are not.

In 1962, Abbott reported a method of utilizing volunteer attending staff members, organized as a group, to cover the emergency department.[1] Initially, the group was comprised of surgeons, internists, general practitioners and a few other specialists. Abbott's group began this service at Pontiac (Michigan) General Hospital, and the method has been referred to as the Pontiac Plan. The physicians under the Pontiac Plan provide care to patients in the emergency department and subsequent to hospital admission, if the patient's problem is within the area of the doctor's qualifications. The physician may, at the same time, maintain a private practice outside of the hospital.

Mills, in 1963, wrote of success with another method of coverage, in which a physician group entered into a contract with the hospitals that utilized full-time emergency department staffing. As opposed to the Pontiac Plan, these physicians have no other private practice and do not have the privilege to admit and care for patients in the hospital. This arrangement has been called the Alexandria Plan following its inception in the Alexandria (Virginia) Hospital.[21]

As experience has been gained and emergency department utilization has continued at a high rate, the position of "emergency physician" is emerging, and the specialty of emergency medicine is being developed. A new national medical organization, The American College of Emergency Physicians, was founded and has grown at a steady rate. Residency training programs in emergency medicine are being established in increasing numbers across the country. Specialty board certification is being sought.

Whatever the future may hold, it can be stated that one *sine qua non* of a good emergency department is the availability of adequate, qualified physician coverage at all times. (See Table A-2, pp. 33–35.) Specialty back-up must be available for consultation and definitive management of the seriously ill or critically injured patient. The emergency physician must possess a broad capability to provide optimum care and must be familiar with various agencies in the community which provide supportive services to emergency patients on referral. The physician should encourage interprofessional educational programs for emergency personnel and actively participate in them, himself.

Physicians' extenders

As previously noted, the trained ambulance attendant may be logically considered the extended arm of the physician at the site of the emergency during the prehospital phase of care. But, in the hospital emergency department as well, physicians' assistants are being used to perform a variety of tasks which the physician would otherwise do, if he had time.

The physician's assistant, or PA, is a new career in the field of health care. Training programs for PAs vary around the country, from a course of weeks or months provided by an individual hospital on the basis of local need, to a 2- or 4-year college-level experience leading to an associate or baccalaureate degree. The PA may suture lacerations, apply casts, assess patients, initiate intravenous fluid therapy and the like. PAs may perform very important services, under the supervision of a physician, and thus extend the activities of the emergency physician.

The nursing profession has examined this new career very carefully. In some areas, nurses have refused to accept medical orders written by a PA. Caution must be taken that the PA is not exploited. Inappropriate use of such an individual can seriously impair quality health care.

COMMUNICATIONS

A broad communications network which ties together all the agencies and personnel forming the emergency medical services system (EMS) is the backbone of an EMS system. The agencies which may become involved in the emergency care of a single acutely ill or injured patient are many and varied and may include, among others, the police, fire department, ambulance company, specialty unit (CCU, burn center, trauma center) and/or support service (poison control, blood bank). All act interdependently in the management of emergency victims, and it is the communications network that provides for the coordination of these agencies.

Hospital-to-hospital and hospital-to-ambulance voice linkage are vital aspects of an emergency care system, providing the ambulance attendant with physician or nurse consultation by radio at the site of incident. It also allows the hospital advance notice of the arrival of a patient, so that special preparations may be made as needs dictate or the ambulance can be directed to another emergency department if necessary.

In some areas of the country, voice linkage is combined with telemetry of biomedical data, such as the electrocardiogram, allowing for continuous monitoring of the patient by the physician or trained nurse during transport and for verbal orders to trained ambulance attendants capable of starting an intravenous line, giving certain drugs and defibrillation. The value of such a system is well documented. Local implementation requires the identification of need and the development of an emergency medical services system plan in the area to be served.

The United States Department of Transportation has mandated an emergency medical service communications system, which combines the hospital-to-hospital and hospital-to-ambulance capabilities. The Federal Communication Commission has reserved radio frequencies in the UHF and high-band VHF ranges for this purpose. The ultimate goal is that a national emergency medical services radio frequency will allow an emergency vehicle anywhere in the nation to communicate with any hospital in the area it is traveling. By way of example, when such a system becomes operational, an attendant in an ambulance transporting a patient from one state to another will have the ability to call any hospital along his route for information and direction should the patient's condition worsen.

As the radio network is established and all concerned recognize its value, wide utilization is anticipated. Data transmission links are currently being studied as a way to lessen the problem of inadequate "air" time.

SUMMARY

A significant increase in emergency department utilization has occurred since World War II. In many hospitals, the department functions as a community health center. It is apparent that some change must be effected if appropriate emergency care is to be made available to the public. Advances in medical technology, coupled with population migration, make health planning difficult. But with improved methods of transportation, a broad spectrum of emergency services can be made available to every segment of the population by the pooling of resources in a regionalized

system of care. Federal legislation (The Emergency Medical Service Systems Act of 1973, Public Law 93–154) has provided for the development of comprehensive, regionally oriented EMS systems.

Regionalization is a current trend and will be a future reality. All medical services, equipment and personnel will be coordinated to that end. As the emergency nurse will be an important player in both the planning of regionalization and in its realization, she should be knowledgeable of the evolving roles and trends in emergency health care now.

BIBLIOGRAPHY

(1) Abbott, V. C.: "How to Staff a Hospital Emergency Department," *Bulletin of the American College of Surgeons,* 47 (1962):4.

(2) *Accidental Death and Disability, the Neglected Disease of Modern Society* (Washington, D.C.: National Academy of Sciences—National Research Council, 1966).

(3) Andrews, R. B.; Brill, J. C., and Horovitz, L.: "A Socio-Technical Approach to the Planning of Emergency Medical Services," *Journal of the American College of Emergency Physicians,* 2 (1973):416.

(4) Benson, D. M., and Hebsibm, J.: "Elements of a Comprehensive Emergency Medical Service System," *Journal of the American College of Emergency Physicians,* 2 (1973):188.

(5) Boyd, D. R.: "A Symposium on the Illinois Trauma System," *Journal of Trauma,* 13 (1973):275.

(6) Boyd, D. R.; Dunea, M. M., and Flashner, B. A.: "The Illinois Plan for a Statewide System of Trauma Centers," *Journal of Trauma,* 13 (1973):24.

(7) Cosgriff, J. H., Jr.: "The Emergency Medical Care Committee: A Response to the Crisis in Emergency Care," *New York State Journal of Medicine,* 73 (1973):2366.

(8) Cosgriff, J. H., Jr.: "Emergency Nursing," *Supervisor Nurse,* 8 (1974):30.

(9) *Emergency Medical Services,* proceedings of the Airie Conference on Emergency Medical Services, May 5–6, 1969 (Chicago: American College of Surgeons).

(10) *Emergency Medical Services Communications Systems* (Washington, D.C.: U.S. Department of Health, Education, and Welfare, Publication [HSM] 73–2003, 1972).

(11) Ford, Loretta: "Expanding the Role of the Nurse in Maternal and Child Care," paper read at the Obstetric Nursing Conference, Navy Nurse Corps, Naval Medical School, National Naval Medical Center, Bethesda, Md., March 1, 1968.

(12) Gibson, G.; Anderson, D. W., and Bugbee, G.: *Emergency Medical Services in the Chicago Area* (Chicago: Center for Health Administration Studies, University of Chicago, 1970).

(13) Hampton, O. P., Jr.: "A Rating System for Emergency Departments," *Prism,* 2 (1974):28.

(14) Hanlon, J. J.: "Emergency Medical Care as a Comprehensive System," *Health Service Reports,* 88 (1973):579.

(15) Hannas, R. R., Jr.: "Staffing the Emergency Department," *Hospitals,* 47 (1973):83.

(16) Harvey, J. C.: "Categorization of Emergency Capabilities," *Hospitals,* 47 (1973):69.

(17) Harvey, J. C.: "The Emergency Medical Service Systems Act of 1973," *Journal of the American Medical Association,* 230 (1974):1139.

(18) Horty, J. F.: "Categorizations: A Legal View," *Hospitals,* 47 (1973):75.

(19) Huntley, H. C.: "The First Hours Are Critical in Medical Emergencies," *Journal of the American College of Emergency Physicians,* 1 (1972):13.

(20) Lambrew, C. T.; Schuchman, W. L., and Cannon, T. H.: "Emergency Medical Transport Systems: Use of ECG Telemetry," *Chest,* 63 (1973):477.

(21) Mills, J. D.: "A Method of Staffing a Community Hospital Emergency Department," *Virginia Medical Monthly,* 90 (1963):518.

(22) Murphy, S. P.: "San Diego Plan for Emergency Services," *American Journal of Nursing,* 72 (1972):1615.

(23) National Commission for the Study of Nursing and Nursing Education: *An Abstract for Action* (New York: McGraw-Hill Company, 1970).

(24) ——: *From Abstract into Action* (New York: McGraw-Hill Book Company, 1973).

(25) Nesbitt, W. R.: "Emergency Medicine and Family Practice," *Journal of the American College of Emergency Physicians,* 3 (1974):98.

(26) *Roles and Resources of Federal Agencies in Support of Comprehensive EMS* (Washington, D.C.: National Academy of Sciences—National Research Council, 1972).

(27) Romano, T.: "Trauma Nurse Specialist," *American Journal of Nursing,* 73 (1973):1008.

(28) Romano, T., and Boyd, D. R.: "Illinois Trauma Program," *American Journal of Nursing,* 73 (1973):1004.

(29) "Standards for Cardiopulmonary Resuscitation and Emergency Cardiac Care," *Supplement to the Journal of the American Medical Association,* 227 (February 18, 1974):833.

APPENDIX A

Categorizing hospital emergency departments

TABLE A-1 SCOPE OF HOSPITAL EMERGENCY SERVICE CAPABILITIES, BY CATEGORY

Category	Scope of capabilities
Category I Comprehensive emergency service capabilities	The hospital shall be fully equipped, prepared and staffed to provide prompt, complete and advanced medical care for all emergencies, including those requiring the most complex and specialized services for adults, infants and children, including newborns. It shall have a capacity adequate to accommodate the direct and referred patient loads of the region served and be capable of providing consultative support to professional personnel of other hospitals and health facilities in the same region.
Category II Major emergency service capabilities	The hospital shall be equipped, prepared and staffed in all medical and surgical specialties to render resuscitation and life-support for adults, children and infants, including newborns. It shall also supply definitive care for all such patients, except for the occasional patient who requires follow-through care in very specialized units. Transfer may be necessary and shall be under prior agreement with other hospitals.
Category III General emergency service capabilities	The hospital shall be equipped, prepared and staffed in the medical and surgical specialties necessary to render resuscitative and life-support care of persons critically ill or injured of all ages. The availability of supplementary specialty services shall be prearranged with non-staff specialists. Transfer of patients for specialty care shall be by prior agreement with other hospitals.
Category IV Basic emergency service capabilities	The hospital shall be equipped, prepared and adequately staffed to render emergency resuscitative and life-support medical services for patients of all ages. Transfer when necessary shall be under prior agreement with other hospitals.

Source: The 3 tables comprising this appendix are taken from the article "A Rating System for Emergency Departments," by O. P. Hampton, Jr., reprinted from *Prism* magazine, pp. 31, 54–55 and 56, respectively. Copyright © 1974 by the American Medical Association.

TABLE A–2 ABSTRACTS OF GUIDELINES FOR CATEGORIZATION OF HOSPITAL EMERGENCY SERVICE CAPABILITIES

Specifications	I Comprehensive	II Major	III General	IV Basic
Emergency department				
Responsibility	Full-time medical staff physician director with status equal to that of other hospital department heads.	Same as Category I recommended; otherwise a physician participating in ED staffing.	Not specified.	Not specified.
Essential staff	Staffed at all hours by physicians in at least third postdoctoral year; physicians, RNs and allied health personnel all have broad training in emergency life-saving measures.	Same as Category I except physicians in at least second postdoctoral year; All ED personnel have same special training as in Category I.	Staffed by physician(s) on call from in house at all hours, an RN and other trained personnel; all ED personnel have same special training as in Categories I and II.	Physician(s) on call at all times from inside or outside hospital; RN, LPN or other on call at all times from inside hospital; all ED personnel trained in emergency life-saving procedures.
Essential capabilities and equipment	Capability to care for all direct admissions and transfers; equipment for airway maintenance, ventilation, suction devices, CVP monitoring, IV fluids, sterile surgical sets of all kinds, gastric lavage equipment, cardiac monitor-defibrillator, pacemakers, drugs and supplies.	Same as Category I.	Capability to care for all direct admissions; equipment same as for Categories I and II.	Capabilities not specified; equipment same as for Categories I, II, III, less monitor-defibrillator; access to latter is required.
Psychiatric facilities	For acutely disturbed patients from any cause and a predetermined plan for follow-up and, as necessary, for transfer to specialized facilities.	Same as Category I.	Not specified.	Not specified.
Hospital				
Essential staff	Physicians in third postdoctoral year in each specialty concerned with life-	Physicians in at least second postdoctoral year in each specialty concerned	Physician(s) trained in emergency life-saving procedures in house at	Designated medical staff physician(s) trained in emergency life-saving

(Continued)

33

TABLE A-2 ABSTRACTS OF GUIDELINES FOR CATEGORIZATION OF HOSPITAL EMERGENCY SERVICE CAPABILITIES (Cont.)

Specifications	I Comprehensive	II Major	III General	IV Basic
	threatening conditions in hospital at all hours; other medical staff specialists on call and promptly available to either ED or in-hospital areas.	with life-threatening conditions in hospital at all hours; on call staff specialists as in Category I.	all times; hospital medical staffs available to call from in or outside hospital at all times.	measures on call from in house or outside the hospital; other staff physicians available to call from in or outside hospital at all times.
Blood bank	In hospital; has all conventional types at all times; maintains supplementary storage facilities in or adjacent to the ED.	Same as Category I.	Only blood storage facilities containing all conventional types; ready access to a supplemental supply.	Only access to an established blood bank or to local donors on a hospital list.
Laboratory service	Comprehensive for all tests needed in care of seriously injured or ill by qualified technicians in hospital at all hours.	Same as Category I.	Adequate for most essential tests; qualified technicians in hospital or on call from outside the hospital at all times.	Same as Category III.
Radiological services	Both in hospital and in or adjacent to ED providing all sophisticated services, including angiography and other contrast studies in Radiology Department. Qualified technicians and radiology specialist physicians in hospital at all hours.	Same at Category I except only qualified technicians to be in hospital at all required hours.	Available at all times in Radiology Department by qualified technicians, either in house or on call from outside the hospital.	Same as Category III.
Operating room(s)	Ready for emergent patients at all times with essential OR staff, including anesthesiologists in hospital and available promptly at all hours; cardiopulmonary bypass capability on short notice.	Same as Category I except only nurse anesthetist in house at all times and cardiopulmonary bypass capability not required.	Operating room personnel including anesthesiologists or nurse anesthetists in house or on call from outside hospital at all times.	Except that anesthesiologist is not mentioned, same as Category III.

Postoperative recovery room	In or adjacent to the OR staffed with specially trained personnel at all times when needed for PO emergency patients.	Same as Category I.	Staffing same as Category I when unit has patients; other areas may be utilized at times.	Not specified.
Intensive care units	Separate cardiac, surgical and other units for adults, children and infants including newborns, staffed at all times by specially trained RNs and other personnel; renal and peritoneal dialysis capabilities are required.	Same as Category I.	Medical (cardiac) and surgical, separate or combined; staffed at all hours by specially trained personnel.	Not specified.
Helicopter landing facilities	In close proximity to the ED.	Not required.	Not specified.	Not specified.

35

TABLE A–3 EVERY HOSPITAL CATEGORY MUST MEET THESE GUIDELINE REQUIREMENTS

Category	Requirements
Hospital records	Prompt availability of previous records of emergency patients to the emergency department.
Poison control and drug abuse	Poison control advisory service in-house or ready access to a poison control emergency center; a predetermined plan for the diagnosis and treatment of the alcoholic or drug abuse patient.
Continuing education programs	Provided for all emergency care personnel, professional and sub-professional in both the ED and the hospital.
Audit and review	Performed regularly on the ED services in the same manner as those for other hospital departments, including periodic mortality and morbidity reviews.
Periodic comprehensive review of emergency ambulance services	Conducted jointly by ED personnel, other medical staff members and emergency ambulance personnel; law enforcement and fire department personnel may be included.
Mass casualty preparations	A well-rehearsed plan for natural disasters with ready access to supplemental space, equipment, supplies and drugs.
Emergency care references	Tetanus, burn, poison control, emergency medical identification recognition charts and treatment manuals and texts in the ED.
Responsibility to the public	Acceptance of all patients for treatment in the ED and in the hospital as needed within their capabilities; necessary treatment not be delayed pending financial arrangements.
Accessibility and transportation	ED accessible to ground transportation in all kinds of weather; where practical, the ED has arrangements to receive and dispatch patients using airborne transportation.
Communications equipment	For in-hospital coordination and for direct two-way voice communications between ED and ambulances, dispatchers, law enforcement personnel and other hospitals.

4

Legal aspects of emergency nursing

JANE C. DONAHUE

> The law is the highest inheritance the sovereign people
> has, for without the law there would be no sovereign people
> and no inheritance.*
>
> *Roscoe Pound*
> *Dean Emeritus, Harvard Law School*

To suggest to the emergency department nurse that she add legal philosophizing to her already taxing list of duties would probably be her "last straw." But it is generally assumed that the philosophy of law, the function of law in our society and the legal fundamentals of nursing practice are well known to the nurse searching for guidelines or some standard to adopt to make her practice "safe from *suit.*" † The situation is further complicated by seemingly irrational legal decisions which give the patient, unschooled in nursing and medical matters, the right to decide what shall be done or not done to him and giving him a cause of action for damages if his informed consent is not obtained.

The facts vary from case to case, and the statutory provisions regulating hospitals and the practice of nursing vary from state to state, but there are common denominators: (1) sustaining the natural rights of the patient — his right to be free from injury caused by another, without his own fault (*negligence*) and (2) protecting the patient's right to decide what shall be done with his own body (informed consent).

As Justice William O. Douglas has said: "In our scheme of things the rights of man are inalienable. They come from the Creator, not from a president, a legistlature or a court." ‡ It is this philosophy which determines responsibility in professional practice, the qualifications and right to practice by virtue of licensing laws and the limits of practice by requiring the informed consent of the patient.§ This philosophy of man's rights is embodied in the U.S. Constitution, the "yardstick" which determines the validity of both *statutes* and case decisions.

The discussion which follows will hopefully be understandable and acceptable to the nurse if viewed from this perspective — that statutes, regulations and case decisions are meant to achieve patient safety (freedom from

---

* *Time,* May 5, 1958, p. 14.

† In this chapter, the italicization of a word generally indicates that it is defined in Appendix B, which follows this chapter.

‡ *Time,* May 5, 1958, p. 17.

§ Licensure, "Physicians, Surgeons and Other Healers," 61 *American Jurisprudence* 2d, §9–14; Consent, "Physicians, Surgeons and Other Healers," 61 *American Jurisprudence* 2d, §152–161.

injury) and to secure the patient's natural and inalienable rights.

THE AGENCY

The authority of a nongovernmental hospital to operate and the requirements to be met by each of its departments vary from state to state, in accordance with the statutory provisions of the law. In greater or lesser detail, the regulations of the state commissioner of health make certain requirements of each hospital department concerning staffing, equipment and operating procedures.[3, §1-13] (See Appendix C, at the end of this chapter.)

If the statutes are mandatory in nature and if the regulations for the departments are mandatory also, it is imperative that the departments conform to prevent revocation of the hospital operating license.[3, §4] (See Appendix C.) If the hospital is a governmental agency, federal, state or local, the statutory provisions for operation must be incorporated. In addition, a hospital wishing to participate in the health insurance program for the aged (Medicare) must comply with the "Conditions for Participation." (See "Medicare Participation," Appendix C.)

The standards of the Joint Commission of Accreditation of Hospitals are not statutory, but requirements for accreditation of a hospital may be made compulsory by incorporating the necessity for accreditation in the state requirements for an operating license.

Secondarily, noncompliance with statutes, codes and regulations may, in addition to affecting the agency's right to operate, impose *liability* for negligence.[14, §234-273] The bases of liability fall into 3 different categories: (1) statutory violations resulting in absolute liability without regard to negligence; (2) statutory violations amounting to negligence *per se;* and (3) a violation of an administrative rule which may be evidence of negligence.*

* "Negligence," 57 *American Jurisprudence* 2d, §234-273; "Negligence," 41 *New York Jurisprudence,* §41-46.

Staffing the agency

Requirements for staffing the emergency department will vary with the demands made upon it, generally dependent on the density of population in the area and the availability of other emergency services or private services. Again, statutory and code requirements and state licensing requirements for practice must be observed. Some discussions emphasize the requirement that only a physician may diagnose in the emergency department. It is premature to say what effect the expanding role of the nurse will have on this requirement or exactly how the nurse practitioner will function in this area.†

The proper use of allied personnel (the assignment of duties to licensed practical nurses, aides and orderlies) is always a difficult problem. It is analogous to the situation of the licensed professional nurse carrying out the legal orders of a duly licensed physician or performing acts which might be otherwise characterized as within the practice of medicine. In staffing and in assigning duties, it must be remembered that (1) the right to practice is derived from the licensing law; and (2) the scope of practice is dependent on the scope of practice contained in, or reasonably implied in, the definition of practice or, in some instances, from custom of the practice. In an emergency situation, the rules are relaxed to the end that a life may be saved by action which might otherwise be prohibited to the practitioner. An emergency is not a "chronic" situation. It is a sudden, unexpected event which does not allow for orderly preparation. However, neither economics practiced by understaffing nor staffing with unlicensed persons are defenses to unlawful practice of a profession.[16, §9-43, 78-84]

The emergency department

Generally speaking, there is no obligation for a private hospital to maintain an emer-

† Charles U. Letourneau, "Legal Aspects of the Hospital Emergency Room," 16 *Cleveland-March Law Review* 50 (1967); "Proof of Facts," 26 *American Jurisprudence,* p. 356.

gency ward.[3, §16] However, statutes or codes for the state may *mandate* the maintenance of an emergency department. (See Appendix C.) The liability of a hospital to admit or treat a patient seems to be dependent on various factors. Some cases have held there is a duty; some have held there is no duty except in emergency situations; and some predicate liability on the dependence of the patient on the customs of the hospital to provide emergency care.[10]

Summarizing, the law does not impose a duty on a hospital to admit every person seeking care. This is a harsh rule, and an exception has been carved out by case decisions which find emergency situations analogous to the termination of gratuitous services, which termination results in *injury*.* If there are emergency facilities, the refusal of care by either a physician or a nurse may result in liability. But this is rationally qualified by making the necessity for care a medical decision, a valid exercise of medical or nursing judgment. Minimally, the judgment must be based on the taking and evaluating of a history and on attempting a diagnosis.[10]

LIABILITY FOR TREATMENT

The principle to be understood with regard to *tort* liability, whether for failure to admit, failure to treat or injury in treatment due to acts or omissions of personnel or from defective equipment, is that liability is predicated on the departure from the standard of care observed by others in the field. Each case is dependent upon the facts in the case. The use of precedent cases as authority for a particular incident of liability is the accepted technique of attorneys in preparing briefs and of authors in writing articles on tort. While this technique is proper, seldom are the facts in cases the same; thus, this method fails when the goal is to apprise a particular group of what is expected of it in order to avoid liability.

* *Restatement of the Law of Torts,* 2d, §323.

Specifically, nurses in the emergency department, as in any other department or agency, in order to avoid liability must adhere to the standards of good nursing practice. Conversely, a patient making a claim for injury must prove, if he is to succeed in his claim, that the nurse departed from professionally accepted standards of nursing practice and that some act or failure to act resulted in his injury.[16] This indicates that the nurse must know what the standards of accepted nursing practice are at all times, which implies the necessity of keeping current in education and practice, as well as adopting new and better standards as they evolve. It implies also a setting of standards by the profession.

Occasionally, when the result of negligence is obvious, the patient may be freed from proving negligence by *res ipsa loquitur.*

Hospitals are more frequently named in liability torts than are nurses. The "acts of the hospital" are often referred to. The nurse's responsibility in liability torts is illustrated by the following decisions.

(1) Judgment for the *plaintiff* was affirmed where the nurse in charge of the emergency department left a patient on an examination table 2½ to 3 feet wide without sides, and the patient fell from the table. (*Petry* v. *Nassau Hospital,* 48 N.Y.S. 2nd 277, App. Div. 50 N.Y.S. 2nd 173)

(2) The court held that there was a question for the jury as to the liability of the hospital where the wife of the deceased informed the nurse in charge of the emergency ward that she thought her husband was having a heart attack. After failing to obtain the services of doctors associated with the husband's insurance plan, the nurse refused to have the husband examined or treated at the hospital, and the husband died shortly after arriving home. (*O'Neil* v. *Montefiore Hospital,* 202 N.Y.S. 2nd 436)

(3) In another case, recovery was denied, where after superficial examination by two nurses, 48 hours after the deceased had suffered myocardial infarction, on the grounds there was no evidence presented that the actions or inaction of the hospital staff was the *proxi-*

mate cause of the death. (*Ruvio* v. *North Broward Hospital Dist.* [Fla.] 186 So. 2nd 45)

(4) In an aspirin poisoning death, the court held that the hospital's negligence in not having a registered nurse on duty in the emergency ward at 2:00 A.M. was not the proximate cause of the death, since the nurses's aide took the history just as a nurse would have done and advised the father to tell the doctor the child had ingested aspirin, which he failed to do. (*Johnson* v. *St. Paul Mercury Ins. Co.* [La. App.] 219 So. 2nd 524)

(5) Another leading case applied the rule that liability of a hospital may be predicated on the refusal of service to a patient in case of an unmistakable emergency, if the patient relied upon a well-established custom of the hospital to render aid in such a case. The court, in affirming the trial judge's refusal to grant *defendant's* motion for summary *judgment*, pointed out that the nurse on duty informed the parents that the hospital could not give care because the infant was under the care of a physician, and there was danger of conflict between medicine given by the attending physician and what the hospital physician might prescribe. Although the infant had a temperature of 102°F., the nurse did not examine the child, take his temperature, feel his forehead or look down his throat. Assuming it is the duty of the emergency room nurse to make such a determination, the court said in this case whether her determination was within the reasonable limits of judgment of a graduate nurse, even though mistaken, appeared to be a question requiring *expert* opinion at trial. (*Wilmington General Hospital* v. *Manlove* [1961] 54 Del. 15, 174 A 2nd 135; *Stanturf* v. *Syres* [Mo.] 447 S.W. 2nd 558)

To summarize, the nurse must adhere to the standards of practice followed by nurses (her *duty of care*). But she must also know what the law and accepted practice are in her state and in her type of facility (private hospital, governmental hospital) regarding the obligation to render emergency care, when and if it can be refused and, of paramount importance, what examination and diagnosis must be made in this situation before refusing care. Uniformly, articles and statutes, codes and standards require the physician to make the examination and diagnosis and strongly disap-

prove of allowing a nurse to do so. However, case decisions imposing liability will do so based on the failure of the nurse to examine, her failure to take the history or, having done so, her failure to obtain the necessary medical care.

Currently, nursing is being redefined so that the role of the nurse will be extended and expanded. It is safe to predict that her obligation as the primary contact of the patient will be at least as broad as these case decisions and that her responsibility in the emergency department will include history taking, examination and diagnosis limited to determining the necessity for medical care or treatment.

A comprehensive understanding of professional negligence which will support a claim for damages should include an understanding that "negligence" in practice does not necessarily imply incompetence or an intent to injure. It may be accidental, inadvertent or perhaps the result of the nurse's inability to do 2 things at once (perhaps due to inadequate staffing). The patient's right to make a claim for damages is based philosophically on his inherent rights to be free from injury and to have his integrity, his "wholeness," protected. In other words, the patient's right to care, consistent with good professional standards and as indicated by his needs, is independent of poor staffing patterns or incompetent personnel.

Claims by patients for injuries are not always indefensible. Defenses such as the *contributory negligence* of the patient to the injury, assumption of risk by a patient, errors in judgment and, although not defense in the strict interpretation, the expiration of the *statute of limitations* should be known and understood so that certain practices, especially record keeping and documentation of defenses, will be done routinely in the emergency department. In some jurisdictions, such as New York, contributory negligence of the claimant is a complete bar to suit. The difficulty arises in proof: Was the patient capable of being contributorily negligent? What were his age and mental capacity? Was he under medication, intoxicated, psychotically disturbed? In other jurisdictions, where the *comparative doctrine of negligence* applies, proof of contributory negligence must still be supplied, and here it will reduce damages, not bar them.

While statutes of limitations are not defenses to suits for damages, by restricting the right to suit as time-barred, they do in effect defeat a claim. Statutes of limitations define the time within which suit must be commenced, that is, a summons served. If the time has expired, the suit will be dismissed on motion to dismiss by counsel for the defendant. The time within which suit must be commenced is determined by the statutes in each state, and it begins to run with the date of injury or, in some instances, the date the injury was discovered. The expiration date may be extended in cases involving minors or others under disability.

Accurate dating of patient records is thus imperative. Having a record is imperative—even if the patient leaves the agency without treatment or leaves indicating he will return or seek aid from his family physician.

Error in judgment is a most frequently used defense. For this defense to be available and succeed, the judgment associated with treatment or care must be based on proper professional evaluation, such as history taking, examination (including x-rays or other tests where indicated) and diagnosis. For example, a superficial examination and no treatment based on noting the odor of alcohol on a patient's breath could result in liability if there are injuries unnoticed and treatments not given.*

Consent for treatment

It is a well-established and universal law that consent for treatment must be obtained before giving treatment. Treatment without consent is a *technical assault* which, if proven, will sustain an action for damages.[15, 16, §157–161]

There are few situations in which patient consent is not required, such as in prisons where treatment may be ordered to protect all inmates or, to a limited extent, in emergency situations. In an emergency, where consent cannot be obtained, consent limited to actions required to save the life is implied, on the grounds that the reasonable person would wish to have his life saved. But only what is necessary to save the life may be done. Anything additional, even though beneficial and even though without negligence, may not be done.

Emergency situations often involve unconscious patients, minors whose parents cannot be reached and similar situations in which it is impossible to get consent "before it is too late" to save a life. Most of the law concerning consents is common or case law, but in some jurisdictions, there are statutes regulating ages for consent in certain situations.† There is a presumption of sanity in the law which stands, so that the patient may consent for treatment unless it is known that he is incompetent.[16, §157] In some jurisdictions, where statutes so provide, even the patient who is known to be incompetent may have the right to consent, nonetheless.‡

Consent for treatment may be implied by conduct or may be expressed orally or in writing. To be valid, it must also be an "informed" consent and be given by a person who is legally competent to consent. "Implied consent" is indicated by the conduct of the individual presenting himself for treatment, volunteering symptoms, asking for help. In situations where the treatment involves only those minimal risks inherent in all interference with the body, implied consent given by a competent adult should be sufficient. However, a written consent, be-

---

* *O'Neil* v. *Montefiore Hospital, 202 N.Y.S. 2d 436.*

† Examples of state law: New York, Public Health Law, §2305 (2), Minors right to treatment for venereal disease without consent *or knowledge of parents;* New York, Public Health Law, §2305, Enabling certain persons to consent for certain medical, dental, health and hospital services. (Section permits consent by minors for themselves and their children in a wide variety of circumstances.)

‡ New York State, Mental Hygiene Law, §15.63 (b)4.

cause it is tangible, preservable evidence, should be the rule. "Express consent" involves an exchange in which what is to be done to the patient is discussed and the patient assents to the discussed treatment.

Repeatedly, the courts have held that to be valid a consent must be informed, and that an "informed consent" is one in which the patient knows what is to be done, the expected result of the proposed treatment, alternatives to the proposed treatment and, most importantly, the risks involved in the proposed treatment. These requirements for informed consent are minimal. Some discretion is allowed the physician regarding how much to tell a specific patient based on that patient's condition and the necessity of not arousing unwarranted fears; however, consents obtained by fraud or misrepresentation are not valid.

To be valid, a consent must be given by a person legally competent to consent. The adult of sound mind is competent to consent. An adult is defined as one who has reached the age of majority, which varies from state to state. In the past, 21 years was the age of majority, and in some states the age differed with the sex of the individual. Today, 18 years is most commonly the age of majority, and where 18 is not the age of majority, specific statutes, such as the *Uniform Anatomical Gifts Act,* may make it such for certain purposes.

Minors

As a matter of policy, few agencies are willing to accept the consent of a minor, although cases have decided that persons of 15 years or even younger may give valid consent if of sufficient capacity to understand what is being done. There is risk in accepting this, especially where statutes specify that parents are the natural guardians with rights to care, to custody and to name a *testamentary guardian.* In emergency situations, signed consent of such a minor, where a parent or guardian cannot be reached, would be better than no consent.

In instances where treatment is necessary to preserve the life of a minor and consent is refused by a parent or guardian, a court order stating the child is medically neglected and requires treatment may be necessary. Since speed may be essential in such situations, procedures for contacting the proper judicial officer should be well established by every emergency department.

Currently, some organizations interested in problems of children are urging a pediatric bill of rights on the grounds that medical treatment for children turns, not upon the grounds of the child's best interests, but on the parents' willingness to consent to treatment. In view of the adoption of requirements for legal representation of minors and other due process safeguards, as well as the enactment of statutes reducing the age required to consent in a variety of matters,* it is safe to predict that some form of the proposed pediatric bill of rights will be adopted eventually. If this occurs, since the statutory law is in *derogation* of case law, it will be necessary to revise hospital rules concerning consent for minors to conform to the regulations found in the statute adopted.

Motor vehicle operators

In many states, the operator of a motor vehicle on the state's highways is presumed to have given his consent to a chemical test of his blood, breath, urine and saliva for the purpose of determining alcoholic content whenever he is taken into custody for any offense involving operating a motor vehicle while intoxicated.

The validity of such statutes has been upheld against a variety of contentions, such as violating due process of law and infringement upon the *guarantee against self-incrimination.* If the patient refuses to submit to such a test, he may not be forced to do so, but his license may be revoked. Where the state's statutes so provide, the test must be made by a physi-

* *Ibid.*

cian.* The state's statutory provisions should be known to the emergency department staff, and provision for notification of changes in the law should be made.

Refusal of treatment

The attempted suicide patient, who not only refuses but actively resists treatment, presents the staff with a complex problem. If retained against his wishes and forcibly treated, he may consider a suit for *false imprisonment* and assault. If allowed to leave untreated and serious injury or death results, he or his family may consider a suit in negligence. There is no easy answer. The best approach is to treat each case as a medical decision, basing judgment on examination and diagnosis and keeping in mind those factors that constitute an emergency which will sustain implied consent. If the patient can be allowed to go without harm, he should be allowed to do so after signing a refusal of treatment form; if not, a decision based on the facts must be made.†

Since the patient has the right to consent or to withhold consent, refusal in some situations must be accepted. Where treatment is refused, a refusal of treatment form should be obtained. If the patient refuses to sign, this fact should be noted on the form and witnessed.

Those states adopting some form of protection as suggested in the American Law Institutes Model Penal Code (Sec. 3.08 [4]) exempt a duly licensed physician, or person acting under his direction, from prosecution for assault in administering a recognized form of treatment which is reasonably believed to promote the physical or mental health of the patient if administered with valid consent or if administered in an emergency when the physician reasonably believes that no one competent to consent can be consulted and

that a reasonable person, wishing to safeguard the welfare of the patient, would consent.‡

PROTECTION FROM LIABILITY

Staff liability coverage

Each person is responsible for his or her own negligence.[14, §§32–65] The question is: If a patient makes a claim and proves it successfully, and there is a money verdict, who must pay? Situations vary, and each emergency department nurse is well advised to seek consultation to determine her potential liability and, when indicated, obtain professional liability insurance.

Ordinarily, the emergency department nurse is an employee of an agency, usually a hospital. Under the *respondent superior* doctrine, the employer must respond to acts occurred in the course of their employment, that is, to pay damages for the negligent acts of its employees. What is the course of employment, that is, what are the duties of the employees in question? Proving the fact of employment should present no problem; proving "course of employment" and that the act causing injury was in the course of employment may present a problem. Thus, written position (job) descriptions are not only valuable but imperative.

While suits by employer hospitals against professional employees to recover damages paid to patients are uncommon to date, it seems possible, in view of the consistently increasing number of suits by patients and amounts paid in damages, for *indemnification suits* to become a necessity if insurance companies are to continue to write coverage for hospitals and remain solvent. To protect oneself in this situation, the nurse employee must have her own professional liability policy.§

* "Automobiles and Highway Traffic," 7 *American Jurisprudence* 2d, §259, 260; "Criminal Law," 21 *American Jurisprudence* 2d, §364.

† "Hospitals and Asylums," 40 *American Jurisprudence*, §19; 22 *American Law Review* 353.

‡ New York State, Penal Law, §35.10 (5).

§ *Maccri* v. *Parsons Hospital*, Pessar M.D. 271 N.Y.S. 2nd 1009.

Not all hospitals are required to pay damages; those which have *charitable immunity* can avoid payment. Government hospitals enjoy *sovereign immunity* except when waived by virtue of statute, such as the Federal Tort Claims Act and State Tort Claims Acts. To avail herself of the protection afforded government employees from payment for negligence in course of employment, the nurse must know what the statute in her jurisdiction provides she must do: e.g., deliver summonses served on her to certain officials; the time in which it must be delivered; acts of cooperation in defense she must perform. She should determine, also, if the statutory protection is sufficient or if she should supplement it by private coverage.

The agency's policy may insure the nurse, thus giving her the benefit of defense if she is named in the suit. However, unless the policy is so written, it may not insure her, and the nurse, named as a defendant, would then be obliged to retain and pay her own defense counsel. This should be investigated, and if not covered, the nurse should arrange coverage under the agency policy or obtain her own coverage.

Equipment requirements

In considering equipment for the emergency department, certain factors must be noted: what equipment is required, its "working" condition, liability for injury due to defective equipment and liability, if any, for failure to have sophisticated equipment or to order transfer of patient to a facility having such equipment.

Frequently, statutes and codes will require certain equipment and, in general, a hospital is required to supply, for the patient's benefit, such equipment as is usually and customarily used in the locality for the diagnosis or treatment of the condition in question.* The physician using the equipment will be liable, also, if he has failed to use reasonable skill, care

and diligence in operating the equipment.† A hospital owes its patients only the duty of exercising ordinary care to furnish equipment suited to uses intended and as are in use by other area hospitals.‡ Where the defect in the equipment is latent and could not be discerned by inspection, hospitals could avoid liability if employees were not negligent in routine checking or inspection.

A hospital is not required to have the latest or most sophisticated equipment,§ but a question arises if the patient or his *distributees* allege it was negligent not to transfer the patient to equipped facilities. Reasonably, the question is one of medical judgment, and if such judgment is based on examination, indicated tests, consultation and diagnosis, there should be no liability.

Medical records

The medical and legal effect of the document must always be kept in mind. Minimally, it should be tangible evidence that the patient received treatment in accordance with the standards of good emergency department care; in other words, it should prove a defense to allegations of negligence. The contents will vary with statute, code and accreditation standards and requirements. (See Appendix C.)

The importance of the accuracy of the dating, including the year, is imperative if the statute of limitations is to be used to move to dismiss untimely and old claims. The availability of this defense will depend on the provisions of the statute in each jurisdiction.‖

---

† "Attending Physician's Liability for Injury Caused by Equipment Furnished by Hospital," 35 *American Law Review* 3d 1068.

‡ "Hospital's Liability to Patient for Injury Sustained from Defective Equipment Furnished by Hospital for Use in Diagnosis or Treatment of Patient," 14 *American Law Review* 3d 1254.

§ "Hospital's Liability to Patient for Injury Allegedly Sustained from Absence of Particular Equipment Intended for Use in Diagnosis or Treatment of Patient," 50 *American Law Review* 3d 1141.

‖ "Limitation of Actions," 51 *American Jurisprudence* 2d, §103; "Hospitals and Asylums," 40 *American Jurisprudence* 2d, §39.

---

* "Hospital's Liability to Patient for Injury Allegedly Sustained from Absence of Particular Equipment Intended for Use in Diagnosis or Treatment of Patient," 50 *American Law Review* 3d 1141.

Not only the date but the time of death may be crucial if a question arises concerning the *order of death* in determining estate questions. Today, novel legal questions may arise when a patient is apparently dead on arrival, and resuscitation measures are successful, and death occurs later. Accurate recording might help to resolve the questions.

In insurance policy cases, where the issue in double indemnity claims revolves around the cause of death (that is, whether or not death resulted from the injuries), the accuracy of the history, examination and diagnosis as recorded may be the only evidence in these cases, especially in the absence of autopsy findings. The cases are not in harmony concerning the admissibility of the record.[3, §43] Admissibility in evidence depends on both the state statute and the provisions of such law.* Where the intoxication or sobriety of the patient is an issue, again the provisions of each state's statute and cases rule.†

CONFIDENTIAL RELATIONSHIPS

Both the medical and nursing professions are, by their respective codes of ethics, prohibited from revealing information concerning patients. This rule of confidentiality has found limited expression in the state's codes by prohibiting testimony by physicians and nurses which was gained in caring for a patient and of information necessary to care. Statutes are in derogation of common law and are strictly construed. For testimony of a physician to be admitted, the patient must waive the personal privilege, in other words, give authorization for the release of information.[16, §101] The statute may also provide exceptions, allowing testimony without the patient's consent, if, for example, a crime is involved.

A problem arises when the state has both a confidential communications statute and statutes mandating the report by physicians and institution personnel of gunshot and other wounds, other results of assault, suspected battered children and communicable diseases. These are often a part of the penal or criminal code. In each type of mandated reporting, the statutes must be studied together. Neither the provisions of the statutes nor the cases are in harmony.‡ [16, §161]

SUMMARY

In the final analysis, the broad general rule is patient safety and all it implies. Further, observance of the various codes and statutes as they apply to the patient situation is needed.

Periodic in-service programs are needed with consideration being given to statutes and hospital code provisions regulating the agency, negligence in the emergency department, the medical record, confidential communication, requirements for consent for treatment and statutory provisions concerning mandated reports such as for crime, gunshot wounds and battered children. Provision must be made to advise all personnel of statutory changes as they occur.

BIBLIOGRAPHY

(1) Bergen, Richard P.: "Who Should Provide Emergency Care," *The Best of Law and Medicine '68–'70* (Chicago: American Medical Association, 1970).

(2) Donahue, Jane C.: "Symposium on the Nurse and the Law," *The Nursing Clinics of North America,* 2:1 (1967).

(3) "Hospitals and Asylums," 40 *American Jurisprudence* 2d.

(4) "Hospital's Liability as to Diagnosis and Care of Patients Brought to Emergency Ward," 72 *American Law Reports* 2d 396.

(5) Hoyt, Emanuel; Hoyt, Lillian R., and

---

* "Admissibility of Hospital Record Relating to Cause or Circumstances of Accident or Incident in which Patient Sustained Injury," 44 *American Law Review* 2d 553.

† "Admissibility of Hospital Record Relating to Intoxication or Sobriety of Patient," 38 *American Law Review* 2d 778.

‡ "Applicability in Criminal Proceedings of Privilege as to Communication Between Physician and Patient," 7 *American Law Review* 3d 1458.

Groeschel, August H.: *Law of Hospital, Physician and Patient* (New York: Hospital Textbook Company, 1952).

(6) Hoyt, Emanuel; Hoyt, Lillian R., and McMullan, Dorothy: *Law of Hospital and Nurse* (New York: Hospital Textbook Company, 1958).

(7) Kerr, Avice: "Emergency Care Records," *Nursing '73,* 73 (August 1973): 40–43.

(8) Lesnik, Milton J., and Anderson, Bernice E.: *Nursing Practice and the Law* (Philadelphia: J. B. Lippincott Company, 1962).

(9) Letourneau, Charles U.: "Legal Aspects of the Hospital Emergency Room," 16 *Cleveland-March Law Review,* 50 (1967).

(10) "Liability of Hospital for Refusal to Admit or Treat Patient," 35 *American Law Reports,* 3d 841.

(11) Martin, William F.: "Hospital Emergency Room Liability Cases," *The Best of Law and Medicine '68–'70* (Chicago: American Medical Association, 1970).

(12) Martin, William F.: "Professional Negligence in Hospital Emergency Rooms," *The Best of Law and Medicine '68–'70* (Chicago: American Medical Association, 1970).

(13) Murchison, Irene A., and Nichols, Thomas S.: *Legal Foundations of Nursing Practice* (New York: The Macmillan Company, 1970).

(14) "Negligence," 57 *American Jurisprudence* 2d.

(15) Office of the General Counsel of the American Medical Association: *Medicolegal Forms with Legal Analysis* (Chicago: American Medical Association, 1973).

(16) "Physicians, Surgeons and Other Healers," 61 *American Jurisprudence* 2d.

(17) Smith, Kelly: "Must a Private Hospital Be a Good Samaritan?" 18 *University of Florida Law Review,* 475 (1965).

APPENDIX B

A glossary of legal terms

(1) *Charitable immunity* is the doctrine that a charitable hospital is not responsible for the negligence of its physicians and nurses in the treatment of patients. This doctrine has been overturned in some states.

(2) *Comparative doctrine of negligence* is one in which the plaintiff is not necessarily barred from recovery, by his own negligence.

(3) *Contributory negligence* is an act or omission on the part of a person, injured or ill, which contributes to that person's injury or death. It is an act or omission which a reasonably prudent person under the like or similar circumstances would not allow.

(4) A *defendant* is the person(s) the suit was filed against, *e.g.,* accused of neglect.

(5) *Derogate* means contrary to or militate against. It may also mean partial repeal of a law or statute, as opposed to *abrogate* which means full repeal of a law or statute.

(6) *Distributees* are a deceased's heirs.

(7) *Duty of care* is the legal duty of the nurse to the patient, to have and use skills in care used by other prudent nurses under similar circumstances.

(8) *Expert* defines special training or special knowledge acquired from extensive experience.

(9) *False imprisonment* is wrongful restraint of an individual against his will.

(10) *Gratuitous* describes a service provided without recompense or compensation.

(11) *Guarantee against self-incrimination* is the principle that one is not required to testify or give evidence against oneself.

(12) *Indemnification suit* is one by which an employer (hospital) seeks to recover a loss by bringing action against its employee(s).

(13) *Injury* in malpractice is the legal loss a patient suffers and claims was caused by the negligence of the nurse. The loss can be physical, mental, monetary.

(14) A *judgment* is the court's determination, or the court's and jury's determination that damages are or are not due, and if due, the amount due.

(15) *Liability* is the legal responsibility (that established by law) to account for any damages which may result from one's wrongful or negligent actions (as determined by law), by paying damages to the injured party.

(16) *Malpractice* is one part of the law of negligence when it is applied to a professional person's misconduct, lack of reasonable skill or omission of a duty, when a person, or his property is injured.

(17) *Mandatory* means obligatory.

(18) *Negligence* is doing something that a reasonable, prudent nurse would not do, or failing to do something that a reasonable, prudent nurse would do in carrying out the nursing care of the patient. (See also, *comparative doctrine of negligence* and *contributory negligence*.)

(19) *Order of death* is involved in a common disaster or multiple deaths (involving husband and wife, for example). It refers to the time sequence of each death and may be important in terms of property rights and testamentary (will) disposition.

(20) *Plaintiff* is the person who files a suit.

(21) *Proximate cause* of an event is that which in a natural sequence, unbroken by any new cause, produced that event and without which that event would not have happened.

(22) *Res ipsa loquitur* is a rule of evidence in courts. In certain injury situations, "the thing (the injury) speaks for itself." The plaintiff does not then have the burden of proving the negligence.

(23) *Respondent superior* is the legal principle that the employer (the "superior") is liable for (responsible for) the negligence of his employee.

(24) *Sovereign immunity* is the right of a governmental agency to be free from liability and suit unless it consents otherwise. (New York State, among others, has waived this immunity.)

(25) A *statute* is a law enacted by a legislature.

(26) *Statute of limitations* is the state law that sets forth a time limit within which a legal action must be started before the right to bring the action is lost.

(27) A *suit* is the legal litigation between a plaintiff and a defendant. The court, with or without a jury, litigates or decides the respective rights of the parties. A *civil suit* is filed by an individual for restitution (money) for an injury. A *criminal suit* is filed by the state for violation of a law.

(28) *Technical assault* is touching another without his consent, express or implied.

(29) *Testamentary guardian* is a person appointed by a will to act as guardian of a minor.

(30) A *tort* is a legal wrong committed upon the person or property of another. A negligent act resulting in injury is a tort.

(31) *Uniform Anatomical Gifts Act* is a law which provides that an individual may, during life, request in writing that upon death one or more body organs may be used for transplantation or other medical purposes.

APPENDIX C

Examples of state and federal statutes

Frequently unknown to the nurse are the specific requirements of the state for her department. To illustrate the comprehensive detail of the requirements, part of the Statute and the Emergency Room State Hospital Code requirements for New York State are given, with the suggestion that a copy of the appropriate state statutes and code be obtained by each nurse. Federal requirements for Medicare participation are also included, at the end of this appendix.

New York State

Public Health Law, Sec. 2805-b: Admission of patients and emergency treatment of non-admitted patients.

(1) Every general hospital shall admit any person who is in need of immediate hospitalization with all convenient speed and shall not before admission question the patient or any member of his or her family concerning insurance, credit or payment of charges, provided, however, that the patient or a member of his or her family shall agree to supply such information promptly after the patient's admission.

(2) In cities with a population of one million or more, a general hospital must provide emergency medical care and treatment to all persons in need of such care and treatment and applying to such hospital therefor. Such care may be provided or procured by the general hospital at a location other than the general hospital if, in the opinion of the attending physician, the general hospital does not have the proper equipment or personnel at hand to deal with a particular medical emergency.

Nothing in this act shall be construed to deny to the attending physician the right to evaluate the medical needs of persons applying to the hospital for emergency treatment and to delay or deny medical treatment where, in the opinion of the attending physician, no actual medical emergency exists. However, no person actually in need of emergency treatment, as determined by the attending physician, shall be denied such treatment by a general hospital in cities with a population of one million or more for any reason whatsoever. (Eff. June 11, 1973)

Public Health Law, Sec. 2806: Hospital operating certificates; suspension or revocation.

(1) A hospital operating certificate may be revoked, suspended, limited or annulled by the commissioner on proof that: (a) the hospital has failed to comply with the provisions of this article or rules and regulations promulgated thereunder; or (b) a general hospital has refused or failed to admit or to provide for necessary emergency care and treatment for an unidentified person brought to it in an unconscious, seriously ill or wounded condition.

[(2), (3), (4): Provisions re hearings for above.]

Pursuant to the Public Health Law (New York State) the Code must also be observed.

Chapter V: State Hospital Code. 720.17 Emergency Department: The hospital shall maintain an emergency department and shall comply with the following:

(a) The governing authority shall appoint a physician who shall serve as physician-in-charge of the emergency department. He shall be responsible for the prompt and efficient treatment of emergency patients and the co-ordination of physician coverage according to a plan to be established by the medical board and approved by the governing authority. Such plan shall require that any hospital having 40,000 or more emergency room visits annually shall have a full-time attending or resident physician-in-charge and he or a physician-designee shall be accessible 24 hours a day. A contract arrangement acceptable to the commissioner providing similar coverage shall be deemed to meet this requirement.

(b) Hospitals having less than 40,000 emergency room visits annually shall devise a schedule to provide prompt medical attention for all emergency patients as the need may dictate. This plan shall provide for reception, evaluation and treatment of emergency patients and for specialist consultation where required. A roster of "on-service" coverage by members of the medical staff shall be maintained.

(c) A registered professional nurse shall be assigned to emergency department duty at all times. Such assignment need not be exclusive of other duties, but must have priority over all other duties whenever a patient is brought to the emergency department. Alternates shall be assigned in order that coverage shall be continuous. Regular and alternate personnel, if assigned to other duties, shall be stationed within easy reach of the emergency department.

(d) All nursing personnel assigned to the emergency department shall receive such orientation and training in the reception and treatment of emergency patients as deemed advisable by the physician-in-charge and by the hospital administrator. Such training shall include at least the equivalent of a Red Cross first aid course. An outline or check list covering such instruction shall be maintained in a current form.

(e) The emergency suite shall be provided with appropriate equipment for rendering emergency patient care including but not limited to:
    (1) examining table;
    (2) wheeled stretcher;
    (3) wheel chair;
    (4) resuscitation devices with oxygen supply;
    (5) inhalator attachments or accessories, including masks;
    (6) mechanical suction devices, including stomach pumps;
    (7) spotlight;
    (8) irrigation stands;
    (9) pressure sterilizers unless this procedure is performed elsewhere;
    (10) a refrigerator; and
    (11) complete trays for catheterizations, cutdown, lavage, intubations and tracheotomies, blood pressure sets, ophthalmoscopes, percussion hammers, surgical instruments, needles, syringes, drains, assorted splints and miscellaneous equipment, as specified by the medical board and the physician-in-charge.

(f) The following items or classes of items shall be immediately available, subject to specification in each case to be determined by the physician-in-charge and the medical board:
    (1) local anesthetic and analgesic agents;

    (2) antibiotics;

    (3) antidotes to poisons;

    (4) antiseptics;

    (5) immunizing agents;

    (6) blood;

    (7) blood plasma, fibrinogen;

    (8) parenteral fluids, including blood plasma expanders;

    (9) sedatives;

    (10) stimulants, cardiac and respiratory; and

    (11) others as determined by the medical staff.

(g) The medical staff shall formulate complete lists of standard equipment and supplies for emergencies, including those required to be available in the emergency suite. Copies thereof shall be posted in the emergency department and shall indicate the location of each item or class of items.

(h) An emergency department procedure manual shall be compiled, composed of procedures for use of house staff physicians and other personnel regarding initial handling of various types of injuries including poisonings, names of staff physicians on call, etc. This manual shall not serve in lieu of training requirements for emergency department personnel.

(i) Provisions for prompt care of emergency patients shall include, as a minimum, a 24 hour call schedule and procedure applying to the following services and departments: general surgery and surgical specialties, anesthesia, departments of medicine, obstetrics-gynecology and pediatrics, central supply, delivery room, laboratories, operating rooms, pharmacy, radiology department, and blood bank.

(j) A record shall be made and maintained of each patient examined and treated in the emergency room, including date, name, address, age, place of injury, diagnosis, treatment, disposition, and name of treating physician; the originals of such records shall be filed in the medical record unit.

(k) Assignment schedules, names, addresses and telephone numbers of all physicians and other personnel including alternates on emergency call duty, shall be maintained at the hospital switchboard and in the emergency department. Switchboard operators shall have readily available written instructions for the handling of outside calls requesting aid or advice in emergencies.

(l) The location and telephone number of the local poison control center, if any, shall be maintained at the telephone switchboard and in the emergency department. In any event, a list of poison antidotes shall be maintained in the emergency department and in all nursing stations. A list of persons on call for poison emergencies shall be posted in the emergency department and at the telephone switchboard.

(m) Except in the case of a medical or surgical emergency, no pregnancy may be terminated in the emergency room or emergency department.

(n) All anatomical parts and tissues removed at operation, including but not limited to those resulting from an induced termination of pregnancy in the emergency room, shall be delivered to a qualified pathologist and a report of his findings shall be filed on the patient's medical record. Microscopic sections of such tissue shall be retained by the hospital.

Medicare Participation

Sec. 405.1033: Condition of Participation; Emergency Service or Department

The hospital has at least a procedure for taking care of the occasional emergency case it might be called upon to handle. Participation is not limited to hospitals which have organized emergency services or departments, but if they are present, there are effective policies and procedures relating to the staff, functions of the service, and emergency room medical records and adequate facilities in order to assure the health and safety of the patients.

(a) *Standard: organization and direction.* The department or service is well organized, directed by qualified personnel, and integrated with other departments of the hospital. The factors explaining the standard are as follows:

(1) There are written policies which are enforced to control emergency room procedures.

(2) The policies and procedures governing medical care provided in the emergency service or department are established by and are a continuing responsibility of the medical staff.

(3) The emergency service is supervised by a qualified member of the medical staff and nursing functions are the responsibility of a registered professional nurse.

(4) The administrative functions are a responsibility of a member of the hospital administration.

(b) *Standard: facilities.* Facilities are provided to assure prompt diagnosis and emergency treatment. The factors explaining the standard are as follows:

(1) Facilities are separate and independent of the operating rooms.

(2) The location of the emergency service is in close proximity to the exterior entrance of the hospital.

(3) Diagnostic and treatment equipment, drugs, supplies, and space, including a sufficient number of treatment rooms, are adequate in terms of the size and scope of services provided.

(c) *Standard: medical and nursing personnel.* There are adequate medical and nursing personnel available at all times. The factors explaining the standard are as follows:

(1) The medical staff is responsible for insuring adequate medical coverage for emergency services.

(2) Qualified physicians are regularly available at all times for the emergency service, either on duty or on call.

(3) A physician sees all patients who arrive for treatment in the emergency service.

(4) Qualified nurses are available on duty at all times and in sufficient number to deal with the number and extent of emergency services.

(d) *Standard: medical records.* Adequate medical records on every patient are kept. The factors explaining the standard are as follows:

(1) The emergency room record contains:

(i) Patient identification.

(ii) History of disease or injury.

(iii) Physical findings.

(iv) Laboratory and x-ray reports, if any.

(v) Diagnosis.

(vi) Record of treatment.

(vii) Disposition of the case.

(viii) Signature of a physician.

(2) Medical records for patients treated in the emergency service are organized by a medical record librarian or her equivalent.

(3) Where appropriate, medical records of emergency services are integrated with those of the inpatient and outpatient services.

(4) A proper method of filing records is maintained.

(5) At a minimum, emergency service medical records are kept for as long a time as required in a given State's statute of limitations.

5

Clinical assessment

BARBARA BATES
JOAN E. LYNAUGH

Wherever and whenever a nurse practices, her first function is clinical assessment of the patient. Assessment is a dynamic and continuous process. It consists of gathering both reported data (which may come from the patient himself, his family or his friends) and observable data (which the nurse gathers for herself) and of extracting from these data the substance of the problem confronting the patient. Assessment also includes ascertaining what the problem means to the patient, to his family and to other significant persons.

The assessment process must also consider what can be done about the problem. Can it properly be dealt with by the nurse and the patient? Should the nurse refer the patient to someone more able to address the problem and deal with it? Will she decide to ignore the problem? Would delay be the best tactic? Whatever decisions are made, the fact remains that the assessment process is not complete until some intervention has begun.

Assessment is undertaken for 3 main purposes, the first being triage. It is critical that an accurate and rapid assessment of patient needs be carried out so that the patient can be directed to the most appropriate source of care. Triage decisions are determined by the degree to which the problem is life-threatening, the risk of complications over the short run, the salvageability of the patient and the efficacy of treatment.

The second purpose of assessment is to define the problem adequately and accurately so that definitive diagnosis is reached and treatment is carried forward. The third purpose of assessment is to provide comfort for the patient and his family. An adequate and accurate assessment provides psychological, physical and sometimes even social comfort. The patient with a fairly benign problem can often achieve comfort through adequate assessment by a competent nurse. It is thus important for the nurse (assessor) to convey assurance to the patient, through touch, explanation and demonstration.

BARRIERS TO ASSESSMENT

It may be easy to define what assessment is and why it is done, but there are many barriers to adequate assessment of patient needs and to the successful establishment of patient care priorities. These barriers may be categorized into 3 groups: patient-related, institutional and professional. Recognizing these obstacles may help the nurse to overcome them.

When the patient presents himself for care, he may be met by the health care provider, have his problem quickly determined and efficiently dealt with and leave satisfied with his care, his problems resolved. On the other hand, the encounter between the nurse and the patient may not be so smooth. Communication between nurse and patient may be undone by differences in language, mores, ethnic group or social class. The patient may be suffering from mental confusion, including intoxication, senility, delirium or fatigue. The patient's behavior may be deviant in some way, including nudity, drunkenness, aggressiveness or hypochondriasis. The nurse may perceive that the patient is not sick enough to need her attention. The patient may talk too much or not be able to talk at all. At times, the nurse's view of the problem is at variance with the patient's view. For example, the patient presenting with what the nurse assesses as a simple tension headache may believe that he has the "same thing" his cousin died of three weeks ago. The degree to which these patient-related barriers in fact do obstruct assessment depends on the sophistication of the nurse (assessor), the resources available to her and the attitude she brings to the problem of giving care.

Institutional barriers also obstruct assessment. An imbalance between the number of staff available and the number of patients requiring care may preclude effective and adequate patient assessment. Or, an overadequate staff which is poorly organized may be just as ineffective as too few staff. Adequacy of staff to load is quantitative and qualitative. To deal with some of the patient barriers mentioned above, it is necessary to have adequate staff resources, including interpreters, social service and laboratory and radiologic services.

Professional inadequacy is yet another barrier to assessment. A nurse may have inadequate knowledge to apply to a patient's problem, or she may have inadequate drive to carry out this function or may simply not want to evaluate certain patients' problems. In some cases, nurses fail to perceive assessment of the patient as part of their work. Such persons prefer to let someone else do the decision making.

STEPS IN ASSESSMENT

In the emergency department, assessment of a patient bears a singular burden. The assessor must focus quickly and efficiently on the presenting condition and at the same time be sensitive to clues of unrelated serious problems, for which the patient can at least be referred elsewhere. But the assessment, itself, although more sharply focused than in most other settings, proceeds by the same 6 essential steps:

(1) Quick overview of the patient.
(2) History.
(3) Physical examination.
(4) Data analysis and problem definition.
(5) Evaluation of the patient's reaction to his illness.
(6) Establishing a plan of management.

Urgency demands efficiency and may limit the scope of diagnosis and management. It rarely, however, justifies the omission of any of these steps.

Quick overview

Assessment of the patient begins with a quick overview, designed to determine the patient's complaints, why he came to the agency and whether his immediate survival is threatened.

The patient's complaints should be noted, if possible, in his own words, e.g., "a terrible pain in my chest when I breathe." Interestingly, the complaint itself may not be his reason for coming. For example, the patient with chest pain may have been sent in by his doctor for laboratory work, not for full assessment. He may want reassurance that he is not having a heart attack—a worry perhaps engendered by a recent family death. Management is influenced both by the problem and the reason for seeking care.

Of course, management will be useless if the patient fails to survive the early minutes of the encounter. The nurse should quickly observe the patient, with the following questions in mind:

(1) Is he breathing freely? (If not, clear and maintain his airway.)

(2) Is he bleeding severely? (If so, control it, e.g., with a pressure dressing.)

(3) Is he in shock? (If so, get him into bed and start intravenous fluids.)

(4) Is he conscious and able to give his own history? (If not, detain and question the person who brought him in.)

(5) Are there signs of fracture or other serious injury? (If so, take special precautions in handling him.)

History

The focused interview technique should be used to elicit the history of the problem that brought the patient to the emergency department. This technique concentrates on rapidly delineating the nature of the problem from the patient's point of view.

At the beginning of the encounter, the nurse clarifies the nature of the interaction. She tells the patient who she is, and what she is doing there and what she will do for him. The nurse must also give the patient guidelines about the kind of information that she requires. The patient should have a firm understanding of the necessity and goal of the questioning.

It is possible that the patient himself cannot be interviewed and that the information instead must be obtained from a family member or someone who has accompanied the patient. If this is the case, the source of the information should be duly noted, so that it will always be clear that the history is from a secondary source.

In outlining the dimensions of the problem presented by the patient, it is important to help the patient tell all he can about his symptoms, within the limits that circumstances permit.

(1) Most patients can *localize* their symptoms to some specific body region. The nurse should try to help the patient be as specific as possible by having him point to the area or act out the symptom.

(2) Patients will often be able to describe the *quality* of the symptom by comparing it with something else. For example, the description of chest pain as "a great weight on my chest" is typical of the chest pain of myocardial infarction. The nurse should try to get the patient to describe the quality of his symptom in a framework that has meaning for him.

(3) The provider is also interested in the *limitation of everyday functions* caused by the symptom or problem.

(4) Patients need to be encouraged to report the exact *chronology* or sequence of development of symptoms. The nurse should help the patient to report the exact time of the beginning of the symptom and of each subsequent occurrence. Onset can often be associated with significant dates like holidays, birthdays or anniversaries. Intervals between symptoms should be noted, as well as their duration. The nurse should establish how often the symptom occurs and how long it lasts in terms of minutes, hours, days, weeks or months. The symptoms or problems that patients present usually have a pattern of variation, and the periodicity of symptoms should be noted, especially as the symptom might relate to times of eating, sleeping, exercise or social activity. The patient should be questioned as to the course of the symptom, i.e., whether the pain or other symptom grows better or worse over time.

(5) It is worthwhile to inquire about the *setting* in which the illness or symptom has been experienced. The patient may be at home or at work; he may be sleeping, bending over or reading a book. He may be discussing something with his boss or his wife. He may be in a work or play situation in which he is exposed to noxious substances or other dangers.

(6) Unless the symptom is of very recent onset, the patient will have learned *what makes the symptom better and what makes it worse,* e.g., food or activity.

(7) Often symptoms or problems that patients present are accompanied by *other expressions of dysfunction.* It is important to know whether the chest pain is accompanied by nausea, whether loss of weight has been associated with the presenting symptom and so on.

Exploring the symptom or problem with the patient may be done with either rapidity or great deliberateness. Depending on the time available and other circumstances of the interview, it is preferable to allow the patient to explain his problem in his own words and in as open-ended a way as possible. However, it is sometimes necessary to compress the time in which the subjective information is collected. This can be done by outlining for the patient the general dimensions of his problem which are important. The nurse can also whittle down the range of data collection by considering the risk factors appropriate to the patient. Questions testing the possibility of a myocardial infarction, for example, may be omitted when the patient with chest pain is a 16-year-old girl.

The focused interview in an emergency department situation will be more compressed than in other settings. The demands for efficiency may limit the range of alternatives considered and, therefore, limit the depth of the interview. People provide better information when anxiety does not interfere with their capabilities for communication. However, the nurse can elicit good quality information even under high-pressure circumstances. She can help the patient to control his anxiety by forcing herself to move slowly and to speak distinctly, by providing privacy for the patient and by making the patient as comfortable as possible, including relief of pain when possible. The patient can also be helped to accurate answers by repeating or rephrasing questions.

Although the focused interview is primarily a data collection tool, it is important to remember that it, as all interactions, can be therapeutic. An adequate interview can be, at the same time, a reassuring experience for the patient. In fact, a thorough elicitation of a detailed description of the symptom is the first step to reassurance. Thus, in completing an interview, it is important to determine the affective meaning of the symptom to the patient. The nurse should try to find out what the symptom means to the patient and what the patient thinks is wrong.

Physical examination

Like the focused interview, the physical examination does not always follow the same steps but varies with the needs of the patient. The patient with a simple laceration of the finger obviously requires an entirely different assessment from the patient with fever or coma of unknown cause. The examination pattern outlined below is thus not intended as a guide for routine performance. It is too detailed for some purposes and hopelessly sketchy for others. The outline is intended to give an overview of the examination process and its sequence.

General survey

Complete the observation of the patient initiated in the quick overview and continued through the interview. Note any *signs of distress,* for example, the wheezing, cough and labored breathing of cardiorespiratory distress or the trembling, fidgety movements and cold, moist palms of anxiety. Observe the patient's *skin and nails,* noting for example, the clammy pallor of shock, the presence of cyanosis, bruises, rashes or fever. Observe his *position, motor activity* and *gait* for signs such as the writhing restlessness of renal colic or the quiet guarded position of peritonitis; the tremor of alcohol withdrawal; the paralysis of a limb. Observe the patient's *dress, grooming* and *personal hygiene.* Note any odors, such as acetone (diabetic acidosis), uremia, melena, alcohol. Watch the patient's *expression* for signs of anxiety, depression, pain or panic; and note his *manner, mood and relationships* to persons and things around him. Listen to his *speech*, and evaluate his state of *awareness* and *rationality*.

Specific examinations

Vital signs Take the patient's pulse, respiratory rate, blood pressure and temperature.

Head Inspect and palpate for tenderness, lumps, bleeding.

Eyes Note their position and alignment. Observe the conjunctivae for redness (e.g., due to inflammation, marihuana use) and the sclerae for jaundice. Note the size and shape of the pupils, their reactions to light and their accommodation. Observe the range of extraocular movements. If indicated (e.g., by neurologic disease or severe hypertension), examine the fundi with an ophthalmoscope, observing especially for papilledema, hemorrhages and exudates.

Ears Inspect the ear canals and drums for inflammation.

Nose Inspect the external nose for deformity. Inspect the nasal mucosa for swelling, and note its color (e.g., the redness of inflammation, the greyness of allergy) and the presence of any discharge or bleeding. Press on the frontal and maxillary sinuses to detect tenderness (as in sinusitis).

Mouth Inspect the tongue and buccal mucosa for color and signs of dehydration. Look at the throat and pharynx for swelling, inflammation, exudate.

Neck Palpate the neck for enlarged or tender lymph nodes, for tracheal deviation (which may signify a mediastinal shift) and for thyroid enlargement or tenderness.

Lungs and thorax Inspect the thoracic cage, noting the rate and rhythm of breathing, the excursion and symmetry of the chest wall. Palpate any lesions, and identify any areas of tenderness. Percuss the chest for abnormal areas of dullness (produced, e.g., by pleural effusions or pneumonia). Listen to the lungs for the quality and symmetry of breath sounds and for the presence of abnormal sounds, such as rales, wheezes, rhonchi and pleural friction rubs.

Breasts Inspect for masses and inflammation; palpate for nodules.

Axillae Palpate for enlarged or tender lymph nodes.

Heart Inspect the precordium for the apical impulse and for abnormal pulsations. Identify the location of the apical impulse. Palpate for enlargement of the right and left ventricles. Listen to the heart, identifying the 2 heart sounds. Count the rate and identify the rhythm: Is it fast, normal or slow; regular or irregular? If it is irregular, in what pattern? Are there abnormal heart sounds or heart murmurs? If so, describe them.

Abdomen Inspect the abdomen. If indicated, watch for the exaggerated peristaltic waves of intestinal obstruction. Listen to the abdomen with a stethoscope, noting the frequency and character of bowel sounds. Palpate the abdomen in all 4 quadrants, at first gently, then more deeply. Note any areas of tenderness or guarding. Identify any enlargement of liver, spleen or kidneys.

Male genitalia Examine the penis, noting any urethral discharge. Inspect and palpate the scrotal contents, noting any swelling, masses, tenderness or hernias.

Female genitalia Inspect the external genitalia, noting any swelling, inflammation or discharge. With a speculum, inspect the vagina and cervix, noting inflammation, tenderness or discharge. Palpate the uterus for enlargement and tenderness. Palpate the adnexa, noting any tenderness or masses.

Anus and rectum Inspect the anus, noting any lesions or bleeding. Palpate the anal canal and rectum, noting any masses, tenderness or blood.

Limbs Inspect the limbs for signs of peripheral vascular disorders (e.g., pallor, cyanosis, ulcers), musculoskeletal problems (e.g., deformities of arthritis, fractures) and neurological conditions (e.g., atrophy, abnormal position or movement). Palpate the legs and feet for edema. Check the dorsalis pedis and posterior tibial pulses.

Neurological If indicated by evidence of neurological disease, check motor function by inspection, testing muscle tone, strength and coordination. Check sensory perceptions of pain, light touch, position, vibration and discrimination. Test the superficial and deep tendon reflexes. Observe the meningeal signs (as in meningitis).

Mental status Throughout the interview and examination, observe the patient's appearance and behavior, his mood, his thought processes and perceptions and his cognitive functions (e.g., orientation, attention, concentration, memory and judgment).

Data analysis and problem definition

The history and physical examination comprise the basic tools of clinical assessment. They are time-consuming and clearly visible to both patient and examiner. Sound management depends not only on good data collection, however; it also demands the logical analysis of data. As the skilled examiner performs, this process seems to take place instantly, unconsciously, invisibly. But it must not be overlooked, performed hastily or carelessly. Although snap judgments are sometimes correct, and often dramatic, they tend to breed error.

The analytic process can be separated into the following 6 steps:

(1) *Identify abnormal findings.* From the patient's initial history and examination, and sometimes from existing laboratory work, identify those symptoms, signs or other abnormalities that must be explained.

(2) *Localize these findings anatomically.* What structures are involved? It may not be possible to take this step when the only findings are nonspecific, such as fever or fatigue. Nevertheless, it is usually possible to localize the problem to a body region (e.g., the abdomen), more specifically to an organ system (e.g., the gastrointestinal tract) or to an organ (e.g., the colon).

(3) *Interpret the findings in terms of the probable underlying process.* This may be a pathologic process (e.g., neoplastic, inflam-matory, metabolic, traumatic or toxic), a physiopathologic process (e.g., increased gastrointestinal motility) or a psychopathologic process (e.g., a depressive reaction).

(4) *Make a hypothesis about the specific nature of the patient's problem.* This step requires all the clinical knowledge the examiner can muster and itself has 4 components. (a) *Select the most specific and central problems* presented by the patient. (b) Using your inferences about the anatomic sites involved and the process going on, *match these problems* against conditions known to produce them. The list so developed will depend upon the examiner's knowledge. In some situations the nurse may have sufficient knowledge to continue on her own through the analytic process. In other situations, this step will mark the point of referral, consultation or transfer of responsibility of another professional. (c) *Eliminate those diagnostic possibilities which fail to explain* the patient's central findings or with which data are incompatible. For example, a patient's chest pain might be matched against myocardial infarction but eliminated because it does not explain the associated pleurisy and purulent sputum. Here again, and in subsequent steps of both problem definition and management, professionals other than the examining nurse may participate or take primary responsibility. (d) From those diagnoses which can explain the patient's findings, *select the most likely,* on the bases of the match itself and the statistical likelihood of this diagnosis in a person of this age, sex, race, geographic location and so on.

(5) *Test your hypothesis by further data collection.* This may include more history, further maneuvers on the physical examination or selected laboratory studies. In fact, the process of hypothesis formulation and testing guides the skilled examiner throughout the initial patient encounter.

(6) *Establish a working definition of the problem.* This definition should be made at whatever level of precision and certainty the data allow. For example, one might be limited

to "pleuritic chest pain, cause unknown" or be able to state quite precisely "pneumococcal pneumonia, right lower lobe." Any definition of the problem is, of course, subject to further modification as the patient progresses.

Evaluation of the patient's reaction to his illness

Labeling the patient's disease may be both essential and gratifying, but alone it too frequently provides an inadequate data base for patient management. Clearly, the central goal of care is to help the patient retain or attain a healthy state. The working definition of the problem should be complemented by a clear picture of the patient's understanding of and reaction to his situation.

The first strategy is to ask the patient what he understands about his symptoms or illness. His answer will usually reveal not only his grasp of the facts but the attitude he has adopted to help him get through the experience. If, for example, the patient with chest pain says, "I don't know anything; you tell me what to do," he is clearly adopting a passive, dependent attitude until he can mobilize himself. On the other hand, some persons find it necessary to deny symptoms or illness temporarily. In the emergency situation, one is usually dealing with the first line of defense the patient can muster; it can be passivity, withdrawal, denial or anger. Such defenses make it possible for the patient to conserve his energy and avoid overt decompensation. They should be evaluated and supported by the nurse.

Explanation of the symptom or illness should be clear and repeated several times. Similarly, if the patient is expected to do anything, he should be shown how and reminded frequently. Time to adequately evaluate the patient's understanding of and response to his situation must be planned. Too often, historical and physical data about the illness are carefully collected and no attention is given to the impact of both the illness and the assessment process on the patient.

The nurse is ordinarily the care provider best trained for estimating the patient's response to illness. Adequate assessment by her makes possible more effective management.

Establishing a management plan

A management plan may include, for example, triage, referral, further diagnostic procedures, definitive therapy, counselling, support, comfort and involvement of the family. Although appropriate management is the ultimate goal of all the preceding steps, it is beyond the scope of this chapter.

AN ILLUSTRATIVE CASE OF CLINICAL ASSESSMENT

A 19-year-old female college student comes to the health service complaining of a sore throat and "feeling bad." She wants relief of symptoms so that she can take her examinations next week.

This is the patient's statement of her problem and of her reason for coming to the emergency department. A quick overview shows that she is breathing freely, is not overtly hemorrhaging, is not in shock, is conscious and able to communicate and does not look seriously injured. The fact that she does not seem to be a "real emergency" might be a barrier to her care, but not in this institution and assessment proceeds.

History: Her illness began 1 week ago, when she first noted fatigue and malaise. These increased gradually, and 3 days ago she developed soreness of her throat: on both sides, moderately severe, increased with swallowing, partially relieved by aspirin. The pain is getting worse. For 3 days she has also felt feverish but has had no chills. She has not taken her temperature. She has been anorexic, without nausea or vomiting, and has had no change in the color of her urine or stool. She recalls no exposure to similar illnesses. She has no other symptoms.

Physical examination: On examination, she is thin, looking tired and somewhat flushed. Her skin is warm and moist, her hair straight; she wears no makeup. Although coherent in her history, she is somewhat impatient and irritable and prefers to lie down.

Pulse 110, respirations 20, blood pressure 120/75, temperature 102.4° (oral). Head and scalp are normal. Sclerae and conjunctivae are clear. Pupils are round, regular and equal, reactive to light and accommodation. Extraocular movements are intact. Fundi are normal. The nose is clear and the sinuses nontender. Ear canals and drums are normal. The tonsils are moderately enlarged, red and show a small amount of white exudate. The pharynx is moderately reddened. The tonsillar, superficial cervical and posterior cervical lymph nodes are enlarged to about 2–2.5 cm. in diameter; they are slightly tender, mobile, discrete and firm. The lungs are clear. Bronchovesicular breath sounds are present in the right interscapular area. The heart is normal. The abdomen is negative, except that the area of splenic dullness is enlarged, and a spleen tip is just palpable below the left costal margin on deep inspiration. The remainder of the examination produces no abnormal findings.

This completes the first 3 steps in clinical assessment: quick overview, history and physical examination. The examiner is now ready to analyze her data and formulate an explanatory hypothesis. First she identifies the abnormal findings as:

(1) Symptoms: fatigue, malaise, sore throat, feverishness, anorexia.

(2) Signs: tachycardia; fever; red throat with exudate; enlarged tonsils; enlarged, slightly tender tonsillar, superficial and posterior cervical nodes; splenomegaly.

Obviously it is impossible to localize some of these findings anatomically, for example the fatigue, malaise and fever. Nevertheless, there is good reason to believe that the patient's problem involves her pharynx, tonsils, lymph nodes and spleen. The rationale includes the fact that although normal lymph nodes may be palpable in the neck, they are not usually so large or tender. A palpable spleen in an adult indicates splenic enlargement. Bronchovesicular breath sounds may normally be heard in the right interscapular space; therefore, there is no reason to include the lungs in the list of abnormal findings.

In postulating the process involved in the patient's disease, note that she has had an acute febrile course. There are 3 classic manifestations of inflammation present: redness, swelling and pain. An acute infectious process is, therefore, most likely.

In making a specific hypothesis on the cause and nature of the patient's disease, the nurse should review in her mind all the conditions that can cause this clinical picture. Since pharyngeal exudate narrows the possibilities considerably and therefore is a central finding, she might first list the causes of pharyngeal exudate with which she is familiar: monilia infection (thrush), adenovirus infection, streptococcal pharyngitis, infectious mononucleosis and diphtheria.

Then the examiner matches this patient's abnormal findings against the patterns of these diseases. Monilial infections of the mouth do not usually cause acute febrile illnesses and are, therefore, discarded. The only one of these diagnoses that readily explains the posterior cervical adenopathy as well as the splenomegaly is infectious mononucleosis. Diphtheria is unlikely on clinical grounds and is also statistically very rare (but not impossible) in the community. The tentative hypothesis is thus infectious mononucleosis.

The examiner will probably choose to test this hypothesis by laboratory work, including a white blood count, a differential white count and heterophil (or related) test. Since streptococcal pharyngitis can sometimes cause serious complications, such as rheumatic fever, the examiner may wish to take extra caution in ruling out this diagnosis by culturing the patient's throat.

If the tests are confirmatory, the assessor has a working definition of the patient's problem, which in this situation is a definitive diagnosis of infectious mononucleosis.

Going back now to the patient's reason for seeking care, the nurse is confronted with the problem of helping her manage this problem. Her goal was symptom relief. In reevaluating her goal she needs information about the course, treatment and prognosis of infectious mononucleosis. She will also need, perhaps, permission to adopt "the sick role" for the time being. It will probably be useful to help her talk through and evaluate her school situation and necessary life adaptations during her illness. Perhaps she will need written confirmation of her illness if she does not recover sufficiently by examination time. Reasonable self-care measures should be suggested, and follow-up should be planned.

BIBLIOGRAPHY

(1) Avila, Donald L.; Combs, Arthur W., and Purkey, William W. (eds.): *The Helping Relationship Sourcebook* (Boston: Allyn and Bacon, 1971).

(2) Bates, Barbara: *A Guide to Physical Examination* (Philadelphia: J. B. Lippincott Company, 1974).

(3) Enelow, Allen J., and Swisher, Scott N.: *Interviewing and Patient Care* (New York: Oxford University Press, 1972).

(4) Harvey, A. McGehee: "The Approach to Diagnosis," *in* A. McGehee Harvey *et al.* (eds.), *The Principles and Practice of Medicine* (New York: Appleton-Century-Crofts, 1972), pp. 39–42.

(5) Levinson, Daniel: "Teaching the Diagnostic Process," *Journal of Medical Education,* 43 (September 1968):961–968.

(6) Morgan, William L., Jr., and Engel, George L.: *The Clinical Approach to the Patient* (Philadelphia: W. B. Saunders Company, 1969), pp. 16–79.

(7) Peplau, Hildegard E.: *Interpersonal Relations in Nursing* (New York: G. P. Putnam's Sons, 1952).

(8) Sapira, Joseph D.: "Reassurance Therapy: What to Say to Symptomatic Patients with Benign Diseases," *Annals of Internal Medicine,* 77 (October 1972):603–604.

6

Establishing priorities of care

HARRY W. HALE, JR.
CATHY GRAY

The role of triage nurse, though not new, is rapidly gaining popularity in many emergency departments, and in some hospitals it is a most important function. But the exact responsibilities of the triage nurse are not standardized and vary widely from one institution to another. Occasionally, the triage nurse will do little more than assure that those patients most urgently in need of care are seen promptly by a physician, while providing some comfort to other patients and distraught relatives while they wait.

On the other end of the spectrum, the triage nurse may do a highly sophisticated job of evaluating patients in order to establish priorities of care. The triage nurse may also refer patients to other clinics, services or physicians for care, as well as serve as liaison officer between the emergency service and agencies outside the hospital, such as the police, fire department, other hospitals and various facilities and physicians.

The nurse selected for triage duty should be an experienced emergency care nurse, who can tolerate the stresses inherent in the wide variety of acute problems presented in the emergency department. She must be able to remain calm, herself, and to reassure and settle excited patients and relatives. Special training in physical evaluation is also essential to the good triage nurse. Indeed, some training in physical evaluation should be given any nurse asked to do triage. No matter how great or small the scope of triage in any given hospital, the triage nurse is the primary care officer, and this responsibility weighs heavily on the person serving this function. Many nurses are reluctant to take a triage assignment, because they have inadequate tools and preparation to do the job properly.

Particularly in the hospital with a large, active emergency service, a continuing annoyance to patients, relatives and attendants is the long wait that people with minor complaints must undergo, as they are repeatedly bypassed in favor of more acutely ill patients. If facilities are available or can be established, a separate "walk-in" or convenience clinic should be set up for patients with minor and less urgent ambulatory care problems. Such an arrangement proves beneficial to patients and attendants alike, by keeping the less ill patients away from the excitement and bustle that always accompanies the care of the badly injured or acutely ill. Several small rooms adequately equipped for routine examinations will allow a physician or properly prepared nurse to care for a large number of patients with minor problems.

The triage nurse should be stationed close to the patient entrance and should have access to a place where the patient can be questioned and/or examined in quiet and privacy. This facility should include the necessary accessories: examining table, thermometers, sphygmomanometer, stethoscope, flashlight and any other diagnostic equipment the nurse might use.

As she is the patient's first contact with the agency, the triage nurse must project a picture of calm, professional assurance and interest in the patient. The patient may be hostile, drunk, belligerent, in pain and frightened and is almost always apprehensive, anxious and concerned about who is going to see him and how soon. He is familiar with but not reconciled to the long waits in hospital emergency facilities and the other problems widely publicized in the media. The triage nurse is thus working against the odds to establish rapport with the patient and his relatives. This often calls for restraint and always for a positive desire to help the patient. Regardless of his condition or manner, the nurse should never give a patient the impression of passing judgment on him, his behavior or his background.

STEPS IN TRIAGE

The whole process of clinical assessment, as covered in Chapter 5, is involved in deciding the severity and acuteness of illness, as well as the more precise nature of the disease process. In this chapter, the aim is to give some guidelines that may be useful in separating patients into general categories as to their relative need for immediate care. The trauma patient will be discussed separately from and in somewhat more detail than patients with other problems.

The triage nurse should note all information that has been elicited. Data can be recorded on a separate sheet or, preferably, directly on the medical record, so that it will be seen promptly by the physician evaluating the patient. In addition to the primary function of triage, the nurse making initial contact with the patient may be the only staff person to talk with friends, relatives, ambulance attendants or others who brought the patient to the hospital; she thus may obtain information of great importance to the further care of the patient. In most situations, however, the evaluation process will be limited to selective history taking and some general observations of the physical condition of the patient, both processes being carried out more or less simultaneously.

General overview and history

The initial step in this process is to note the patient's general appearance (overview) and, at the same time, to inquire about the principal symptoms that brought the patient to the emergency department (history). It is not always possible to categorize and quantitate features of a patient's physical condition in such a way that he can be labeled as well, mildly acutely ill, severely acutely ill, moderately chronically ill and so on. However, when an experienced nurse observes a patient and concludes that he is severely ill, even though she cannot precisely give reasons for her conclusion, it is wise to assume she is correct.

As a minimum, the triage nurse must make a general inquiry about the nature of the illness or injury and take the patient's temperature, pulse, respiration and blood pressure. Simultaneously, a number of observations can be made and questions asked which will help in the overall evaluation of the patient's condition.

In inquiring about the problem, some of the facts to be noted are the time and mode of onset of the patient's problem and *the patient's own opinion as to the severity and acuteness of his symptoms*. Oftentimes, the patient may report some information which will put the listener on guard to a possibly serious condition not immediately apparent. He may even describe the condition so clearly that the diagnosis is obvious. The wise surgeon has learned that when a patient says, "I gave a hard cough and felt as if my incision ripped," that even though the surface of the wound may look sound, the patient is usually right, and the deeper layers of the wound have, indeed, "ripped." Similarly, the healthy-appearing, slightly hyperpneic male, who, while engaging in normal activity, noted something "snap" or "let go" accompanied by a sharp pain in his chest, may be the victim of a spontaneous pneumothorax.

On the other hand, an apprehensive patient with a minor problem, greatly exaggerated by his own fears and fully voicing those fears, may only need someone to explain his condition and somewhat allay his fear. Unusual bleeding is frightening to most people, and they tend to exaggerate losses. It is important to get the patient to quantitate his loss as accurately as possible. Certain items of history are important, and if the patient is not able to give a reliable history himself, anyone with him who can give a history must be questioned at the earliest possible moment to obtain all possible historical information before he disappears.

Physical observation

A good deal of useful information may be obtained by an experienced nurse taking a short history and at the same time making general observations of the patient.

(1) The *general appearance* of the patient and his awareness of his surroundings is important. His *state of consciousness,* to some degree, can be graded between the extremes of being alert and well oriented to being in profound coma. He may be somewhat apathetic or dull, drowsy or sleeping but easily rousable, rousable only with difficulty by shouting or shaking, responsive only to painful stimuli, comatose and unresponsive or in the latter state with widely dilated pupils unresponsive to light stimulation. Not only is it necessary to estimate the degree of disturbance of consciousness but also any change in this state during the period of observation. For example, a person developing an epidural

hematoma from intracranial arterial bleeding may enter the emergency department in a fairly lucid or drowsy state, then show rapidly progressive loss of consciousness in a period of minutes. Prompt assessment and treatment could save the patient's life and insure complete recovery.

(2) *Restlessness* or unusual activity is an important sign and should be recorded. It is frequently the result of hypoxemia and may indicate that the patient with blood loss or a pulmonary or cardiac problem is closer to decompensation than other signs would indicate.

(3) Any *abnormality of color* should be noted, such as cyanosis or jaundice, both of which can best be observed in the mucous membranes or lines of the palm in dark-skinned people. *Abnormalities of speech* (slurring, hesitation) may be the earliest or most obvious sign of neurological damage. If the observer is not certain of the color or speech patterns of the patient, consultation with a friend or relative can often settle very quickly whether or not either or both are normal. This applies to other possible aberrations in behavior or appearance, as well.

(4) A few words are in order concerning the vital signs recorded in the emergency department. Normal *pulse rate* is generally considered to be 65 to 80 per minute. With the nervous tension felt by many patients in the emergency department, rates of 80 to 90 or higher may reflect nothing more than excitement or apprehension. On the other hand, some patients, most particularly well-conditioned athletes, have normal pulses of 60 to 64 or lower and even after trauma have very little increase in pulse rate.

Rates of 50 to 60 by themselves do not indicate any particular pathologic condition. However, slowing of the pulse is a frequent accompaniment of spinal cord injury and, when present in a patient in coma, may be a sign of serious brain damage. Pulse rates below 40 almost always indicate heart block, which is clearly abnormal and demands further study. Although pulse rate characteristically rises in traumatic shock, this is not always the case and occasionally patients with all other evidence of profound shock will exhibit pulse rates of 75 to 80 per minute.

(5) Similarly, *blood pressure* must be interpreted wisely. Normal values range from 110 to 140 mm. Hg systolic and 70–90 mm. Hg diastolic, but there are some exceptions. Occasionally, individuals maintain blood pressures of 110/60, especially when reclining. Moreover, a blood pressure of 120/70, normal in most people, may represent shock level in a person who usually has a blood pressure of 190/120. Allowing a low level of blood pressure to exist untreated for extended periods in someone with longstanding hypertension may result in kidney shutdown. For individuals with usual blood pressures above or below the normal range, either the patient himself or a relative may be able to give the patient's "normal" or usual values.

(6) Careful observation of *respiration* may be revealing. Dyspnea may indicate cardiac decompensation or that a simple upper respiratory infection has become pneumonia. The patient with rapid, deep respiratory effort while at rest and with a healthy pink color (Kussmaul breathing) may be a diabetic in acidosis.

(7) Another item of *history* important to note, particularly when the only available respondent is a relative, is the possibility of previously diagnosed chronic diseases, such as diabetes, heart disease, kidney disease, chronic lung disease and cancer. Abnormal bleeding tendencies comprise important information. Allergies or sensitivities to any substance, but particularly to those involved in medication, should be recorded. Nervous or emotional disorders, family problems or other acute social problems must be known. Finally, of greatest importance is knowledge of drug usage, whether for medication or in the form of abuse, in particular, cardiac drugs, antihypertensive drugs, tranquilizers or other sedatives, narcotics, steroid hormones, anti-inflammatory drugs, aspirin, anticoagulants and antibiotics.

TREATMENT PRIORITIES

In order to illustrate the role of triage, certain clinical symptoms or conditions will be grouped in order of importance. In the first group are problems for which the patient should be seen immediately by a physician.

Highest priority

(1) *Acute respiratory difficulty* with cyanosis and/or inspiratory stridor in the undiagnosed patient may rapidly lead to death. In the patient with acute respiratory infection and acute laryngitis, breathing may be noisy and coughing episodes frequent, but when this patient is working hard at breathing and exhibits a high-pitched inspiratory crow, his respiratory functional balance may decompensate rapidly, with coma and death following in minutes. One of the commonest problems seen in today's emergency department is chronic obstructive pulmonary disease. Frequently, patients with this problem are well known in their nearest emergency departments. Personnel become accustomed to them and to judging just how serious their respiratory distress is at each visit. Occasionally, such situations lead to a somewhat relaxed approach to their care. Nevertheless, acute respiratory distress, especially when accompanied by cyanosis or stridor, is a high-priority emergency.

(2) A person in *seizure* should be given immediate attention. Even the known epilepsy patient in a typical seizure pattern should be watched and protected from injuring himself. The patient in seizure with no previous history or diagnosis has an even more urgent need for careful and immediate consideration. Is his seizure the result of cerebral injury, anoxia or some other cause that needs diagnosis and treatment? This patient's condition may rapidly worsen.

(3) The problem of the patient in *coma* needs little elucidation. The imminence of death in any patient in undiagnosed coma necessitates prompt initiation of diagnostic and therapeutic measures.

(4) The person in *shock* obviously should have high priority for treatment of both the shock state and the underlying cause or causes. Shock is a dynamic and very unstable state, which may worsen very rapidly. Untreated shock may result in damage to brain, kidney, liver, heart and can result in death quite suddenly, even when the patient's general condition appears fairly good up to the point of cardiac arrest.

(5) The patient with *chest pain, acute dyspnea and/or cyanosis* may have an acutely threatening condition, such as a tension pneumothorax or severe myocardial infarction. This is particularly true if his blood pressure is below his normal baseline blood pressure.

(6) *Severe hemorrhage* from whatever source especially when accompanied by pallor and the restlessness that goes with oxygen hunger is a high-priority condition. Blood pressure may be normal or slightly higher than normal with a widened pulse pressure. A patient in this condition may progress to shock rapidly if not given prompt care.

(7) The patient with *obvious multiple injuries* must be examined promptly to detect evidence of impending shock and initiate measures to prevent or treat it. Diagnostic procedures and treatment for any potentially life-threatening injuries must also be initiated immediately or as soon as possible.

(8) Persons with *excessively high fever* (over 105°F.) may soon experience seizures or exhibit delirium and require prompt attention.

Secondary priority

The following conditions are somewhat less urgent than those described above, but nevertheless require treatment promptly or as soon as possible.

(1) Patients in whom the *state of consciousness is dulled* or obtunded require observation. If these patients show evidence that their condition is deteriorating, they must have more urgent priorities of care.

(2) *Chest pain,* especially if suggestive of myocardial ischemia (squeezing, crushing, vice-like substernal pain with radiation to the neck, shoulder, arm or hand), like any undiagnosed chest pain, should be considered a sign of a potentially urgent condition.

(3) *Dyspnea and/or cyanosis* are signs of respiratory decompensation. Although the patient's condition may otherwise appear to be good, the underlying cause should be recognized and treated as soon as possible, since in many situations deterioration may progress rapidly.

(4) *Active bleeding,* unless readily and promptly controlled, should require prompt attention even though the patient shows no evidence of shock. This includes active gastrointestinal bleeding, the precise amount of which is always difficult to estimate, and severe bleeding from incomplete abortions. Such patients may seem relatively stable when first seen, then rapidly develop shock.

(5) Continuous or repeated bouts of *emesis or diarrhea* demand care without delay, to make the patient comfortable and to correct fluid and electrolyte imbalance, which may cause shock if untreated.

(6) Patients with *severe pain* of any type need prompt attention because of the potential threat of the underlying cause (e.g., perforated ulcer, pancreatitis, dissecting aneurysm in abdominal pain). Also, humane treatment demands relief of this pain *as soon as* adequate steps have been taken leading to diagnosis; analgesia can obscure findings necessary to making an accurate diagnosis.

(7) Finally, persons with high fever (102°–105°F.) deserve attention as soon as possible. Although some of these patients will have a readily treatable low mortality condition, others can be dangerously ill. All deserve prompt diagnosis and treatment.

Caution indicators

Some presenting symptoms should alert the triage nurse to the possibility of danger for the patient. Patients with such symptoms require close observation until medical attention is available.

(1) Any *disturbance of orientation* or state of consciousness or sudden onset of severe headache in a previously well patient fall into this category.

(2) Any *chest or abdominal pain* can be symptoms of many conditions, from mild to mortal. Often the most dangerous disease has an insidious onset, so that when the patient first seeks care, pain may be mild and other symptoms may not have surfaced. Yet, in a relatively short time the patient's condition can worsen. For example, the patient with onset of a spontaneous pneumothorax may have mild pain and no interference with respiratory efficiency, *at first*. In a period of minutes to hours he may develop a tension pneumothorax and be in extreme distress from hypoxia.

(3) Patients having a *pulse of 120 per minute or over at rest* and for no apparent reason deserve careful consideration. Tachycardia may be due to incipient cardiac failure, "silent" myocardial infarction, hyperthyroidism or other serious but obscure conditions.

(4) A history of *recent abnormal bleeding* should alert the nurse to possible danger. A patient often finds it difficult to estimate the amount of blood lost or the external evidence of his bleeding. For example, bleeding from the gastrointestinal tract tends to be intermittent, and often the appearance of the patient belies the actual blood loss. It is true, on the other hand, that patients frequently exaggerate the extent or danger of hemorrhage, but in the interests of safety, one can only assume the cautious attitude of suspecting the more dangerous possibilities until a careful history has revealed the problem.

(5) *Marked pallor* should alert the examiner to the possibilities of severe and sometimes occult blood loss. If the patient is restless, the presence of hypoxia is strongly suggested and makes the need for thorough examination and treatment more immediate.

The above classifications of clinical situations illustrate some degrees of urgency. It cannot be comprehensive, because the number of potential clinical problems is infinite.

Rather, it is designed to give some guidance and to indicate some of the commonest problems in which the examiner may be misled if not alert. The watchword of anyone treating patients in the emergency department should be *caution*. Manage the patient as if the most serious possible problem exists until it is treated or ruled out.

Emergency departments and personnel get into trouble by assuming the patient has the simpler, less dangerous disease. It is much safer to assume the worst until sure. When in doubt, observe further or admit rather than discharge. Emergency department personnel should be afraid to discharge a patient unless sure he does *not* have a dangerous condition. One particular result of error in judgment is becoming all too frequent: A middle-aged man, in otherwise excellent health, enters because of new, sudden substernal pain (perhaps not severe) and is found to have normal blood pressure and electrocardiogram; he is discharged and dies suddenly in traffic out of proximity to the hospital.

THE TRAUMA PATIENT

The problem of the patient with serious or potentially serious injuries is somewhat unique. The management of the multiple-injured patient can never follow a fixed pattern. The infinite variety of combinations of injuries, with varying relative importances, makes it impossible to follow a single pattern of diagnostic workup and treatment. Indeed, in most severely injured patients treatment and diagnosis proceed concurrently, and, at any moment, plans may be interrupted by a new development in the patient's condition. However, priorities of treatment can be established in a general way, so that the most urgent conditions are treated first. Certain guidelines can help in planning the management of these most challenging patients.

General guidelines

In general, the priorities of care for trauma patients are simply stated in the following order of decreasing urgency:

(1) Airway problems.
(2) Hemorrhage.
(3) Shock.
(4) Open wounds.
(5) Closed fractures.

It must be obvious to anyone with even moderate experience in emergency care that all things are relative, so this list serves only as a general guideline. In complete obstruction of the airway, the patient will survive only a few minutes, and therefore this condition takes top priority over all other conditions. Severe hemorrhage takes second place because of the threat to life and because at least temporary control of external bleeding is usually simple and can be accomplished quickly.

However, a patient with labored breathing because of chest injury may be in more immediate danger from a laceration of the femoral artery, and control of the bleeding is then of prime importance. Or, exsanguination may occur as the result of occult injuries to major arteries, in the abdomen or chest, for example. This may necessitate bypassing all other diagnostic or therapeutic measures except blood and fluid replacement, in order to get the patient to the operating room promptly so that bleeding can be controlled by operative means.

Third in order of importance is the treatment of shock. How long the injured patient can survive in uncontrolled shock is entirely unpredictable. Shock leads to inadequate perfusion and therefore reduced oxygenation of vital body tissues. Since the precise magnitude of this deficit at the tissue level at any given time cannot be measured and indeed may be changing constantly, it is impossible to know at what point serious or irreversible damage occurs in the kidney, brain, heart or liver. From the clinical point of view, it is a common experience to see a patient in shock from blood loss maintain a barely adequate blood pressure to assure consciousness as well as some urine output and then suddenly collapse and expire within a few minutes.

Much less urgent than the first 3 conditions is the care of open wounds. While cleansing, debridement and closure of wounds should be done as promptly as possible to minimize the danger of infection. A delay of several hours may not appreciably increase the risk of infection in many instances, depending on the amount of soft tissue damage and contamination. Wounds involving bones and joints are more susceptible to infection than other wounds of the extremities; their early care, therefore, is a somewhat more urgent matter. Saving the patient's life comes before saving his limb, but usually both can be accomplished.

Definitive care of closed fractures can be deferred for days, if necessary, as long as there is no circulatory or neurological compromise to a limb. When gross displacement of fracture or dislocation produces obvious interference with circulation or neurological deficiency to the distal part of a limb (elbow, ankle and knee are likely problem areas), the limb can usually be grossly placed in an approximately normal position restoring circulation in a few seconds and without anesthesia. If this maneuver does not result in restoration of blood flow, consideration must be given as soon as possible to the need for an operation on the injured vessels. Splinting to prevent further damage and pain can be done quickly and need not interfere with the care of other more urgent conditions.

Head injury deserves mention in the priority of care. Generally speaking, head injuries are somewhat less crucial than the first 3 top-priority conditions. However, if open fractures of the skull are present, debridement and cleansing should be done as promptly as possible. There is one situation in head trauma that demands speedy action: the patient, who, after a blow on the head, has a lucid period then shortly afterward begins to lose consciousness and progressively worsens, may have an epidural hemorrhage, and decompensation and death may ensue rapidly. Prompt decompression and control of intracranial bleeding may avert this tragedy.

It may be best to think of the early management of the multiple-trauma patient in 3 phases: overview and urgent treatment; history and initial treatment; complete review, examination and treatment.

In the initial phase of management, a very rapid appraisal is made of the patient's condition, looking for the following: obvious respiratory difficulty, gross evidence of hemorrhage, state of consciousness, gross deformity or swelling sites of pain, sensory or motor loss and, finally, blood pressure and pulse. This initial and very cursory evaluation should take but a few moments and may be followed or interrupted by caring for one of the most urgent priorities mentioned above, such as controlling a bleeding artery.

The second phase should include taking a brief history, if possible, covering at least the time and mechanism of injury, any loss of consciousness or memory, location of any areas of pain, numbness or anesthesia and a brief history of concurrent disease or drug usage. Somewhere in the first or second phase of management of the patient who apparently has or may have major injuries, at least one or possibly 2 large caliber needles or, preferably, catheters should be inserted intravenously, and when the need for monitoring fluid load is apparent, an indwelling catheter should be inserted. An indwelling nasogastric tube should be considered at this point and baseline studies obtained, which would minimally include a complete blood count including hematocrit, as well as blood typing, serum electrolytes, arterial blood gases, urinalysis and electrocardiogram.

At this point, when the most urgent problems have been dealt with, the third phase of the initial management of the severely injured patient is in order: a complete reappraisal of the patient, with a more detailed history and physical examination, followed by whatever x-ray examinations and laboratory studies seem indicated.

Treatment priorities

The list of some of the clinical conditions met in the care of the injured patient presented below will indicate to some degree the relative urgency of each. The list, however, cannot be complete, and it must be remembered that the word *relative* is significant. Hemorrhage means abnormal bleeding. Bleeding from a cut finger, while occasionally frightening to the patient, is rarely of significance to his health; yet in the hemophiliac the same injury assumes much greater importance. Further, bleeding from a severed femoral artery poses a very immediate threat to life until it is controlled. Keeping this relativity in mind, some problems in the care of the trauma victim can be considered in the context of the general order of priorities discussed above.

Highest priority

(1) *Progressively increasing dyspnea* requires immediate attention. Acute cessation of respiration or total obstruction of the airway is incompatible with more than a few minutes of life. But many patients exhibit some degree of difficulty in breathing after injury, ranging from mild limitation because of pain from one or 2 fractured ribs to more acute problems related to other serious chest wall, oral or cervical injuries. These more obvious injuries usually get the prompt attention they demand. However, the patient who comes to the emergency department with little or no respiratory difficulty and then has respiratory difficulty of increasing severity may be developing a tension pneumothorax or compression of the trachea from hematoma. Astute observation should insure immediate diagnosis and care.

(2) *Shock unresponsive to adequate fluid replacement therapy* [rapid infusion through 2 or 3 large intravenous needles or catheters] is an urgent situation. This patient most often has massive bleeding, usually concealed, and a decision about an immediate operation must be made at once.

(3) *Progressively declining pulse pressure and rising venous pressure,* the latter often obvious from distended neck veins, indicate probable cardiac tamponade. Here, too, speed in making a diagnosis and instituting treat-

ment is life-saving, and the time available may be short.

Secondary priority

Situations of a slightly lower order of urgency but still calling for very careful observation and prompt attention are the following.

(1) *Airway or chest wall problems producing dyspnea or cyanosis of a minor degree* may not appear to be serious when first seen but, coupled with continued blood loss and fatigue from the effects of bleeding and other injuries, may result in rapid decompensation and deterioration. The basic mechanical problem must be evaluated promptly. In the meantime, the patient needs support for his overloaded respiratory function. When available, blood gas studies are invaluable in following the progress of treatment of such problems.

(2) *Neck injuries producing stridor and dyspnea* need immediate care. Increasing edema around an injury of the larynx or trachea may produce rapid changes in the patient's ability to breathe.

(3) *Hypotension with no obvious hemorrhage* should lead to prompt search for sites of potential occult bleeding. These may include abdominal injury producing splenic or hepatic damage or fractures of the pelvis, femur or other long bones. A myocardial contusion interfering with cardiac function may produce hypotension, often with few other symptoms of heart injury. Brain injury does not produce hypotension until the very final stage of decompensation, just before death. Hence, the patient who is semicomatose, or even comatose but still showing at least some reflex response, and then develops hypotension must be considered to have some injury in addition to his head injury.

(4) The patient whose shock responds at first to replacement therapy only to develop *hypotension without apparent cause* almost certainly has undiscovered bleeding. Further diagnosis and treatment becomes an urgent need.

(5) Evidences of *continued intrathoracic bleeding* (physical findings, x-ray evidence or thoracostomy tube drainage) call for very close observation of patients. If profuse or obviously from arterial sources, such continued bleeding demands open operations.

(6) *Gunshot wounds in the vicinity of large vessels* should be treated with the greatest caution. Even though distal pulses are apparently normal, serious damage may have occurred, and such patients should be watched carefully for changes in color, temperature and pulse, as well as for external bleeding or hematoma formation at the site of injury.

(7) *Progressive or unusual swelling* in the presence of already apparent or obscure injury should be noted. Its presence will give a clue as to massive bleeding. This can occur with few other symptoms in intra-abdominal injury. It can also be seen as a result of pelvic fractures or fractures of the femur, when massive swelling of hips or thighs reveals extensive hemorrhage. Appropriate blood replacement may consist of many units of blood, and oftentimes surgical intervention is needed at once.

Caution indicators

Finally, there are a number of "caution indicators" to take note of. These are situations in which the observer must be doubly cautious in examining, reexamining and carefully observing the patient.

(1) *The person who has been subjected to a great force* needs close watching, for example, the pedestrian who is struck by a car, the person who has fallen from a considerable height (15 feet or more) or one who was in a car that crashed at high speed and initially appears to have no injuries. Such patients must be assumed to have all manner of injuries and must be examined carefully and repeatedly over a period of hours. It is fortunate for the patient that in such circumstances he is often rushed to the hospital within minutes after his accident. But the nurse or physician who first sees the patient may have too little time to observe for symptoms of shock, respiratory distress or coma to

develop, and the temptation is great to do a quick examination and discharge the patient. If this is done, occasionally a serious injury may be overlooked, and eventual definitive treatment is delayed or too late.

(2) Any person with a history of *loss of consciousness* must be treated seriously. This situation may require a long period of observation, 12 to 24 hours or more.

(3) The "frightened boy" who may have been injured doing something he should not have been doing may tend to *minimize his symptoms and thereby obscure a serious injury.* Indeed, the young boy of 8 to 10 years is often trying to preserve his machismo by denying pain or other symptoms which could help the examiner find obscure and often serious injuries.

(4) The *injured alcoholic* is often a problem in diagnosis, because the effects of alcohol may obscure or confuse the diagnosis of all types of injuries. There frequently is no way to rule out serious injury (especially head injury) in the intoxicated patient except by a period of observation long enough for the acute stupor and analgesia of the alcohol to wear off.

(5) Special consideration is necessary concerning *the injured patient in coma.* First, since the patient can give no history, it is of paramount importance that the first emergency department staff member who sees the injured person obtains as much history as possible from those who accompanied the patient to the hospital.

Secondly, until ruled out by appropriate means, the comatose patient should be assumed to have injuries which can be aggravated by injudicious handling. This means that this patient must be moved as if he had cervical or other spinal injuries until they are ruled out by x-ray. Fractures of the extremities must be ruled out by careful examination, and x-ray if indicated. Appropriate splinting or support must be used in moving such patients until the exact nature and extent of the injuries are known.

Physical findings such as tenderness may be altered by coma, but only in the most deeply comatose patient is tenderness completely obliterated. Moreover, muscle spasm created by adjacent injury is not obliterated by head injury and is revealed by careful examination.

Special caution should be exercised in comatose patients who may or are known to have been taking various drugs, including alcohol, or who have diabetes. Discovering the precise cause of the coma in these patients may be difficult but can be done if all possibilities are considered and appropriate studies carried out.

SUMMARY

An outline for the critical consideration of the emergency patient has been presented in this chapter. It should be kept in mind, however, that nothing takes the place of careful listening to each patient's complaints, thorough and, if necessary, repeated examinations and, if doubt still exists, a period of observation. A final warning in managing emergency patients: maintain a high level of suspicion and when in doubt assume the most serious possible diagnosis, until it has been ruled out.

BIBLIOGRAPHY

(1) Hart, P. F.: "Emergency Triage," *Hospital Administration in Canada,* 14 (1972):60.

(2) Larsen, K. T.: "Triage: A Logical Algorithmic Alternative to a Non-system," *Journal of the American College of Emergency Physicians,* 2 (1973):183.

(3) Murphy, H. T.: "Nurses in Triage? These Brooklyn Emergency Department Nurses Are Ready," *Library Education,* 36 (1973):OR-12.

(4) Nelson, D. M.: "Triage in the Emergency Suite," *Hospital Topics,* 51 (1973):39.

(5) O'Boyle, C.: "A New Era in Emergency Services: Triage Nurse," *American Journal of Nursing,* 72 (1972):1392.

(6) Vayda, E.: "Triage Model Based on Presenting Complaints," *Canadian Journal of Public Health,* 64 (1973):246.

7

Psychiatric emergencies

M. KATHLEEN PENDLETON
R. BRIAN PENDLETON

GENERAL CONSIDERATIONS

The intrusive behaviors associated with varying degrees of anxiety can and do hinder emergency department staff in fulfilling their primary responsibility of saving lives. The result of these intrusions can be fatal. The patient, the family (or others accompanying the patient), the emergency department staff or any combination of these persons may be the source of intrusive anxiety and its demanding behaviors.

The emergency department staff, by role and by definition, has the responsibility of coping with and beginning treatment of these psychiatric emergencies. Such action entails several tasks: (1) keeping calm in order not to add to the anxiety; (2) recognizing and assessing behaviors provoked by anxiety; (3) successfully intervening in these behaviors; and (4) learning from each situation how better to deal with the next psychiatric emergency.

Attempting to find an exact definition of a psychiatric emergency is like trying to find an exact definition of "love." Each definer uses his own theoretical and experiential background to choose the words which best describe his experience with the phenomenon.

Some common threads do appear in the available definitions, one being the *suddenness* of the event: "a sudden serious disturbance"; [5, p. 931] "an urgent condition." [27, p. 457] Another commonality among definitions refers to the *overwhelming nature* of the event: "an obstacle seen as unsurmountable"; [7, p. 1] "unable to cope with life forces"; [26, p. 43] "exceeds an individual's adaptive capacity." [27, p. 457]

The implied, but seldom stated, third thread is that the person needs *psychological assistance* during this time of high stress. These 3 threads unite in a simple and pragmatic definition: A psychiatric emergency exists whenever "some person's anxiety has increased to the point that immediate aid is requested." [19, p. 401] By using this definition, with its focus on the patient and on the present level of anxiety, guidelines for sound interventions are readily available.

Anxiety is highly contagious; at any given moment the emergency department staff can be faced with anxiety in self and anxiety in a patient. Staff members must be able to understand, accept and handle their own level of anxiety in a tense situation and be able to intervene successfully into the patient's anxious behaviors. This is crucial, because the most powerful intervention strategy the emergency department staff has is competent self-assurance. As Rogerson states:

> The composure of the emergency room staff in knowing how to handle psychiatric emergencies is an extremely valuable asset in dealing with such emergencies—especially when it is coupled with an accepting attitude and prompt decisive action.[27, p. 475]

Long experience has shown that the insecurities of a staff in handling psychiatric emergencies decrease markedly with a good prescription of well-tested, specific interventions. Self-confidence and composure increase with each instance of successful intervention. This chapter, therefore, is designed to make explicit the strategy and tactics of handling psychiatric emergencies and to make clear some of the reasons behind them, so that successful intervention can be accomplished even by the novice.

The behaviors associated with anxiety can be considered in many ways. For this chapter, the concept of anxiety will be viewed as a horseshoe-shaped spectrum, with "too little anxiety" and "too much anxiety"[4] approximating each other at the ends. Viewed this way, a person can be seen as able to react to stress in a variety of ways, depending on personality characteristics, life experiences and the immediate environment. One person may exhibit the behaviors associated with panic and another, the behaviors associated with feelings of severe depression. The quantity of subjective anxiety (known only to the person) involved in either reaction can closely approximate the other. (See Figure 7–1.)

This chapter is organized around 4 identifiable levels of *visible* anxiety: (1) little or no visible anxiety; (2) mild or moderate anxiety; (3) severe anxiety; and (4) panic. No one of these levels exists completely by itself, since the behaviors more frequently associated with one level can slide in and out of various other levels. As it is difficult to discuss the staff's responses to clinical situations without considering the situations, the patient will be the primary focus in this discussion, with suggestions for the staff's implementation of the ideas presented. The last few paragraphs of the chapter will be directed to staff alone.

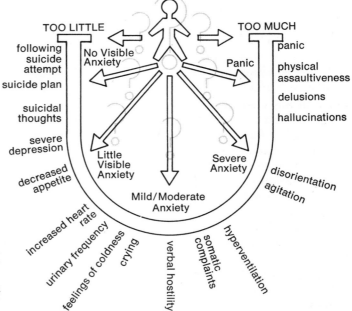

Figure 7–1 The horseshoe of anxiety. This model illustrates: (1) that a person exhibiting little or no anxiety is not the complete opposite of the person exhibiting panic, and (2) that any one person can respond to stress in a variety of ways.

PATIENT CONSIDERATIONS

Little or no visible anxiety

Some level of anxiety is necessary to function. Each person usually learns when his own level of anxiety is exceeded and the resulting feeling of being without the energy to lift a finger. Because each person is usually in touch with his own fluctuating levels of anxiety, he should be able to assess when levels of anxiety in others are too low to be functional. The most reliable clue is when the seriousness of a situation and the person's response do not match. Thus, when a person shrugs off a 30 pound weight loss or responds, "Oh, yeah," to having come very close to a successful suicide, health care professionals' antennae should start scanning. The most frequent occurrence of this incongruent lack of anxiety is in depressed persons or in persons being treated following an attempt to commit suicide.

A patient most distressing to health care professionals is the person who has attempted suicide. Emergency department staff frequently interpret the attitude of a suicidal person as saying, in effect, "What you value so highly isn't worth much." Sometimes it is difficult to remember that the primary consideration is to save that person's life.

Life-saving procedures depend upon the type and severity of the means used to attempt suicide; as these procedures have been outlined in other chapters, they will not be developed in this chapter. But something needs to be added here, namely the reasons the staff must carry out those procedures with an accepting, nonpunishing attitude.

Health professionals have long known that people are more inclined to talk when they believe they will be heard and that more information can be collected from a verbal than from a nonverbal person. It logically follows that behaviors on the part of the professional staff which indicate ability and desire to listen to another person will increase that person's verbal output, increase the information collected, increase the likelihood of appropriate referral and decrease the probability that this person will return to the emergency department following another attempt at suicide.

So, while following procedures for gastric lavage, suturing or other trauma-directed measures, the nurse should keep the tone of her voice well-modulated, and avoid being shrill or sharp or moving suddenly. She should not cram the lavage tube down the patient, rather take time to talk reassuringly while working, explaining what is being done. She must also watch what is being said; no punishing comments, such as, "This will teach you a lesson" or "Do a better job next time," are indicated in such a situation. The patient knows what has been done and feels bad enough without having more guilt and feelings of worthlessness added.

Emergency department staff members are *the* health care profession as far as the patient is concerned. If he gets the message that he is not being heard, that it really does not matter what happens to him, that he should not be taking the staff's time away from someone who really needs it, it is highly unlikely that he will seek help from another health care professional, *i.e.*, a psychotherapist. If psychotherapy is mandated and follows punishing treatment in the emergency room, it will take longer for a trusting relationship to be established between patient and therapist. This deprives the troubled person of support and help during those 3 most dangerous months following a suicidal crisis [12] and increases the chances that this person will return to the emergency room after a second suicide attempt. An accepting attitude lets the patient know that the staff cares about *the person*, regardless of feelings about the behavior of the person.

Too frequently, after the hectic atmosphere of the initial life-saving procedures, the patient is left alone. On the surface, there appears to be little need to spend any additional time with him, since he is apparently no longer in danger of dying, and there is no behavior indicating that anxiety is present. It seems as if the suicidal act has drained all of the anxiety out of him.[6] Now is the time for the staff to start inquiring as to "What specifically happened right before you took the pills?" While talking and listening, the staff should ask the following questions of themselves:

(1) Did the staff member have to be insistent to get an answer from the patient?

(2) Does the patient respond slowly? (If the staff member waits quietly, the patient will eventually answer the question.)

(3) Is the patient highly verbal? (If so, he needs only to be given a few open-ended questions, "How did this evening start?" or statements, "Tell me how this happened," and the whole story unfolds.)

(4) How does the patient respond to touch? By holding out his hand to the staff member? By accepting a staff member's hand when offered? By withdrawing from touch?

(5) Is it easier for this patient to talk with a particular staff member?

This information can be jotted on a card and kept in a specified place, available only to staff members who are fully aware of their responsibility in patient confidentiality. Then, if this person is seen following another suicide attempt, the available information can be built upon instead of repeated.

The actions discussed above serve 3 purposes. They plainly say, "I (a staff person) care enough about you (the patient) to take this extra time." They provide the staff members with something other than a "here we go again" focus for a patient who attempts suicide more than once. And they provide human contact for someone who desperately needs it.

Among possible difficulties involved in taking extra time with a depressed patient is that the staff person is vulnerable and may risk painful rejection by the patient. Another is that the staff's attention may be misused by patients who use suicide attempts as a means of controlling those around them. However painful the rejection or the feelings of being "used," it is helpful to remember that pure suicidal manipulators are few, and it is better for the nurse, as well as for the patients, to provide attention than to withhold the caring.

Assessment and Prevention

Saving lives is the primary consideration of the emergency department staff. With persons who have attempted suicide, the life-saving role is rather well defined; but in *preventing* suicides, yet another aspect of saving lives, the role is less well defined. One reason that the preventive role is less explicit is the common feeling of emergency department staff that they never see anyone *before* he attempts suicide.

Certain concepts are now known about suicide, however: (1) 65 percent of all persons who commit suicide have had some contact with a health care facility or professional within the 3 to 6 month period previous to the suicide attempt;[31] (2) in no research study on suicide has there been shown to be a positive relationship between good health and suicide;[17] (3) the second most frequent warning about suicide (after direct expressions of suicidal intent) is a discussion of depressed feelings;[26] (4) these depressive feelings are frequently masked by a variety of physical complaints;[19,26] and (5) suicide-prone persons are more likely to respond to any stress as a crisis.[17]

It is reasonable to expect that an emergency department staff sees a higher percentage of persons who are suicide risks than do other health care professionals. The persons in this anxiety category may come to the emergency department because of expressed or inferred feelings of depression, which may be viewed as either the cause of or the result of physical symptoms.

The severely depressed person (referring to a feeling tone, not to a diagnostic category) will probably be brought to the emergency department by family or friends. This person will be sad, and the emergency department staff will feel sad, not tense, around this person. He will move slowly, be apathetic, be unable to initiate any activity and will show the effects of decreased appetite, lack of sleep and poor grooming.

Exploring this person's thoughts about suicide is critical. Few people commit suicide while feeling and acting severely depressed. Suicide is a more frequent occurrence as they start to feel better, but the staff does not know where this person is on the depression scale, until someone asks. A direct inquiry in a matter-of-fact voice (no sense of the dramatic), such as, "Have you thought of taking your own life?" "Have you felt that you wanted to kill yourself?" or "Have you wished to be dead?" is necessary. If the answer is "No," the staff member has shown that she cared enough to ask and that it is acceptable to talk about suicidal thoughts, thus leaving the door open should suicidal thoughts occur later.

This is often hard for a nurse to do because of the fear of putting ideas into someone's head. It is extremely rare that a depressed person has not considered suicide. The thought of suicide has usually been entertained at least long enough to reject it. Staff members should assume they will not be mentioning an unthought of topic.

If the depressed person expresses any sort of "Yes," to the above questions (e.g., "I've thought about ending it all" or "They would be better off without me" or "I can't stand any more of this"), the next question to ask and get an answer to is: "How do you think you might kill yourself?" or "Did you think about how you might do it?" The staff should then find out if the person has the necessary items for carrying out the proposed plan. The more specific and detailed the plan, the greater the risk of successful suicide. The more easily available the means for carrying out the plan, the greater the risk. The more violent and the greater assurance of success there is in the

chosen method, the greater the risk; thoughts of shooting and jumping are considered more lethal than cutting oneself or swallowing pills.[28]

When the data point to a high suicidal risk, any one or all of the following are appropriate actions, depending upon the situation:

(1) Inform those persons with the patient (*e.g.*, family or friends) of your concerns and suggest further immediate evaluation. If there are no family or friends to notify, the risk of suicide increases.

(2) Notify an available crisis counselor (*e.g.*, a member of an on-call crisis team connected with your emergency department, the suicide/crisis telephone team, or the psychiatric outpatient clinic). Explain your concerns, and request someone to come to the emergency department to do further evaluation.

(3) If the community does not have a crisis team or a mental health/psychiatric worker available and the risk of suicide is too high to let the person leave, try any of the following until it is possible to reach the patient's personal physician.

If the person can move and perform some tasks, put him to work under direct supervision. (How long has it been since there has been time to sort out the cupboard where the record forms are kept?) Keep in mind the patient's proposed method of suicide, and avoid allowing him contact with the instruments of the expressed method. Someone who has talked about cutting his wrists is not ideally suited to sorting and wrapping suture sets.

If the person cannot muster the motivation for such tasks, find a place for him to sit where he can be readily seen. Explain to him the concern for his safety. Make a point of frequent contacts with him, about every 15 minutes. Offer him a magazine, coffee, an ash tray; empty the ash tray; and give of your time. Let him know that he is not alone. Get a doctor, preferably his personal physician, to the emergency department as quickly as possible.

The big "don't" is *don't* make promises which are impossible to keep, such as, "I won't let you kill yourself." This is false reassurance. It immediately sets up a power struggle between the staff and the patient, one that the staff can never win.

Try to remember that the emergency department is probably the only place open. There is nowhere else for the depressed person to go. He is undecided whether suicide is the answer, or he would not have sought help. No matter how ridiculous it may seem, considering suicide is often a way of getting feedback about oneself: "Am I worthy enough as a person to even consider continuing living?" A staff member's concern can swing the patient's feelings toward life.

Patients with undefined anxiety

The next group for consideration falls into that shadowy area between "little or no visible anxiety" (see Table 7–1, below) and "mild to moderate anxiety" (see Table 7–2, page 79), the group of patients who come to the emergency department for any of a wide range of physical complaints. This is not to say that everyone who comes to the emergency department with a headache or an ingrown toenail is contemplating suicide but that the emergency department staff can develop the skills to differentiate between the headache which requires an aspirin and the one which needs further exploration.

Again, the first question to be asked is some form of "Why now?" It can be phrased as, "What made you decide you had better come to the hospital?" or "What happened right before this pain started?" or "What went on today which led up to this?" This can be asked while the preliminary procedures for assessing the physical complaint (e.g., measuring vital signs, having the patient undress or collecting blood or urine specimens) are being done. Then listen closely while the patient relates what happened, especially for any statements which hint at sadness, indicate a grim future, mention being better off dead or indicate any thought of suicide or dying. If a statement pertaining to any of these areas is made, follow it up with, "Something you said concerned me. [Repeat the statement of concern.] Can you tell me more about that?"

TABLE 7–1 LITTLE OR NO VISIBLE ANXIETY

Behaviors observed	Common interpretations	Expected staff behaviors
(1) Complaints of a wide variety of physical problems, ranging from an ingrown toenail through pneumonia to cancer (2) Somatic complaints of: difficulty falling to sleep; early morning awakening; fatigue; loss of appetite; constipation/diarrhea; decrease in sexual functioning or desire; aches and pains; strange taste and/or burning sensation in mouth	(1) Neurosis, depressive (2) Involutional melancholia (3) Schizo-affective, depressed (4) Hypochondriacal	(1) Listen and take him seriously. (Do you know for an absolute fact that this person is "pretending"?) (2) Do an assessment of suicidal potential. (3) Make no derogatory remarks. (4) Show calm, reassuring acceptance of *the patient,* not necessarily acceptance of his behavior.

The answer may be, "Oh, I didn't mean that," or it may be a sudden outburst of feelings and/or tears, at which time an ear and a tissue are needed *plus* getting answers to those questions mentioned earlier, in reference to the severely depressed patient.

Keep in mind that the suicidal risk increases with applicability of each of the following patient characteristics.*

(1) White male between the ages of 45 and 60 years.

(2) Nonwhite male between the ages of 20 and 35 years.

(3) Female between the ages of 20 and 30 years.

(4) Married and under the age of 20 years.

(5) Single, divorced, or widowed.

(6) Has made a previous suicide attempt.

(7) Has been treated within the past 6 months for any psychological problem.

(8) Has suffered a recent loss (in the past 6 months to one year) of anything *regarded by the patient* as important (e.g., home, job, a person, a pet or health).

(9) Firearms or hanging is the method of suicide being considered.

Mild to moderate anxiety

This is probably the most common of all levels of anxiety. Everyone has experienced that flush of exhilaration when faced with an exciting, challenging task. And, at least once, everyone has been gripped with that sudden tight feeling inside that would not let go, sweaty palms, pounding heart in throat, working to breathe, knees like a not-quite-set aspic and wanting to go to the bathroom so badly that there was no way it could be reached soon enough. The former level provides that extra "oomph" to get over an obstacle or the fortitude to stay with a task until it is done,

*For a more complete rating scale, see the "Suicide Prevention Center, Assessment of Suicidal Potentiality" from the Los Angeles Suicide Prevention Center and the Institute for Studies of Self-Destructive Behaviors, 1041 S. Menlo Ave., Los Angeles, Calif. 90006.

like the parent who is reassuring and calm until all of the stitches are in his child's scalp. More intense anxiety creates obstacles, such as hyperventilation and respiratory alkalosis or verbal hostility, anger and retaliation.

It is highly unlikely that an 8-hour shift in the emergency department can pass without the presence of at least one of the above characteristics of moderate anxiety. The manifestations of mild to moderate anxiety are visible in 9 out of every 10 persons who come to the emergency department and are easy to handle if recognized and responded to quickly. Time does not allow a personality assessment of everyone who comes to the emergency department, which would help the staff to predict which persons will move from mild anxiety to more severe and less adaptive anxious behaviors. Therefore, a few precautionary steps should be applied to everyone.

(1) Provide a waiting room out of the mainline of emergency traffic. Anxiety breeds anxiety. If a mildly anxious person is continuously reminded of the trauma and fear associated with the emergency department, his own anxiety will be reinforced, and he will spend much of his energy controlling this escalation of anxiety, leaving no reserve strength to cope with changes, for example, in the condition of a family member being treated.

(2) Make sure that the person (secretary, nurses' aide/orderly, nurse or doctor) who first sees the patient and/or family is friendly, warm, listens well and respects people. These qualities are demonstrated by paying attention to people when they talk, looking at them, calling them by name and title, trying to pronounce names properly and graciously accepting corrections when a name is mispronounced.

Other nonspecific but preventative measures are: (3) Offer a hot drink or food. This can be done by actually handing a person a cup of coffee, tea or cocoa or by having a vending machine in the waiting room. (4) Have restrooms close to the waiting room, obviously marked and well maintained. (5) Have blankets available for use and the waiting room seating out of drafts. (6) Have facial tissues or washcloths available, and offer them when someone is crying. (7) Make sure that people know of the availability of the staff. This can be done by the staff circulating in the waiting room and the treatment rooms.

The consistent application of any or all of the above measures will reduce the anxiety of all persons involved. These measures support the current coping behaviors of the family and/or patient and make the emergency department staff's job easier.

Hyperventilation

The front-line staff member should also be able to assess dizziness, complaints of being "light-headed," sweating and shallow breathing as signs of less adaptive anxiety and be able to take action or summon help. These symptoms are indicative of hyperventilation and respiratory alkalosis and may be the presenting complaint of a patient or may develop in anyone in the waiting room. The appropriate actions include doing a physical examination, establishing normal respirations and teaching.

The physical examination serves to reassure the patient that he is being taken seriously and that his heart and lungs are functioning properly. Rebreathing his own exhaled air increases the CO_2 content of the lungs and increases the effectiveness of the person's breathing. This is done by providing the patient with a paper bag (or using the synthetic bag and mask especially designed for this purpose), instructing him to place the bag over his nose and mouth and to breathe with the bag in place. A staff member must stay with the patient until regular breathing has returned.

The next step is to spend a few minutes teaching the patient how to hyperventilate. Instruct the patient to breathe rapidly for approximately 2 minutes which reestablishes respiratory alkalosis, and then have him again use the rebreathing bag.[19] This demonstrates to the patient that he can control the situation if or when it next occurs.

Coping with anger and hostility

When anger and verbal hostility are the result of building anxiety, the emergency department staff needs all the patience and objectivity it can muster. There is nothing comfortable about being yelled at, sworn at or constantly criticized for the care being given. This anxiety turned to anger may stem from the patient's feelings of frustration (e.g., the staff's apparent preoccupation with filling out forms) or from the patient's unmet expectations of the staff (e.g., the direct and immediate resolution of his problem). The anger is a substitute for anxiety and is being used to exert some control in a situation where the patient feels powerless. The verbal content may connote hostility, but the nonverbal message is fear: "I am afraid something will happen to me. Are you doing everything you can to help me?"[9]

Staff members must respond to the nonverbal message, in a reassuring and nonretaliatory manner. Returning a patient's angry comment with sarcasm, withdrawal or placating statements only adds to the feelings of powerlessness and makes the situation more tense. Openly recognizing the feelings of anger, their relationship to anxiety and that there is nothing wrong with these feelings helps the patient. A not infrequent exchange might be:

Patient's Wife: You never do any work. You just sit there and write. . . . It seems you could find something better to do with your time.
Emergency Nurse: Yes, I'm writing. It must be hard to sit and wait without knowing exactly what is happening to your husband. Is there anything I can do?

The staff nurse must look beyond the surface hostility and respond to decrease the anger and the anxiety, and not with words which will be regretted later. It is useful to remember that the anger is not directed at anyone personally; it just needs a place to be dumped.

Table 7–2 summarizes the characteristics of mild to moderate anxiety and how an emergency department staff should cope with it.

TABLE 7–2 MILD TO MODERATE ANXIETY

Behaviors observed	Common interpretations	Expected staff behaviors
(1) Hyperventilation, peripheral paresthesia, "pins and needles" in extremities, breathlessness	(1) Anxiety (2) Hypochondriacal (3) Anxiety reaction (4) Neurosis: hysterical (5) Adjustment reaction of adult life	(1) Rule out organic basis. (2) Reestablish normal respirations. (3) Make sure restrooms are clearly marked.
(2) Sweating		(4) Friendly, noncoercive *attentions.*
(3) Urinary frequency and/or diarrhea		(5) Good listening skills.
(4) "Butterflies" in stomach		(6) Offer hot drink or food.
(5) Nausea		(7) Separate from other anxious persons.
(6) Increased heart rate		(8) Do not take verbal hostility personally; answer the content (the words being said), and do not respond to the feeling tone (anger); recognize the feeling, but do not respond in kind.
(7) Silence or talking all of the time.		
(8) Feels cold		
(9) Verbal hostility		
(10) Paces the waiting room		
(11) Taps fingers		

Severe anxiety

The manifestations of severe anxiety may be primary or secondary in nature. Consequently, the behaviors of severe anxiety may be the reason for a person's coming to the emergency department or may follow the onset of some other problem, such as diabetes, hepatic dysfunction, renal failure, degenerative disease or the effects and/or withdrawal of drugs, including alcohol. Whatever the reason behind the occurrence, the behaviors are the same.

This person is confused. He is little able to attend to his surroundings and thus is disoriented to time, place and person. He is incoherent and agitated, with restless and aimless movements while mumbling to self, slamming doors and swearing or physically striking out. He is incapable of doing any abstract thinking, including problem-solving; so, the feeling of "I need to urinate" may result in his urinating in a corner of the treatment room instead of following the process of the less anxious person, who thinks: "I need to urinate. I wonder where the bathroom is. I'll ask. I'll go there." He may exhibit a variety of emotions and move quickly from one to another, for example, being angry for 5 minutes, then crying for 5 minutes, laughing for 5 minutes and soberly seductive for the next 5 minutes.

The severely anxious person's internal controls are minimally functioning. The cerebral cortex is responding to a wider than usual variety of stimuli, with the result that the person is out of touch with or distorts reality. A person at this level of anxiety can easily go either to calmness or to panic. And since this person has very little control left, persons in his environment have the greatest influence on which direction he takes.

The emergency department staff's task is to eliminate the source of the loss of control while providing the control which is lacking until the patient can reinstitute his own control. This usually boils down to the staff preventing the patient from hurting himself and/or others while treatment for the specific etiology is begun. The exact procedures related to diagnosis are detailed in Chapter 5 and need not be repeated.

The patient will need to be reoriented to time, place and person frequently, perhaps as often as every 5 minutes. The emergency nurse should use simple language with wide applicability, such as, "I am a nurse" instead of "I am Mrs. Jones, the evening supervisor" and "You are in a hospital" instead of "You are in Metropolitan General Hospital on 76th Avenue East" and "Your name is _____." [26] The nurse must keep the irritability out of her voice; it can be "heard" even when cognitive functions are minimal. If the temper fuse starts getting short, it is wise to go out into the hall and take a few deep breaths.

The room should be well lighted. A balance should be found between soft light and glaring light. The first creates unwanted shadows, adds to illusion and makes reality testing difficult. Glaring light is harsh, uncomfortable and not conducive to relaxation. Well-balanced lighting helps the patient reassure himself, "I am seeing things. They will go away" or "They (the staff) can see me, so they won't forget me." Similarly, the environment should be kept as simple as possible.

A staff person must explain each and every procedural step before touching the patient and talk while facing the patient. Seeing the staff member's lips move leaves very little room for doubt as to the origin of the voice. A calm, reassuring voice and simple words should be used. If the patient demonstrates increased anxiety (pulling away, folding arms around self, looking desperately around the room) the nurse should ask, "Is this procedure absolutely essential to this patient's well-being?" If the answer is "No," then, "Why am I running the risk of pushing this person into a panic?" If the answer is "Yes, this procedure is essential," then, "Must I do it right now, or can I take some more time to explain and help decrease his anxiety?" If it must be done immediately and the confusion has increased, get assistance. This will decrease the probability of the patient hurting himself or a staff member—either of which creates in the patient a loss of self-respect, an increase in guilt and a fear of retaliation.

A nurse should stay with the patient or have another responsible staff or family member stay with him. If he *must* be left alone, leave the door of the treatment room open at least halfway, decreasing or eliminating any feelings of being trapped. Someone should check *with,* not check *on,* the patient every 15 minutes. This means recognizing his presence, announcing one's own presence and orienting him to time, place and person; it does not mean peering through the window on the door.

It is also wise to remember that family members and/or friends may well be in the throes of mild or moderate anxiety, and using a few of the aforementioned intervention strategies can help them gain extra ability to stay calm in the presence of their confused relative or friend. In turn, this will decrease the patient's anxiety and decrease pressures on staff members.

At times medication is necessary for a confused patient. The inherent risk is that most sedatives increase the degree of confusion and disorientation, either by their direct action or by creating within the patient a sensation of losing the little control he has left. The constant presence of another person is the best restraint possible and usually precludes the use of any physical (cloth or leather wrist restraints or a Posey belt) or chemical restraints.

The intoxicated patient

The person most frequently in need of all the preceding interventions, who is frequently difficult to treat, is the "drunk." Each emergency department has its own group of returning alcoholics, ranging from simple disorientation that sleep will cure to delirium tremens (DTs) or Korsakoff's syndrome.

Little else is as discouraging to an emergency department staff as spending time and effort to get a person on his feet and have him leave only to be back the next night, week or month. The anger ("Why doesn't he shape up?"), the pity ("How can he live that way?"), the fear ("I wonder exactly what started the drinking?") and the professional sense of injustice ("This money and skill could be used to help someone who is really sick and who will get well!"), all combine to make the staff want never to see or to treat another person with acute alcohol intoxication. But treatment must be started, for without treatment, 3 out of 5 persons who experience delirium tremens will die, thus defeating the purpose of the emergency department.

Alcoholics fit no one personality pattern, belong to no one particular occupational group and come from no one socioeconomic background. They do share a low tolerance for tension and a low self-esteem. So while administering the necessary intravenous fluids, vitamins and/or medications, an emergency nurse should try to focus on the patient's current acute distress and should not dwell on thoughts of how and why this distress is present. She should offer acceptance and reassurance by making sure that all details of his physical comfort are met. There is no need to reinforce his worthless feelings about self with thoughtless remarks. A sense of humor is valuable, both for the staff's well-being and

as a tool for encouraging a patient to stay in bed or not knock over the intravenous fluids.

Be patient.

Table 7-3 summarizes how emergency department staff should cope with severe anxiety.

Panic

The fourth level of anxiety, panic, is the most awesome. In panic there exists a lack of coordination in behavior and the disappearance of rational thought. The self is completely without control. Fear is overwhelming and emergency department staff must expect the unexpected. Panic creates fear in staff. Whether this fear is due to the panic touching off their own aggressive feelings or to its bringing forth the staff's uncertainties about being able to handle the situation is unimportant for this chapter. What is important is to answer the question, "How do I, a staff member, provide control where there is none?"

TABLE 7-3 SEVERE ANXIETY

Behaviors observed	Common interpretations	Expected staff behaviors
(1) Incoherent (2) Disoriented to time, place, and person (3) Memory loss (4) Loss of judgment (5) Decreased ability to attend to surroundings (6) Hallucinations (7) Emotional liability, sadness, apprehension, euphoria (8) Agitation: pacing, muttering, swearing, random striking out, picking at things	(1) Acute brain syndrome (2) Delirious intoxications: metabolic toxins, direct trauma to the brain, alcohol, drugs, infections (3) Organic brain syndrome, arteriosclerotic, psychotic or nonpsychotic. (4) Drug dependency (5) Alcoholism	(1) Remove the source (through gastric lavage, hemodialysis, medications). (2) Reality orientation: identify self; use simple words; tell person he is in a hospital; tell simply, repeatedly and reassuringly who, what and where. (3) Simplify the environment: use well-lighted room; move slowly; explain procedures; keep door of treatment room open; use one consistent staff member. (4) Avoid extra medications, physical restraints, mechanical restraints.

A panicked person may be brought to the emergency room by the police, family, friends, companions or strangers. The reason for bringing him to the emergency room may be "He drank too much" or "He took too much and is on a bummer" * or "He just flipped out." This panicked patient might also be the drunk in Treatment Room 3, whose delirium tremens' butterflies just turned into giant scorpions, or the kid in Treatment Room 1, who "dropped" street acid (LSD_{25}) and is alternating between deep, meaningful insights and intense sensations of his body dissolving; or it could be a person at the admitting desk who starts yelling about how everyone is part of a plot to make sure he dies and that is the reason he is being refused treatment by a doctor.

Whatever the circumstances, the staff must stay calm and remember that the patient is afraid and wants help, that people are more important than property, that it is their responsibility to act *before* someone is hurt and that panic episodes are transient. It will end.

The panicked person has 2 choices: to strike out at others or to attack himself. His fear and pain may be so acute that his only thought is to escape or end his life. This person may jump out of a window, run through a plate-glass door or break a medicine jar and start slicing himself. In striking out at others, the patient may put his fist through a wall, destroy furniture, hit people. He may be acting in a delusional system, obeying auditory hallucinations, trying to stop threatening visual hallucinations or struggling for *any* definitive action that will stop this horrendous fear and powerlessness.

A staff member should start talking to the patient. A good rule of thumb to remember is if the person is talking, he will probably be able to listen. If he is someone being treated in the emergency department and thus is

in contact with a staff member, that person should do the talking. A familiar face, no matter how recently familiar, can do wonders to decrease fear and confusion.

Someone should go for assistance. A minimum of 3 persons and a maximum of 6 are needed to physically restrain one panicked person. Someone should also see that these extra persons do not burst upon the scene like a cavalry charge. They should wait immediately close by until given directions on how to proceed. Too big and too sudden a show of power will only increase the person's feelings of helplessness and anxiety and breed more assaultive behavior. A single staff member should never try to restrain an adult patient.

Other patients and all other persons not directly involved with the panicked person, including his family, should leave the room. A person with homicidal tendencies is more likely to attack members of his family than strangers.[27]

The person in contact with the patient should keep talking, the voice calm and low. Whispering is not called for, and there is no need to yell. In simple words, the patient should be given the option of giving up a weapon, piece of furniture or whatever else he has which may be used as a weapon. This same person should *constantly* reassure the patient of the staff's awareness of how frightened he is and that everything possible is going to be done to *help* him. Be convincing with the statement, "I don't want you to hurt anyone."

It is important to keep talking and listening to anything the patient says. It may be possible to find a clue as to what started the "fight" behavior, and information or reassurance may then be realistically offered about it. Very few incidents of aggressive behavior start for absolutely no reason at all. The reason may appear to be insignificant to an outside observer, but it is a reason. In talking with the patient, do not worry about being repetitious. Making contact with the patient is what is important, not being a good conversationalist. Do not censure or repri-

---

* Bummer: A term used to describe unpleasant and very frightening experiences following the ingestion of psychedelic drugs. (For definitions of other drug terms, see Table 12–2.)

mand; this is not the time to teach more appropriate behaviors.

Physical Restraint

If the talking is unsuccessful, then physical restraint must be used. The staff person with the most rapport with the patient should direct all activity involved in physically restraining him. This is not the time to haggle over strategies and rationales; save it for a staff evaluation conference. Anything gained in discussing a more therapeutic approach will be lost by the patient's recognition of the staff not working together for him, and the disagreement will only add to the chaos.

Helpless inconsistency ("Here, let me do this" or "No, you do that, not this" or "No, that won't work") gives the patient the message that he is in control of the situation by creating so much anxiety in everyone else. The panicked person does not need this extra burden. In addition, the staff then feels helpless and intimidated and may retaliate in anger to regain its status, self-control and power. The patient responds to this anger with anger, and the entire situation is out of control.

Panicked males will strike with an arm, a leg or an object. Females will use and do anything. Each team member should be assigned a specific task, arms, legs or head. The team should approach the patient from the sides and/or rear; a direct frontal approach is a nonverbal invitation to fight. They should move calmly and quickly, then stay as close to the patient as possible; the less space between a staff member and the patient, the less momentum can be put into a swing or a kick. *Never* grab someone by the throat, mouth or nose. This is threatening to anyone and can only add to panic. If the patient's head must be restrained to prevent biting or banging his head, a staff member should put one hand under his chin and one hand at the back of his neck and support his head against her body. (See Figure 7–2.) If his arm must be restrained, it should be held with one hand over his elbow and the other over his wrist in such a way that the staff person's arms naturally move in the same direction as the patient's. (See Figure 7–3.)

The nurse should keep talking in a reassuring voice, explaining what she is doing and why. By standing to the side and the back of the patient, staff members can place one hand on his far elbow and the other on his wrist, for control and safety. Figure 7–4 illustrates this hold. If two staff members are available for restraint of the patient's arms, each can take one arm, using the hold shown in Figure 7–5. Then try to get the patient against a wall or on the floor. Getting him to sit on the floor with his back against the wall is most useful in utilizing the support of a solid structure with the least threat to the person. This position allows for direct eye contact and ease in administering oral or intramuscular medications and requires fewer staff members for restraining.

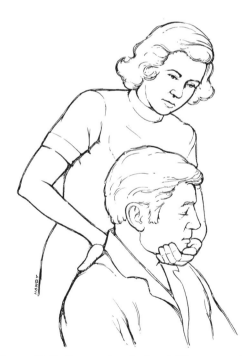

Figure 7–2 Supporting the head. The nurse places one hand under the patient's chin, the other hand at the back of his neck and supports the patient's head against her body.

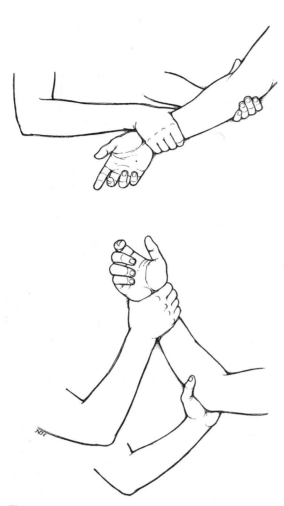

Figure 7–3 Correct and incorrect methods of restraining the arm of an individual out of control. In the correct method (top), one hand is placed over the elbow and the other over the wrist in such a way that the staff person's arms flux in the same direction as the patient's arm. With incorrect placement (bottom), the patient cannot be controlled by the nurse.

Gentle but firm pressure is required when restraining a patient. Staff members should practice with each other, to get an idea of what this means. Slowly squeeze a fellow staff member's arm, and have her report how each degree of pressure feels, especially when it causes pain.

Pressure which can be gradually released

while still maintaining the position of restraint is desirable. A staff member then has the option of either allowing a person to control his own behavior or quickly providing necessary control. It is imperative that the person be allowed as much control as is safely feasible.

A staff member must *never* strike a patient unless it is the only action determining life or death. Striking a patient only reinforces assaultive behavior as a means of coping with stress. If a staff member feels as though she is starting to lose control, she needs to get out of the situation. It is much more valuable for the staff member's self-esteem and the patient's well-being to be able to recognize her own limitations and leave than to stay and add to the tension of the situation.

Sedation

Sedation will most likely be required. Someone who is not a member of the team physically restraining the patient should be avail-

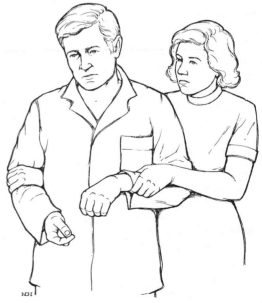

Figure 7–4 Restraining a panicked patient. The nurse grasps the patient's near wrist and far elbow as shown, for maximum control.

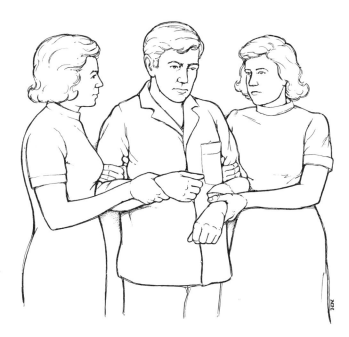

Figure 7–5 Patient restraint by 2 staff members. When greater patient control is needed, 2 nurses may become involved, each using on one arm the hold illustrated in Figure 7–4.

able to prepare the medication. Choice of medication depends on the known or inferred basis for the behavior. Phenothiazines are used when the patient is delusional or hallucinating. An exception is when the hallucinations are induced by hallucinogenic drugs. Then the drug of choice is diazepam (Valium); phenothiazines tend to bring a person down too quickly and increase the likelihood of flashbacks.*

When acute alcohol intoxication appears to underlie the behavior, chlordiazepoxide (Librium), chloral hydrate or paraldehyde may be used, with chlordiazepoxide preferred. There are times when amobarbital (Amytal) can be used. It makes sense to have all available and ready for use.

It is easier to keep other people away from the patient until the sedating medication has started working than to try and move the patient away from others. If he must be moved,

Figure 7–6 illustrates the safest way. The staff restraining the patient should stay with him until the desired effect of the medication is evident. Someone should expect to spend time with this person; he needs human contact.

Hallucinations and delusions

All of us hear our own thoughts, but we do not answer. A hallucination † is really a thought becoming so loud and so persistent that it has to be answered, verbally and/or nonverbally. Indications that a person is hallucinating include:

(1) Head tilted as though listening to someone.
(2) Lips forming words or moving with no sound.
(3) Talking aloud to what appears to be himself.
(4) Ears stuffed with cotton in an attempt to keep the voices out.

---

* Flashback: The reliving of a previous drug-induced experience, frequently a bad one, without the ingestion of additional drugs.

† Hallucination: A perceptual disorder wherein "an inner experience is expressed as though an outer event." [12]

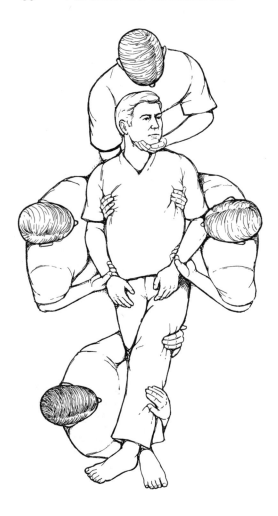

Figure 7–6 Safe method of moving an agitated patient by a 4-person lift. One staff member supports the patient's head, neck and upper back. The trunk is supported by 2 staff members, crossing their arms beneath the patient's trunk and grasping his arms. The fourth staff member clutches the patient's legs in adduction.

(5) Describing an object or person not being seen by anyone else.

If the patient is actively hallucinating, a staff person should state her view of reality to him in simple, nonderogatory terms, for example, "No, I don't hear voices (or see snakes)." But the patient's reality in seeing the objects or in hearing the voices should never be denied; it is very real to him. It is possible to state one's perception of reality without telling the patient he is wrong or that the snakes/voices do not exist.

At the same time, it is not wise to admit to seeing or hearing something just to placate a patient. This is destructive and not reassuring to the patient. A staff member's admission of such indicates to the patient that he can expect these voices will never go away and that the rest of his life will be as horrible as it is right now. If the hallucinations are not particularly frightening nor urging destructive behaviors, leave them alone.

As for delusions,* the best approach is to be a calm, somewhat interested and friendly person. Do not waste time arguing; arguing

---

* Delusion: A false, fixed belief about something which has no basis in fact and which requires certain behaviors from the person having them.

shows the patient the discrepancies in his delusional system, which he will then proceed to correct, thereby strengthening the delusional system. If the patient directly asks, "Do you believe me?", tell him, "I believe that your feelings are true and that you are telling me the truth as you see it." Listen without agreement or disagreement.

Avoid any behavior which could be construed as suspicious by the patient: (1) Do not talk to the patient's family or friends outside of his presence. (2) Do not get into a power struggle with the patient as to who is wrong or right. (3) Do not be overly sweet, solicitous and supportive. (The patient knows the staff member does not know him well enough to know the whole story, so too much support only increases his suspicion of some-

one trying to get something from him.) (4) Do not use the pronoun "we"; use "I." ("We" could be interpreted as an indication of a conspiracy.) *Gentle* honesty goes a long way.

If the hallucinations and/or delusions plus the panic state are related to the ingestion of psychedelic drugs, the nurse or other staff member should continually remind the patient that he has taken a drug, that what is going on is due to the drug and that the effects of the drug will eventually wear off. Then repeat, repeat, repeat! Little will be heard the first time.

A time of crisis is a time of openness to change for the patient. If the crisis is handled well by the emergency department staff, it can give the patient a strong start on a rapid recovery. (See Table 7–4.)

TABLE 7–4 PANIC

Behaviors observed	Common interpretations	Expected staff behaviors
(1) Physically aggressive: homicidal or suicidal (2) Delusions: sees and hears things as others do but interprets them differently; talks about "They are going to do such-and-such" (3) Hallucinations: eyes move as though watching something; is preoccupied, does not hear you; tilts head in a listening manner; talks to self; lips move with no sound	(1) Schizophrenia, paranoid type (2) Manic-depressive, manic type (3) Schizophrenic reaction, undifferentiated (4) Organic brain syndrome, acute or chronic (5) Acute alcohol intoxication (6) Fatigue (7) Psychotic reaction, undiagnosed (8) Drug dependence	(1) Stay calm. (2) Act with confidence and assurance. (3) Remember the behavior is not directed towards anyone personally. (4) Use assistance (persons, drugs, mechanical restraints) *only* to *protect* the patients from harming self or others. (5) Never try to physically restrain an adult alone. (6) Talk; be repetitious and soothing. Give directions ("Do not bite") without anger. (7) Medicate. (8) Reinforce reality, don't insist on it.

STAFF CONSIDERATIONS

Considering the details on anxiety presented in this chapter, it seems that the emergency department staff member must be a model of patience, calmness, clear thinking, nonirritability and lack of frustration. How can a staff member achieve all this? No *one* person can. One person may not be able to work with alcoholics, no matter how hard she tries. Another staff member may be incapable of working with a person who has a long list of physical complaints without seeing the word "hypochondriac" continuously flash before her eyes. Still another staff member may freeze if a patient yells and threatens. These different capabilities will not be detrimental to the quality of emergency care if the staff members can work together and support each other. Such support can be developed in several ways.

First, *learn from each other.* Plan regular staff in-service seminars — a minimum of once a month, preferably more often. Vary the responsibility and the format. A nurses' aide may be responsible for one seminar and decide that the focus should be on the incident with Mr. Z. last week and the reasons behind specific staff interventions. A resident may need help with some paperwork procedures; the ward secretary can help him and everyone else learn just what happens to all of those pieces of paper. Some seminars could be of the didactic, information-giving type by current staff or guest speakers. The hospital in-service educator should be available for consultation and assistance.

Help each other practice the physical restraint holds. The first time to try these holds is not with a panicked patient. Work so that each staff member knows what "firm and gentle holding pressure" means in relation to his own strength.

Consider the possibility of having a camera with a videotape recorder available, much like the type used in banks to record robberies. A flick of a switch could start the camera during a tight situation. The tape could later be played back, evaluated, with suggestions made for similar situations in the future, and erased.

Second, *support each other.* Pat each other on the back when something is done well. Listen to each other, and when an emergency has been especially traumatic for a staff member (a battered child, a baby dead on arrival due to sudden infant death syndrome or an injured neighbor/friend), the support can be genuine and instantaneous.

Compile a flip-card file of names and phone numbers of agencies (e.g., Alcoholics Anonymous, Sudden Infant Death Syndrome Foundation, Suicide/Crisis Center, Poison Control Center, Women Against Rape) and people who can provide on-call assistance or for immediate referrals.

Third, *develop and use a sense of humor.* Laugh with and at yourselves. Joke about situations and behaviors. It is well known that much of the gallows humor experienced in scenes of personal stress, such as in the operating room or during autopsies, is the easiest and most natural way to avoid screaming. Screaming may relieve a staff member's anxiety temporarily, but it will yield a rich but unwanted harvest of anxiety in others.

BIBLIOGRAPHY

(1) Aguilera, Donna C., and Messick, Janice M.: *Crisis Intervention: Theory and Methodology,* 2nd ed. (Saint Louis: C. V. Mosby Company, 1974).

(2) Allison, Colin, and Bale, Roderick: "A Hospital Policy for the Care of Patients Who Exhibit Violent Behavior," *Nursing Times,* 169 (March 22, 1973):375.

(3) Bartolucci, Giampiero: "An Overview of Crisis Intervention in the Emergency Rooms of General Hospitals," *The American Journal of Psychiatry,* 130 (September 1973):953–960.

(4) Bower, F. L., and Pendleton, M. K. (eds.): *Theoretical Foundations of Nursing,* 1 (San Jose, Calif.: Nursing Faculty Publications, Department of Nursing, San Jose State University, 1972).

(5) Brunner, Lillian Sholtis, *et al.: The Lippincott Manual of Nursing Practice* (Philadelphia: J. B. Lippincott Company, 1974).

(6) Choron, Jacques: *Suicide* (New York: Charles Scribner's Sons, 1972).

(7) Davis, John W.: "Opportunity and Techniques in Crisis Therapy," unpublished manuscript.

(8) Dorpat, Theodore; Anderson, William F., and Ripley, Herbert S.: "The Relationship of Physical Illness to Suicide," in H. L. P. Resnik (ed.), *Suicidal Behaviors: Diagnosis and Management* (Boston: Little, Brown & Company, 1968).

(9) Enelow, Allen J., and Wexler, Murray: *Psychiatry in the Practice of Medicine* (New York: Oxford University Press, 1966).

(10) Farberow, N. L.: "Personality Patterns of Suicidal Mental Hospital Patients," *Genetic Psychology Monographs,* 42 (1):3–79.

(11) Frost, Monica: "Violence in Psychiatric Patients," *Nursing Times,* 68 (June 15, 1972):748.

(12) Gravenkemper, Katherine H.: "Hallucinations," in Shirley F. Burd and Margaret A. Marshall (eds.), *Some Clinical Approaches to Psychiatric Nursing* (New York: The Macmillan Company, 1963).

(13) Hendin, Herbert: *Black Suicide* (New York: Harper & Row, 1971).

(14) Johnson, Roger N.: *Aggression in Man and Animals* (Philadelphia: W. B. Saunders Company, 1972).

(15) Kavalier, Frederick: "The Violent Patient: HMC Publishes New Guidelines," *Nursing Times,* 69 (May 24, 1973):656.

(16) King, Joan M.: "The Initial Interview: Basis for Assessment in Crisis Intervention," *Perspectives in Psychiatric Care,* 9 (1971):247–256.

(17) Lester, Gene, and Lester, David: *Suicide: The Gamble with Death* (Englewood Cliffs, N.J.: Prentice-Hall, 1971).

(18) Lieb, Julian; Lipsitch, Ian I., and Slaby, Andrew Edmund: *The Crisis Team: A Handbook for the Mental Health Professional* (New York: Harper & Row, 1973).

(19) MacKinnon, Roger A., and Michels, Robert: *The Psychiatric Interview in Clinical Practice* (Philadelphia: W. B. Saunders Company, 1971).

(20) MacMahon, B., and Pugh, T.: "Suicide in the Widowed," *American Journal of Epidemiology,* 81:23–31.

(21) Meerlo, Joost A. M.: *Patterns of Panic* (New York: International Universities Press, 1950).

(22) Menninger, Karl: *Man Against Himself* (New York: Harcourt, Brace & Company, 1938).

(23) Parkes, Colin Murray: *Bereavement: Studies of Grief in Adult Life* (New York: International Universities Press, 1972).

(24) Pokorny, Alex D.: "Myths About Suicide," in H. L. P. Resnik (ed.), *Suicidal Behaviors: Diagnosis and Management* (Boston: Little, Brown & Company, 1968).

(25) Reid, Jean A.: "Controlling the Fight/ Flight Patient," *The Canadian Nurse,* 69 (October 1973):30.

(26) Robinson, Lisa: "Coping with Psychiatric Emergencies," *Nursing '73,* 3 (July 1973):42–44.

(27) Rogerson, Kent E.: "Psychiatric Emergencies," *Nursing Clinics of North America,* 8 (September 1973):457–466.

(28) Shneidman, E. S., and Farberow, N. L. (eds.): *The Cry for Help* (New York: McGraw-Hill, 1965).

(29) Sullivan, H. S.: *Conceptions of Modern Psychiatry* (New York: W. W. Norton & Company, 1953).

(30) Susser, M.: *Community Psychiatry, Epidemiologic and Social Theories* (New York: Random House, 1968).

(31) Yolles, Stanley F.: "Suicide: A Public Health Problem," in H. L. P. Resnik (ed.), *Suicidal Behaviors: Diagnosis and Management* (Boston: Little, Brown & Company, 1968).

8

Death in the emergency setting

RITA E. CAUGHILL

Death is an unwelcome topic at any time, yet it is a life event that will come to all of us. The feelings aroused by thoughts of death are intangible and frightening; they make us feel lost and uneasy. It is far easier to deny the fact that death is an inevitable part of life. Especially if one is young and full of life, it is preferable to view death as something that happens to other people, but never to oneself.

Western society has developed in such a way that it is difficult for its members to face death or to relate to dying people in a meaningful way. Urbanization has been a major factor in removing people from contact with death. In a simpler society, children grow up close to nature, experiencing the cycle of life and death in the changing of the seasons and the shorter survival spans of plant and animal life. Not only does urban living separate people from the basic laws of nature, it actually fosters feelings of independence from nature and the inevitability of death. The increased longevity resulting from rapid advances in science in the last few decades also promotes the notion that man has mastered death.

Fifty years ago, American family life was built around a large, close-knit structure, which included aunts and uncles as well as grandparents. Typically, close relatives lived within a few miles of each other, if not in the same household. If the mother of young children died, loving aunts or grandmothers were available and willing to step in as parent-substitutes. The nuclear family units of today, however, are likely to consist only of father, mother and children. This tends to increase family members' emotional investments in each other, so that the death of any one member causes a far greater sense of loss in the others, and there is no one to fill the void. The threat of such an overwhelming disaster is too terrible to think about; the average person finds denial of the possibility of death his best defense.

The removal of old people from the family home, where they were loved and respected by children and grandchildren, has contributed in other ways to Western death-denial. Many, of their own choosing, move to retirement communities. Others, physically or financially unable to make it on their own, are shunted off to nursing homes. Out of sight and all but forgotten, their deaths hardly create a ripple in the hurried flow of life.

As a result of all these factors, there is less need to develop a philosophy of life which takes both life and death into consideration.

Very often, no concept of death is established at all, nor a means of dealing with it. Death, then, is viewed merely as the opposite of life, the complete end of everything, the extinction of self—a frightening phenomenon, indeed, with no significance but catastrophic annihilation.

With this as the typical Western attitude toward death, it is hardly surprising that when death is dealt with, the goal is to remove its sting. Literature, drama, television and movies portray death frequently, but it is usually depicted as heroic or tragic, accidental or violent, rarely due to old age or chronic illness. Death is portrayed as an external power, a catastrophic force that happens to people against their will.

Denial of death also occurs quite naturally in the hospital situation and negatively influences the behavior of professionals caring for the dying. The fact that nurses and doctors are uncomfortable in the face of death is not surprising, since they are members and products of a society that fears death and taboos open and frank discussion of it. It is easier to avoid the situation than meet it, to spend as little time as possible with the dying person, to avoid talking about it.

SUPPORTIVE CARE OF THE PATIENT

Death in the emergency department differs from death in most other areas of the hospital, and so do the problems it creates and the ways in which the staff tries to cope with them. In the emergency area, death usually *is* a sudden, catastrophic event caused by an outside force. Whether that causative force is a traumatic accident or a coronary occlusion, it is sudden, unexpected and overwhelming.

The nurse in the emergency department has little opportunity to know her patients as individuals or to become emotionally involved with them. If the patient survives the emergency phase of his situation, he is quickly transferred to another area in the hospital for continued care; if he dies, this, too, happens in a relatively short time. In either case, his critical condition while in the emergency department requires the total involvement of the personnel. The skilled efforts, the teamwork and the very "busyness" of the task help the staff maintain composure in tense situations. Saving lives is the primary function of the unit. The physical needs of the patient are so urgent and demanding that there is no time to think about his psychological needs.

What, then, are the emotional risks for the emergency department nurse relative to dying and death? According to practicing nurses, themselves, the victim dead on arrival is never a real shock, *per se;* this is a common enough occurrence that the seasoned emergency nurse is psychologically prepared to handle it. Any reaction to the DOA comes rather from the severity of the injuries, the type and degree of mutilation and the like.

However, the patient admitted alive but in imminent danger of death presents a different problem. If he is unconscious or semiconscious, this makes it easier for everyone in terms of interacting with him. He may be in a state of physical and emotional shock and not really aware of what is happening to him. If the patient is conscious but seems confused, he should be oriented in a calm way and in simple language that he can readily understand. The nurse should explain that he has been in an accident and that he is in the hospital, tell him who she is and assure him that she and everyone else is giving him the best possible care. This can be done without lengthy explanations or false reassurances; tone of voice and manner of speaking should provide the assurance of care and help. Empty phrases, such as, "You'll be O.K.; don't worry," should be avoided. They may make the nurse feel better, but they do nothing for the anxious patient.

The patient who is aware and concerned about his prognosis creates another kind of problem. He may not say anything, only plead with his eyes for some answer, for reassurance. Even if he asks directly, "Am I going to die?", he may not really want the answer. What he does want to know for certain is, first, that he is getting the best possible care and, then, that you are not going to leave him alone.

One of the greatest fears of a dying person, or a person who suspects he may be dying, is the fear of dying alone. The nurse should stay with him, and if she has to leave the room, see that someone else remains there with him. More than just being there, the nurse can share herself, meet his eyes, smile, touch him, hold his hand, make him feel that she cares about *him,* not just his I.V.'s or the myriad other gadgets that one tends to become absorbed in, to avoid that human contact that means so much to the dying patient.

It is unfair to try to fool the patient who suspects the truth. But it is also cruel to answer "Yes" to the question, "Am I dying?" More than cruel, it is devastating, because it takes away hope, and the patient who has been stripped of hope never does as well as the one who has a degree of hope held out to him. It is much better to respond to the effect that you are all there fighting for him, and you need to have him fight too. If he then persists in the assertion that he is dying, you can agree that that is a possibility, but that you are doing everything you can to prevent it.

Kubler-Ross [15] maintains that a patient should never be told he is dying. Only when the patient himself offers the information that he is fatally ill should the nurse talk openly to him about his dying. In the emergency department, of course, patients are less likely to *tell* the nurse they are dying but more likely to *ask* her, and their questions may be prompted by fear, pain, suspicion or by self-conviction when they get no sensible response to their anxious queries. The nurse must try to assess what is behind the patient's questions, and, of course, her knowledge of what is actually happening to him pathologically will also influence her reply. It is essential that she be very alert and sensitive to each individual as she assesses his need. Is he aware of what is happening to him? How much does he want to know? How much is he able to hear? Be honest in your reply, yet keep in mind that the whole truth may destroy him.

An important source of help and comfort for many patients is spiritual support. The Roman Catholic patient who is in danger of death should always have a priest called. Patients of other faiths may or may not wish to have a clergyman attend them, but they should be given the choice. An appropriate time to suggest this might be when the patient is expressing concern about his possible death. For the patient who does not verbalize such fears, the nurse must use her judgment about when to offer him this option. Some nurses are reluctant to suggest a clergyman to patients who do not mention it themselves, fearing that the suggestion will alarm the patient and thus do more harm than good. It is largely a question of weighing advantages against disadvantages. It would seem unfair to deprive the patient who would gain great comfort and strength from spiritual support but might be reluctant to request it of professional people who are obviously busy with physical care. The patient of opposite convictions, who has no interest in spiritual affairs, might be alerted to his precarious status if offered this option, but the staff can then reassure him in keeping with his emotional response.

While religion may or may not be important to a patient, it cannot be known unless he tells someone. For the patient who does have strong religious convictions, it becomes far more important to him when his life is in danger. In the event that the patient dies, knowing that spiritual guidance and support were provided will be a source of comfort to the family.

SUPPORTIVE CARE OF THE FAMILY

One of the most important aspects of emergency department care and one which is most frequently neglected is support of the family. While the patient is still living and the nurse is absorbed in the many tasks necessary to try to save his life, contact with the family is minimal. Although this is not necessarily desirable, it is more important at that time that all energies be directed to the patient himself. Afterwards, the nurse may be exhausted, emotionally drained, wishing to go off by herself to pull her thoughts together, even cry, but then there is the family to cope with. And it is then that the real emergency occurs for the survivors. It is urgently important that the nurse give them all the help she can as they face this crisis.

It is not easy to do. The death has come as a terrible shock to them; the nurse can imagine how she might feel in the same situation, and she feels very sympathetic, but it is hard to take their reaction, anyway. Especially if they become highly emotional and noisy or angry and unreasonable. You just wish they would sign the necessary papers and leave, to do their grieving at home.

It will help to understand them and accept their behavior, even to assist them more effectively, if the nurse is aware that grief is a definite syndrome, with characteristic and predictable symptoms. Early investigation into the grieving process was done in the 1940s by psychiatrist Erich Lindemann, who studied large numbers of survivors of a disastrous nightclub fire.[16] His observations have been substantiated and augmented through the years by numerous others,[4,10,13] but the simplest and clearest delineation of the progressive steps of grief was outlined by George Engel.[9]

The grieving process

Grief is an experience so common to human beings that hardly anyone can move into adulthood without experiencing it. Parkes [18, p. xi] defines grief quite simply as, "a reaction, emotional and behavioral," which is set in motion "when a love tie is severed." Since many of the familiar objects in our lives are loved objects (e.g., our home, our job, our parents, a spouse, a pet), the loss of any of these interrupts our sense of security and continuity and constitutes a threat to our psycho-logical well-being. The familiar phenomenon we call homesickness is a typical example of such a severance. The death of a loved person, since it is a complete and irrevocable severance of a love tie, creates a far greater threat to the self-system and evokes an acute grief response.

Engel compares the grieving process with wound healing.[9] He compares the experience of grief to a wound and subsequent psychological responses to the tissue healing process. Successful grieving follows a foreseeable pattern, as does successful tissue healing, by which one can judge if healing is taking place normally. But like physical healing, the grieving process takes time and cannot be hurried.

The series of reactions characterizing grief, as described by Engel, should be helpful in understanding what constitutes a *normal* response to grief.[9] The first reaction to knowledge of death is usually shock and denial. The person cries out, "No! It cannot be. I can't believe it!" He may try to disavow the fact in other ways, by throwing himself on the body, for example, as though this will somehow restore life, or as though he believes life is still there.

This initial reaction is frequently followed by a numb state of mind which permits the individual to shut out conscious acknowledgment that the death has indeed occurred. He acts as though he is in a daze. He may force himself to carry out automatic activities as though nothing happened, or he may actually sit motionless, turned in upon himself, so that it is difficult to get through to him.

Some people, however, may be able to carry on in a seemingly normal way, after the initial shock response. They immediately begin to make the necessary arrangements, comfort and support other members of the family and seem in general to be able to accept the death as a reality. It is important to realize that while this type of person may have accepted it intellectually, he has also suppressed the emotional impact of the loss and is still in a state of partial denial. "The mind knows, but the heart cannot accept." Very often this state persists through the funeral preparations and rituals. These people are described as "taking it well" or "holding up well" and are generally admired for what is seen as a stoic reaction. It must be admitted, too, that staff members are pleased to see such a reaction in the hospital situation, since it relieves them of the stress of having to cope with overt grief.

This first stage, then, is characterized by the bereaved person's attempts to protect himself from overwhelming grief. He does this by denial, blocking out either the *reality* of the event or the painful emotions aroused by it. The stage of shock and denial is most intense when the death is sudden and unexpected, and therefore is of special importance to emergency department personnel.

The grief-stricken survivor may move into the second stage within a matter of minutes after learning of the death, or it may take as long as 14 days or more.[18] But, since it frequently develops very quickly, the emergency nurse is quite likely to see this stage of grieving in the emergency department setting.

A conscious awareness of the death begins to develop, and an acute feeling of anguish ensues as the true meaning of the loss sinks in. It is during this phase, in fact, that the greatest depths of anguish and despair are reached. In addition to emotional distress, the grieving person may feel intense pain in the chest or epigastrium, a painful lump in his throat, choking sensations, feelings of weakness or faintness or sighing respirations. Crying is a typical response in this stage and should be encouraged, as it plays an important role in the grieving process. Cultural patterns determine to some extent the amount of public crying and lamentation people will indulge in; some ethnic groups are very open in their expressions of emotion, while others tend to be more restrained. At a time of acute grief, cultural practices are extremely important and should never be discouraged, criticized or belittled in any way.

Regardless of race, ethnic background *or sex,* crying is a legitimate release in the presence of death. We not only accept crying, we expect it; and we are not—or should not be—shocked at the sight of a man's tears under these circumstances. Crying may be a form of regression to the helpless days of childhood, and it does serve to evoke sympathy and support. The grieving person can cry and still retain his self-respect, while acknowledging that he wants and needs the help and support of others.

Another very important emotion which may be openly displayed in this second stage of grieving is anger. Anger may be directed at the doctor, the nurse, the hospital or at someone the grieving person feels must have "botched the job" and allowed his loved one to die. The nurse should be aware that this anger is rarely directed at anyone personally, although it may appear to be; it is more a manifestation of the individual's feelings of frustration and helplessness, his inability to *do* anything about it. Anger might also be felt toward another family member, who somehow failed in an obligation toward the deceased. Or it may be directed against the self, if he feels himself to be at fault. Parents, especially, tend to feel guilt over the death of a child and may berate themselves or each other; they may even injure themselves in an impulsive gesture of aggression or self-destruction. Guilt, in fact, is probably felt to some degree by all bereaved persons, as they search their minds for ways in which they may have failed the loved one, when it is now too late to make amends.

Engel's third stage of grieving is the "work of mourning." It may begin during the funeral rites or shortly after; therefore, it is rarely seen in the emergency setting. During this final stage, which may go on for a year or more, the bereaved one works through his feelings toward his loss in a series of halting steps, until he finally is able to resume a normal life revolving around new interests.

These 3 stages of grieving are not clear-cut; rather, one merges into the other, and regression into an earlier phase may occur at times throughout the grieving process. With these normal manifestations of grief and grieving in mind, let us consider some ways emergency nurses can help the survivors at the critical time of loss.

Staff responsibilities

Who announces the death to the family and how? If at all possible, it is helpful to give the family some advance warning that things are not going well, that death seems imminent and inevitable. In one instance, an operating room nurse, shocked at an unexpected death on the table, made several trips out to the family in the waiting room, first warning them that the patient had taken a turn for the worse, on the next trip that there wasn't much hope but they were still trying and so forth—all this when the patient was already dead! Finally, she made one more trip and told them the truth, that he had expired. She made this series of trips because she could not bring herself to tell them the terrible news until she had gradually built up the courage to do it. While her method was decidedly questionable, she actually softened the blow for the family by giving them a little time to prepare themselves for this unexpectedly bad turn of events. This is referred to as preparatory grief or anticipatory grief, and it is helpful because it allows the survivors to work through some of their feelings before the final blow, death, actually arrives.

Families of patients who die a lingering death have time to go through a good deal of their grief work beforehand, so that when the patient finally dies, they may already be into the third stage, the restorative stage. When death is sudden and unexpected, however, there is little or no time for preparatory grieving, and the shock is then much greater. Emergency department staff can help, perhaps, by using the approach of the operating room nurse—not, of course, to lie, as she did, if the patient is already dead—but if there is time, a periodic reporting of progressively bad news, rather than holding out too much

hope in an attempt to be kind. Sudden death is a fact which must be accepted; avoiding the family or offering false hope is not helpful.

It is almost always better if the physician tells the family of the death. He is the person the relatives see as the primary authority. They have the opportunity to ask him questions if they wish and to ask his advice about immediate problems they may have. Even if the physician has never had any previous contact with the family, which is often the case, he can still establish a meaningful relationship with the survivors in a very short interval of time. Asked later about how they had been informed by the doctor, relatives' comments range from, "He used such technical language that we could not understand what he was talking about" to the other extreme, "The doctor was so kind. He had bad news to tell us, but he tried to be helpful. He made us feel that he really cared about us."

Many doctors defend the position that they should not have to become involved with the family after a death, maintaining that their responsibility is to the living and when the patient dies, their responsibility ends. But the grieving relatives *are* living and urgently in need of support.

Emergency department nurses often maintain that they are better equipped to inform families than physicians are, that their "nurturing" role enables them to show their concern and sympathy more effectively and that they are more supportive of the grief-stricken kin. This may be true, and if the task does fall to the nurse and she is comfortable in the role, the family surely benefits from her touch. Nevertheless, it is still important that the family have contact with a physician who has been in attendance with the deceased patient. If no physician is in evidence, they will be left to speculate whether a doctor was actually present, and the thought that their loved one might have been saved if a competent doctor had been available may torment them for all time. The physical presence of a physician with whom they can talk and ask questions will reassure them that everything possible was done. The nurse can certainly accompany the physician if she wishes, can temper his remarks if she feels that is necessary and can stay with the family after he leaves, to explain, amplify and reinforce his information.

When the family is not present and must be summoned by telephone, the problem is somewhat different. Most authorities maintain, and personal experience verifies, that if the death has been sudden and completely unexpected, the family should never be notified by phone. It is impossible to estimate, on one end of the line, the situation on the other end. Heart attacks have been precipitated, acts of self-injury or even self-destruction have been attempted by distraught survivors who are alone when the devastating news comes. In addition, the harried relatives, in their haste to reach the hospital, may themselves become the victims of an automobile accident en route.

The all-important factor when phoning the family is to keep calm. The caller sets the stage for the way in which the family reacts. If it can be quietly conveyed that there has been an accident and that they should come to the hospital as soon as they can, with no urgency in the voice, chances are they will be able to avoid panic. They will, of course, be alarmed and may immediately suspect the worst; but even if they ask if it is "serious" or if he is dead, one can still avoid the truth without denying, by saying, perhaps, "He has been badly injured, but he is receiving excellent care and everything possible is being done. There is no need for you to rush." When they arrive, and there is face-to-face contact, the nurse should again try to control the situation by being very composed and calm in approach. She should explain what has happened clearly and in terms they can understand, emphasizing the quality of care given. Again, the physician should speak with the family, even if he has to wait there for their arrival.

It is always better if another member of the family or perhaps a close friend is also present. They provide support for each other, and grief that is shared is somehow easier to bear. In any case, the bereaved should not be left alone. If it is the nurse who breaks the news to the family, and she is *really* too busy to remain long with them (not simply looking for an excuse to escape from this uncomfortable situation), some reasonable substitute must be found, a chaplain or spiritual advisor, perhaps. Even an aide who is a warm, concerned individual can fill this role with a little training and a lot of support.

Many authorities recognize the pressing need in the emergency department for some sort of psychological consultation service for families. Quint and others [8] see this as possibly a social worker's role, but they ask, realistically, who would pay for the 24-hours-a-day services of such a person? Is the public ready to assume the cost? While in some instances a chaplain may fill the role of comforter to the bereaved, it is important to realize that the mere fact of being a clergyman does not necessarily equip one to meet the needs of people in the acute stages of grief. He, too, needs adequate preparation, often not provided in his training. Kubler-Ross suggests that specially trained volunteers might be utilized effectively.[14] They would have the advantage of being uninvolved in the efforts to save the patient, which is so emotionally draining, and could therefore devote all of their energies to comforting the family. Volunteers who have experienced grief in their own lives are ideal and can readily be trained in basic psychological and communication techniques. They could be available on a round-the-clock basis, with no added cost to the hospital.

Another essential element, too often lacking in hospitals, is a room where grieving relatives can be provided privacy. Every area of the hospital should be able to provide such a room, but certainly in high-risk areas it is indispensable. To give the family shocking news in a corridor or in a waiting room filled with curious and perhaps anxious observers is heartless and inexcusable. If no space can be found in the emergency department itself, a nearby chapel or any small empty room might be utilized. Hopefully, emergency departments now in the planning stages will include one or more such "crying rooms."

Survivors must be allowed, indeed encouraged, to express their acute grief in whatever way it comes out. Whether noisy or subdued, accept their tears, their anger without comment. Touch is extremely effective in conveying sympathy and concern, an arm around the shoulders, a handclasp. A simple offer of services is comforting: "Can I get you a glass of water?" "How about a cup of hot coffee?" "Can I phone your sister to come and be with you?" What you say is not as significant as how you say it. What you do is not as important as being there.

Sociologist David Sudnow did a detailed study of death practices in a large county hospital in California. One of his particularly sad observations was this:

> In none of the cases I have observed did the physician touch the relative or attempt to say anything while the relative was crying. No sympathy remarks or gestures of sorrow were offered during the earliest period following his announcement [of death].[23, p. 141]

In this study, the "physicians" were almost always young residents. It is not professionally demeaning to say, "I'm sorry," or even to shed a tear with the bereaved if you are so moved. All professionals are human beings first.

The following case presentation illustrates the kind of thoughtlessness in some professional people which results in a brutal confrontation with family:

> Mr. H., age 49, was admitted to the emergency department at 11 P.M., where he was immediately pronounced dead. He had been discharged from the same hospital only 2 weeks previous, following a lengthy hospitalization with a myocardial infarction. Earlier that evening, he had encouraged his wife to go to a party at the home of friends, since he was feeling fine and could manage quite well alone.
>
> Subsequently he had developed chest pain,

went to the phone to call a neighbor for help, said a few words and collapsed. The neighbor immediately came to the house and found him lying on the floor. An ambulance was summoned, and Mr. H. was rushed to the hospital but was dead on arrival.

> Mrs. H. arrived at the hospital soon afterward, obviously dressed in party attire, concerned about her husband but with no thought of death on her mind. She immediately approached a nurse with a multitude of questions: "How is he? Is he able to talk? How sick is he? Can he sit up?" The nurse detected alcohol on Mrs. H.'s breath and responded coldly: "Your husband is dead. There are papers here that have to be signed right away. We would also like to know what undertaker to call."

This nurse may not have meant to be cruel, but she did not feel that undue kindness was in order, either. She judged Mrs. H. on the basis of her party attire, the fact that she had been drinking and, worst of all, the fact that she had gone off to a party and left her husband to die alone. Without doubt, Mrs. H. would be tormented by feelings of guilt for the very same reasons, even though her motives were innocent. The nurse reinforced her guilt, added to the hurt and delayed a healthy resolution of the grieving process.

Sedating grieving relatives is not always a good idea. Physicians and nurses have to be very honest in looking at their own actions and reactions, especially in practices that "have always been done this way, and for this reason." Sedation does quiet the sobbing and appears to help the person "get hold of himself." Actually, though, it only serves to delay the grief reaction. It would be far better to allow him to cry and express his rage and frustration right there where there is a shoulder to cry on and where he can vent his anger without injuring himself. It is difficult to help people who are irrational with hurt and anger; it is far easier to send them home, get them "out of your hair." If someone can be patient and understanding and perhaps agree that she would probably feel the same way, the bereaved may be able to recover to the point that they can safely be sent home.

A survivor should never go home alone. The person who is utterly alone in the world, with no relative, no friend, no minister, not even a neighbor who can stay with him, is a very real problem. Many people in acute states of anguish are suicidal for a time. It would be better to admit this person overnight, in the care of nurses who are warm and compassionate, with the hope and expectation that he will be able to cope tomorrow. Is this idealistic? Perhaps, but why should ideals always be brushed aside as impossible? It would be possible, if we really believed it was important and necessary.

Viewing the body

Should the family be allowed to see the body? Nurses often feel that if there is severe mutilation, especially of the head or face, it is too shocking a sight for the family to endure. Difficult as it is, it is necessary if the family is to accept the death as a reality. Studies have shown that survivors who have the most difficulty resolving their grief are those who never see the body, because of drowning, an airplane crash or other tragedy where the body was never recovered. In the emergency department, the body can be cleansed, cleared of tubes and other resuscitative devices, and made as presentable as possible. At least some identifiable part should be visible for the relatives, to confirm the loss. Prepare them ahead of time so that they will have some idea what to expect, but they should always be given the option of seeing the deceased. It is a form of reality orientation the numbed survivor needs.

Two practicing nurses clearly illustrate the difficulties of working through the grieving process when they have not viewed the dead body. One lost a much-loved brother due to an automobile accident. His body was sent immediately across the country to the city where their parents lived, and he was buried there. This young woman never saw his body and has never seen his grave. Although many years have passed, she still resents her mother "taking Donny away from me." She feels he should have been buried "here," but when asked if she has thought of going there to visit his grave, she resists the idea and still irrationally blames her mother for the loss.

The other young nurse states that her father died when she was about 12 years old and was cremated. She did not even see him while he was sick and hospitalized. His death is unreal to her, despite the fact that his ashes sit in an urn on the home mantelpiece. The family plans to sprinkle the ashes from a plane (which was his wish), and then there will not even be ashes to confirm the fact of his death. This girl is in a state of partial denial of her father's death. She knows he died, yet she has never had any proof of that fact and cannot wholly accept it.

SUDDEN INFANT DEATH SYNDROME

With increased recognition of Sudden Infant Death Syndrome (SIDS) as a disease entity, we are becoming more aware of the special problems these hapless parents face. These babies, discovered dead in their cribs without any previous hint of illness, are sometimes rushed to the emergency department in the arms of the distraught parents. Their experience there, unfortunately, has not been a source of comfort to them but rather has added to their misery.

The concomitant increase in child abuse cases has made hospital staffs suspicious in the face of any sudden, unexplained death of a child. SIDS babies frequently exhibit areas of ecchymosis on the head and body, due to pooling of blood in dependent areas at the time of death, which resemble the bruises of a battered child. The staff's natural feelings of revulsion and dismay when faced with an abused child seem to outweigh rational thought, and they react to the parents with hostility and suspicion.

The following excerpts from an interview with a mother of an SIDS baby bring out some of the feelings and reactions emergency department staff should be aware of.

Q: What was your first reaction when you discovered your baby dead in his crib?

A: Panic. At first I told myself he was just sound asleep, even though I could tell right away that something was terribly wrong. I picked him up, and I kept saying, "No! No! He can't be dead, he can't be!" I remember I kept hoping it was all a bad dream, that he would wake up in a minute and start to cry.

Then my husband phoned the rescue squad. We knew nothing could be done, really, but we couldn't just give up. I kept hugging the baby, patting his back, rocking him with my body.

Q: What did the rescue squad do?

A: They gave the baby oxygen with a mask on his face. I think they knew it was hopeless, but they kept giving him the oxygen. They wouldn't say he was dead. I guess they can't do that. Anyway, they took us to the hospital, my husband and me and the baby, and they kept giving him the oxygen.

Q: How did they treat you? What was their reaction to the situation?

A: They were all right. They were concerned about the baby, and they really tried. They didn't say much to us, but they were polite, and I got the feeling they really felt bad when they couldn't bring the baby around with the oxygen.

Q: What happened when you got to the hospital?

A: Well, they took us to the emergency entrance, and of course, we were taken care of right away. By that time, I was practically in a state of shock, but I remember that the police arrived about the same time we did. One of the policemen whispered to the doctor something about the baby being dead, or was he going to pronounce him dead, or something like that. Then they began to ask us all kinds of questions, like what had we done to the baby? Had he fallen recently? Had he been sick? Had either of us ever hit him? I was shocked when I realized what they were driving at. It had never occurred to me that anyone would think we had tried to hurt our baby. We loved him! We had wanted him for such a long time. My husband had doted on him — his little son! And I had waited for what seemed like ages to have a baby, because I had to work a few years after we were married. I just couldn't believe that everybody didn't *know* we adored our baby.

It was then that I really began to go back over things and wonder if I had done anything wrong, if maybe I hadn't burped him enough after his last bottle before I put him to bed. He had had a little cold the week before, but he seemed to be all over that. Then I began to wonder if my husband was suspicious of me too, if *he* thought I had neglected the baby somehow.

Q: Did anyone support you at this time?

A: No. No one. I really felt that they were all just suspicious of us, that they thought we were some kind of abnormal parents, child-beaters or something. A nurse came in and told us we would have to sign for an autopsy, and I couldn't. I didn't want my baby cut up. She said if we didn't sign, the coroner would do the autopsy anyway, so then my husband signed the paper. I was crying by then, and my husband was shaking all over, and we just clung to each other because there was nothing else we could do.

In a situation like this, what should be done to help this distraught couple? The same principles of supporting grieving relatives apply here as elsewhere. First, it is imperative that the staff not attempt to judge the parents in this situation. No one can possibly know how or why this infant died. No one can know whether the parents are guilty of neglect or abuse or whether they are completely innocent. Even if it is found later that kindness and support have gone to parents who did abuse their child, nothing has been lost by the effort. In fact, such parents may be genuinely remorseful by that time, their grief augmented by their guilt.

Parents of SIDS victims need repeated reassurance that nothing they have done has caused their child's death nor that anything they failed to do caused it. It is helpful if the nurse is informed on the characteristics of SIDS, its incidence and some of the theories on etiology, so that she can use some factual information in reassuring parents. While the cause of the syndrome is not yet known, much information is available about it, and a national lay organization * provides professional counseling for parents, among other services.

The initial stages of grief are coped with in the emergency department, and the nurse can

* The National Foundation for Sudden Infant Death, Inc., 1501 Broadway, New York, N.Y. 10036. Local chapters exist in many cities throughout the country.

help best by understanding the parents' ordeal, accepting their behavior, assuring them that they are in no way to blame for the death and comforting, supporting and showing willingness to help in any way possible. Keep in mind that these parents are acutely sensitive to the critical atmosphere they encounter at almost every turn. It is one of the cruelest aspects of their ordeal, and it compounds their grief and guilt.

GAINING PERMISSION FOR AUTOPSIES

One cannot ignore the unpleasant task of obtaining permission for an autopsy. Responsibility for this depends on the individual institution, the hour of the day or night death occurs and probably many other factors. All too often, the burden falls on the nurse, and if this is the case, there are a few points she may utilize to make the task a little easier and success in obtaining permission a little more likely.

The following case history clearly illustrates the wrong approach to a touchy situation, and then the successful encounter.

Hours earlier, the grief-stricken woman had been happily married, enjoying a quiet evening at home with her husband and two small children. Now she was in the waiting area outside the hospital's emergency rooms, recently informed that her 42-year-old husband had died of acute myocardial infarction. The family physician was called but arrived after the patient had died. As he entered the room he found the wife sobbing uncontrollably while a resident she had never seen before asked her for permission to perform an autopsy. She immediately refused and when he started to pursue his request further, she became extremely angry and refused to discuss the subject.

The family physician discovered that the wife had not yet been given a sedative, so he offered this and other practical assistance soon after he arrived. He shared her grief and gave her the solace and encouragement she needed at this tragic moment. Before long, after the initial impact of sudden death had started to wear off, the physician brought up the subject of autopsy once again. After he

told her the reasons behind the request and the benefits to be gained by the autopsy, she gave the physician her permission without hesitation.

Why did the family physician succeed where the resident failed? Two of the most obvious reasons are that, unlike the resident, he knew the family and had a satisfactory doctor-family relationship. Also, he waited until the shock had started to wear off before making the request. But perhaps the most important reason behind his success was the way in which he made the autopsy request.*

Let's review the steps in requesting an autopsy recommended by a panel of thanatologists,[11] which were used by the family physician in the above illustration.

(1) Wait for the proper moment. This means waiting until the initial shock has worn off, offering meanwhile sympathetic support and some practical assistance (coffee, phone calls).

(2) Make the request in a positive manner, rather than in the form of a question. Instead of saying, "Mrs. Smith, would you be willing to sign permission for an autopsy on your husband?" you might say, "I'm sure you'll want us to perform a postmortem examination. There are many reasons why it should be done." Terms such as postmortem examination or examination after death are much more acceptable to the lay person than the word "autopsy."

(3) Give the relative some valid reasons why the examination should be done. For example, it is the last chance to learn all the facts about the accident or illness that caused the death; it is easier to accept death when we know it was inevitable; the exact cause of death is often necessary for settling insurance or legal matters. Families are more receptive to the idea that *people* will be benefited by the findings in an autopsy. They are not too concerned about advancing the cause of science.

(4) If the family members still resist, they

* From *Patient Care,* May 31, 1970. © Copyright, 1970, Miller and Fink Corp., Darien, Conn. All rights reserved.

should not be bullied or badgered into giving permission. But their voiced objections should be answered, and to do this without seeming to pressure is tricky and requires tact. As an example, a frequent objection is this: "No, my husband has suffered enough already." Of course, the autopsy will not cause him any more suffering, and the family knows this, but they need to be told. It might also be added that, in the long run, autopsies actually reduce human suffering.

If the relative has strong guilt feelings about the deceased, he is less likely to grant permission. Psychologists have found that relatives who had abandoned the patient during the dying process or who had sloughed him off were the least likely to grant autopsy permission.[24]

Finally, if the nurse, herself, is convinced of the importance of the autopsy, she is much more likely to succeed in gaining permission. If she feels that it will accomplish nothing more than satisfying curiosity or raising the hospital's quota, she is not likely to convince the family it is important. Above all, the nurse's manner in interacting with the family will greatly influence the decision. A warm and understanding approach, even admitting that it is hard for you to discuss the matter, too, will do much to gain the family's cooperation.

STAFF SELF-SUPPORT

In the emergency department, geared as it is to saving the lives of the critically ill and the critically injured, the death of a patient, despite all efforts, is like a defeat. Even when the staff is convinced that the death was inevitable, there is still the lingering doubt, the thought that maybe it was their fault, that there must have been something else that could have been done.

Feelings are more acute when the victims are young: the child killed in a fall, the teenager caught in the shattered wreck of a collision, the young father with a fatal coronary. We are a youth-oriented culture, and we place a high value on the young. In earlier days, death of children was common; parents were lucky to raise even 3 out of 7 children to adulthood. Now we have conquered most of the childhood diseases, and the death of a young person is seen as a terrible, senseless waste.

In much the same way, we attach a greater social value to success, beauty, education, responsibility. We are far more devastated when the young mother with a toddler dies, than we are, for example, if it's "old George, a worthless bum, who is of no earthly use to anyone." People who become nurses and doctors bring with them the set of social values they grew up with and have lived with all their lives. The fact that they view other people, including their patients, in the light of these values is nothing to be ashamed of. But it *is* something to be aware of and to guard against its influencing the kind of care given. Awareness of personal response to social loss can also give one the courage to face a tragic situation with more composure than otherwise.[11]

The following case history demonstrates the way in which an overwhelming social loss factor can influence the staff to act in direct opposition to their objective professional judgment:

It was a quiet Sunday afternoon when Wendy W., age 12, was rushed to the emergency room of a small suburban hospital. Struck by a speeding car, she had been thrown 500 feet in the air.

The staff was shaken at the sight of her. Every bone in her body appeared to be broken. Her bloodied limbs sprawled at grotesque angles, jagged pieces of bone protruding at several sites on legs and arms. Her skull and neck were fractured, the head twisted at an odd, unnatural angle. There was no pulse, no blood pressure. But there was still a weak heart beat.

Everyone knew she didn't have a chance, that it would be kindest to let her die. But everyone knew, too, that this child's younger brother had lost his life in the very same way in the very same emergency room less than 2 years ago. Everything in them rebelled against this horror, and they reacted accordingly. When the cardiologist said, "It's no use. Let her go," one of the nurses cried out in anguish: "Do something! Can't you do *something? Anything.*" Who could refuse? They all went to work with one accord, and the next 2 hours were filled with feverish activity. Yet in the end, the child died, just as they had all known she would. When at last the staff gave up their efforts, there was not a dry eye in the room. No one said anything to anyone else. There was nothing to say.

It is very hard not to attempt to resuscitate a young person. In this situation, the physician made a very difficult decision. Yet he was easily swayed by the more emotional and less rational reaction of a young nurse. Staff members need help in overcoming their own fears of death and finding satisfactory ways of coping with their hang-ups. This would help to prevent some of the desperate efforts which are clearly doomed to failure and are so emotionally exhausting for the staff.

Nurses and physicians are exposed to other kinds of emotional trauma, too. Often they identify closely with the patient or with a member of the family. A woman who is the same age as the nurse, a child who is as young as her own child, an older person who reminds her of her father—these are the ones who bring the tragedy closer to her own life and heighten the impact of death upon her.

Many patients are warm and magnetic and involve the staff in a deeper emotional attachment than is ordinarily developed. One attractive, middle-aged woman comes to mind. She was admitted to the emergency department with severe chest pain, which was subsequently determined to be a coronary occlusion. She remained in the emergency department for 3 hours before a bed was available on a unit, and in this time became much more comfortable. She was very friendly and likeable, and since the staff members were not busy, they spent a lot of time with her. When she was finally transferred to another unit, they discussed her chances of recovery and all hoped she would get along well, "since she was such a lovely person." About an hour later, a "code 5" was sounded. The

emergency staff sensed it could be "their patient" and waited anxiously to find out. When they learned it was, indeed, this lovely lady and that she had died, the staff was overcome with gloom. For the remainder of the shift, everyone went about her own duties in silence, deep in her own thoughts.

Sometimes it is family members who upset the staff as much as the patient. They may be excessively demanding, hysterical and noisy in their lamentations. Possibly the hardest to tolerate is the family that accuses the staff of negligence or even of causing their loved one's death. Adding to the dilemma is the staff members' difficulty in coping with their own feelings after a death. They are tired, frustrated and drained by their unsuccessful efforts. What they really need is a chance to ventilate their own feelings, but instead they must maintain their composure and attempt to calm the family.

Members of the staff who have suffered a recent bereavement of their own may have great difficulty coping with dying patients and their families. They need help in handling their own problems, an opportunity to discuss their own recent crisis, as well as the emergency department experiences which have upset them.

Staff need to support and aid each other in the crises that develop, so that each member of the team can grow in his ability to cope with his own feelings and to provide thoughtful care. Sociologists Glaser and Strauss [13] suggest that members of *every* hospital unit, but especially the high-risk units, should sit down and examine closely the typical dying trajectory in their unit and the reaction patterns of various staff members when a death occurs: who does what, who should do what, where the problems are, how they might be solved. Who is the strongest member of the team and the weakest? How can they help each other to improve not only the care but the emotional climate of the unit?

In fact, all staff members should sit down together and get out their feelings and emotions, support each other, help each other.

This means doctors, nurses, aides, orderlies, everyone who is part of the emergency scene. All need to talk together as human beings, forgetting the hierarchy which for years has prevented physicians from sharing their feelings with nurses and has made nurses feel they must maintain an air of cool detachment as a part of their professionalism. All experience grief, anger, shock, frustration in emergency care. All need support. And all will be surprised at how much it helps to admit it openly and share feelings with each other. In every group in which discussions of death and dying are initiated, the reaction expressed after only a few sessions is usually, "I thought I was the only one who felt this way! I never knew other people had the same feelings I had." And all feel better just knowing it.

In addition to team conferences, role play has been found to be a very useful tool in improving communication with the dying and the bereaved. Emergency staff may need assistance in getting this started, but it should be available from the continuing education department. It is difficult initiating any of this activity, and the first attempts will be painful and may appear futile. One particular situation may require some psychiatric counseling, or one may benefit from pastoral counseling. Help is always available, but ultimately the greatest strength will come from each other.

After a time, as each staff member gains perspective into her feelings about death, she can look at ways in which she can best help her dying patients and their surviving relatives. It is only by working together in this way that each can come to grips with her anxieties about death, integrate death into the process of living and help those who truly need help at a time of great personal crisis.

BIBLIOGRAPHY

(1) Bergman, Abraham B.: "Sudden Infant Death," *Nursing Outlook,* 20 (December 1972):775–777.

(2) ——: "Unexplained Sudden Infant Death," *The New England Journal of Medicine,* 287 (August 3, 1972):254–255.

(3) Bergman, Abraham B.; Pomeroy, Margaret A., and Beckwith, Bruce: "The Psychiatric Toll of the Sudden Infant Death Syndrome," *GP,* 40 (December 1969):99.

(4) Brewster, Henry H.: "Grief: A Disrupted Human Relationship," *Human Organization,* 9:19–22.

(5) Committee on Infant and Preschool Child, American Academy of Pediatrics: "The Sudden Infant Death Syndrome," *Pediatrics,* 50 (December 1972):964–965.

(6) Curran, William J.: "An Enigma Wrapped in Swaddling Clothes: Congress and 'Crib Death,'" *New England Journal of Medicine,* 287 (August 3, 1972):235–237.

(7) Emery, John L.: "Unexpected Deaths in Infants," *Nursing Times,* 69 (April 12, 1973):474–475.

(8) ——: "Welfare of Families of Children Found Unexpectedly Dead ('Cot Deaths')," *British Medical Journal,* 1 (March 4, 1972):612–615.

(9) Engel, George L.: "Grief and Grieving," *American Journal of Nursing,* 64 (September 1964):93–98.

(10) ——: *Psychological Development in Health and Disease* (Philadelphia: W. B. Saunders Company, 1962). Chapter 26, "Psychological Responses to Major Environmental Stress," concerns grief and mourning.

(11) Glaser, Barney G., and Strauss, Anselm L.: "The Social Loss of Dying Patients," *American Journal of Nursing,* 64 (June 1964):119–121.

(12) ——: *Time for Dying* (Chicago: Aldine Publishing Company, 1968).

(13) Jackson, Edgar N.: *Understanding Grief* (New York: Abingdon Press, 1957).

(14) Kubler-Ross, Elisabeth: *Lessons from the Dying Patient* (Flossmoor, Ill.: Ross Medical Association, 1973). Taped lecture series.

(15) ———: *On Death and Dying* (New York: Macmillan, 1969).

(16) Lindemann, Erich: "Symptomatology and Management of Acute Grief," *American Journal of Psychiatry,* 101 (September 1944):141–148.

(17) The National Foundation for Sudden Infant Death, Inc.: *Clinical Pediatrics,* 11 (February 1972):83.

(18) Parks, Colin Murray: *Bereavement* (New York: International Universities Press, 1972).

(19) Pomeroy, Margaret R.: "Sudden Death Syndrome," *American Journal of Nursing,* 69 (September 1969):1886–1890.

(20) Quint, Jeanne C. (panelist): Symposium on "Managing the Dying Process," *Patient Care,* May 31, 1970.

(21) Salk, Lee: "Sudden Infant Death: Impact on Family and Physician," *Clinical Pediatrics,* 10 (May 1971):248–249.

(22) Steinschneider, Alfred: "Prolonged Apnea and the Sudden Infant Death Syndrome: Clinical and Laboratory Observations," *Pediatrics,* 50 (October 1972):646–654.

(23) Sudnow, David: *Passing On* (Englewood Cliffs, N.J.: Prentice-Hall, 1967).

(24) Symposium: "Managing the Dying Process," *Patient Care,* May 31, 1970.

(25) Vaughan, D. H.: "Families Experiencing a Sudden, Unexpected Infant Death," *Journal of Royal College of General Practitioners,* 16 (November 1968):359–367.

Shock

JAMES S. WILLIAMS

Even today, shock is thought of by many as a clinical state manifested by rapid pulse and low blood pressure. In reality, the simple term "shock" denotes a complex series of alterations of physiological processes associated with reduced blood flow and resulting in a syndrome manifested by a variety of clinical findings. For years, shock was a well-recognized but poorly understood chain of events which, if allowed to proceed unaltered, became irreversible and terminated fatally. Today, a certain percentage of shock patients die; however, the therapeutic modalities available allow for a significant salvage rate. Much of this progress is due to the persistent and innovative work of a large number of dedicated medical scientists applying the sophisticated methods possible with modern technology.[2, 3, 8, 9, 11, 12, 13]

It has been shown that the shock state is a dynamic one, with a stress-response pattern. This invariably is associated with a deficiency of peripheral blood flow combined with lowered tissue perfusion, which if prolonged or untreated produces alterations in cellular metabolism which may eventually impair physiologic processes.[7] To manage the patient in shock properly, one must have knowledge of these processes in order that appro-priate intervention techniques be applied to interrupt and reverse the abnormal chain of events.

A multitude of factors play a role in the shock state. The material covered in this chapter alludes to many of these factors. An effort will be made to elucidate the basic changes in the homeostatic mechanism which occur in the shock state as the result of lower tissue perfusion and alteration in cellular metabolism.

DEFINITION

Shock is present when there is reduced perfusion of body tissues leading to cellular hypoxia and damage of vital organs. If the state is uncorrected and allowed to continue, eventually a critical number of cells will be injured beyond repair, resulting in cessation of vital organ function and progressive unrelenting death of the remaining cells in spite of treatment. This is the state of "irreversible shock."

CLASSIFICATION

The circulation system can be divided into 5 parts: arteries, capillaries, veins, heart and blood. Using these divisions, with the exception of arteries, shock can be classified as to etiology into oligemic (blood loss) shock, capillary shock, venous "pooling" shock, and myocardial (heart) shock. (See Figure 9–1.)

(1) *Oligemic shock* (blood loss or hypovolemia): Oligemic shock results from loss of whole blood or its parts from the circulatory system at a rate sufficient to produce reduced effective circulating blood volume and inadequate tissue perfusion.

(2) *Capillary shock:* Capillary shock is that which occurs when circulating blood volume is sequestered in the capillary bed. This results in an inadequate tissue perfusion.

(3) *Venous pooling shock:* Venous pooling shock is that which results when circulating blood volume is sequestered on the venous side of the heart.

(4) *Myocardial shock* (pump failure or cardiogenic): Myocardial shock is the result of cardiac action being unable to deliver a circulating volume at a rate sufficient to produce adequate tissue perfusion.

PATHOPHYSIOLOGY

Oligemic shock

The acute loss of blood volume stimulates the volume baroreceptors in the aortic arch and carotid arteries resulting in vasoconstriction through increased sympathetic nervous system tone. In addition, adrenalin is released from the adrenal cortex aiding the vasoconstriction and causing tachycardia by direct action on the heart. If loss is rapid enough, the oxygen carrying capacity of the blood is lessened. This is marked by shortness of breath (air hunger) and is frequently associated with cerebral symptoms. There may not be enough circulating blood volume for the patient to manifest cyanosis.

Depletion of circulating volume may involve either whole blood or merely the fluid portion (plasma). Examples of whole blood loss are major vessel damage associated with internal or external bleeding. Examples of loss of parts of whole blood would be the decrease in plasma fluid as a result of protracted vomiting or diarrhea and fluid loss from burns or peritonitis. (See Table 9–1, page 108, for other secondary causes.)

The clinical signs and symptoms are characterized by pallor, clammy extremities, hypotension, tachycardia and apprehension. As time progresses, cold, pale or cyanotic extremities and lips are noted, and the victim eventually succumbs.

Capillary shock

There are some 70 miles of capillaries in a normal adult and only 10 percent of these are open at one time. If a major percent of the capillary beds were to open up, a large quantity of circulating volume would be easily sequestered.

Causes of capillary type shock are numerous. Examples include septic shock, spinal cord shock, neurogenic shock, types of anesthetic shock, anaphylactic shock, drug shock (antihypertensives and tranquilizers) and adrenal insufficiency. (See also Table 9–1.)

Initially, the extremities are warm, and the patient is hypotensive, usually without tachycardia. As time passes, the sustained inadequate circulating volume stimulates the sympathetic nervous system through baroreceptor mechanisms, and vasoconstriction becomes a prominent feature. The cardinal symptoms and signs of shock ensue (see page 115).

Venous pooling shock

The veins are normally very distensible; they have a considerable reservoir capacity and thus can harbor large quantities of blood volume. Anything that mechanically prevents blood from entering the heart chamber will cause blood to accumulate in the vast area of the venous reservoir. Effective circulating volume will drop sharply, and inadequate tissue perfusion will ensue.

Examples of venous pooling shock would

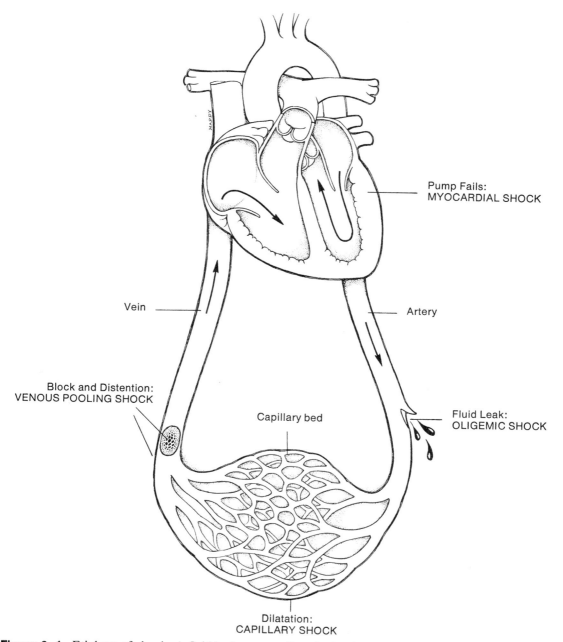

Figure 9-1 Etiology of shock. A fluid leak causes oligemic shock; excessive capillary dilatation results in capillary shock; blood trapped in the venous system causes venous-pooling shock; and when the heart pump fails, myocardial shock ensues.

Source: Adapted from material of the Photography Unit of the University of Rochester Medical Center, Rochester, New York.

TABLE 9–1   PRIMARY AND SECONDARY CAUSES OF SHOCK, BY ETIOLOGY

Etiology	Primary cause	Secondary cause
Oligemic	(1) Loss of whole blood (2) Loss of plasma (3) Loss of fluid	(1) Internal or external bleeding (2) Burn or peritonitis (3) Crush injury (4) Dehydration, vomiting (5) Diarrhea (6) Bowel obstruction
Capillary	(1) Dilatation of the capillary bed, with sequestration of whole blood	(1) Vasodilator damage (2) Spinal cord "shock" (cord transection) (3) Septicemia (4) Addisonian crisis (5) Anesthetic agents (6) Drug overdose
Venous pooling	(1) Entrapment of whole blood on the venous side of the heart	(1) Massive pulmonary embolus (2) Air embolism (3) Cardiac tamponade (4) Tension pneumothorax
Myocardial	(1) Failure of the heart muscle to pump adequate blood	(1) Myocardial infarction (2) Myocarditis (3) Extensive arteriovenous shunt (4) Pericarditis

be that associated with a pulmonary embolus obstructing the pulmonary arteries; a tension pneumothorax with mediastinal shift, causing obstruction of the vena cava due to kinking as it enters the thorax through the diaphragm; an air embolus, whereby blood is churned into froth in the right heart chambers, preventing normal flow of blood through the heart; and pericardial tamponade, whereby pressure in the pericardial sac collapses the atria, preventing filling.

The clinical manifestations are precipitous with increased venous pressure, rapid pulse, marked drop in blood pressure, cyanosis and rapid onset of the other cardinal signs and symptoms of shock (see page 115).

Myocardial shock

In pump failure shock, the heart is not strong enough to pump blood into the arterial tree with sufficient force to maintain adequate perfusion pressure, and therefore it backs up into the pulmonary circulation and subsequently into the systemic venous and capillary circulation. The victim experiences shortness of breath due to venous distention of the atrium, pulmonary circulation and vena cava. Fluid accumulates outside the capillary beds and in the alveoli of the lungs and other extravascular tissues. Examples of this type of shock include acute or chronic myocardial infarction and any cause of acute or chronic myocardial degeneration. (See Table 9–1.)

The clinical signs and symptoms are related to the rate of onset as well as the degree and locale of the myocardial damage. The usual cardinal symptoms are pain, dyspnea, restlessness leading to venous distention, edema and finally the classic signs of shock (see page 115).

Table 9–1 summarizes the pathophysiology of the 4 types of shock described above.

Disseminated intravascular coagulation

Any discussion of the shock state would not be complete without mention of this entity. Disseminated intravascular coagulation (DIC) has also been known by a number of other terms: consumption coagulopathy, defibrination syndrome and intravascular coagulation fibrinolysis syndrome. Basically, it involves alterations in the blood clotting mechanism, initially hypercoagulability followed by hypocoagulability. It occurs in a variety of clinical situations,[1,4,6,10,15] but of particular interest to the emergency nurse is its association with the shock state, in patients with multiple injuries and in patients with bleeding in the last trimester of pregnancy.

Experimental studies have shown it to occur particularly in shock due to hemorrhage or sepsis.[14] It is described as a functional state with intravascular clotting caused by activation of the normal coagulation system. The fibrinogen-fibrin reaction is accelerated, with the result that fibrinogen elements in the blood are reduced. Other factors, especially the blood platelets, are depleted. The results are: (1) clot formation in the microcirculation, with subsequent impairment in flow and (2) a hemorrhagic diathesis. Thus, in the same patient, the result can be abnormal hemorrhage and/or thrombosis.

The most dramatic result of DIC is the acute generalized hemorrhagic state. Diagnosis is difficult and depends on the clinical picture combined with adjunct studies, a number of laboratory tests which include, among others, a partial thromboplastin time, peripheral blood smear for study of red cells, platelet count and evaluation of various clotting elements in the blood. An excellent review of the subject was prepared by Damus and Salzman.[10] The reader is referred to this article for more in-depth study of this dramatic problem.

EFFECTS ON CELL METABOLISM (ENERGY PRODUCTION)

Cells must have oxygen in sufficient quantity to produce energy for maintaining normal cell function. Since shock, by definition, results in inadequate tissue perfusion and cellular hypoxia, it is not surprising that cellular energy production is impaired during shock.

Normally, cell energy is supplied by adenosine triphosphate molecules (ATP). Every time the alpha phosphate bond is split, 7,000 calories of energy are released for cell use. The ATP molecules are manufactured primarily by the use of glucose (see Figure 9–2). Glucose, either from ingestion or split from glycogen stores in muscle or liver, is converted into high-energy phosphate via the Krebs–Tricarboxylic Acid (TCA) cycle. During this process, hydrogen ions accumulate and must be carried away. Normally, in the presence of oxygen, they are transported via the cytochrome system. With hypoxia, however, they accumulate and are stored as lactate. As long as there is oxygen deficiency (debt), manufactured pyruvate is converted into lactate in order to store the ions. Energy production is drastically reduced and lactate accumulates in excess as lactic acid.

The major source of lactate is the muscle mass. It is normally metabolized in the liver and heart. During shock, more lactate is produced than can be utilized by these organs. The excessive accumulation of lactate as lactic acid, as well as other acid metabolites, results in acidosis, which has an unstabilizing effect on cell membranes.

Normally, the cell membranes which are lipoprotein in nature are maintained by ATP (see Figure 9–3). It is evident that if ATP production is faulty, membrane stability will be in jeopardy. Indeed, as shock progresses, membrane function is impaired. Normal transfer of sodium and potassium in and out of the cell (the so-called sodium pump) is impaired, and water accumulates within the cell. The hydrolytic enzymes normally contained within the lipoprotein lysosomal membrane leak into the cell cytoplasm and begin the digestion of the cell components. Eventually, they enter the general circulation and act on distant cells. If treated in time, cell membrane damage is reversible. If not, death occurs.

If shock progresses untreated, tissue levels of ATP decrease progressively as stores are used up. The PO_4 ion released during ATP

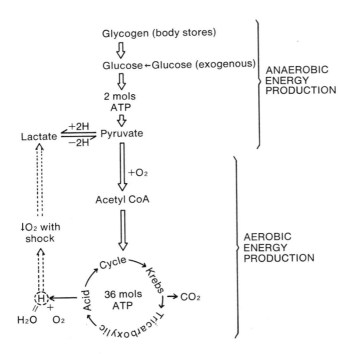

Figure 9–2 Anaerobic and aerobic energy production. Glycogen and exogenous glucose are converted to pyruvate. Two mols of ATP are formed and (without oxygen) represent the sole source of high energy phosphate to sustain cell function. Excess hydrogen ions generated in this process convert pyruvate to lactate. In the presence of oxygen, lactate can be converted back to pyruvate, which in turn is changed to a 3-carbon molecule, acetyl CoA. This material enters the Krebs' cycle and results in the formation of CO_2, H_2O and 36 mols of high energy ATP. If insufficient O_2 is present, excess hydrogen ions are stored as lactate.
Source: Adapted from material of the Photography Unit of the University of Rochester Medical Center, Rochester, New York.

breakdown accumulates in the serum. Likewise, glycogen stores, in the liver particularly and in the body in general, are depleted. In severe experimental shock models, after 2 hours, glycogen was virtually absent, and ATP was reduced as much as 75 percent, depending on the organ.

EFFECTS ON SPECIFIC SYSTEMS

The effect of shock stress on specific body systems varies and is related to several factors. Considered must be: (1) general health prior to shock; (2) age of the victim; (3) duration and degree of shock; (4) preexisting specific organ system disease; (5) coexisting illness or injury; and (6) drugs or medications.

Central nervous system

Since blood flow to the brain and spinal cord is regulated by metabolic needs and not by the sympathetic nervous system, blood flow to these areas in shock is maintained above all other organs. The one exception is the heart, which shares equal-flow priority. An elevation in pCO_2 or a drop in blood pH will increase cerebral flow. If the patient has been hyperventilating, a respiratory alkalosis may be present and the pCO_2 reduced. In this case, blood flow to the brain may decrease and oxygen disassociation from oxyhemoglobin be reduced, with a resultant degree of anoxia. Anoxia may also result from intra- or extracranial vascular disease or perfusion pressure of less than 50 mm. of Hg.

Peripheral nervous system

Although peripheral vasoconstriction is a prominent part of most shock cases, peripheral nerves, as organ structures, are extremely resistant to shock.

Circulatory system and myocardium

Adaptation of the heart muscle to changes in pressure and volume is regulated by Starling's law and mediated through the sympathetic and myocardial catecholamines. Regulation can occur in 2 ways: (1) homeometric adaptation, by which the heart puts out an increased volume, but the end diastolic blood volume in the ventricle remains unchanged and (2) heterometric adaptation, by which the end diastolic volume increases to accommodate the increased volume. The second method is quicker but less efficient, since the heart muscle is more dilated and contraction requires more work.

In myocardial pump failure shock, the heart muscle is unable to handle the increased blood volume, and quickly a heterometric adaptation occurs. This may be followed by a homeometric adaptation through increased sympathetic stimulation of myocardial catecholamines and result in a temporary decrease in the end diastolic volume. Extra cardiac catecholamines may help during this phase.

However, hypoxia and depletion of myocardial catecholamines soon result in an un-

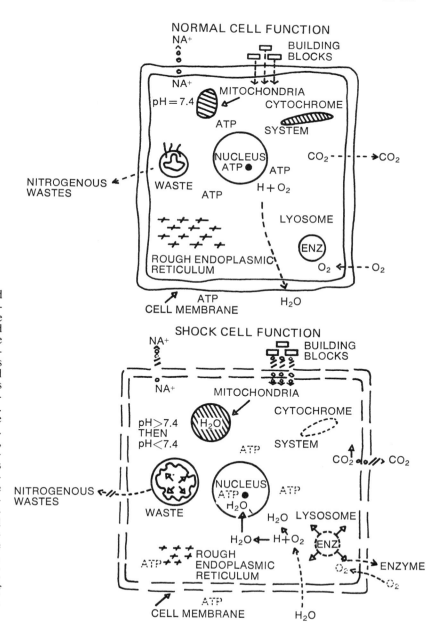

Figure 9–3 Normal and shock cell function. Normally, ATP maintains the cell. Excess Na⁺ is pumped out, and building blocks are brought in. The endoplasmic reticulum uses this material to produce integral cellular parts. CO_2, excess water and wastes are expelled. O_2 enters the cell. In shock, ATP stores are depleted and not replaced. H⁺ ions, Na⁺ ions, CO_2, H_2O and wastes accumulate. Cell membranes deteriorate. Hydrolytic enzymes escape from the lysosomes. Important intracellular systems disintegrate. pH rises early and then drops to severely acidotic levels. Eventually, the cell digests itself and dies. Source: Adapted from material of the Photography Unit of the University of Rochester Medical Center, Rochester, New York.

responsiveness of the myocardium to sympathetic activity, and adaptation reverts back to heterometric, resulting in an increasing end diastolic volume heralding myocardial decompensation. Energy for maintenance of myocardial function is gradually reduced. The myocardial fibers become disarranged; the heart wall dilates; and irreversible arrhythmias occur. Subendocardial hemorrhagic necrotic areas have been observed, due to either anoxia or circulating lysosomal hydrolytic enzymes. One fraction of these enzymes from the gut and pancreas have been labeled "myocardial depressant factor" (MDF), but their clinical significance is uncertain.

Arterial system

With blood volume depletion, the elastic arterial wall constricts in an attempt to accommodate. Aided by arterial constriction, particularly in the periphery (extremities), blood pressure is maintained. As volume continues to decrease, arteriovenous shunts open, and blood bypasses peripheral capillary beds. Eventually, the same process occurs in the splanchnic and renal beds. The blood in these beds moves slower and slower, finally sludging. Anoxia results in increased capillary permeability and in interstitial and intracellular edema. When arteriolar constriction can no longer be maintained, dilatation occurs, with additional fluid loss. A pressure sufficient to reestablish venular flow cannot be generated. Stagnant anoxia persists, and cell death progresses.

If restoration of volume is attempted at this point, the tissue edema will be picked up in the lymphatics, along with acid metabolites. This lymph volume added to the circulation is generally inadequate to reverse shock.

In capillary shock, the early capillary dilatation gives way to increased sympathetic tone, and the same path as described above is followed.

Respiratory system

Of all systems, the respiratory system is most vulnerable to the subtle changes of shock and its treatment. Multiple external and internal stresses are brought to bear on the lungs. (See Figure 9–4.)

Early in shock, because of pain or apprehension, the victim splints the chest or breathes rapidly and shallowly. Deep breathing does not occur, and atelectasis results. With an increased respiratory rate, the effective alveolar ventilation decreases. Arteriovenous shunting occurs through the nonventilated atelectatic lung. Arterial oxygen saturation falls. The problem is compounded by an increased pulmonary vascular resistance, in response to local pulmonary vascular compression, acidosis, hypoxia and humoral and neural factors. CO_2 accumulates systemically. Being unable to diffuse out of the lung, CO_2 contributes to the acidosis and provides additional drive for hyperventilation by stimulating brain, carotid body and aortic arch receptors. The distensibility or compliance of the lung is lost as it "stiffens," and the work of respiration increases.

Progressive respiratory deterioration during and following shock is enhanced by other contributing factors.

(1) *Preexisting pulmonary disease,* such as chronic bronchitis, congestive heart failure, emphysema or pneumoconiosis, leave the shock victim little pulmonary reserve.

(2) *Pulmonary trauma* or injury to the chest wall results in early alteration in pulmonary function.

(3) *Aspiration of gastric contents* or blood may result in extensive damage to cilia activity and bronchial mucosa.

(4) *Overzealous fluid replacement* with blood, colloid or crystalloid can produce pulmonary edema more readily in the shock-stressed lung than in the normal lung.

(5) *Embolization of fat particles* after long bone fractures or soft tissue trauma results in conversion of the neutral fat to fatty acids that are toxic to pulmonary tissue.

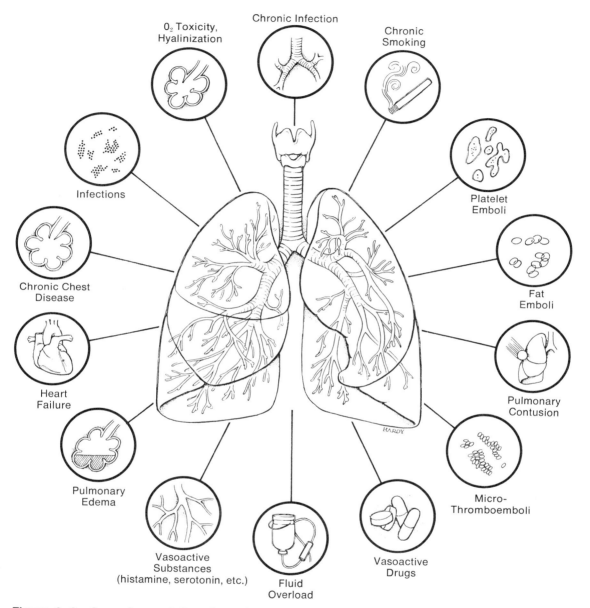

Figure 9–4 Some factors influencing "shock" lung. Pulmonary infiltrates and congestion occur in shock. No one single factor is to blame; rather many stresses are brought to bear on the lung and contribute to the so-called "shock" lung.
Source: Adapted from material of the Photography Unit of the University of Rochester Medical Center, Rochester, New York.

(6) *Microemboli* are common, as platelet aggregates secondary to sludging, as thrombi from traumatized veins or intravascular coagulation and as particulate matter from transfusion.

(7) *Oxygen toxicity,* characterized by intra-alveolar transudation and hyalinization, results from prolonged exposure to high concentrations of O_2.

(8) *Supervening pulmonary infection* severely compounds the already stressed respiratory system.

(9) *Cardiac failure* superimposed on the shock situation results in pulmonary congestion and elevated pulmonary vascular pressure.

(10) *Vasoactive substances* released during shock, such as serotonin, catecholamine, bradykinin and histamine, cause pulmonary venous constriction and vascular congestion.

(11) *Surfactant activity* is markedly reduced due to inadequate phospholipid production secondary to ischemia and thus contributes to atelectasis.

(12) *Massive head injury* has been associated with progressive pulmonary insufficiency, perhaps secondary to respiratory neuroregulatory dysfunction.

(13) *Iatrogenic causes,* such as intravenous air, incompatible medication (allergens, depressants, vasoactives), anesthesia and the like, must be included as contributing causes for progressive pulmonary insufficiency.

Digestive system

During shock, there appears to be a redistribution of blood flow away from the gastrointestinal tract secondary to sympathetic activity causing splanchnic vasoconstriction. The anoxia which ensues results in reduced energy, producing oxidative phosphorylation, injury to the intestinal mucosal cells, release of hydrolytic enzymes from the lysosomal membrane and sequestration of fluid in the gut from increased capillary permeability due to local acidosis and hypercarbia. The vasoconstriction affects the liver, as well, but is well tolerated unless there is preexisting liver disease.

Excretory system

With decreased perfusion pressure, renal blood flow decreases. Glomerular filtration drops, and although renal venous oxygen saturation decreases only slightly, urine oxygen tension falls drastically, indicating that oxygen dissolved in urine may be an important source of renal parenchyma oxygen supply. The excretory regulatory function of the kidney is impaired. If the decreased perfusion is sufficient in degree or duration, i.e., if this ischemic injury to sufficient nephrons has produced acute tubular necrosis, the kidney ceases to function.

Endocrine system

With stress there is an increased output of adenocorticotropic hormone (ACTH) from the anterior pituitary gland. This results in release of glucocorticoids from the zona fasciculata cells of the adrenal. They have glucogenic effects, increasing the release and manufacture of glucose. They keep vascular smooth muscle reactive to catecholamines. In addition, they are necessary for the conversion of norepinephrine to epinephrine in the adrenal medulla.

From the zona glomerulosa of the adrenal cortex, aldosterone is released. This salt-retaining hormone is released in response to renal hypotension. (The proteolytic enzyme renin, coming from the juxtaglomerular apparatus in the glomerulus of the kidney, causes the formation of angiotensin I in the plasma. This, in turn, is changed to angiotensin II, which initiates the release of aldosterone.) Aldosterone then acts on the proximal tubule of the nephron to increase sodium retention.

Catecholamines are released from the adrenal medulla in response to increased sympathetic nervous system tone. Epinephrine predominantly is released, as well as some neorepinephrine. They increase vasocirculation tone and result in the conversion of glycogen to glucose.

CLINICAL SIGNS AND SYMPTOMS

The clinical signs and symptoms of shock are dependent on the etiology and the physiological compensatory mechanisms the body employs to counter the shock. The classic clinical picture of shock is related to the increased sympathetic activity which eventually predominates regardless of the cause of shock. The symptoms of shock which the patient relates are the cornerstones not only to the etiology of the shock but also to the diagnosis.

(1) *State of consciousness:* Early in shock, the victim may be lucid, restless and anxious, in response to the increased circulating catecholamines. As anoxia sets in, the patient becomes quite restless, agitated and irrational. Continued deterioration results in an obtunded, depressed and stuporous individual. It must be kept in mind that age plays a role, and therefore it is not uncommon to find a lucid youngster in profound shock without obtainable blood pressure or an elderly person restless and obtunded in mild shock.

(2) *Skin temperature:* Sympathetic hyperactivity causes vasoconstriction of the skin vessels, stimulation of the sweat glands and contraction of the erector pilae muscles. Thus, the skin is pale, cool and clammy, and the hair is "standing on end." If the insult is severe enough, the skin may be cyanotic or exhibit patchy cyanosis (livor). Early in capillary shock, such as septic shock, it is not uncommon to find the skin warm, pink and dry from capillary dilatation. As time passes, sympathetic tone increases, and this situation is reversed.

(3) *Mucous membranes:* These membranes undergo vasoconstriction, become pale and are a good index of carboxyhemoglobin level.

(4) *Nail beds:* Vasoconstriction affects the nail beds. Therefore, their color and cap-

illary refill times are a reasonably good index of the degree of peripheral vascular "clamping."

(5) *Peripheral veins:* Since peripheral veins collapse with volume depletion and sympathetic venoconstriction, they are of value in evaluating the degree of shock. Distended veins, on the other hand, signify obstruction of the venous return, as in venous pooling shock or heart failure.

(6) *Pulse:* The pulse increases from catecholamine effect on the heart. As intravascular volume decreases and vasoconstriction increases, the quality of the pulse weakens, becoming thready. An irregular pulse signifies a diseased or severely stressed myocardium.

(7) *Respiration:* Epinephrine release causes a fear response and hyperventilation. With decrease in effective circulating blood volume and/or a marked reduction in oxygen-carrying capacity, gasping respiration occurs, called "air hunger." Labored or tugging respiration is indicative of obstructed airway from bronchospasm, lung collapse or foreign material.

(8) *Blood pressure:* Blood pressure is maintained by peripheral vasoconstriction and by increased cardiac output from the epinephrine inotropic action on the heart until circulatory collapse is imminent. In some instances, a peripheral blood pressure cannot be obtained because of such severe sympathetic "squeezing" and yet a central pressure is near normal.

DIAGNOSIS

Appropriate treatment is based on an accurate diagnosis. Historical data will establish a diagnosis in over 80 percent of all cases. Physical examination will increase the percentage to about 90 percent. Laboratory data (including x-ray), monitoring and observation will reveal the diagnosis in the remaining cases.

(1) *Historical data:* A time sequence from the minute the patient was last stable to the present should be developed. Previous ill-

ness, infirmity or disease should be noted. Any drugs the patient takes and allergies should be recorded. Accident data and pain characteristics are important.

(2) *Examination:* The level of consciousness is observed and vital signs recorded. Regional examination is then done as rapidly as the situation indicates.

(3) *Laboratory studies:* Blood samples are drawn at the time of the intravenous catheter placement. Electrolytes, hematocrit, white blood count and differential and arterial blood gases are important. A blood type and crossmatch should be obtained, as well as any additional indicated studies. Important roentgenograms should be taken, including a chest film to establish a baseline cardiopulmonary status. During this period, the care of the patient must not be relegated to the x-ray technician who is not trained in patient care.

(4) *Electrocardiogram:* An early heart conduction tracing (ECG) will be useful in evaluating the myocardial status and should be repeated when indicated.

(5) *Cultures:* Blood and pertinent cultures should be obtained early and pus or sputum smear stained and examined under a microscope for early tentative diagnosis.

(6) *Monitoring:* Vital signs, urine output, central venous pressure, ECG, blood gases and laboratory studies should be followed. The patient's clinical course should be documented in the chart as it evolves.

THERAPEUTIC CONSIDERATIONS

Most shock, when treated early, will respond and be successfully reversed. When the insult producing the shock has been massive or prolonged, reestablishment of a normal physiological state is much more difficult and less successful. The therapeutic goal in the treatment of shock is to reverse the inadequate tissue perfusion. In order to accomplish this goal, the defects in the oxygen delivery cycle must be recognized and corrected.

Volume replacement

Hypovolemia occurs in all types of shock. Anoxia is followed by capillary dilation and tissue edema. Therefore, early fluid replacement in the form of lactated Ringer's solution or normal saline has therapeutic merit. One liter administered within a 30-minute period frequently stabilizes vital signs.

When whole blood or plasma is lost, it should be replaced volume for volume, realizing that additional fluid is still necessary. Administration is monitored by central venous pressure (CVP) and urine output. A CVP of 15 mm. of H_2O is indicative of incipient pulmonary edema. Dextran, albumen or plasma, because of their osmotic qualities, may be used to hold fluid in the intravascular space until whole blood or packed red cells are available.

Dextran given as a 10 percent solution is a polymer of glucose with a molecular weight of 75,000 and helps to restore normal osmotic pressure. Excessive use, however, may promote a bleeding tendency.

As a 5 percent solution of stabilized human plasma protein in normal saline, plasma protein fraction is an excellent temporary substitute for whole blood. Formulas are available for determining the rate of fluid administration, particularly in burns (Brooke Army and Evans Formula). Volume replacement may result in pulmonary congestion or edema due to sequestered extravascular fluid being drawn into the intravascular space by the increased osmotic pressure. If so, it should not be allowed to progress without continuous supervision.

Oxygenation

The availability of oxygen to the tissue is dependent on airway patency and lung function. An obstructed airway or damaged lung will result in inadequate oxygenation. To maintain a clear airway, an endotracheal tube or tracheostomy may be required. If pulmonary congestion, trauma or edema is present, constant positive pressure ventilation (breathing) (CPPB) may be necessary to drive the fluid back into the circulatory system and keep it out of the gas exchange area of the lung.

Restlessness and hyperventilation are the first clinical signs of poor oxygenation but late in comparison to arterial oxygen pressure (pO_2). Assisted ventilation, using a volume ventilator, should be started early. When arterial pO_2 fails to rise significantly with 100 percent oxygen ventilation, it is indicative of physiological shunting through unaerated segments of lung tissue. The shunt may account for 15 to 30 percent of the cardiac output and aggravate cardiac compensation.

If improvement in cardiac function is not associated with improvement in arterial pO_2, it suggests the insult to the lung may be so great that progressive pulmonary insufficiency has developed. Eventually, oxygen can no longer enter the circulatory system, and carbon dioxide cannot escape. The arterial pO_2 falls, and the pCO_2 rises. Metabolic acidosis and lactic acidemia herald a terminal situation.

Drug therapy

Cardiotonics

The cornerstone of adequate tissue perfusion is a smoothly functioning myocardium. During shock, the heart muscle adjusts to the stress with its own intrinsic mechanisms. Eventually, these mechanisms may fail. If there is clinical evidence this is indeed occurring, medication can be given to improve cardiac function.

(1) *Digitalis glycosides:* Digitalis acts to slow ventricular rate by decreasing conduction through the arterioventricular node, decreasing myocardial irritability and thus preventing attacks of supraventricular tachycardia. In addition, it has a positive inotropic action on the heart, strengthening cardiac contractions.

(2) *Steroids:* Massive doses of steroid preparations, given as a "slow push," have a direct inotropic effect on the heart and increase coronary artery flow. In addition, steroids counteract the effects of bacterial endotoxin, promote peripheral vasodilatation, stabilize the lipoprotein membranes of the cell and increase the flow of lymph back into the circulation.

(3) *Lidocaine:* Lidocaine, a potent smooth muscle relaxant with vagal blocking action on the atrioventricular node, also reduces myocardial irritability. It increases refractoriness of the myocardium without affecting the conducting system and is therefore useful in the treatment of ventricular arrhythmias.

Diuretics

Maintenance of renal function during shock is important for regulation of fluid and electrolyte balance. Diuretics are used in this effort.

(1) *Mannitol:* This osmotic diuretic is of great value in shock, because it produces an obligatory urine flow by interfering with the nephron transport mechanism. It is postulated that the dissolved oxygen in the urine prevents anoxic tubular cell damage and acute tubular necrosis.

(2) *Furosemide:* This powerful diuretic inhibits the active reabsorption of sodium in the proximal tubule and should be used after blood volume has been restored. It acts rapidly and is effective in treating pulmonary edema.

Vasopressors

Vasopressor drugs have 3 effects, consisting of central inotropic effects, chronotropic effects and peripheral vasoconstriction. They should not be used until blood volume is restored, for fear of reducing tissue perfusion. These drugs are useful in capillary shock states.

(1) *Metaraminol* (Aramine): This medication significantly increases myocardial contractibility by increasing the efficiency of heart beats while reducing heart rate. It is a moderate vasopressor.

(2) *Isoproterenol:* This medication is a beta-adrenergic blocking agent which increases myocardial contractibility and heart rate but produces vasodilatation.

SUMMARY

In the emergency setting, the patient with shock should receive the highest priority of care. Early, thorough evaluation should be done to make the proper diagnosis and determine the etiology of the shock state. Appropriate treatment is instituted to stabilize vital signs and functions, ideally within a 30-minute time period. In some patients, particularly those with massive bleeding, stabilization may not be possible without operative intervention, and rapid and shorter work-up should be done, with early institution of therapeutic measures and transfer to the operating theater. In other patients in shock, stabilization may require many hours of intensive care, with close observation and utilization of a variety of laboratory aids and monitoring techniques, in addition to numerous therapeutic modalities.

In the shock state, because it is dynamic and because of the nature of the therapy, more than one mechanism may be involved. For example, an elderly patient in oligemic shock may, as a result of fluid replacement, develop cardiogenic shock. Thus, those caring for the shock patient, particularly the nurse (likely to be in more constant attendance), must be familiar with the parameters used in assessing the patient's response to therapy in order to detect any deviation from the desired or anticipated course.

There is a great temptation on the part of some physicians and nurses to make a premature judgment as to the prognosis for the shock patient, which may result in a rather strictured approach to therapy. This can have an adverse effect on the eventual outcome. One must guard against this thinking and outline a plan of management designed for survival, until it is apparent that death is imminent or cerebral death has occurred. While it is important to prolong useful life, it is also important not to prolong death. This judgment may be the most difficult in caring for the shock victim.

It must be readily apparent that the shock state is indeed a complex one, which may tax the expertise and judgment of the nurse. The newer concepts of human shock have been discussed, to give the reader knowledge of the stress-response pattern that occurs in the patient in shock. The management of specific causes of the shock state is discussed in the appropriate chapters.

BIBLIOGRAPHY

(1) Attar, S.; Kirby, W. H., Jr.; Masaitis, C.; Mansberger, A. R., and Conley, R. A.: "Coagulation Changes in Clinical Shock," *Annals of Surgery,* 164 (1966):34.

(2) Baxter, C. R.; Canizaro, P. C.; Carrico, C. J., and Shires, G. T.: "Fluid Resuscitation in Hemorrhagic Shock," *Postgraduate Medicine,* 48 (1970):95.

(3) Border, J. R.: "Advances and New Concepts in the Management of Shock: Kidney" *in* P. Cooper, ed., *Surgery Annal* (New York: Appleton-Century-Crofts, 1969), pp. 108–109.

(4) Bounous, G.; Sutherland, N. G.; McArdle, A. H., and Gurd, F. N.: "The Prophylactic Use of an Elemental Diet in Hemorrhagic Shock and Intestinal Ischemia," *Annals of Surgery,* 166 (1967):312.

(5) Clermont, H. G.; Adams, J. T., and Williams, J. S.: "Effect of Cross-Cir-

culation in Hemorrhagic Shock," *Surgery Gynecology and Obstetrics,* 135 (1972):593.

(6) Clermont, H. G.; Adams, J. T., and Williams, J. S.: "Source of a Lysosomal Enzymes Acid Phosphatase in Hemorrhagic Shock," *Annals of Surgery,* 175 (January 1972):19–25.

(7) Clermont, H. G., and Williams, J. S.: "Lymph Lysosomal Enzyme Acid Phosphatase in Hemorrhagic Shock," *Annals of Surgery,* 176 (July 1972): 90–96.

(8) Clermont, H. G.; Williams, J. S., and Adams, J. T.: "Liver Acid Phosphatase as a Measure of Heptocyto Resistance to Hemorrhagic Shock," *Surgery,* 71 (June 1972):868–875.

(9) Crowell, J. W., and Read, W. L.: "In Vivo Coagulation—A Probable Cause of Irreversible Shocks," *American Journal of Physiology,* 183 (1955):565.

(10) Damus, P. S., and Salzman, E. W.: "Disseminated Intravascular Coagulation," *Archives of Surgery,* 104 (1972): 262.

(11) deDuve, C.: *Lysosomes: A New Group of Cytoplasmic Subcellular Particles* (New York: Ronald Press Company, 1959).

(12) Deykin, D.: "The Challenge of Disseminated Intravascular Coagulation," *New England Journal of Medicine,* 283 (1970):642.

(13) Drucker, W. R.: "Shock and Metabolism," *Surgery, Gynecology and Obstetrics,* 132 (1971):234.

(14) Fitts, C. T.: "Vasoactive Drugs in Treatment of Shock," *Postgraduate Medicine,* 48 (1970):105.

(15) Glenn, T. M., *et al.:* "Circulatory Responses to Splanchnic Lysosomal Hydrolases in the Dog," *Annals of Surgery,* 176 (July 1972):120–127.

(16) Guenter, C. A., and Hinshaw, L. B.: "Comparison of Septic Shock Due to Gram-Negative and Gram-Positive Organisms," *Proceedings of the Society of Experimental Biology and Medicine,* 134 (1970):780.

(17) Hardaway, R. M.: "The Role of Intravascular Clotting in the Etiology of Shock," *Annals of Surgery,* 155 (1962):325.

(18) Hinshaw, L. B.; Archer, L. T.; Black, M. R.; Greenfield, L. J., and Guenter, C. A.: "Prevention and Reversal of Myocardial Failures in Endotoxin Shock," *Surgery, Gynecology and Obstetrics,* 136 (1973):1.

(19) Hinshaw, L. B.; Shanbour, L. L.; Greenfield, L. J., and Coalson, J. J.: "Mechanism of Dumased Venous Return: Subhuman Primate-Administered Endotoxin," *Archives of Surgery,* 100 (1970):600.

(20) Hopkins, R. W.: "Septic Shock: Hemodynamic Cast of Inflammation," *Archives of Surgery,* 101 (1970):298.

(21) Horwitz, D. L.; Moquin, R. B., and Herman, C. M.: "Coagulation Changes of Septic Shock in the Subhuman Primate and Their Relationship to Hemodynamic Changes," *Annals of Surgery,* 175 (1972):417.

(22) Knisley, M. H.: "Intravascular Erythrocyte Aggregation (Blood Sludge)," *in* sec. 2, vol. III, "Circulation," *Handbook of Physiology* (Washington, D.C.: American Physiological Society, 1965), p. 2257.

(23) Mayer, G. G.: "Disseminated Intravascular Coagulation," *American Journal of Nursing,* 73 (1973):2067.

(24) Sarnoff, S. J., and Mitchell, J. H.: "The Control of the Function of the Heart," *in* W. F. Hamilton and P. Don, eds., *Handbook of Physiology: Circulation* (American Physiological Society) (Baltimore: Williams & Wilkins, 1962), vol. 1, pp. 489–532.

(25) Shires, G. T., *et al.:* "Alterations in Cellular Membrane Function During Hemorrhagic Shock in Primates,"

Annals of Surgery, 176 (September 1972).

(26) Shires, G. T.; Canico, J., and Canizara, P. C.: "Pulmonary Responses: Shock," *in* J. E. Dunphy, ed., *Major Problems in Clinical Surgery* (Philadelphia: W. B. Saunders Company, 1973), pp. 62–64.

(27) Somenschien, R. R.: *Physiology of the Central Circulation Blood Vessels and Lymphatics,* Abramson, E. I., ed. (New York: Academic Press, 1962), pp. 241–245.

10

Management of wounds and bites

JAMES H. COSGRIFF, JR.
DIANN ANDERSON

A wound is one of the most common reasons a person seeks emergency treatment, and in many instances, the emergency nurse is required to render primary or even total care. This is especially true in smaller emergency departments and in school and industrial health service settings.

Wounds may be classified in 4 ways:

(1) *Etiology:* surgical, accidental, self-inflicted.
(2) *Appearance:* incised, crushing, abraded.
(3) *Mechanism of injury:* blunt, penetrating, perforating.
(4) *Presence of gross contamination:* clean, dirty, infected.

The site of injury and the nature of the incident are important to total patient assessment. They may give clues to more serious injury to deeper structures. Airway maintenance, control of hemorrhage and treatment of shock are the initial steps of management when indicated.

The objective of wound care is to achieve primary healing with a cosmetically acceptable scar and a minimum of disability. The methods by which this is accomplished depend on numerous factors, such as: (1) type and site of the wound; (2) degree of contamination and presence of foreign substances; (3) injury to other structures, muscles, blood vessels, nerves, tendons; and (4) general status of the patient. These factors will be considered later, as specific wound management is discussed.

PHYSIOLOGY OF WOUND HEALING

When a wound occurs, the body responds with a pouring of tissue fluid and blood cells into the area, forming a fibrin network. Fibroblasts and capillary buds penetrate this network form to bridge the defect. As the capillaries increase in number, more blood cells are brought to the area, giving the tissue a red color. This is referred to as *granulation tissue* and is present to a greater or lesser extent in every wound. As the granulation tissue matures, the fibroblasts increase in number, adding strength to the healing wound and gradually squeezing out the blood vessels, thus forming scar tissue. This process takes place in the deep portions of the wound;

as the defect is being bridged below, epithelial cells proliferate to cover the surface of the granulation tissue. Depending on the site and depth of the wound, its tensile strength is usually sufficient for sutures to be removed in 7 to 10 days; however, wound healing contin-ues for 6 to 12 months until a mature scar is formed.

For practical purposes, wound healing occurs in one of 3 ways, by first intention, by second intention or by third intention. The mechanisms of healing in first and second intention are applicable to all body tissues (skin, fat, muscle, bone, tendon, nerve). Variations in the process result from the special characteristics of each tissue.

Healing by first intention

First intention (primary closure) is the ideal method of wound healing. It occurs in most clean, incised wounds, the best example being a surgical incision. The various layers of tissue which have been opened by wounding are coapted, insuring that dead space is obliterated so that serum and hematoma collections are not likely to occur; and the skin is carefully approximated. Thus, the damaged tissues are restored to as near normal alignment as possible. In this type of healing, the least amount of granulation occurs, because the tissue defect is small, the scar is small and wound healing is most efficient. Figure 10–1 illustrates the steps of wound healing by first intention.

Healing by second intention

Second intention healing occurs in wounds involving a loss of tissue, so that the tissue layers of the wound edges cannot be accurately approximated. An example is the exit wound of a gunshot injury or an avulsion injury wound, in which skin and underlying tissue are absent. In addition, when a wound which was sutured previously (as in first intention) is complicated by hematoma or abscess formation, it is drained and usually allowed to heal by second intention.

The granulation tissue in this method of healing necessarily occurs in greater amounts, in order to bridge the tissue defect from below to the surface. As the granulations reach the surface, the epithelial cells grow in from the periphery and provide cover. The

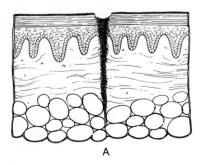

A

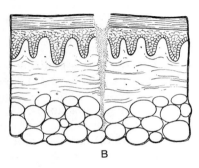

B

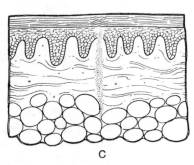

C

Figure 10–1 Wound healing by first intention. The defect produced by a wound (A) develops a minimal amount of granulation tissue (B). Healing is completed (C) as the epidermis grows over the defect. A fine line scar is produced.

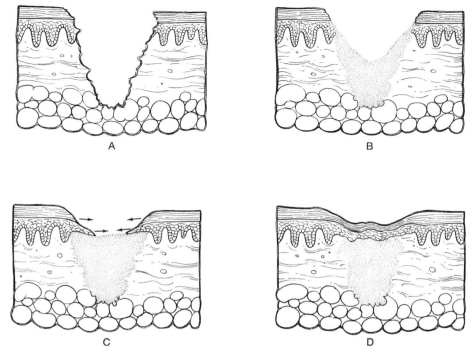

Figure 10–2 Wound healing by second intention. The defect (A), created by a wound or debridement, involves tissue loss. Granulation tissue fills the defect from below (B). As the granulation tissue develops to the surface, the epithelium (epidermis) grows across the surface from the wound edges until complete coverage is obtained (C, D). Varying degrees of scarring result.

amount of granulation tissue, which varies with the size of the defect, determines the scar size. Figure 10–2 illustrates the steps in wound healing by second intention.

Healing by third intention

Wounds allowed to heal for a period of time by secondary intention and then closed surgically to produce a lesser scar and more rapid healing are examples of healing by third intention. The most common example is a contaminated surgical incision, such as that associated with a perforated appendix. In this instance, the peritoneal and muscle layers are closed, but the subcutaneous fat and skin tissue remain open, allowing for drainage and formation of granulation tissue. These layers are then sutured 5 to 7 days later. This method is also referred to as healing by secondary suture.

SPECIFIC MANAGEMENT OF SURFACE WOUNDS

Wound history is very important to determining the mechanism of injury. For example, an accidental, incised wound caused by a clean kitchen knife is vastly different from a laceration made by a farm implement; a human bite is usually more serious than a dog bite. A lapse in time between wounding and treatment of more than 6 to 8 hours usually contraindicates primary closure (healing by first intention).

Physical assessment should include a rapid, complete evaluation of the patient. Once the patient's general status has been evaluated and found to be stable, attention should be directed to the wound site. However, it may be seen immediately that a major wound of an extremity with involvement of a large artery and/or vein is leading to severe blood loss and hypovolemic shock or that lesser injuries, especially of vascular areas visible to the patient, such as a hand or fingertip, are causing an apprehensive patient to faint due to neurogenic shock. Such acute situations must be resolved before time is taken for a complete physical assessment.

Complete assessment includes not only the characteristics of the wound itself, but also its effect on the function of the part involved if an extremity. Injuries involving the distal portions of a limb may damage tendons and nerves; therefore, active motion of fingers and wrist or toes and ankle should be tested and compared with the opposite, noninjured limb. Sensory perception should be evaluated to determine any nerve damage. Findings consistent with tendon, nerve or major vascular damage indicate a complicated injury which should be properly treated in the operating room. But control of hemorrhage, stabilization of the patient and primary wound care should be accomplished prior to transport of the patient to the surgical suite.

The injured part should be immersed in and thoroughly cleansed with a hexachlorophene soap (pHisoHex), tincture of green soap or similar antiseptic preparation (Betadine). The irrigating solution should be warm, avoiding extremes of temperature. Excess hair about the wound site should be shaved, except in the case of the eyebrow, which should *never* be removed, since it may not regenerate. After such cleansing preparation, the area is dried with a sterile towel, and an anesthetic solution and instruments are readied for exploration and closure of the wound.

Dealing with anxiety

Anticipation of pain during wound care arouses a degree of fear in any patient. Explanation of when and what kind of pain the patient can expect during the procedure does much to allay his fear and, at the same time, increase his confidence in those attending him. Even young children can become much more cooperative when approached in this honest, forthright manner. The presence of a reassuring person, whether it be the nurse, attendant or a parent or relative who has also been prepared for the procedure, is immeasurable in allaying the patient's anxiety.

In some patients, with an unstable emotional or physical status or of a young age, some sedation may be needed. A short-acting barbiturate, given early in the treatment period, may relax the patient sufficiently so that wound care, including suturing, can be accomplished with minimal trauma. For children, secobarbital sodium, one milligram per pound of body weight, may be given intramuscularly. Some emergency departments specify the use of a combination of drugs in a formula similarly based on patient weight. Adults may require diazepam or a similar preparation.

For children who need restraining, a Papoose Board is useful, especially in treating facial injuries which require time-consuming, meticulous care. Figure 10–3 displays the Papoose Board and degrees of restraint with its use. Except for the very young, an explanation of the strange and foreign apparatus and why it is needed is important in allaying the child's fear. When feasible, permitting the child to handle an unfamiliar object will help him become more cooperative when the object is used.

Local anesthesia

A variety of local anesthetic agents is available. Those most frequently used are lidocaine hydrochloride and procaine hydrochloride. The solutions found in most emergency facilities vary from 0.5 percent to 2.0 percent solutions; i.e., they contain from 5 to 20 mg. per cc. of anesthetic. In general, the weakest effective solution should be used, to minimize the incidence of reactions, especially when a large volume is needed.

The emergency nurse should be familiar with the pharmacologic effects of these drugs: the minimum lethal dose (MLD 50), diffusibility and duration of action. Lidocaine hydrochloride has a wider diffusibility and lower

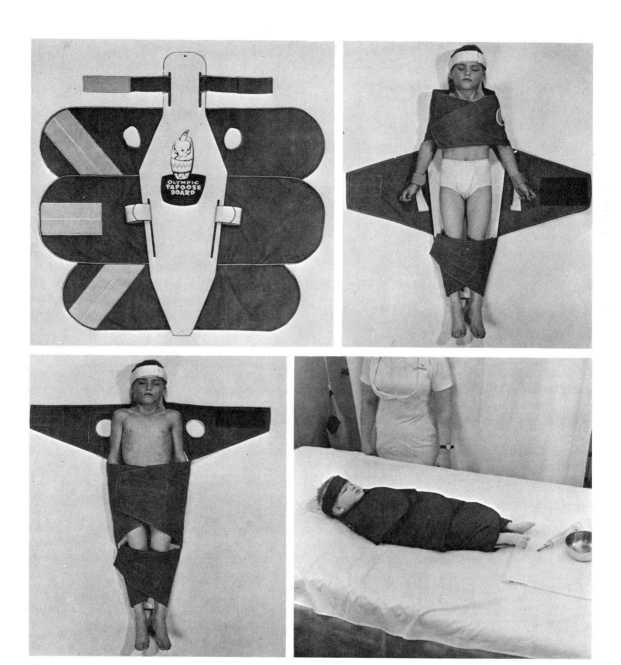

Figure 10–3 Papoose Board and various applications. Various sizes are available, depending on patient size and needs. The flaps can be used all together or in any combination, depending on the body area injured and in need of work.

Source: All photos courtesy of Olympic Surgical Co., Inc., Seattle, Washington.

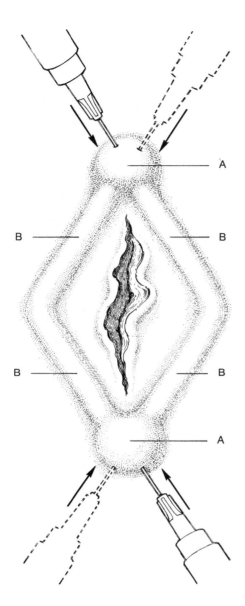

sensitivity rate than procaine hydrochloride, but is somewhat delayed in onset of action. These solutions are also available with epinephrine added, which causes local vasoconstriction, thus lessening blood loss and prolonging duration of anesthetic action by delaying its absorption. Solutions containing epinephrine are thus especially useful in vascular areas, such as the face and scalp. But because of this vasoconstrictive action, caution is advised in using such solutions with the elderly, with hypertensives, for wounds that are severely contused or for wounds located on the digits, as they are supplied by end arteries.

After preparing the skin with a topical antiseptic solution, a short, small-bore needle (25- or 26-gauge) should be used to raise a skin wheal in normal tissue at each end of the wound or in each quadrant of the wound area. Then anesthesia is broadened by injecting subcutaneously through each wheal toward the adjacent one, using a longer, larger needle (22-gauge). (See Figure 10–4.) Thus, the entire field of injury is surrounded by the anesthetic agent, and the area within the field is insensitive to pain.

Injection into the dermis (when raising the wheal) causes a painful, burning sensation. Though one is tempted to inject the agent into the open wound edges because it is less painful, this is poor technique, since it is possible to force contaminated material into adjacent, noninjured tissue. In certain areas, such as the face and fingers, specific nerves are infiltrated rather than using the technique of regional infiltration described above.

Wound exploration and closure

Once anesthesia is effected, the wound should be carefully and thoroughly explored, using instruments which produce a minimum of trauma to the already damaged tissues. Adson-type toothed forceps and/or skin hooks are ideal for this. Figure 10–5 displays and itemizes basic instruments needed for exploration and closure. Grossly visible foreign bodies and devitalized tissue should be removed by sharp dissection using scissors

Figure 10–4 Technique of field block anesthesia. Using a small-bore needle (25- or 26-gauge), an intradermal wheal is raised at either end of the wound, in normal skin (A). A longer, larger needle (22-gauge) is placed on the syringe and passed through each wheal into the subcutaneous fat. The anesthetic solution is injected slowly into the subcutaneous tissue lateral to the wound, until the site of injury is completely surrounded (B). The entire field within the perimeters of the injection is thus anesthetized. This method is applicable for repair of wounds or excision of lesions of the skin or subcutaneous tissue.

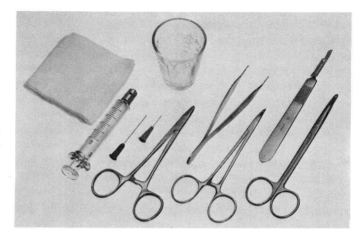

Figure 10–5 Basic instruments needed for repair of lacerations. Shown above are: medicine glass, syringe (Luer-lok), needles (22- and 25-gauge), needle holder, toothed Adson forceps, curved hemostat, scalpel handle (#3) with #15 blade, small dissecting scissors. A sufficient number of gauze sponges and towels should be included.

or a scalpel blade. (See Figure 10–6.) Hemostasis may be accomplished by pressure or by clamping and tying bleeding points. The interior of the wound is then irrigated with sterile saline and prepared for closure when possible.

Closure should be done in layers (muscle, fascia, fat, skin) to obliterate dead space and thus prevent collections of serum (seroma) or blood (hematoma) which may interfere with wound healing (see Figure 10–7). The skin margins should be sharply freshened and carefully coapted to provide proper alignment and insure a minimum of scarring.

The selection of suture material is a matter of individual choice. There is a large variety of

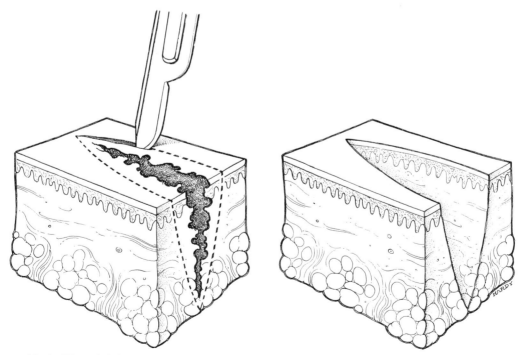

Figure 10–6 Wound debridement. Jagged tissue edges are excised to provide clean, sharp tissue margins before closure by suture.

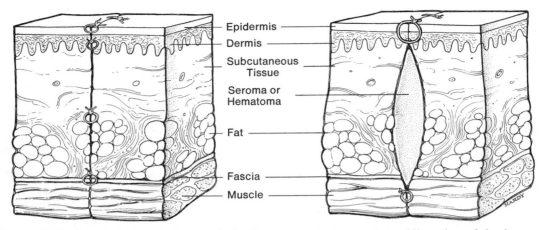

Figure 10-7 Layered wound closure. Left: Correct method; complete obliteration of dead spaces. Right: Incorrect method; deeper layer not sutured, with formation of seroma or hematoma to fill the dead space.

absorbable and nonabsorbable types in most emergency facilities. In general, absorbable sutures are used to approximate the deeper layers of wounds and nonabsorbable sutures for the skin. The choice of absorbable suture will depend on the strength necessary to approximate the tissue and maintain the integrity of the suture line. Chromicized catgut is stronger and takes a longer period to be absorbed by the body than plain catgut; however, it is more irritating to the tissues and produces a greater inflammatory response. Synthetic absorbable suture (polyglycolic acid suture) is available and may be preferred.

Nonabsorbable sutures in common use for skin closure include silk and a variety of synthetic materials (Mersilene, Prolene, Dermalon, Ethiflex). The smallest suture and finest needle adequate to accomplish the task should be used, to promote good healing while provoking a minimum tissue response.

Many superficial wounds, after cleansing and careful evaluation, may be closed by application of sterile butterfly dressings. This is especially true for lacerations of the incised type, with sharp, straight edges.

Grafts

In more complicated wounds involving extensive damage or loss of tissue or when proper debridement causes a defect and edges cannot be approximated, healing by first intention may not be possible. If the resulting defect is small and in an unexposed area such as the trunk, arm or legs, healing may be permitted to proceed by second intention. If the injury involves the face, neck or hands, immediate coverage by skin graft is mandatory.

For the face and neck, sliding or rotational pedicle flaps may be used; while on the hand, immediate split-thickness grafts are usually applied. These procedures are not commonly carried out in the emergency department; management in the emergency setting consists of cleansing, application of a sterile dressing and preparation of the patient for transfer to the operating suite.

Fingertip amputation (loss of the full-thickness skin) is a common and potentially disabling injury, and grafts usually can be applied in the emergency department. Such grafts are of the full-thickness type, containing sensory nerve endings, thus allowing for some sensory perception when fully healed. Grafts should *not* be taken from hair-bearing areas, since the hair follicles will continue to function in the transplanted skin. The preferable site of such donor grafts is the inner aspect of the arm or forearm.

Dressings

Wound care is not complete until a proper dressing has been applied. The dressing should protect the wound from external contamination, keep tension on the suture line to a minimum and immobilize the part. Dressings should be applied firmly but should not be constrictive. When wrapping an extremity in a circumferential manner, caution must be used not to apply the dressing too tightly, or it may interfere with venous return and cause distal swelling. Nonadherent pads (Telfa) may be used directly on the wound to lessen discomfort at the time of dressing change. However, such dressings absorb very poorly, and their use when drainage is expected is questionable.

Joints should be wrapped in a slightly flexed position, using a "figure 8" technique (see Figure 10–8). Dressing the scalp or face may be difficult. At times, meticulous wound closure may negate the need for dressings in those areas. In other cases, a plastic aerosol dressing, such as vibesate (Aeroplast), or a collodion applied with a sterile applicator is sufficient.

Tissues which are elastic and swell readily (e.g., the eyelid) should be protected with a bulky pressure dressing, such as folded or fluffed gauze pads or sterile mechanic's waste, to apply gentle but firm, diffused pressure. Conforming gauze (such as Kerlix or Kling) is applied as an outer dressing. In the case of the eyelid, the gauze should be wrapped around the head, like a turban. To prevent slippage off the head, the outer dressing must cover the entire proximal ear, extending below the lobe. The pressure of such a dressing on the cartilage in the pinna of the ear may be painful, but placing a folded gauze pad behind the pinna will relieve such discomfort.

When dressing a wound of a hair-bearing region (arm, trunk, leg), especially when adhesive tape is to be used, the skin should be clean-shaven to provide for better adherence of the tape to the skin surface and to minimize pain at the time of tape removal for dressing change. The very young and elderly

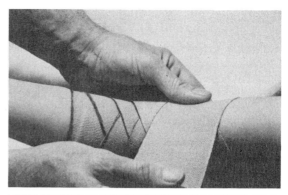
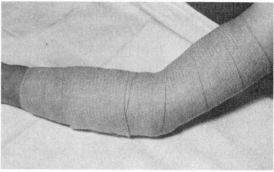

Figure 10–8 Wrapping a joint. Top: This method of wrapping a joint may be used for the larger joints (elbow, wrist, knee, ankle). (Edge of Ace bandage was colored to indicate method of overlapping.) Bottom: Joint should be in position of moderate flexion for application of circumferential dressing.

have delicate skin which may be sensitive to ordinary adhesive tape. Nonallergenic tape or ordinary scotch tape may be used very effectively in such patients, as well as in those with a known allergy to adhesive.

When applying tape, it should be placed smoothly on the skin, free of wrinkles. In taping a movable area, such as the skin of the breast or flank, extreme caution must be taken to prevent pulling or traction of the skin by the tape. Painful blebs, equivalent to a second-degree burn, may result and heal with a permanent unsightly scar. When, however, such traction may be necessary, a thin layer of tincture of benzoin, applied to the skin and allowed to dry prior to applying the tape, will frequently provide a protective, adhering surface and prevent this complication.

In injuries of the wrist, hand and/or fingers, careful attention to dressings is important. If the wound requires that the entire hand be enclosed, it should be placed in the "position of function," that is, the wrist in mid-extension and the thumb and fingers in mid-flexion (see Figure 10–9). A form-fitting aluminum splint may be used to maintain this position. Fluffed gauze pads should be placed in the interdigital spaces of the fingers. When an occlusive dressing is applied to a foot, cotton placed between the toes will absorb perspiration and prevent maceration of the skin. When a wound is localized to a finger and immobilization is required, a padded aluminum splint, available in variable widths, may be bent in the desired position and applied. It is usually more comfortable for the patient if at least one adjacent finger is included in the dressing. Thus, if the small finger is lacerated, the ring finger might also be immobilized in the dressing. This prevents unnecessary motion of the injured finger and thus lessens pain. Tubular gauze dressings are available in a variety of sizes and are extremely useful in dressing digits. Adequate lengths are cut to secure the tube dressing about the wrist, to prevent slipping.

Swelling and throbbing pain are not uncommon, especially when the injury involves an extremity. It may occur after the anesthesia has worn off, within the first few hours or days

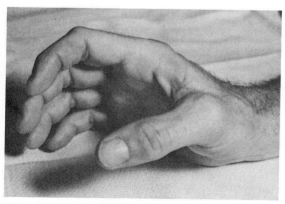

Figure 10–9 "Position of function" of hand. This position is used for occlusive dressings.

after injury and repair. It is best to advise the patient of this possibility and that elevation of the part will usually alleviate the symptoms. When the injury involves an area above the waist, the arm affected or proximal to the injury may be placed in a sling prior to discharge from the emergency department; the immobilization will decrease pain. The patient should further be advised that in the event of any undue pain, redness, swelling, paresthesia or drainage from the wound, he should return, promptly, for evaluation.

Barring unforeseen complications, the dressing need not be disturbed for 5 to 7 days, depending on the site and nature of the injury. Skin sutures are removed in 7 to 10 days as determined by the location and severity of the injury.

TYPES OF WOUNDS

Abrasions

Abrasions (brush burns) are painful wounds involving the epidermis and occasionally the upper layers of the dermis. Because of the nature of the injury (usually a sliding fall), imbedded foreign bodies may be present.

Extreme patience must be taken to remove all imbedded foreign material. This can frequently be done without anesthesia in small abrasions, using a sterile needle point, a scalpel with a number 11 knife blade or a fast-action water spurting device, such as the Water Pik. In more extensive injuries, local or general anesthesia will be necessary, and a surgical hand brush will be required to clean out the foreign bodies. If they are not completely removed, tattooing may occur.

Puncture wounds

The puncture wound is a form of penetrating wound, in which a sharp, narrow, pointed object, such as a nail, is forced through the skin. Since the surface seals readily, the wound rarely bleeds enough to wash out the pathogens which may have been introduced.

The wound should be *thoroughly* cleansed. A history of the type of injury is important to determining further management. If the object which caused the injury was a rusty nail or similar object, complete excision of the puncture tract should be done and the wound allowed to heal by second intention. Tetanus prophylaxis should be provided as recommended.

Imbedded foreign bodies

Imbedded objects are often a source of consternation in that the patient may not be certain that an object is in the tissue or where. A history of the direction of entry may be helpful in locating the foreign body when it is not easily palpable. When the object is metal or glass with a high lead content, x-rays of the area, with radio-opaque markers placed on the skin at the wound site, are very helpful in localizing the foreign material.

Foreign bodies which lie close to or protrude from the skin in the subcutaneous tissue may be removed by careful traction, without anesthesia. If the object is deeper in the subcutaneous tissue or difficult to localize by palpation, careful thought must be given to removing it. A needle, in particular, may be difficult to find in the deeper tissues. One must calculate the chances of recovering the object and compare them to the amount of dissection and opening of tissue planes needed to locate it. If the odds are that further damage may be done by surgical intervention, a wait-and-see approach is advisable: the patient is told to wait for signs of further localization or continued symptoms.

When a foreign body is recovered, it should be affixed to the patient's record with transparent tape to serve as a permanent part of the chart. The recommended guidelines for tetanus prophylaxis must be followed. In the absence of patient sensitivity, nitrofurazone (Furacin) gauze with an outer compression dressing may be applied to the wound and left undisturbed for 5 to 7 days.

Splinters

Wood splinters in the skin or beneath a fingernail require careful removal technique.

Special pointed "splinter" forceps may be necessary to remove the foreign body. Gentle pressure on surrounding skin while trying to extract the splinter may assist in the removal.

When the splinter is lodged beneath the fingernail, it may be easily removed by gentle traction with splinter forceps. When the trailing end of the splinter does not extend beyond the end of the nail bed, it can sometimes be reached by carefully inserting the forceps in the track formed by the foreign body. At other times, the nail may have to be split longitudinally with a sharp scissors and a narrow V-shaped segment excised to remove the splinter. Local anesthesia may be required in the more complicated situations.

Fish hooks

Wounds from imbedded fish hooks occur most commonly on the extremities, particularly the digits, which can be snared in the process of extracting the hook from a fish. If the barbed end is imbedded in the deeper tissue, an incision should be made over the tip of the barb and the tip forced through. The shaft of the hook should then be cut close to the skin with a wire cutter and the remaining hook pulled, barbed end first, through the incision. (See Figure 10–10.) When both ends of the hook are protruding from the skin, the same technique should be utilized, preferably cutting off the barbed end.

TETANUS PROPHYLAXIS

Tetanus is a grave complication of any injury and can occur following seemingly minor wounds. It is caused by the *Clostridium tetani,* an anaerobic spore-forming organism which thrives in devitalized tissue and produces a neurotoxin. Even today, this disease, once established, has a 50 percent mortality rate. The best treatment is prevention. Strict adherence to the proper management of wounds is the best prophylaxis available. Thorough cleansing and complete surgical debridement of devitalized tissue are most effective in preventing tetanus.

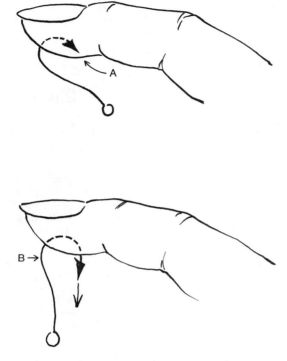

Figure 10–10 Ideal method of removing an imbedded fish hook. After the part is anesthetized, the barbed point of the hook is pushed through a small incision in the skin (A). A wire cutter is used to cut the shaft of the hook (B). The barbed end may then be pulled through the subcutaneous tissue and removed.

In addition to proper surgical technique, biological preparations are available to provide immunity against this organism. The 2 in most common usage today are tetanus toxoid, which provides active immunity, and human immune globulin, which produces passive immunity. Until the 1950s, tetanus antitoxin was the biological agent used almost exclusively for prophylaxis in civilian hospitals. It is prepared from the serum of horses or cows and produces an extremely high rate of sensitivity reactions in humans. Tetanus toxoid was developed and came into wide usage and effectiveness during World War II in the U.S. armed forces. Only 12 cases of tetanus occurred among 2,500,000 wounded American servicemen. And of these 12, 8 had an incomplete tetanus inoculation series.

The tetanus toxoid series consists of an initial intramuscular or subcutaneous dose of 0.5 cc. and booster doses 0.5 cc. one month and 12 months later. In children, it is frequently given in conjunction with diphtheria and pertussis vaccines (DPT). For young adults, it may be administered with diphtheria vaccine (DT) or alone. Once the basic immunization has been established, subsequent booster shots are required only at 10-year intervals in the absence of wounding. A booster dose may be given at the time of injury but not within 5 years of a prior injection, except under certain conditions.

In grossly contaminated wounds where the risk of tetanus is significant or in the absence of prior immunization, 250 units of tetanus immune globulin should be given intramuscularly in addition to 0.5 cc. of toxoid, with the restriction noted previously. The globulin provides an immediate protective antibody titer, until the toxoid can produce a recall of antibodies to a protective level. Antibiotics may be used in special circumstances. The recommendations of the Committee on Trauma of The American College of Surgeons are summarized in Figure 10–11.

While reactions to the globulin are rare, incidence of reactions to the toxoid is increasing. Generally, they take the form of local erythema and induration at the injection site, frequently accompanied by a febrile response as high as 105° F. Local applications of cold or ice packs, combined with analgesics and antipyretics, provide symptomatic relief.

Each patient receiving tetanus prophylaxis should be given a wallet-sized immunization card prior to discharge from the emergency department, as a record of his immune status. Figure 10–12 depicts such a record.

BITES

Bites are among the most common injuries of humans, by all kinds of insects, reptiles and animals, including humans. Bites represent a type of abraded or penetrating wound, which may be complicated by infection from the bacterial flora of the attacker.

Specific measures for patients with wounds

I. Previously immunized individuals

A. When the patient has been actively immunized within the past ten[2] years: 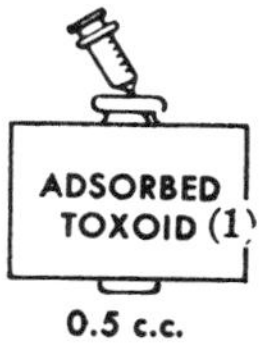
1. To the great majority, give 0.5 cc of adsorbed tetanus toxoid[1] as a booster unless it is certain that the patient has received a booster within the previous five years.
2. To those with severe, neglected, or old (more than 24 hours) tetanus-prone wounds, give 0.5 cc of adsorbed tetanus toxoid[1] unless it is certain that the patient has received a booster within the previous year.

B. When the patient has been actively immunized more than ten[2] years previously: 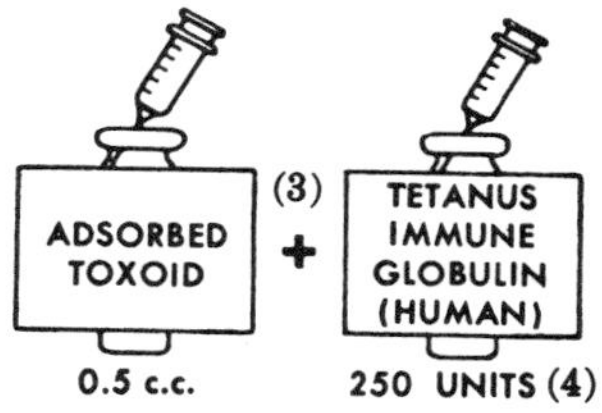
1. To the great majority, give 0.5 cc of adsorbed tetanus toxoid[1].
2. To those with severe, neglected, or old (more than 24 hours) tetanus-prone wounds:
   a) Give 0.5 cc of adsorbed tetanus toxoid[1] [3],
   b) Give 250 units[4] of tetanus immune globulin (human)[3],
   c) Consider providing oxytetracycline or penicillin.

II. Individuals NOT previously immunized

A. With clean minor wounds in which tetanus is most unlikely, give 0.5 cc of adsorbed tetanus toxoid[1] (initial immunizing dose).

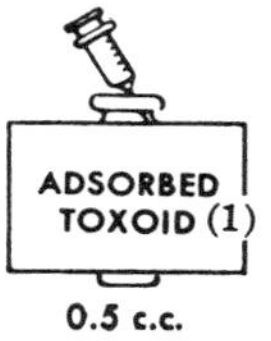

B. With all other wounds:
1. Give 0.5 cc of adsorbed tetanus toxoid[1] (initial immunizing dose)[3], 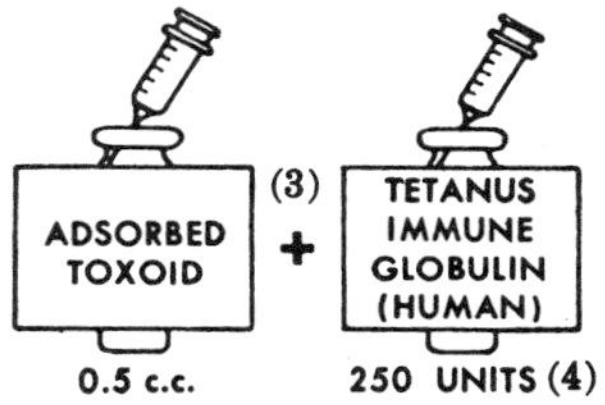
2. Give 250 units[4] of tetanus immune globulin (human)[3],
3. Consider providing oxytetracycline or penicillin.

NOTE: With different preparations of toxoid, the volume of a single booster dose should be modified as stated on the package label.

---

(1) The Public Health Service Advisory Committee on Immunization Practices in 1972 recommended DTP (diphtheria and tetanus toxoids combined with pertussis vaccine) for basic immunization in infants and children from two months through the sixth year of age, and Td (combined tetanus and diphtheria toxoids: adult type) for basic immunization of those over six years of age. For the latter group, Td toxoid was recommended for routine or wound boosters; but, if there is any reason to suspect hypersensitivity to the diphtheria component, tetanus toxoid (T) should be substituted for Td.
(*Morbidity and Mortality Weekly Report, Vol. 21, No. 25, National Communicable Disease Center*)

(2) Some authorities advise six rather than 10 years, particularly for patients with severe, neglected, or old (more than 24 hours) tetanus-prone wounds.

(3) Use different syringes, needles, and sites of injection.

(4) In severe, neglected, or old (more than 24 hours) tetanus-prone wounds, 500 units of tetanus immune globulin (human) are advisable.

PRECAUTIONS regarding passive immunization with tetanus antitoxin (equine):

If the patient is not sensitive to tetanus antitoxin (equine), and if the decision is made to administer it for passive immunization, give at least 3000 units.

Do not administer tetanus antitoxin (equine) except when tetanus immune globulin (human) is not available within 24 hours, and only if the possibility of tetanus outweighs the danger of reaction to heterologous tetanus antitoxin.

Before using tetanus antitoxin (equine), question the patient for a history of allergy and test for sensitivity. If the patient is sensitive to tetanus antitoxin (equine), do not use it, as the danger of anaphylaxis probably outweighs the danger of tetanus; rely on penicillin or oxytetracycline. Do not attempt desensitization, as it is not worthwhile.

Figure 10–11 Tetanus table. This table outlines appropriate doses for different situations.
Source: Reprinted from the *Bulletin of the American College of Surgeons,* December, 1972, from the Committee on Trauma of the American College of Surgeons.

IMMUNIZATION and HEALTH RECORD

Name ______ Phone ______

Address ______

Birth Date ______ Blood Type ______

Family Doctor ______ Phone ______

Notify in an Emergency ______ Phone ______

Served in U. S. Armed Forces from ______ to ______

TETANUS TOXOID IMMUNIZATION DATES			
Initial Series			
Booster Shots			

CARRY THIS CARD IN YOUR WALLET

I AM ALLERGIC TO: Horse Serum ☐ Penicillin ☐

Other ______

I HAVE: Heart Disease ☐ Diabetes ☐ Epilepsy ☐

Other ______

MEDICINES TAKEN REGULARLY: Anticoagulants ☐

Insulin ☐ Other ______

ADDITIONAL MEDICAL INFO: ______

N. Y. STATE HEALTH DEPARTMENT

Figure 10–12 Immunization card. Front and back sides are shown.

Human bites

Of all bites, that of the human is one of the most serious. It may be considered in several categories: (1) the attacker actually sinks his teeth into the victim's skin, causing a perforating wound or loss of skin; (2) an individual strikes his fist against another's teeth and incurs a laceration of the knuckles; and (3) the individual bites himself, as in the tongue lacerations occurring during an epileptic seizure.

The introduction of bacteria-laden saliva into these wounds, some with crushed or contused tissue, may have serious consequences. Because of the multiplicity of organisms present in the human mouth, these infections are mostly of the mixed type and may be unusually severe. This constitutes the main complication of human bites.

Careful assessment for possible injury to deep structures by evaluating sensory and motor function is most important. In knuckle wounds, the extensor tendon may be divided. The wound can be carefully spread with skin hooks or the patient asked to make a fist and a careful examination made in that position. It is recommended that a culture of the wound be taken and be followed by thorough cleansing and debridement of contused or devitalized tissue. Primary closure is usually not recommended. Healing by secondary intention is preferable until evidence of infection is absent; then, secondary suture of tendons or nerves may be done. Adequate doses of a broad-spectrum antibiotic should be started immediately.

Self-inflicted bites of the tongue may be deep and are prone to bleed profusely. When the injury is deep, suturing is usually required. The tongue is very sensitive to injection, so use of a topical anesthetic agent, such as tetracaine hydrochloride, prior to infiltration is helpful. After closure, the patient should be placed on antiseptic mouthwashes and a liquid or soft diet, as tolerated, until healing occurs.

Animal bites

A large number of animal bites are recorded annually. When the bite has been inflicted by a domestic animal previously immunized for rabies, the wound can be treated in the usual manner with cleansing and debridement. All devitalized tissue should be excised and the wound allowed to heal by secondary intention. In bites involving exposed areas, such as the face, head, neck and hands, serious consideration must be given to primary suture. Closure of these wounds demands meticulous cleansing and debridement.

The use of prophylactic antibiotics will depend on the severity and location of the injury and are not required routinely. Tetanus immunization should be given according to recommendations outlined previously.

Rabies

When the bite was made by an animal that may have rabies, special precautions must be taken to avoid this deadly disease in the victim. Children under 12 years of age seem more susceptible to the disease than older children or adults. The incidence of this disease in humans has declined over the years, with rabies vaccination of domestic animals. The disease in wildlife, however, especially in skunks, foxes and bats, has become increasingly prominent and now constitutes the most important source of rabies infection in both domestic animals and humans today.

History is of particular importance in determining if the victim was bitten by a rabid animal and if anti-rabies treatment is needed. Attention should be given to the following considerations:

(1) *Species of the biting animal:* Carnivorous animals and bats are more infective than other animals.
(2) *Circumstances of the biting incident:* An unprovoked attack is more likely to occur from a rabid animal.
(3) *Type of exposure:* Since the disease is transmitted by infectious saliva through a break in the skin, the nature of the wounding is important.
(4) *Vaccination status of the biting animal:* A properly immunized animal has a minimal chance of developing and thus spreading the disease.
(5) *Presence of rabies in the region:* Local health officials can provide data regarding the prevalence of the disease and of rabid animals in the locale.

In most localities, animal bites should be reported to police agencies. The offending animal, if domestic or able to be trapped, is placed under surveillance until the 10 to 14 day incubation period for rabies has passed. If the animal is not identified or located or if it is found to be rabid, anti-rabies treatment is necessary.

Wound management is the same as for nonrabid animal bites. Particular attention must be given to cleansing and debridement. Closure of these wounds is *not* advisable, because of the high incidence of secondary infection.

Rabies prophylaxis

Although the incidence of rabies disease in humans is extremely low, many thousands receive rabies prophylaxis annually in the U.S. The decision of when vaccination is necessary must be based on careful evaluation of the patient and his history.

When indicated, rabies prophylaxis is effected by use of duck embryo vaccine given subcutaneously for 14 to 21 consecutive days, depending on the severity of exposure. A variation of this routine is to give 2 daily doses of the vaccine for a 7 to 14 day period, completing the last week of prescribed treatment with single doses. A single booster injection is given 10 to 20 days following the completion of the daily injection routine. Since the vaccine causes a regional lymphadenitis, it is best given in the anterior abdominal wall, lower back or lateral aspect of the thighs, varying the site each day.

In severe exposures, anti-rabies serum is injected around the bite site and is also given intramuscularly for immediate passive immunization. This serum is of equine origin and must be given with the usual precautions. Recently, the development of a rabies vaccine derived from human sera has been developed and is being used in controlled studies. This vaccine is said to be more potent, requiring a total of only 3 injections and is associated with a lower incidence of patient sensitivity.

Bites of snakes, insects and marine animals

Snakebites

Although snakebite is not considered a common injury, several thousand Americans are bitten each year. Of those so injured, 10 to 20 people die. There are 2 principal groups of poisonous snakes native to the United States. These are the family *Crotalidae* (rattlesnake, cotton-mouth and water moccasin, copperhead) and the family *Elapidae* (coral). Coral snakes rarely bite man, accounting for only one to 2 percent of venomous snake bites. By contrast, pit vipers (family *Crotal-*

idae) strike promiscuously, often without provocation.

Outdoorsmen and unsuspecting children are most likely to be bitten by snakes. In areas where bites are common, the populace is usually knowledgeable of the immediate management of the injury and carries snakebite kits. This is particularly important, since the injury often occurs in a remote area, and several hours may elapse before the patient is seen in an emergency facility.

Upon arrival of a bite victim, the nurse should make a rapid assessment of the patient and the wound site. The presence of fang marks, bleeding, progressive swelling and discoloration are local signs indicative of snakebite. Generally, a bite by a poisonous snake leaves 2 large puncture wounds where the fangs enter the skin, and in the case of pit viper bites, is very painful.

Reactions to a pit viper bite will occur within the first 15 to 30 minutes. If there is no reaction within 30 to 60 minutes, envenomation has most likely not occurred. Systemic responses, occurring in addition to the local signs, include tingling around the mouth, face and scalp and painful, enlarged lymph nodes. More advanced signs include nausea, vomiting, ecchymosis and evidence of shock. The venom consists of proteolytic and other enzymes causing local destruction of tissues.

In coral snake envenomation, definitive symptoms may not occur for as much as 18 hours following the bite. Initial signs usually include moderate discoloration and swelling, paresthesia and muscle twitching around the bite and *transitory* pain. Systemic responses, such as blurred vision, ptosis, slurred speech, dyspnea, nausea and increased salivation, occasionally occur.

First aid for venomous bites

Initial emergency measures entail localizing and/or removing as much of the toxic agent as possible and keeping it from entering the systemic circulation. Administration of antivenin, if available, treatment of symptomatic responses and care of the wound are further measures which may be accomplished at an emergency facility or near the location of injury, provided the materials are available.

Initiating first aid measures at the earliest moment is crucial. The victim should be at rest with the affected part immobile. A tourniquet is applied both proximal and distal to the bitten area and should be tight enough to impede subcutaneous venous and lymphatic circulation, but not so tight as to affect arterial circulation. Palpation of a pulse distal to the tourniquets is indicative of unimpaired arterial circulation. The tourniquet should not be loosened, lest it cause shock from the sudden release of toxic factors into the blood stream. Application of cold to the area may aid in controlling pain and slowing blood circulation to and from the part, but should not be unduly prolonged to already hypoxic tissues. Some feel cryotherapy is contraindicated.

The efficacy of incision and suction to remove venom has been questioned. If properly performed within the first 30 minutes, it may be of some value. However, if the victim can reach a treatment facility promptly, such surgical intervention is best left to the physician or trained personnel. If incisions are made, they should extend longitudinally through each fang mark and be approximately 1/4 inch deep. Suction is applied and continued for an hour or until the patient arrives at the medical facility.

Emergency department treatment

The cardinal signs of snakebite are fang marks, swelling, pain, ecchymosis and paresthesia in and around the area of envenomization. Envenomization may cause diminished prothrombin activity and lowered serum fibrinogen levels. Therefore, baseline clotting studies should be done, including prothrombin time, partial thromboplastin time, platelet count and serum fibrinogen level. A peripheral blood smear may show "burring" of red cells, which is helpful in making the diagnosis.

Should any indication of bleeding develop, close observation of the clotting mechanism is warranted. Definitive treatment of the site of injury is surgical removal of the entire ecchymotic area, including full thickness of the subcutaneous tissue. Because of the hypoesthesia or anesthesia, this may be performed without benefit of local infiltration anesthesia.

Antivenin for bites of the pit viper (Polyvalent Crotalidae) and the coral snake (North American Coral Snake Antivenin) is available. (See Figure 10–13.) Since it is prepared from horse serum, testing for hypersensitivity is essential before administering the therapeutic dose. The antivenin can be administered intramuscularly or intravenously, as indicated. (It is usually reserved for patients with systemic reactions.) Further chemotherapy, in terms of analgesics, antibiotics and tetanus prophylaxis, may also be necessary.

The patient should be kept at complete rest, sedated as needed and admitted for further observation and managment.

Black widow spider

Of the biting spiders, the black widow (*Lactrodectus Mactans*) is the most common. It is usually found in wood and brush piles, barns and garages. It has a coal-black body and is about 1½ inches long. The mature female has a red or orange hourglass marking on its belly; the immature female has three similarly colored spots on its back.

Frequently, the patient will be unaware of the bite but may complain of intense pain at the bite site. This area may become pale or congested. The victim remains comfortable until abdominal cramps occur 15 to 30 minutes later. Abdominal muscular rigidity, becoming boardlike, is associated with the cramps and may be confused with an acute abdominal episode. The spider venom is neurotoxic and causes an ascending motor paralysis and destruction of peripheral nerve endings leading to weakness, tremor and severe pain in the extremities. Later, the victim may develop bradycardia, feeble pulse, and difficulty in breathing and speech. Stupor, delirium and confusion are common, especially in children.

Accurate assessment and prompt institution of supportive therapy is important in reversing the effects of the black widow bite. In addition to the first aid measures discussed under snakebite, further management consists of administration of specific antivenin, relieving muscle spasms and pain and providing emotional support to the patient and family.

Antivenin for the treatment of black widow spider bite is prepared from horse serum and must be given with the usual precautions. To reduce muscle spasms and pain, intravenous calcium gluconate is indicated. Curare, a muscle relaxant, may be useful. Morphine or sodium phenobarbital is needed at times to control excruciating pain. Because of the

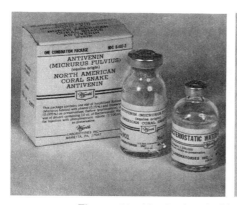
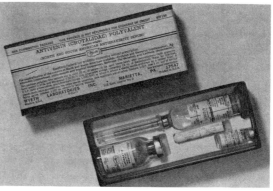

Figure 10–13 Antivenin kits for coral snake and crotalidae.
Source: Photos courtesy of Wyeth Laboratories, Philadelphia, Pa.

severity of the victim's response to the spider venom, he is usually admitted for further observation and supportive care.

Brown house spider

The brown spider (*Loxosceles Reclusa*), also known as the brown recluse, is about 2½ inches long and lives in the mid-western and mid-southern states. Its habitat is clothes closets and other dark locations in and around the house. The bite produces a necrotoxin; therefore, the bitten area may develop an ischemic center and ulcerate.[15] Severe local pain, restlessness and fever may be associated symptoms.

No antivenin is available. However, if the patient seeks treatment within 24 hours, the prognosis is good. Prompt administration of antihistamines and corticotropin will limit the effects of the necrotoxin to the bitten area and reduce systemic reactions. Further management consists of pain control and local wound care. Wide ulceration can result, and in some anatomical areas, such as the pretibial region, delayed healing occurs and secondary grafting may be required.

Scorpion stings

Scorpions are nocturnal arachnids, lying hidden during the day beneath debris of all kinds, as well as under buildings and lumber piles. Of over 300 species known, only a limited number are considered lethal to man. The poisonous scorpion, which lives mainly in the arid southwestern United States, is the *Centruroides sculpturatus.*

The scorpion's venom is present in a bulb-like enlargement at the tip of its tail. While more toxic than most snake venom, the injected quantity is minute. Thus, fatal scorpion stings are infrequent; almost all reported deaths from scorpion stings have occurred in children under 6 years of age.

Local evidence of the sting may be minimal or absent. The first symptom is mild tingling or burning at the site. This may be followed by excessive salivation, drowsiness, nausea, vomiting, mydriasis and photophobia. The poison acts on the nervous system, producing

fatality by its effect on the cardiac and respiratory centers.[11] Rapid progression of symptoms within the first 2 to 4 hours indicates a poor prognosis.[6]

Emergency measures are as outlined for snakebite. Covered ice packs may be applied for the first few hours to slow absorption. Scorpion antiserum is the specific antidote.

Stings from wasps, bees and hornets

Stings from wasps and bees are the most common injuries caused by insects. While they rarely cause severe reactions, their toxins do contain histamine and in sensitive persons can cause symptoms of anaphylaxis. Initial care consists of gentle cleansing of the wound. In the case of a bee sting, the stinger should be removed carefully, by holding the forceps flat against the skin, to avoid squeezing more toxin into the wound. Other measures include applying a baking soda paste, ammonia in water solution (10%) or calamine lotion to relieve itching. An ice pack applied to the bite site will frequently reduce local reaction.

Some persons experience systemic or severe local reactions to insect stings. If these responses occur within 20 minutes of the sting, epinephrine is given. Follow-up therapy may include antihistamines, steroids or a long-lasting epinephrine (epinephrine in oil). These persons should be prescribed an emergency treatment kit, to be carried with them whenever exposure to insects causing their sensitivity is possible.

Stings from marine animals

Bathers in tropical and subtropical oceans occasionally are stung by marine animals, the commonest being the jellyfish and Portuguese Man-of-War. They pose a particular threat when washed ashore by storms or changing ocean currents, and it is wise to avoid swimming and to wear shoes when walking on the beach at such times. Both possess tentacles which can discharge a varying quantity of toxin into a victim's skin.

The Portuguese Man-of-War has numerous

string-like tentacles, extending for many yards, and floats by means of a colorful air bladder. The victim, once in contact with a tentacle, will instantly receive many sharp stings accompanied by circular, reddened patches in the affected areas.

In contrast, the sting of the jellyfish is less likely to produce distinctive local marks. More often, pain, edema and redness will occur to the affected part. Systemic effects resulting from *extensive* stinging become apparent within an hour and include anxiety, muscle pain and cramps, dyspnea, tightness in the throat, cardiac weakness and prostration. Some sensitive victims will evidence an anaphylactic response.

Systemic symptoms' may be alleviated by the parenteral administration of a 10 percent solution of calcium gluconate, benadryl or epinephrine. Untreated systemic symptoms usually subside within a few hours or days. Topical applications of a weak alkaline solution, such as diluted household ammonia, and an analgesic ointment relieve local symptoms. The pruritis resulting from the stings may persist for weeks. Papain-containing meat tenderizers (Adolf's) sprinkled liberally on the affected area (wetted) will relieve the stinging sensation.

SUMMARY

The objective of wound care is to achieve primary healing with a cosmetically acceptable scar and a minimum of disability. Proper management of the patient with a wound thus requires assessment skills and a knowledge of wound healing. To develop a plan of treatment for a patient with a specific type of wound, consideration must be given to the etiology, site and severity of the injury and to the general condition of the patient.

The principles of wound care include complete exploration of the site of injury, adequate debridement, control of hemorrhage and primary closure, when possible or as indicated. An appropriate dressing must be applied to protect the area of injury and immobilize the part, as conditions require. At times, inge-

nuity is the key to successful treatment of wound injuries.

BIBLIOGRAPHY

(1) "A Guide to Prophylaxis Against Tetanus in Wound Management," *Bulletin of the American College of Surgeons,* 57 (1972):32.

(2) Auld, M. E., *et al.:* "Wound Healing," *Nursing '72,* 2 (1972):36.

(3) Beeson, P. B., and McDermott, W.: *Cecil-Loeb: Textbook of Medicine* (Philadelphia: W. B. Saunders Company, 1968).

(4) Derbes, V. J.; Falliers, C. J.; Fine, S. R.; Itkin, I., and Shaffer, J. H.: "Insect Stings: Emergency Therapy for Severe Reactions," *Patient Care,* 6 (1972):46.

(5) Dowling, H. G.; Minton, S. A.; Parrish, H. M., and Russell, F. E.: "Snakebite: Poisonous Until Proven Otherwise," *Patient Care,* 5 (1972):76.

(6) Driesbach, R.: *Handbook of Poisoning,* 7th ed. (Los Altos, Calif.: Lange Medical Publications, 1971).

(7) Glass, T. B., Jr.: "Early Debridement in Pit Viper Bite," *Surgery, Gynecology and Obstetrics,* 136 (1973):774.

(8) Huang, T. T.; Lynch, J. B.; Larson, D. L., and Lewis, S. R.: "The Use of Excisional Therapy in the Management of Snakebite," *Annals of Surgery,* 179 (1974):598.

(9) Hunter, G.; Frye, W., and Swartzwelder, J.: *A Manual of Tropical Medicine,* 3rd ed. (Philadelphia: W. B. Saunders Company, 1960).

(10) Loder, J. S.: "Treatment of Jellyfish Stings," *Journal of the American Medical Association,* 226 (1973):1228.

(11) Mackie, T.; Hunter, G., and Worth, C.: *A Manual of Tropical Medicine,* 2nd ed. (Philadelphia: W. B. Saunders Company, 1957).

(12) Myers, M. B.: "Sutures and Wound Healing," *American Journal of Nursing,* 71 (1971):1725.

(13) Paton, B. C.: "Bites — Human, Dog,

Spider and Snake," *Surgical Clinics of North America,* 43 (1963):537.

(14) "Recommendation of the Public Health Service Advisory Committee on Immunization Practices: Rabies Prophylaxis," *Morbidity and Mortality Weekly Report,* 16(19), May 13, 1967.

(15) Resnick, S.: "Necrotic Arachnidism," *Journal of the American Medical Association,* 198 (1966):957.

(16) Russell, F. E.: "Injuries by Venomous Animals in the U.S.A.," *Journal of the American Medical Association,* 177 (1961):903.

(17) Thomson, H. G., and Sitek, V.: "Small Animal Bites: The Role of Primary Closure," *Journal of Trauma,* 13 (1973):20.

(18) United States Public Health Service, *Morbidity and Mortality Report* (Washington, D.C.: USPHS, 1972).

11

Drug reactions and interactions

GREGORY M. CHUDZIK

GENERAL CONSIDERATIONS

The use of medications is, for many, central to treatment of a symptom or illness. It is not unusual for a person to see a physician for the sole purpose of obtaining a medication to alleviate his symptoms. If the doctor tells him none is required, the patient may feel that he has not been adequately treated. Trends exist towards an increased use of both prescribed and over-the-counter medications. Self-medication has increased, as well as treatment with drugs by a variety of medical specialists who may be unaware of a patient's drug history.

Drugs, singly or in combination, can exert a number of responses within an individual, which can be expected or unique. A variety of physical and emotional factors also determine the extent to which an individual responds to any given drug. Thus, it is important that the nurse understand how drugs may act and interact to produce symptoms which bring a patient to the emergency department setting.

Gathering information regarding drug usage assumes increased importance in the patient who presents with symptoms that are undiagnosed or unexplained in terms of past history. In collecting a history of drug usage, the nurse must determine:

(1) *What drugs the patient is currently using and how frequently.* Knowledge

of primary drug actions and side effects can often explain the patient's presenting complaint.

(2) *What medications he has taken within the past 6 to 8 months.* Some symptoms resulting from drug therapy are insidious and late in onset; the medication may be discontinued before the effects of its use become manifest.

(3) *Drug allergenicity.* Responses of an individual to any drug can be infinite and life-threatening. Before any medication is administered, a history of drug allergy *must* be ascertained.

(4) *How the patient uses drugs.* Does he use a variety of drugs simultaneously and frequently? Does he take medications only as a last resort?

Responses to these queries will reveal attitudes toward drug therapy that can be helpful in analyzing the patient's problem and the need for patient education and in predicting the degree of success of a treatment regimen involving drug therapy. The history is then duly recorded and reported to the physician.

Resource materials on drug reactions and interactions should be a part of every primary care setting; some are listed in the bibliography. Further, access to a poison control center is helpful. Such centers have a wide variety of informational material which is indexed, cross-referenced and comprehensive.

The purpose of this chapter is to increase the emergency nurse's awareness of the types of responses a patient may experience to a drug or combination of drugs. Mechanisms that influence drug activity are discussed, as they have many implications regarding the administration of medications.

ADVERSE RESULTS OF DRUG ADMINISTRATIONS

Administration of a drug results in: (1) the desired drug activity and/or (2) a drug reaction, manifest by additional effects which are not primarily sought through the administration of the drug. It is this second group of results which will be discussed here. It must be remembered that no drug is so specific or so special that it achieves its effects in exactly the desired manner in every patient to whom it is given. No drug is absolutely free of some capacity or ability to produce unsought or unexpected reactions in a certain percentage of patients receiving it. These reactions may be harmless; some may even be of benefit; but those that cause some concern to the patient and which may best be considered as harmful deserve careful consideration.

Adverse drug reactions may be divided into "major" and minor" adverse reactions depending on their severity. Examples of major and minor drug reactions are listed in Table 11–1. Drug interactions may vary in their significance depending on their nature or the circumstances which accompany them. They may be adverse; they may be beneficial; they may be significant or insignificant; they may be apparent or hidden, severe, mild, acute, chronic; they may be immediate (such as anaphylaxis) or delayed (such as cirrhosis of the liver). In this chapter, consideration will be given mainly to those which are emergent, most adverse, apparent and usually acute and more immediate than delayed.

All drug reactions, either serious or minor, may be termed or classified as side effects,

extension effects or drug interaction effects. These, in turn, may be identified as localized or systemic.

A "side effect" is an effect different from that primarily sought. It is one in which differing pharmacologic mechanisms are involved or perhaps in which an organ other than the "target" organ may be involved with the original pharmacologic mechanism. A familiar example of this is the production of diarrhea during the use of antibiotics. This diarrhea may result from a number of factors, including direct irritation of the mucosal wall of the intestines or perhaps a destruction of the normal flora of the gut. Side effects usually occur when the drug has more than one pharmacologic action. It may influence more than one body system or have a multiplicity of sites of action or a multiplicity of organs of action, thus producing a number of pharmacologic actions usually unwarranted or unsought in the administration of the drug.

An "extension effect" is that primary pharmacologic activity which is normally sought but is more pronounced and/or extended. As an example, idiosyncratic reactions to a particular drug may be due to a hypersusceptibility of certain people to the drug, producing pronounced overdose effects with normal doses. Overdosage of a drug produces an extension effect, as does hypersensitivity or accumulation of the drug in the body due to a lack of normal detoxification or excretion mechanisms.

Often, those reactions considered minor adverse drug reactions or minor signs of drug toxicity serve a very useful and informative role. They inform the observer of either (1) adequate effect at this time, or (2) an impending major adverse effect. It is important to remember these minor reactions or initial signs. They may be precursors of more serious impending toxicities. They can serve the nurse in patient observation and aid in the diagnosis of adverse drug reactions.

Drug-induced diseases include the entire spectrum of undesirable conditions that have been reported in man. They may affect any

TABLE 11-1 EXAMPLES OF ADVERSE DRUG EXPERIENCES

Major drug reactions	Minor drug reactions
(1) Addiction (physical or psychological dependence)	(1) Acidosis
(2) Allergic reactions (hypersensitivity)	(2) Anorexia
(3) Anaphylactic shock	(3) Chromatopsia
(4) Atrophy of any organ or tissue	(4) Cramps
(5) Blood dyscrasias (agranulocytosis, aplastic anemia, bone marrow depression, thrombocytopenia)	(5) Diarrhea (mild)
(6) Blood pressure changes (severe)	(6) Dizziness
(7) Blood sugar changes (severe)	(7) Drowsiness
(8) Cancer (neoplastic disease)	(8) Euphoria
(9) Cardiopathy (arrhythmias, decompensation)	(9) Fatigue
(10) Coma	(10) Fever (low-grade)
(11) Convulsions	(11) Glossitis
(12) Death	(12) Headache
(13) Exacerbation (peptic ulcer, infections)	(13) Hiccup
(14) Hearing impairment (deafness)	(14) Nausea
(15) Hemorrhage (severe)	(15) Paresthesias (mild)
(16) Impairment of psychomotor activity	(16) Pharyngitis
(17) Iodism, Brominism, and the like	(17) Proctitis
(18) Kidney dysfunction	(18) Pruritus ani
(19) Libido enhancement (severe)	(19) Skin rash (mild)
(20) Libido reduction (severe)	(20) Stomatitis
(21) Liver dysfunction	(21) Vaginitis
(22) Mental depression (severe)	(22) Vertigo
(23) Mutation	(23) Vomiting
(24) Ocular damage (blindness)	(24) Weakness
(25) Pancreatitis	
(26) Paralysis	
(27) Peripheral vascular collapse	
(28) Photosensitivity (severe)	
(29) Psychoses	
(30) Resistant organisms	
(31) Respiratory depression	
(32) Superinfections	
(33) Teratism	
(34) Thyroid depression	
(35) Tolerance	
(36) Ulceration	
(37) Withdrawal symptoms (severe)	

cell, tissue or body system and any pharmacodynamic mechanism concerned with absorption, distribution, metabolism and excretion of drugs. Adverse drug reactions frequently mimic dermatologic and many other diseases. Thus, a disease may be diagnosed and treatment initiated, not recognizing the fact that the disease is drug-induced. Instead of giving more drugs, it may only be necessary to remove those drugs which the patient is currently receiving. It is important to realize that almost anything can happen as a result of a drug reaction. Adverse drug experiences are extremely difficult to predict and diagnose. Any number of patients with adverse reactions may be admitted to an emergency department with apparent physical signs or symptoms often leading to treatment with further drug therapy along another line. Drug interaction effects may result.

TABLE 11–2 EXAMPLES OF DRUGS KNOWN TO CAUSE
BLOOD DYSCRASIAS, BY DISORDER

Disorder	Generic drug name	Trade drug name
(1) Agranulocytosis (Granulocyto- penia or Leukopenia)	Methyldopa	Aldomet
	Acetylsalicylic acid	(Aspirin)
	Phenylbutazone	Butazolidin
	Chloramphenicol	Chloromycetin
	Prochlorperazine	Compazine
	Chlorothiazide	Diuril
	Thioridazine	Mellaril
	Tolbutamide	Orinase
	Benzylpenicillin sodium	(Penicillin)
	Propylthiouracil	
	Tripelennamine	Pyribenzamine
	Quinidine sulfate	(Quinidine)
	Streptomycin	
	Sulfonamides	
	Tetracycline	
	Imipramine HCl	Tofranil
(2) Aplastic Anemia	Methyldopa	Aldomet
	Acetylsalicylic acid	(Aspirin)
	Barbiturates	
	Phenylbutazone	Butazolidin
	Chloramphenicol	Chloromycetin
	Chlorpropamide	Diabinese
	Acetazolamide	Diamox
	Chlorothiazide	Diuril
	Sulfisoxazole	Gantrisin
	Sulfamethoxypyridazine	Kynex
	Tolbutamide	Orinase
	Benzylpenicillin sodium	(Penicillin)
	Quinidine sulfate	(Quinidine)
	Streptomycin	
	Trimethadione	Tridione
(3) Hemolytic Anemia	Acetylsalicylic acid	(Aspirin)
	Probenecid	Benemid
	Chloramphenicol	Chloromycetin
	Nitrofurantoin	Furadantin
	Isonicotinic Hydrazide	I.N.H.
	Para-aminosalicylic acid	(P.A.S.)
	Benzylpenicillin sodium	(Penicillin)
	Quinidine sulfate	(Quinidine)
	Sulfonamides	
	Tetracycline	
	Chlorpromazine	Thorazine
	Vitamin K	
(4) Megaloblastic Anemia	Anticonvulsants	
	Barbiturates	
	Diphenylhydantoin sodium	Dilantin
(5) Pancytopenia	Methyldopa	Aldomet
	Acetylsalicylic acid	(Aspirin)
	Barbiturates	

TABLE 11–2, *cont.*

Disorder	Generic drug name	Trade drug name
(5) Pancytopenia, *cont.*	Phenylbutazone	Butazolidin
	Chloramphenicol	Chloromycetin
	Chlorpropamide	Diabinese
	Acetazolamide	Diamox
	Chlorothiazide	Diuril
	Meprobamate	Equanil
	Sulfisoxazole	Gantrisin
	Sulfamethoxypyridazine	Kynex
	Tolbutamide	Orinase
	Benzylpenicillin sodium	(Penicillin)
	Quinidine sulfate	(Quinidine)
	Streptomycin	
	Tetracycline	
(6) Thrombocyto-penia	All of the above.	All of the above.

Blood dyscrasias

Agranulocytosis, aplastic anemia, hemolytic anemia, megaloblastic anemia, pancytopenia and thrombocytopenia are the most frequently observed blood dyscrasias. The actual mechanism for the induction of these disorders is not always the same. The 3 major mechanisms are: (1) bone marrow hypofunction, as a result of direct depression of protein synthesis; (2) immune mechanisms inducing bone marrow hypofunction; and/or (3) interference with other hematopoietic mechanisms.

Agranulocytosis, which may have a mortality rate of 50 percent, often appears with the typical clinical signs and symptoms associated with acute leukemia or aplastic anemia and may often appear to be precipitated by a bacterial infection.

Aplastic anemia is possibly the most serious of all drug-induced blood dyscrasias. Mortality in this disorder may reach 80 to 100 percent if the agent is not identified and withdrawn and appropriate therapy initiated immediately. In some cases, aplastic anemia may appear 6 to 8 months following drug therapy. These cases of insidious and delayed onset occur after the offending agent has already been removed and are often diagnosed as idiopathic. In most cases, one does not think about looking 6 to 8 months back into the medical history of patients to discover any drug use.

Hemolytic anemias are often the result of drug influence on a pharmacogenetic deficiency. Among the more common of these genetic abnormalities is glucose-6-phosphate dehydrogenase deficiency. In these cases, the patient already has a genetic abnormality which allows hemolysis to occur when these drugs are introduced into the system.

Megaloblastic anemia is usually the result of a folic acid (Vitamin B_{12}) deficiency. It is felt that anticonvulsants, such as diphenylhydantoin and the barbiturates, interfere with the mechanism of absorption of folate from the gastrointestinal tract, thus allowing the manifestations of a megaloblastic anemia. This problem can be easily overcome by administering the anticonvulsants several hours apart from folic acid.

Pancytopenia and thrombocytopenia have been caused by an overwhelming number of drugs. Both have a very high morbidity and mortality rate. Thrombocytopenia may present as a bloody nose or excess tendency to bruise. It must be diagnosed and treated as quickly as possible.

Table 11–2 lists examples of some drugs known to cause blood dyscrasias, by specific disorders.

Cardiovascular toxicities

Practically all drugs have the potential to produce some toxic effect on the heart or blood vessels. This may be magnified in the presence of a preexisting cardiovascular disease. Very few if any medications can be given for long periods of time without increasing the potential for cardiovascular damage. As an example, some of the tranquilizer drugs have been given in high doses for many years and are considered to be quite safe in psychiatric circles, but reports of cardiac dysrhythmia, conduction disturbances and electrocardiographic changes suggestive of infarction began to appear in the literature about 1963 or so.

Drugs such as phenylbutazone, penicillin, streptomycin, sulfonamides and chlorpromazine have been known to cause myocardial damage as the result of hypersensitivity reactions. Arsenicals, ethyl alcohol and lead cause a direct toxic effect on the myocardium, while other drugs, such as the anesthetics, atropine, hydralazine and reserpine may damage the myocardium as the result of an overdose or adverse drug interaction. Damage to blood vessels may result from excessive vasoconstriction or vasodilatation which may result from hypersensitivity or overdose.

Problems such as those listed above may lead to an elevation of the blood pressure, possibly progressing to acute pulmonary edema, a cerebral vascular accident or even a myocardial infarction.

Table 11–3 lists 4 cardiovascular toxicities and some of the agents known to cause these toxicities.

Gastrointestinal toxicities

Nausea, diarrhea, vomiting, ulceration, hemorrhage, stomatitis and proctitis are the major signs and symptoms of gastrointestinal toxicity. A list of drugs causing these toxicities would be too long to include here and of no immediate help. Nausea, vomiting and diarrhea are among those minor reactions which are seen with most drugs, but it must be remembered that these minor intestinal ailments may be the initial signs of an impending, more serious reaction.

Aspirin is probably one of the most common ulcerative and hemorrhage-causing drugs known to man. It has been estimated that loss of blood occurs in approximately 70 percent of all people who ingest aspirin. This may be a result of local irritation and also an effect on coagulation due to the reduction of platelet adhesiveness caused by aspirin. Anticoagulants, cancer chemotherapeutic agents and steroids are also well-known inducers of ulcers and gastrointestinal hemorrhage. Other common agents implicated in gastrointestinal bleeding are ethacrynic acid and indomethacin. Potassium chloride when given as a solid was perhaps one of the most ulcerogenic agents. This is the reason it is now dispensed as a solution.

Stomatitis and proctitis are caused by cancer chemotherapeutic agents and high doses of steroids. It is important to remember that the list of drugs which affect the gastrointestinal tract is constantly growing.

Hepatotoxicity

The liver serves as the major site of drug metabolism. At this site glyconeogenesis, glycogenolysis, acetylation, glucuronidation and other major biochemical functions are performed. Any damage to the liver that alters its functions or produces significant insufficiency may have far-reaching effects on the brain, endocrine glands, skin and most other parts of the body. Damage to the drug-metabolizing enzymes of the liver significantly decreases the capacity to detoxify drugs, thereby leading to overdose or extension effects with concurrently administered drugs.

Hepatic tolerance to drugs varies greatly from one individual to another, and liver changes induced by drugs may occur either immediately or be delayed for months following withdrawal of drug therapy. These changes cannot be predicted. Some have a familial component and may not be dose-related; however, most are dose-related and

**TABLE 11–3   EXAMPLES OF DRUGS KNOWN TO CAUSE
CARDIOVASCULAR TOXICITIES, BY DISORDER**

Disorder	Drug generic name	Drug trade name
(1) Arrhythmias	Cardiac glycosides	
	Cardiac stimulants	
	Procainamide	
	Quinidine sulfate	(Quinidine)
	Xanthines	
(2) Dysrhythmias	Nortriptyline	Aventyl
	Amitriptyline	(Elavil)
	Pentofrane	
	Chlorpromazine	Thorazine
(3) Cardiac depression	Barbiturates	
	Procainamide	
	Quinidine sulfate	(Quinidine)
(4) Myocarditis	Arsenicals	
	Ethyl alcohol	
	Lead	
	Phenylbutazone [a]	Butazolidin
	Benzylpenicillin sodium [a]	(Penicillin)
	Streptomycin [a]	
	Sulfonamides [a]	
	Chlorpromazine [a]	Thorazine
	Anesthetics [b]	
	Atropine sulfate [b]	(Atropine)
	Hydralazine [b]	
	Reserpine [b]	

[a] From hypersensitivity.
[b] From overdose.

reversible on cessation of drug administration. Unfortunately, some of these conditions progress irreversibly and may persist for years as a chronic disease eventually terminating in death.

Four results of hepatotoxicity are necrosis, hepatomegaly, jaundice and decreased function. Jaundice, the most observed manifestation of hepatotoxicity, has been classified into 3 main types: (1) cholestatic, (2) hepatocellular, (3) hemolytic.

Cholestatic jaundice, the most common of the drug-induced jaundices, occurs when drugs modify hepatic excretion or secretion. This type of jaundice is characterized by intrahepatic obstructive symptoms and is often accompanied by eosinophilia, fever and rash. Among those drugs known to induce cholestatic jaundice are chlorothiazide, chlorpromazine, erythromycin estolate, some of the sulfa drugs and a few of the oral contraceptives.

Hepatocellular or necrotic jaundice resembles severe viral hepatitis and may produce a mortality as high as 50 percent. This direct cellular destruction has been caused by some drugs, including diphenylhydantoin, halothane, isoniazid, methotrexate, penicillin, the long-acting sulfonamides and oxyphenbutazone.

The exact cause of hemolytic jaundice is not known but thought to be hypersensitivity of or perhaps direct toxic action on the erythrocyte itself. Amphetamines, phenylbutazone and quinine have been implicated in hemolytic jaundice.

Nephrotoxicity

Kidney damage is perhaps one of the most perilous of all hazards of medication. Nephrotoxic drugs or chemicals may damage enough nephrons, directly or indirectly, to significantly alter the urinary excretion rate of the drugs themselves, as well as other constituents of the extracellular fluid. Severe nephrotoxicity may result from direct damage to structure or function, as seen with carbon tetrachloride or mercuric chloride, as well as other mercurial compounds and the crystalluria often seen with sulfa drugs. It may also result from an immune reaction, as evidenced with the amino glycosides, or from a hypersensitivity, as seen with amphetamines and sulfa drugs. Chronic poisoning with lead and other heavy metals has also led to kidney failure. Exacerbation of existing dormant renal diseases has been evidenced with drugs such as cathartics, diuretics, antineoplastics, steroids, narcotics, tetracyclines and vasoactive compounds.

Fluid and electrolyte disturbances as a result of nephrotoxicity are very serious problems. Hyponatremia presents with central nervous system manifestations, including confusion, convulsions, irritability, coma and, possibly, death. Hypernatremia, often accompanied by dehydration and hypertonicity, may be encountered in patients unable to drink adequate quantities of water, since they are stuporous or comatose. Drug toxicities may very easily induce this state. Hypokalemia, often associated with diuretic or cardiac glycoside therapy, can induce cardiac arrhythmias, muscle weakness and, perhaps, paralysis. On the other hand, hyperkalemia may be induced by such potassium-sparing diuretics as spironolactone and triamterene.

Metabolic acidosis has been linked with therapy including salicylates and ammonium chloride, while metabolic alkalosis has been linked to steroid therapy and ethacrynic acid.

Neurotoxicities

Neurotoxicities may manifest either through the central nervous system or peripherally, and can affect a wide range of organs and tissues. Those most commonly affected are the central nervous system, ears, eyes, skeletal muscle innervation, innervation of the vasculature and the heart.

Central nervous system depression is easily induced by a great number of drugs. The effects of analgesics, antihistamines, anesthetics, hypnotics, narcotics, psychotropic agents, sedatives and other central nervous system depressants are very well known. Combinations of such drugs may produce a drug interaction causing serious problems in many patients. The combined depressant effect of one or more of these drugs may lead to respiratory depression, coma and, very possibly, death.

The induction of seizure activity has been linked to a number of agents, including the analeptics, central nervous system stimulants, amphetamines, local anesthetics, antidepressants, antihistamines and even antibiotics, such as cycloserine and the penicillins.

Drugs, such as isoniazid, penicillin, streptomycin, sulfonamides, anticonvulsants, chlorpromazine, phenobarbital and some of the antidepressant drugs, have been implicated in encephalopathy. The phenothiazines, such as chlorpromazine and prochlorperazine, have been well implicated in the occurrence of extrapyramidal effects. These effects consist of cog-wheeling motions of the extremities, along with involuntary neck movements. When exposure to these drugs can be documented, the best treatment is intramuscular diphenhydramine (Benadryl) or benztropine mesylate (Cogentin), which provides almost instantaneous relief.

Peripheral neuropathy resulting from medications is usually manifest by bilateral or unilateral palsies, paresthesias, such as numbness and tingling of the extremities and the tongue, and a variety of other problems, such as fasciculations, muscle twitching, tremor and unsteadiness of gait. Antibacterial agents are very commonly implicated with these reactions, as are antidepressants and antitubercular drugs.

The amino glycosides, kanamycin, neomycin, gentamicin, and streptomycin are well-known inducers of ototoxicity. In addition, ethacrynic acid and salicylates induce ototoxicity.

Oculotoxicity has been manifested in the form of myopia following therapy with hydrochlorothiazide and hydralazine. Blurred vision has been evidenced following therapy with the tetracyclines, chloramphenicol and digitalis glycosides. In addition, further oculotoxicities have been manifested following therapy with agents such as penicillamine, ethambutol and the antimalarial agents.

Alterations in the behavioral patterns of an individual are manifestations of central nervous system effect of a drug. Drugs such as the antidepressants, amphetamines and barbiturates are expected to induce behavioral modification. However, other drugs have been known to induce unexpected changes in behavior. Among these agents are reserpine, guanethidine, penicillin, the sulfa drugs, antineoplastics and steroids.

Dermatotoxicity

It is almost impossible to show definite cause-effect relationships between drugs and dermatological manifestations of toxicity. Perhaps the only method of establishing such a relationship is to "challenge the patient"; that is, withdraw the medication, wait until the reaction subsides and then administer the same medication to the patient. Such a challenge may be extremely hazardous and in most instances should never be attempted.

Dermatotoxicity is probably the most common of all manifestations of drug toxicities and occasionally includes very severe drug-induced eruptions that are life-threatening. Those severe eruptions which have definitely been caused by drugs include exfoliative dermatitis, Stevens-Johnson syndrome (erythema multiforme exudativum), a lupus-like syndrome and toxic epidermal necrolysis. Severe manifestations of these eruptions may permanently handicap the patient or even result in death.

Exfoliative dermatitis is usually characterized by erythema, induration, scaling and thickening of the skin. It is associated with the exfoliative forms of psoriasis and other usually benign skin conditions. Among those common drugs associated with exfoliative dermatitis are para-aminosalicylic acid (PAS), barbiturates, demeclocycline, diphenylhydantoin, diphtheria-pertussis and tetanus toxoids, furosemide, isorbid, penicillin, phenothiazines and sulfonamides.

Stevens-Johnson syndrome, the most common of the severe drug-induced skin eruptions, may be caused by hypersensitivity or immune reactions. It is characterized by high fever and severe headache preceding conjunctivitis, rhinitis, stomatitis and urethritis, which are usually followed in a few days by the appearance of erythematous papules with a hemorrhagic center. Bullae and vesicles may also be present. As this drug reaction progresses, the patient may become extremely ill and manifest many signs of toxicity, including headache, joint pains, malaise, a rapid weak pulse, general weakness and a purulent, ocular exudate. This exudate may eventuate in partial or total blindness. The mouth and lips are covered with erosions having a red face and a grayish-white pseudomembrane exudate, which may also be swollen. Recovery from these advanced states is usually very slow. Among the drugs implicated in Stevens-Johnson syndrome are barbiturates, codeine, diphenylhydantoin, penicillins, salicylates, thiazides and sulfonamides.

Lupus erythematosus-like syndrome resembles systemic lupus erythematosus (SLE) and may be due to a coupling of a drug, acting as a hapten, with body proteins. The drug-induced disease may also be the result of the exacerbation of latent SLE. It is difficult to diagnose by means of the L.E. cells, since L.E. cells are found in many other diseases, such as hemolytic anemia, chronic hepatitis, dermatomyositis, leukemia and miliary tuberculosis. This problem is developed in approximately 10 percent of those patients receiving hydralazine in high doses for long periods of time. It is also a frequent complication of procainamide therapy and has been reported in conjunction with such drugs as diphenylhydantoin, isoniazid, alpha methyldopa, the oral contraceptives, aminosalicylic acid, penicillin, streptomycin, tetracyclines and thiazides.

Toxic epidermal necrolysis is a condition, first described in 1956, which resembles "scalding of the skin." This eruption is most commonly seen in females and is characterized by erythema and tenderness followed by loosening and peeling of large areas of the skin, as well as by confusion, fever and swelling of the eyes. Superficial layers of the skin may be easily removed with gentle rubbing. Many drugs have been implicated in this condition, among them: antihistamines, neomycin, phenobarbital, penicillin, sulfonamides and the tetracyclines.

Photosensitization is the susceptibility to dermatitis caused by exposure to sunlight. A wide variety of drugs have been associated very frequently with this phenomenon, which may be divided into 3 distinct types: (1) photoallergy, (2) phototoxicity and (3) photoaugmentation. Photoallergic reactions occur when the photosensitizing chemical forms a hapten through the absorption of light rays, followed by the hapten forming an antigen by combining with skin protein, followed by an antigen-antibody reaction occurring in the skin when it is rechallenged with an offending agent. Phototoxicity occurs when the photosensitizing chemical absorbs ultraviolet energy and this photoactivated chemical transfers the energy to vulnerable cellular constituents, wherein the cells sustain damage manifested as a severe sunburn. Photoaugmentation occurs when the ultraviolet light potentiates the reactivity of the skin by means of a direct effect on cellular components to make them more vulnerable to contact dermatitis. Among the more common photosensitizers are: salicylates, sulfonamides, demeclocycline, griseofulvin, barbiturates and phenothiazines.

A large number of medications have been implicated in dermatotoxicity and mimic practically every known manifestation of dermatitis. Some of the terms used to categorize the dermatologic reactions are: achromotrichia, acneiform, alopecia, angioneurotic edema, atrophy, bullous, depigmented, ecchymotic, eczematoid, erythematous, exanthematic, fixed, furunculoid, hirsutism, lichenoid, macular, maculopapular, morbilliform, monilial, necrotic, papular, petechial rash, photosensitization, porphyria, pruritus, purpura, scarlatiniform, striae, tumor-like, urticarial and vesicular. As this long list indicates, the most frequently encountered adverse drug reactions are related to the skin.

Pulmonary toxicity

Oftentimes, adverse reactions to drugs may closely resemble respiratory disease, and therefore the true causes in such induced conditions may be overlooked. Again, these cases may see the prescribing of an unnecessary medication rather than withdrawal of an offending agent.

Induction of pulmonary toxicity may be accomplished as the result of an allergic reaction, an idiosyncratic reaction or a toxic reaction to a drug or as the result of a combination of any of these or as the result of a generalized reaction to a drug. As a rule, the pulmonary toxicities, whether induced directly or indirectly, are generally reversible when the offending agent is withdrawn.

Asthma, the most common drug-induced respiratory disease, may occur within 20 minutes after ingestion of a drug by a patient with a history of asthma or nasal polyps. Such an attack may be severe, prolonged and perhaps fatal. The most common drugs shown to induce such asthmatic attacks are: aspirin, anesthetics, griseofulvin, cephalosporins, penicillins, streptomycin, neomycin and tetracyclines.

Pulmonary eosinophilia is characterized by cough, dyspnea and fever, with audible crepitations that are sometimes widespread, but without tachypnea, wheezing or prolonged expiration. It is observed most often following nitrofurantoin thrapy than any other drug. However, some other drugs, such as imipramine, aminosalicylic acid, penicillin and sulfonamides have been implicated in this toxicity.

In general, the lungs are highly sensitive to drugs and chemicals. Oil-containing medications, such as cod liver oil and mineral oil, may induce lipoid pneumonia. Drug-altered respiration may indeed lead to disturbances in fluid and electrolyte balance, and pulmonary emboli have been reported following inadvertent administration of oil medications into the vein, as well as following therapy with oral contraceptives.

The wide variety of manifestations of pulmonary toxicities to drugs should alert the reader to the possibilities of pulmonary diseases being linked to drug therapy. Other manifestations include pulmonary complications of SLE and polyarteritis nodosa and iodism.

SAFE USE OF MEDICATIONS

The safe use of any medication depends on the knowledge and experience of the individual prescribing practitioner. This individual should be adequately familiar with the chemistry and pharmacology of the drugs used. He should be particularly interested in the physical, chemical and biopharmaceutic properties, the metabolic fate and other pharmacodynamic characteristics of every drug he prescribes. A much more cautious, more sophisticated and more thoughtful approach to medication of the patient is urgently needed to decrease the alarming incidences of adverse drug reactions. However, overconcern with safety should not deny the patient the beneficial aspects of drug therapy.

One must remember that adverse drug reactions are not limited to those discussed in this chapter, nor are they limited to those which are well reported in the literature. Drug-induced diseases cross the entire spectrum of undesirable conditions reported in man. They may affect any cell, tissue, organ or body system. While some are predictable because they are frequently extensions of the known phar-

macologic actions of the drugs, others are many times bizarre and impossible to predict. One must be prepared for such unexpected reactions and recognize them once they occur.

Although the mechanisms of action of many drugs have been elicited and their deleterious potentials recognized, the practice of polypharmacy, the inclusion of multiple ingredients in medications, has altered the possible problem of iatrogenic damage with the consideration of drug interactions. It is commonplace today for the patient to take several drugs concurrently. The appeal for the physician to prescribe not just one but a combination of pharmacologically active ingredients is difficult to resist because of the inference that more drugs are necessarily better than fewer drugs. This is further complicated by patient habits of seeing 2 or more physicians concurrently, as well as habits of self-medication.

The past few years have seen development of an awareness that multiple-drug therapy can lead to results which cannot be explained by consideration of the pharmacologic activity of each drug as a separate entity. It has become evident that frequently one drug may alter the effect of another. Reactions such as this may diminish or abolish the intended beneficial effect of one or both drugs; may result in a disproportionate potentiation of one or both; or may elicit an undesirable side effect or toxic manifestation not associated with the respective drugs individually. There is no doubt that many interactions have occurred for years without detection, but as understanding of drug action increases, interactions should be more easily identified and possibly even anticipated. The problem of drug interactions is indeed a complicated one; however an appreciation for potential drug interactions must be ever present in mind.

The vast majority of drug interactions are related to pharmacologic action, that is, to interactions occurring at the site of action of the drug. A thorough knowledge of the pharmacology of drugs involved will aid in the identification and anticipation of drug interactions. However, since the pharmacology or site of action is not the only mechanism involved in drug interactions, awareness of some of the other mechanisms which may influence drug interactions is necessary.

The following helpful hints are in no way all-encompassing. Since the problem of drug interactions is extremely complicated, these considerations are, in effect, an oversimplification of the major mechanisms by which drug interactions occur. An awareness of these mechanisms and how they might affect drug interactions will be extremely useful to the emergency nurse, however.

In general, drug interactions will result in: (1) decrease in drug efficacy or (2) increase in pharmacologic effect and possibly in toxic drug reactions.

Mechanisms which may decrease drug activity

(1) *Absorption:* Drug interactions in the G.I. tract may be due to chemical reactions (chemical and enzymatic), as well as to pH alterations and an absorption type of antagonism.
(2) *Transport:* Displacement of drugs from protein binding sites may result in increased metabolism and excretion.
(3) *Distribution:* Saturation of specific tissue binding sites may decrease activity but increase toxicity of administered drugs.
(4) *Site of action:* Interactions may occur when an agent occupies receptors normally used by an active drug or when an agent acts on another site, either producing an opposite effect or a blocking effect.
(5) *Metabolism:* Enzyme-induction effects of some drugs may result in an increased metabolism of an administered drug, thereby decreasing its effect.
(6) *Excretion:* Changes in urinary pH may increase the excretion of weak acids and bases. Example: basic urine decreases the half-life of acidic drugs, such as salicylates, and acidic urines will decrease the half-life of basic drugs such as amphetamines.

Mechanisms which may increase drug activity

(1) *Absorption:* Soluble salt formation or more rapid dissolution of drugs will increase their absorption. This may be caused by pH changes, wetting agents or organic solvents such as alcohol.
(2) *Transport:* Displacement of drugs from protein binding sites will result in higher free or active form of the drug and possible toxic reactions of the displaced drug.
(3) *Distribution:* An increase in blood flow to tissues will increase the amount of drugs being presented to these tissues.
(4) *Site of action:* Administration of 2 or more agents possessing similar pharmacologic actions or side effects may give rise to drug interaction by the additive effects of these properties.
(5) *Metabolism:* Some drugs may inhibit production or metabolism of a second compound, resulting in prolonged duration and/or intensified action of the second drug.
(6) *Excretion:* Direct competition of some agents for active tubular transport may alter the excretion rates and increase the half-life of drugs. Changes in urinary pH will alter the excretion rates of weak acids and bases. Acidic urines increase the half-life of acidic drugs, and basic urines do the same for basic drugs.

BIBLIOGRAPHY

(1) *Clin-Alert* (Science Editors, Inc., 142 Chenoweth Lane, P.O. Box 7185, Louisville, Ky.). Abstracts from recently published journal articles, with drug reactions.
(2) Dramer, W., *et al.:* "Some Physical and

Chemical Incompatibilities of Drugs for I.V. Administration," *Drug Intelligence and Clinical Pharmacy,* 5 (July 1971): 211–228. Listing of drug, route of administration, pH range, incompatibilities with other drugs.

(3) Elking, Sister M. Paulette, and Kabot, H. F.: "Drug Induced Modifications of Laboratory Test Values," *American Journal of Hospital Pharmacy,* 25 (September 1968):485–519. Tables presented with normal values and effects of drugs on test alteration in various body fluids (urine, CSF, serum, etc.).

(4) *FDA Clinical Experience Abstracts* (U.S. Department of Health, Education and Welfare, Food and Drug Administration, Bureau of Drugs, Medical Library [BD-45], 5600 Fishers La., Rockville, Md. 20852). Monthly reports of adverse drug reactions, side effects, etc.

(5) *FDA Drug Bulletin* (Assistant to the Director for Medical Communications, Bureau of Drugs [BD-40], 5600 Fishers La., Rockville, Md. 20852).

(6) Garb, S.: *Clinical Guide to Undesirable Drug Interactions and Interferences* (New York: Springer Publishing Company, 1971). Tabulation of drugs and drug interactants.

(7) Hansten, P. D.: *Drug Interactions,* ed. 1 (Philadelphia: Lea and Febiger, 1971). Presentation of drug, mechanism of interaction, clinical significance, references.

(8) Latiolais, C. J., *et al.:* "Stability of Drugs After Reconstitution," *American Journal of Hospital Pharmacy,* 24 (December 1967):567–691. Listing of drug, route of administration, stability after dilution, recommended diluent and concentration.

(9) Martin, E. W.: *Hazards of Medicine* (Philadelphia: J. B. Lippincott Company, 1971).

(10) *Medical Letter on Drugs and Therapeutics* (The Medical Letter Inc., 56 Harrison St., New Rochelle, N.Y. 10801). Biweekly journal.

(11) Meyler, L., and Herdheimer, A.: *Side Effects of Drugs,* 6 (Baltimore: Williams & Wilkins, 1968).

(12) Moser, R. H.: *Diseases of Medical Progress: A Study of Iatrogenic Disease,* ed. 3 (Springfield, Ill.: Charles C Thomas, 1969).

(13) Pierpoli, Paul: "Drug Therapy and Diet," *Drug Intelligence and Clinical Pharmacy,* 6 (March 1972):89–99. Food and drug interactions.

12

Care of the patient exposed to drugs or toxic substances

A. J. RICE
DIANN ANDERSON
MARY FURTH

The person who comes to an emergency department with symptoms suggestive of exposure to a toxic substance may be either suicidal or an accident victim. Chapter 7 discussed assessment of suicidal behavior, as well as the crisis treatment and psychosocial or psychiatric follow-up of the suicidal person. This chapter will discuss the emergency management of the person exposed (accidentally or intentionally) to toxic substances or drugs in sufficient amount to bring him to an emergency care setting. Immediate treatment is warranted for such an individual, irrespective of the lethality of the act. In fact, lethality assessment may be invalid at first, particularly in the unconscious patient. Hence, reassessment will be needed later after the more urgent medical aspects of care and treatment are implemented.

A wide variety of substances can be toxic to man when the elements of quantity, sufficient exposure and a susceptible site of exposure are present. Whether or not an agent is toxic depends upon these factors, as well as on the age and size of the individual and other specifics to be discussed later. Because the combination of these many toxic substances can

be infinite, a nationwide network of poison control centers has been set up in or near all major population centers. These centers maintain a detailed file of all potentially dangerous products and provide information on request to health care agencies and, in some instances, to the general population.

INITIAL CARE

General first aid measures for treatment of exposure to potentially toxic substances should be well known to all persons. These measures are determined in part by the substance involved and, even to a greater extent, by the area or route of exposure. Discussion of each determination follows. In all instances, the victim's physician or nearest hospital, poison control center or rescue unit should be called, depending on the patient's needs and what is accessible.

Route or area of exposure

Ingestion

This group includes a wide variety of plants, chemicals, certain contaminated foods and drugs. In general, vomiting should be induced in the patient, *except* if:

(1) He is unconscious or having seizures.

(2) The swallowed substance was a strong corrosive (such as lye or strong acids); these can be as dangerous coming up as going down.

(3) The swallowed substance contained kerosene, gasoline or other petroleum distillates. The major hazard with these is the development of an aspiration pneumonia, which increases in likelihood with emesis. It is advisable to give demulcents such as oil, ice cream or milk to protect the gastic mucosa. One exception is if the petroleum distillate also contained a dangerous pesticide, which must be removed.

The use of emesis and gastric lavage will be discussed in detail later in this chapter.

Some curious, investigative children are prone to put parts of plants into their mouths. While most are quite harmless, a number of plant parts can be quite toxic if taken in a sufficient amount by a small child. The toxic parts of common house and garden plants, along with related symptoms suggestive of toxicity, are outlined in Appendix D, at the end of this chapter.

Inhalation

This group includes fuel gases, auto exhaust, dense smoke from fires and fumes from poisonous chemicals. Particularly if the substance is odorless or the onset of symptoms is slow, exposure can be considerable before the victim is aware of it.

The victim should be moved into fresh air, and measures to facilitate breathing (loosening clothing, mouth-to-mouth resuscitation) should be initiated as indicated.

Toxic substances on the skin

These include pesticides, acids, lye and other caustics, as well as exposure to plants such as poison ivy and oak. The skin should be washed promptly with copious amounts of water and soap, if available. (Dry powders should be brushed from the skin before washing.) All contaminated clothing should be removed.

Substances in the eye

When a foreign substance enters the eye, it should be irrigated immediately under gently running water with the lid held open for a full *10 minutes*. The variety of chemical injuries to the eye and their management is discussed in detail in Chapter 27.

Toxic bites and stings

This group includes bites and stings from snakes, insects, unprovoked animals that may be rabid, as well as poisonous marine animals. Emergency treatment of each is detailed in Chapter 10. Persons who manifest unusually severe reactions to stinging insects should carry emergency treatment kits and emergency identification cards at all times.[21]

Assessment and examination

Gathering pertinent data is necessary to determine the urgency of the incident. Important information includes: (1) the brand and manufacturer of the toxic substance; (2) the amount taken; (3) route of entry or area of exposure; (4) time elapsed since exposure; (5) what, if any, emergency measures have been implemented; and (6) presence of signs or symptoms.

Often, only some of this history is known or revealed. The circumstances surrounding the exposure may give clues as to whether the exposure was accidental or purposeful. The person accompanying the patient should be available for consultation, especially when an accurate history cannot be obtained from the patient himself.

In the acutely ill patient, prompt assessment and intervention may be necessary to support the individual's vital functions. The procedures are those generally applicable to any patient who has an emergency medical problem. Irrespective of the toxic agent, emergency department personnel must be ready to treat the presenting symptoms. For example, if the patient is not breathing, pulmonary resuscitation should be initiated after clearing the airway; if the patient's blood pressure has fallen to a critical level, administration of plasma expanders, fluids and vasoactive drugs should be started, and measures to prompt good kidney and cardiac function should be initiated.

A complete and thorough evaluation of the physical status of the individual is necessary. The physical examination should be guided by the type of exposure and by knowledge of the substance involved. For example, evaluation of a local or topical exposure will differ from that known to cause systemic responses. If there is any suspicion of an ingestion, measures to hasten elimination should be undertaken, but not at the expense of evaluating the total patient. Even in a drug overdose, it is possible that there are underlying factors, such as chronic illnesses or neurological problems, which may distort or mask the acute problem at hand and may also push the individual into a graver and more life-threatening situation.

It is important to recognize the person who may have developed an addiction to either a sedative or narcotic. If an individual has developed dependency and is treated for an overdose by complete elimination of the addicting drug, an acute withdrawal syndrome may be precipitated. This may be a life-threatening situation, especially in the case of barbiturate and other sedative addiction. This cannot be overlooked in any overdose of an addicting drug, and medical personnel should be prepared to treat the withdrawal symptoms.

The unconscious patient must be evaluated for head trauma. Many times, this evaluation will be overlooked when there is clear evidence that a drug has been ingested, especially when alcohol is evident on the breath, or when the individual is known to the emergency department staff because of repeated attempts at suicide.

In evaluating patients with drug overdoses,

qualitatively or quantitatively, it is important to be aware that many areas do not have toxicological analyzing laboratories for emergency screenings. It is therefore important that emergency personnel become astute diagnosticians and be willing to use the presenting symptomatology for instituting treatment. Further treatment can be carried out as needed and determined by continued evaluation and monitoring of the patient.

FOOD POISONING

Foods may cause acute illness by several methods, including contamination by bacteria or their products. Thus, the symptoms of acute food poisoning may be due to food which contains large numbers of microorganisms or preformed bacterial toxins. Only the most common will be discussed here. The reader is referred to a textbook of medicine for more complete information.

Salmonellosis

Salmonella food poisoning is one of the more common communicable diseases in the United States. The greatest single source of the infection is domestic and wild animals, particularly fowl. It is *always* acquired via the oral route, usually from contaminated food or drink. In children, however, pet turtles are a common source of this infection. It seems to occur more commonly in the summer months and may be found as sporadic cases, in a family or as a large epidemic.

The history is quite characteristic, with an abrupt onset of colicky abdominal pain, accompanied by loose, watery diarrhea, with mucus or blood. Nausea and vomiting occur frequently. The symptoms develop 8 to 48 hours after ingestion of the contaminated material.

Physical signs include abdominal tenderness, with increased peristaltic activity. Findings may be confused with those of an acute surgical abdomen. The disease usually runs its course in 2 to 5 days but may extend to 10 to 14 days. The diagnosis may be confirmed by bacteriological studies of the suspected food or of the feces. Fresh stool samples are necessary.

Treatment is primarily supportive and is directed toward correcting dehydration and any electrolyte imbalance by parenteral replacement. Diphenoxylate hydrochloride with atropine sulfate (Lomotil) may alleviate the abdominal cramps and diarrhea. Other useful agents are tincture of paregoric and morphine sulfate. The disease is rarely fatal, except in the very young and very old.

Staphylococcal food poisoning

Some strains of staphylococci produce an enterotoxin which can cause gastroenteritis. These are found primarily in foods which are improperly refrigerated, especially cream-filled pastries, custards, cottage cheese and meats. The disease is spread by nasal droplet from contaminated food workers.

The history is characterized by a short incubation period of 1 to 6 hours, followed by an abrupt onset of severe nausea and vomiting, crampy abdominal pain, diarrhea and prostration. There is usually no fever. Admission is usually not required.

The diagnosis may be confirmed by laboratory examination of the food suspected of being contaminated. Treatment consists primarily of rest and sedation. In more severe cases, parenteral fluid replacement may be necessary.

Botulism

Botulism is an acute form of food poisoning, caused by toxins produced by *Clostridium botulinum*. These toxins are among the most potent known. The organism is a spore-forming anaerobe, which is widely distributed in the United States. The source of this disease in humans is improperly canned foods, especially the home-preserved variety. The toxin is absorbed in the upper gastrointestinal tract.

The average incubation period is 12 to 36 hours after ingestion of the contaminated food, though, rarely, it may be as short as 3 hours or as long as 2 weeks after inoculation. In general, the shorter the incubation period, the more serious the disease.

Symptoms are nausea, vomiting, weakness, lassitude and dizziness, progressing to skeletal muscle paralysis. While the patient appears alert and oriented, speech and swallowing may be difficult. The pupils are dilated and frequently nonreactive. Postural hypotension may be found, along with progressive muscle palsies in a previously healthy person.

The diagnosis may be established rather easily when a group of persons are stricken after ingesting home-preserved food, but if a single individual is involved, the diagnosis may be difficult. Laboratory examination of the suspected food may confirm the diagnosis.

Treatment is directed toward evacuating the gastrointestinal tract by cathartics and enemas. Fluid and electrolyte replacement may be necessary. Perhaps the most serious threat is respiratory paralysis, which requires ventilatory assist by tracheostomy and a volume respirator.

Polyvalent botulinus antitoxin should be given once the diagnosis is established clinically. Since this is derived from horse serum, the usual precautions of skin testing and desensitization should be observed when indicated. Guanidine hydrochloride may be helpful, since it binds the toxin.

The mortality rate, dependent on the particular type of toxin, varies from 10 to 70 percent.

THE DRUG OVERDOSE

The care of patients who have ingested drugs deserves special consideration, since these persons frequently present in an emergency care setting for treatment. Drug overdose continues to be an ever-increasing medical and social problem. In what can be described as the drug-oriented or "pill-popping" society that exists today, it cannot be predicted that the problem will diminish in the near future. While it is difficult to obtain accurate statistics on the true incidence of drug overdoses, it is estimated that approximately 22,000 suicide attempts involving drugs occur in the U.S. per year, with roughly one in 8 being successful. In addition, about 1,000,000 to 2,000,000 accidental poisonings occur per year in the pediatric age group, leading to an estimated 4,000 deaths.[28]

Nursing responsibilities

The emergency nurse has a number of responsibilities when caring for a patient who has overdosed. Initially, she must be able to determine the patient's need for life-support measures and to institute them as necessary. Supportive care is the mainstay in the management of the overdosed patient[12, 13, 30, 40] and takes precedence over any other form of management. Although these measures are detailed in other chapters, their importance must be recognized here, as well. Close, continued monitoring is essential, realizing that the patient's status can change suddenly.

It is also essential that the nurse be aware of the clinical manifestations associated with the commonly abused drugs and the methods by which these drugs can be counteracted or removed from the body. Certain contraindications or precautions exist with each method and will be detailed subsequently.

If the overdose has been self-inflicted rather than accidental, the need for emotional support and follow-up is important. The patient should be treated with respect and with concern for his well-being—an important point, since most suicide attempters have low self-esteem and do not need this self-concept reinforced further. Assessment and intervention, as detailed in Chapter 7, should be done and the patient placed in a therapist's care for follow-up and continued counseling, as indicated.

Treatment methods

A number of measures are used singly or in combination for the treatment of drug overdoses. The selection of method depends upon the drug taken, the time elapsed since ingestion and the presenting condition of the patient. These methods include the use of: (1) inducing emesis, (2) gastric lavage, (3) adsorbing agents, (4) purgatives, (5) antidotes, (6) forced diuresis and (7) hemodialysis. Of these measures, inducing emesis or using gastric lavage is commonly done to remove ingested material from the stomach. The administration of an adsorbing agent and a purgative frequently follows to prevent systemic absorption of a drug that has traveled beyond the stomach. The use of the last 3 methods outlined, antidotes, forced diuresis and hemodialysis, depends largely upon the drug ingested and the patient's condition.

Inducing emesis

Inducing emesis can be accomplished in a number of ways. At home, when syrup of ipecac is unavailable, it is advisable to stimulate the oropharynx with the finger or to give egg white to induce vomiting. Strong salt or mustard solutions no longer are recommended as emetics because of dangers inherent in their use.

For drug-induced emesis, only 2 agents can be used with safety—syrup of ipecac and apomorphine. They should be used only when the patient has a good sensorium and the development of lethargy and coma is unlikely; unless the patient is awake, the cough reflex may be depressed and may lead to aspiration of vomitus.

Syrup of ipecac is given in dosages determined by the patient's age: 15 ml. (1 tbsp.) for children 9 months to 2 years; 20 ml. (1 tbsp. + 1 tsp.) for children 2 years to 10 years; 30 ml. (2 tbsp.) for people over 10 years. Ipecac is a centrally acting drug; its site of action is the chemoreceptor trigger zone in the medulla. Hence, an effect will not be seen for 20 to 25 minutes. If this fact is not appreciated, repeated doses may be given before the effect of the first dose occurs, and this may result in protracted vomiting, an especially dangerous condition for children. For this reason, ipecac should be repeated only *once* and after a sufficient period of time has passed after the initial dose. When a drug with strong antiemetic properties has been ingested (e.g., phenothiazene derivatives such as Thorazine or Compazine), gastric lavage may be the method of choice.

A sufficient quantity of water must be given (one to 10 glasses) to produce emesis. Syrup of ipecac is available without prescription and should be kept in any home with young children.

Apomorphine is a powerful emetic, producing vomiting in about 5 minutes. Again, the patient should be given water beforehand. The drug is administered subcutaneously or intramuscularly in the following doses: 0.5 to 2.0 mg. or 0.03 mg. per pound of body weight for a one to 2-year-old child; 5 to 10 mg. for an adult. The drug is available in 6 mg. tablets, which should be stored in a dark, tightly stoppered bottle. The solution is prepared by crushing one tablet in a 5 ml. syringe and dissolving it in 3 ml. of sterile water.[6]

Apomorphine possesses narcotic properties and causes respiratory depression activity. Thus, it should not be given if a patient has taken a sedative or hypnotic or has respiratory depression. Naloxone hydrochloride (Narcan) is the antagonist to apomorphine; it reverses the emetic and narcotic effect of apomorphine without possessing similar activities itself.[39]

Gastric lavage

This procedure involves passing a large-bore, soft rubber tube (Ewald tube) into the stomach and with it washing the stomach with one to several liters of fluid, usually water or saline. In adults, 200 to 300 ml. should be instilled with each exchange until tablet fragments and dissolved drugs are removed, indicated by clear return of lavage fluid.[25]

This method is most frequently used on lethargic or comatose patients in whom aspiration of vomitus could occur. Hence, 2 precautions must be observed when using this procedure: (1) a cuffed nasotracheal or endotracheal tube must be in place prior to lavage; and (2) the patient should be placed on his left side, with his head hanging over the examining table and with his face down.

Lavage is contraindicated when a caustic or corrosive has been ingested because of possible perforation of the esophagus in passing the tube. Also, when strychnine has been ingested, lavage is contraindicated, since stimulation while passing the tube into the stomach may trigger convulsions.

Lavage may be ineffective for patients brought to an emergency department in a coma several hours after ingestion. Such patients may have very little, if any, drug remaining in the stomach, and lavage is not useful for material in the small bowel.[37] Conversely, if the drug does remain in the stomach, the lavage may actually wash the drug into the small bowel or hasten gastric emptying. Lipid-soluble drugs, such as glutethimide (Doriden), are not readily removed by aqueous lavage. For this reason, some advocate the use of a nonabsorbable oil, such as castor oil,[6] which acts as an adsorbent as well as a cathartic. It should be used with equal parts of water.

Of the two methods for removing gastric contents, inducing emesis has been demonstrated to be more effective than gastric lavage [10, 11, 12] since drug-induced emesis also empties the first portion of the duodenum. Neither gastric lavage nor emesis is very useful for removing a drug which is more distal, in the small bowel. In many instances, the patient is not encountered for many hours after the ingestion, at which point much of the material ingested has already escaped the stomach. Hence, emesis and gastric lavage will be of little benefit.

Several drugs are notorious for remaining in the small intestine for long periods of time and act as a reservoir for continued absorption. Drugs such as aspirin [23] and glutethimide (Doriden) [12] are reported to be absorbed for up to 48 hours post ingestion.

Adsorbing agents and purgatives

For drugs which have passed into the small bowel, the use of adsorbing agents and purgatives is helpful. Activated charcoal, given in a slurry of one ounce charcoal mixed with water, will act as an adsorbent for a wide variety of drugs and chemicals (except cyanide) [8,19] resulting in lower blood levels of the drugs.[3,14,20,35] It is best given alone, not in combination with certain purgatives, for example. Further, if ipecac is used, the charcoal must be given *following* emesis so it will not bind to the emetic and prevent emesis. The charcoal can be swallowed or given via lavage tube.

Purgatives hasten the transit of the ingested substance through the intestine and are especially useful when given concomitantly with charcoal. Commonly used agents are castor oil (one to 2 ounces) or sodium sulfate (one to 2 ounces of a 50 percent solution). Magnesium sulfate or magnesium citrate, while also frequently administered, are less desirable for two reasons: (1) the magnesium ion will bind to the charcoal and take up binding sites and (2) some magnesium ions will be absorbed and may act as a central nervous system depressant.

Purgatives are usually administered in the emergency department, and no further attention is paid to whether an effect is seen or not. Several ingested drugs have rather potent anticholinergic activity and decrease gastrointestinal motility. In patients ingesting such drugs, more than one dose of a purgative may be required.

Antidotes

For most patients who have ingested drugs or harmful substances, one of the 2 methods for removing them from the stomach, followed by administration of activated charcoal and a purgative, is the usual treatment of choice. However, certain drugs or chemicals can be treated by administration of an antidote to reverse or diminish the untoward effects of the offending agent.

An antidote can counteract a toxic substance by preventing absorption, by neutralizing it through changing its chemical nature or by counteracting its effects by producing other effects. For the wide variety of drugs available, there are relatively few specific antidotes. This is especially true for the sedative-hypnotic drugs frequently used in suicide attempts. Antidotes for specific substance ingestion are listed in Table 12–1.

Naloxone hydrochloride (Narcan) is the specific antidote for narcotic agents. It has an advantage over previously used antagonists in that it lacks intrinsic narcotic activity.[26] It is relatively safe and almost immediately effective.

Glucose is included in Table 12–1 as a reminder that patients in insulin shock may present similar to an overdosed patient. Fifty milliliters of a 50 percent solution is given intravenously *after* blood is drawn for glucose determination. As with Narcan for narcotic overdoses, glucose for the patient in insulin shock produces dramatic results within a short period of time.

Several other antidotes will be discussed later as they relate to treatment of specific drug overdoses.

Diuresis and hemodialysis

For removal of absorbed poisons, promoting diuresis and hemodialysis may be the methods to employ. Increased urinary flow can hasten elimination of many drugs which are excreted by the kidneys. Therefore, the use of water diuresis and osmotic diuresis and changing the pH of the urine may aid in elimination of selected types of drugs.

Hemodialysis is a method which may prove useful in some instances. Hemodialysis is not done in emergency departments and is mentioned here as one method which may be employed if more conservative methods fail. It has proven useful for the treatment of methanol detoxification and the renal failure associated with massive aspirin overdose.

Assessment and management for specific drug overdoses

In order to determine what kind of drug the patient has taken, the nurse must understand the syndromes of clinical signs and symptoms

TABLE 12–1 SPECIFIC ANTIDOTES FOR TOXIC AGENTS

Toxic agent	Antidote
(1) Opiates	Naloxone hydrochloride (Narcan)
(2) (Insulin)	(Glucose)
(3) Cholinesterase inhibitors	Atropine and pralidoxime chloride
(4) Methanol	Ethanol
(5) Iron	Sodium ferrocyanide and deferoxamine mesylate
(6) Atropine or scopolamine	Cholinesterase inhibitors (physostigmine)
(7) Warfarin	Vitamin K
(8) Arsenic or mercury	Dimercaprol (BAL)
(9) Lead	Ethylenediaminetetraacetic acid (EDTA)
(10) Cyanide	Nitrites and sodium thiosulfate
(11) Carbon monoxide	Oxygen or hyperbaric oxygen

which accompany overdoses of the various groups of drugs. She must also understand the terminology of the drug user so that the information she gathers from him or those attending him can be meaningful. Some commonly used terms are listed in Table 12–2.

Drugs are classified according to the chemical structure; hence, drugs in a classification have similar actions in the body. The commonly abused drugs are discussed below, as they relate to assessment and specific management of the patient who has overdosed on them.

Sedative-hypnotic drugs

The drugs that are most often used in suicide attempts are the sedatives, the barbiturates being the single most common group. The amount necessary to cause death may vary considerably, depending on the specific drug and the size of the patient. In general, however, the potentially *lethal dose is 10 times the hypnotic dose*. A synergistic effect exists when any of the sedatives are used with tranquilizers and alcohol, such that these substances will potentiate the lethality of the sedative and lower the amount necessary to cause death. Many times, the suicidal individual will attempt to "get up nerve" with a

couple of beers or shots of whiskey before taking an overdose.

Once an individual has taken a large enough dose of a sedative, without intervention, he will eventually become comatose and may succumb. Some of the sedatives, such as the barbiturates, cause hypothermia, respiratory depression, hypotension with decreased cardiac and renal output and decreased muscle reflexes.

The long-term use of prescription sedatives, with increases in amount taken and in tolerance, may become habituating. Treatment of sedative withdrawal, especially that of intermediate- and short-acting barbiturates must be accomplished by constant monitoring and careful decrease in dosage. Addiction to prescription sedatives warrants hospitalization, since an individual may convulse at any time, a consequence which can lead to death. *No individual who is addicted to sedatives should be allowed to withdraw suddenly or "go cold turkey,"* unlike the narcotic addict, who may become suddenly abstinent, and although suffering some discomfort, will generally not succumb.

Glutethimide (Doriden) is one sedative which deserves singular discussion, since patients who overdose on this drug often pre-

TABLE 12–2 COMMONLY USED TERMS OF THE DRUG USER

Colloquial terms	Definitions
Drugs	
(1) Reds (2) Rainbows (3) Yellow Jackets (4) Blue heavens (5) Goof balls (6) Pink lady	"Reds" are secobarbital sodium (Seconal); "yellow jackets" are pentobarbital sodium (Nembutal); numbers 1 through 6 are all barbiturates.
(7) Snow (8) Stuff (9) H (10) Junk (11) Smack	Numbers 7 through 11 all represent heroin.
(12) Bennies (13) Pep pills (14) Footballs (15) Whites (16) Hearts (17) Copilots	Numbers 12 through 17 all represent amphetamines. "Bennies" are specifically benzedrine.
(18) Snow (19) The Leaf (20) Speed ball	Numbers 18 through 20 denote cocaine; "speed ball" specifically denotes cocaine mixed with heroin.
(21) Joints (22) Sticks (23) Reefers (24) Weed (25) Grass (26) Pot (27) Mary Jane	Numbers 21 through 27 are all familiar names for marijuana.
(28) LSD (29) Acid (30) Mescaline (31) STP (32) DMT	Numbers 28 through 32 are common names for hallucinogens.
Drug amounts	
(1) Nickel bag	Five dollars worth of drugs. Formerly, this was 50 tablets, when used in reference to methamphetamine. Inflation has reduced the "nickel bag" to 30 or 40 tablets.
(2) Dime bag	Ten dollars worth of drugs.
(3) Jar	One thousand "whites" or "reds."
(4) Pillow	One hundred "jars."
(5) Spoon	A measurement of powdered drugs.
(6) Tabs	Tablets.
(7) Caps	Capsules.
(8) Lid	One ounce of marijuana.
Other terms	
(1) Score	Succeed in buying drugs.
(2) Busted	Arrested.
(3) Burn out	Lose desire for the drug.
(4) Freak	Drug user.
(5) Freaked out	Irrational on drugs.
(6) Blowing it	Becoming irrational on drugs; "freaking out."

TABLE 12–2, *cont.*

Colloquial terms	Definitions
Other terms, *cont.*	
(7) Stoned	In a stupor with drugs.
(8) Loaded	"Stoned."
(9) Out-to-lunch	"Super-stoned."
(10) Trip	Experience with LSD or other psycheledic drug or amphetamine.
(11) Crash	Sleep.
(12) Party	Get loaded with other drug users.
(13) Come down	Wear off the effect of a drug.
(14) Step on (a drug)	To cut a drug with some other substance, to dilute it.
(15) Strung out	Addicted.
(16) Cold turkey	Kicking a drug habit by total abstinence.

sent with peculiar manifestations. The patient is usually deeply comatose, with fixed, dilated pupils, secondary to the rather potent anticholinergic (atropine-like) activity of this drug. Respirations appear normal, color is good and arterial blood gases are usually normal. Yet this patient may suddenly become apneic when he is manipulated in some fashion.[36, 43] For this reason, *all patients with Doriden intoxication should be intubated prior to any diagnostic or therapeutic maneuver*. Because the body is unable to readily rid itself of this lipid-soluble drug, these patients should be admitted for close surveillance and treatment.

Tranquilizers

The most used minor tranquilizers are the benzodiazepines: chlordiazepoxide (Librium), diazepam (Valium) and oxazepam (Serax). When taken alone, these drugs are rather benign, in that no deaths have been reported. However, when taken in combination with the sedative-hypnotic drugs and/or with alcohol, the benzodiazepines may synergize with the central nervous system depressants to cause severe respiratory depression and hypotension.[11] These patients present in various states of consciousness, including coma, but they are not usually in a life-threatening situation. Important assessment information should include, however, whether the patient had taken other central nervous system depressants, as well.

The phenothiazine derivatives comprise the major tranquilizers, including: chlorpromazine (Thorazine), trifluoperazine (Stelazine), fluphenazine (prolixin), promazine (Sparine), prochlorperazine (Compazine), thioridazine (Mellaril) and perphenazine (Trilafon). An overdosed patient may present with any level of consciousness, including coma. As with the minor tranquilizers, this group also synergizes with other central nervous system depressants.

Other problems associated with tranquilizers occur to varying degrees and include the following.

(1) *Cardiac effects:* The phenothiazine derivatives produce a direct myocardial depression. ECG changes may become prominent, namely prolonged Q-T intervals and widened QRS complexes. Ventricular tachycardia, a life-threatening arrhythmia, may develop.

(2) *Severe hypotension:* This may develop following an overdose, since orthostatic hypotension is not uncommon even in therapeutic doses.[17] This phenomenon is probably secondary to several mechanisms:[33] a central nervous system effect, direct myocardial depression and vasodilation.

(3) *Extrapyramidal effects:* These include parkinsonian responses, spastic torticollis and opisthotonus. Such symptoms are both painful and frightening to the patient. Fortunately, parenteral administration of benztropine mesylate (Cogentin) [27] or diphenhydramine (Benadryl) [4] reverses these symptoms rather rapidly.

(4) *Seizures:* Phenothiazines lower the seizure threshold and thus may precipitate convulsions in the seizure-prone patient.[33]

Tricyclic antidepressants

Tricyclic antidepressants are frequently involved in overdoses. They include: imipramine (Tofranil), amitriptyline (Elavil), desipramine (Norpramin) and nortriptyline (Aventyl). Depressed persons being treated with these drugs comprise a high-risk group for suicide attempts.

These patients usually present with agitation or delirium or in coma. In addition, since these drugs possess potent anticholinergic properties,[18, 29, 38] intestinal ileus, bladder atony (requiring catheterization), dilated pupils and extreme thirst may also be present.

Cardiac arrhythmias, including sinus tachycardia, atrial fibrillation, atrial flutter, atrioventricular block, ventricular tachycardia and ventricular flutter have been reported.[2, 9, 15] If cardiac incapacity is suspected, cardiac monitoring is essential. The patient with an arrhythmia may respond to isoproterenol (Isuprel), electrical pacing and physostigmine (which may also reduce attendant agitation or delirium).

Narcotics

With today's heavy use of narcotics, a frequent visitor to the emergency department is the patient who has accidently overdosed on heroin. Overdoses with heroin are more often accidental than intentional, occurring when a relatively unadulterated quantity of the drug becomes available.

The classic triad of narcotic overdose is (1) stupor or coma, (2) respiratory depression and (3) pinpoint pupils. Pupils may be dilated, however, if other drugs have been ingested or if the patient has been hypoxic for a significant period of time. Additional clues include needle tracks and ice cubes around the groin or milk in the pharynx, representing efforts of friends to revive the patient.

Treatment consists mainly of ventilatory care and the use of the specific narcotic antagonist, naloxone hydrochloride (Narcan). Responses to this antagonist may be dramatic. However, giving Narcan to the heavy, chronic user could precipitate acute withdrawal symptoms and must be administered with caution.

Relapses may occur, since the antagonist's duration of action is shorter than that of the narcotic. This is especially true of methadone intoxication. Methadone activity may persist for 24 to 36 hours. This drug is now the second most commonly abused drug.

Pulmonary edema is not uncommon following acute narcotic overdose. This condition should be suspected in the patient who remains dyspneic after responding to Narcan. Aspiration pneumonia is a frequent sequela.

Amphetamines

The patient seen in the emergency department with amphetamine intoxication is the one who is on a "bad trip"—a toxic psychosis in which the patient suffers visual, tactile and auditory hallucinations and responds to these with systemized paranoid delusions.[5] This end result usually follows chronic overdose, although it may rarely be seen after a single, very large dose.

An aspect of amphetamine activity, better appreciated by the user than by health care professionals, is that amphetamine excretion depends on urinary pH. An alkaline urine favors the reabsorption of the amphetamine from the renal tubules back into the systemic circulation. Hence, many users take sodium bicarbonate along with their amphetamine to prolong their "high."

Management depends on protecting the patient from harming himself or others and reducing the psychotic state. Use of personnel or friends (who are not "high") to "talk down" the patient may be useful. For those who are extremely combative or difficult to manage, chlorpromazine (Thorazine) may be used.[24] Evidence suggests that an alkaline urine favors amphetamine metabolism and that the metabolites may be responsible for the psychosis.[5] An effort to acidify the urine (to a pH of less than 6.6) may be worthwhile to shorten the duration of the psychosis.[5, 10]

The cardiovascular status should also be evaluated, since hypertension and arrhythmias can attend the use of these central nervous system stimulants.

Salicylates

Salicylate overdose (salicylism) is fairly common, especially as an accidental ingestion in children who, unfortunately, are also most prone to develop dangerous metabolic derangements from it.

Acute intoxication produces acid-base disturbances which may differ in the adult and child.[22] The adult usually exhibits a respiratory alkalosis, followed by a respiratory acidosis if a large enough amount has been consumed. In most adults, the acid-base disturbance does not progress beyond this point. However, young children may develop a severe metabolic acidosis, which may be very difficult to treat.

Crucial to accurate assessment is knowing the quantity of salicylate ingested, determining blood salicylate levels and observing clinical manifestations seen in the patient.

Generally, a toxic dose is considered to be *one grain of salicylate per pound of body weight.* While most adult aspirin tablets contain 5 grains of acetylsalicylic acid, it must be remembered that some of the time-release preparations contain as much as 7 to 10 grains per tablet. Hence, determining the brand of salicylate taken is also helpful.

Serum salicylate levels compared to number of hours post ingestion provide a useful criterion in determining how much drug has been absorbed over time. Done's Nomogram (see Figure 12–1) can be applied when a single toxic dose of aspirin has been ingested and

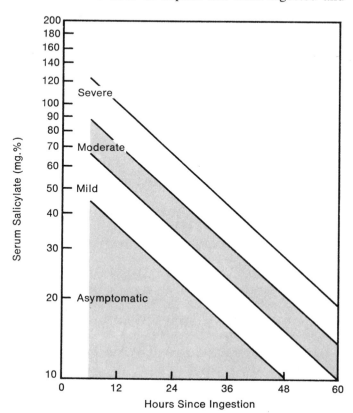

Figure 12–1 Done's Nomogram. The nomogram relates serum salicylate concentrations and expected severity of intoxication at varying intervals following ingestion of *one* large dose of salicylate.
Source: J. Arena, *Poisoning: Toxicology, Symptoms, Treatment,* ed. 2, 1975. Courtesy of Charles C Thomas, Publisher, Springfield, Ill.

sufficient time has elapsed for it to be absorbed. Generally, this period of absorption is at least 6 hours. Periodic comparisons of serum salicylate levels with time post ingestion indicate the amount of salicylate being absorbed. This value, compared with the severity of the patient's symptoms, is helpful in predicting the need for intensive treatment for salicylate intoxication. Values of 40 mg. percent 6 hours post ingestion require hospitalization or close supervision at home. However, hospitalization may be required in patients with values of 30 to 40 mg. percent when attended by symptoms of salicylate intoxication.[6]

Signs and symptoms of early salicylism may include gastrointestinal upset, tinnitus, diplopia, dizziness, lethargy and mental confusion. Later, marked dehydration may ensue due to an increased respiratory rate, sweating, vomiting and urine losses. These fluid losses may be grossly underestimated using the usual clinical criteria.[23, 39]

Marked hypokalemia may also be present. Paradoxically, marked hyperthermia may develop because of the effect of the salicylate level on metabolic rate.[23, 39] The patient may also be in an altered state of consciousness and have a hemorrhagic diathesis, secondary to aspirin's effect on platelets and prothrombin-dependent clotting factor synthesis.

Treatment, following initial removal of the drug from the stomach and use of adsorbing and purgative agents, is symptomatic and supportive and is dependent upon continued assessment of the patient. If a child is sent home from the emergency department, the parents should be instructed in observing their child for possible complications. In such a case, written instruction sheets for parents are invaluable. Table 12–3 offers an example of instructions to parents of a child who has ingested aspirin in a large dose.

Anticholinergic drugs

The anticholinergic drugs resemble atropine in effect and act as competitive blockers for the neurohormone acetylcholine, the

---

TABLE 12–3   INSTRUCTIONS TO PARENTS: INGESTION OF ASPIRIN

Your child has recently been seen in the Children's Hospital Emergency Room because of ingestion of aspirin or an aspirin-like product. Although we do not feel admission to the hospital is necessary at this time, there are several things which we would request you do at home.

Every hour for 8 hours:
(1) Count the number of breaths per minute and mark it on a piece of paper. If they show a tendency to increase in number, call the Poison Control Center for further instructions. Count breaths whether the child is asleep or awake.
(2) Place your hand in front of the child's mouth and measure how far away you can feel his breath. If this is more than 5 inches, please call the Poison Control Center.
(3) Encourage the child to drink as much water, cola, ginger ale, milk or other fluid as he will take.
(4) Let us know if the child persists in vomiting more than 2 hours after he returns home. If at any time you suspect your child is not breathing properly or any other new symptom develops, please feel free to call the Poison Control Center.

Please call the Poison Control Center or your doctor between 6 and 12 hours after you leave; the doctor on duty will instruct you on how much longer you need to continue the above directions.

Take whatever steps you feel will prevent a repeat episode, not just for aspirin, but for any pill or household product. Encourage your neighbors to do likewise.

Poison Control Center telephone:_____.
Call anytime, day or night.

Source: Adapted from Children's Hospital, Columbus, Ohio, protocol.

neurotransmitter for the parasympathetic nervous system.

The most frequently abused drug in this group is scopolamine, an ingredient in numerous over-the-counter sleep preparations. Overdoses of these preparations lead to a characteristic set of symptoms:

> Red as a beet,
> hot as a hare,
> dry as a bone,
> blind as a bat
> and mad as a hatter.

A flushed color to the skin is due to cutaneous vasodilatation; the dryness is caused by its effects on salivary and sweat glands. The patient may have an "anticholinergic fever," due to his inability to perspire, which may reach extreme levels. The central nervous system effects can cause severe hallucinations, agitation and delirium.

Most of these effects can be counteracted by (1) cholinesterase inhibitors (which allow acetylcholine to build up and overcome the competitive blockade) or (2) a direct-acting cogener of acetylcholine, such as methacholine (Mecholyl). The only effective drug for treatment of the central nervous system effects, however, is physostigmine.[32] It is the only drug of its kind which can pass the blood-brain barrier and thus control the cerebral effects. It is given subcutaneously or intramuscularly and shows rapid results. However, its action is shorter than that of scopolamine; so the patient may return to his previous behavior when the effects of the physostigmine subside.

Cholinesterase inhibitors

Cholinesterase inhibitors are most often used in insecticides and in chemical warfare agents; so exposures tend to be unintentional, through environmental or household accidents. Generally considered too toxic for the treatment of systemic disease, its main medical use is in topical administration to the eye for the treatment of glaucoma.

Ill-effects are produced from the accumulation of acetylcholine (since the action of cholinesterase is inhibited and thus cannot break down acetylcholine). Ensuing symptoms are then produced by a variety of mechanisms:

(1) *Overactivity of the parasympathetic nervous system:* This produces symptoms which comprise the SLUD syndrome: salivation, lacrimation, urination and defecation. In addition, bronchoconstriction and increased bronchial secretions occur.

(2) *Stimulation of skeletal muscle:* This leads first to muscle fasciculations, twitching and cramps, followed by fatigue, weakness and paralysis. These processes affect all striated muscles, including the diaphragm and intercostals.

(3) *Central nervous system effects:* These produce confusion, ataxia, slurred

TABLE 12–4   CATEGORIES OF DRUGS, WITH GENERIC AND TRADE NAMES

Drug generic name	Drug trade name
Sedative-hypnotic drugs (the barbiturates)	
(1) amobarbital	Amytal
(2) pentobarbital sodium	Nembutal
(3) secobarbital	Seconal
(4) meprobamate	Equanil, Miltown
(5) ethchlorvynol	Placidyl
(6) glutethimide	Doriden
Minor tranquilizers (the benzodiazepines)	
(1) chlordiazepoxide	Librium
(2) diazepam	Valium
(3) oxazepam	Serax
Major tranquilizers (the phenothiazine derivatives)	
(1) chlorpromazine	Thorazine
(2) trifluoperazine	Stelazine
(3) fluphenazine	Prolixin
(4) promazine	Sparine
(5) prochlorperazine	Compazine
(6) perphenazine	Trilafon
(7) thioridazine	Mellaril
Tricyclic antidepressants	
(1) imipramine	Tofranil
(2) amitriptyline	Elavil
(3) desipramine	Norpramin
(4) nortriptyline	Aventyl
Narcotics	
(1) methadone	Dolophine
Amphetamines	
(1) amphetamine	Benzedrine
(2) dextroamphetamine	Dexedrine
(3) methamphetamine	Methedrine
Other drugs used for treatment	
(1) benztropine	Cogentin
(2) diphenhydramine	Benedryl
(3) naloxone hydrochloride	Narcan
(4) methacholine	Mecholyl
(5) physostigmine	Eserine
(6) isoproterenol	Isuprel

speech, convulsions and central respiratory paralysis.[34]

Fortunately, some rather specific and efficacious antagonists are available for treatment of these formidable agents. Atropine is the first-line treatment and is usually given in heroic doses (up to 50 mg. per day)[34] to block the effect of acetylcholine. If the atropine is not effective, acetylcholine bromide (Pralidoxine) may be given. This drug breaks the bond between the cholinesterase and the inhibitor, thereby regenerating free enzyme. It should only be used if atropine fails, since it can produce severe cardiovascular toxicities.

Table 12–4 summarizes the drugs discussed in this chapter, by category and generic and trade names.

SUMMARY

The person exposed to a potentially lethal substance may be in a life-threatening state when the emergency nurse sees him. Although immediate intervention may be necessary, it must be based on careful assessment of the patient's clinical signs and symptoms, comparison of the signs and symptoms with knowledge of those substances known to cause them, the history of the incident and the specific precautions outlined in this chapter.

Once the patient has been medically treated and is no longer in danger, a determination of those factors contributing to the accident or suicide must be examined, and efforts must be made to reduce the possibility of recurrence in the future. The nurse's efforts may take the form of early crisis management (discussed in Chapter 7) with referral to a mental health professional or facility, patient and family teaching and/or referral or follow-up communication to the appropriate occupational health or public health agency.

BIBLIOGRAPHY

(1) Abdallah, A., and Tye, A.: "A Comparison of the Efficacy of Emetic Drugs and Stomach Lavage," *American Journal of Diseases of Children,* 113 (1967):571.

(2) Alexander, C., and Nino, A.: "Cardiovascular Complications in Young Patients Taking Psychotropic Drugs," *American Heart Journal,* 78 (1969):757.

(3) Alvan, G.: "Effect of Activated Charcoal on Plasma Levels of Nortriptyline after Single Doses in Man," *European Journal of Clinical Pharmacology,* 5 (1973):236.

(4) American College of Neuropsychopharmacology, Food and Drug Administration Task Force: "Neurologic Syndromes Associated with Antipsychotic Drug Use," *New England Journal of Medicine,* 289 (1973):20.

(5) Anggard, E., *et al.:* "Amphetamine Metabolism in Amphetamine Psychosis," *Clinical Pharmacology and Therapeutics,* 14 (1973):870.

(6) Arena, J.: *Poisoning: Toxicology, Symptoms, Treatment,* ed. 3 (Springfield, Ill.: Chas. C Thomas, Publisher, 1974).

(7) Arnold, F., *et al.:* "Evaluation of the Efficacy of Lavage and Induced Emesis in Treatment of Salicylate Poisoning," *Pediatrics,* 23 (1959):386.

(8) Atkinson, J., and Azarnoff, D.: "Comparison of Charcoal and Attapulgite as Gastrointestinal Sequestrants in Acute Drug Ingestions," *Clinical Toxicology,* 4 (1971):31.

(9) Barnes, R., *et al.:* "Electrocardiographic Changes in Amitriptyline Poisoning," *British Medical Journal,* 3 (1968):222.

(10) Beckett, A., and Rowland, M.: "Urinary Excretion Kinetics of Amphetamine in Man," *Journal of Pharmacy and Pharmacology,* 17 (1965):628.

(11) Bell, D. S.: "Dangers of Treatment of Status Epilepticus with Diazepam," *British Medical Journal,* 1 (1969):159.

(12) Chazan, J., and Cohen, J.: "Clinical Spectrum of Glutethimide Intoxication," *Journal of the American Medical Association,* 208 (1969):837.

(13) Chazan, J., and Garella, S.: "Glutethi-

mide," *Archives of Internal Medicine,* 128 (1971):215.

(14) Chernish, S.; Wolen, R., and Rodda, B.: "Adsorption of Propoxyphene Hydrochloride by Activated Charcoal," *Clinical Toxicology,* 5 (1972):317.

(15) Cooll, D., *et al:* "Amitriptyline and Cardiac Disease: Risk of Sudden Death Identified by Monitoring System," *Lancet,* 2 (1970):590.

(16) Corby, D., *et al.:* "The Efficiency of Methods Used to Evacuate the Stomach After Acute Ingestions," *Pediatrics,* 40 (1967):871.

(17) Curry, S., *et al.:* "Factors Affecting Chlorpromazine Plasma Levels in Psychiatric Patients," *Archives of General Psychiatry,* 22 (1970):209.

(18) Davis, J. and Termini, B.: "Attempted Suicide with Psychotropic Drugs: Diagnosis and Treatment," *Medical Counterpoint,* 1 (1969):59.

(19) Decker, W., *et al.:* "Adsorption of Drugs and Poisons by Activated Charcoal," *Toxicology and Applied Pharmacology,* 13 (1968):454.

(20) Decker, W., *et al.:* "Inhibition of Aspirin Absorption by Activated Charcoal and Apomorphine," *Clinical Pharmacology and Therapeutics,* 10 (1969):710.

(21) Derbes, V., *et al.:* "Insect Stings: Emergency Therapy for Severe Reactions," *Patient Care,* 6 (1972):46.

(22) Done, A.: "Treatment of Salicylate Poisoning," *Modern Treatment,* 8 (1971):528.

(23) Done, A.: "Treatment of Salicylate Poisoning: Review of Personal and Published Experiences," *Clinical Toxicology,* 1 (1968):451.

(24) Espelin, D., and Done, A.: "Amphetamine Poisoning," *New England Journal of Medicine,* 278 (1968):1361.

(25) Fane, L.; Combs, H., and Decker, W.: "Physical Parameters in Gastric Lavage," *Clinical Toxicology,* 4 (1971):389.

(26) Foldes, F.; Duncalf, D., and Keswabara, S.: "The Respiratory, Circulatory and Narcotic Antagonist Effects of Nalorphine, Levallorphan and Naloxone in Anesthetized Subjects," *Canadian Anesthesia Society Journal,* 16 (1969): 151.

(27) Grady, G. F., and Kursch, G. T.: "Pathogenesis of Bacterial Diarrhea," *New England Journal of Medicine,* 285 (1971):891.

(28) Gunn, D., and Goldenan, D.: "Extrapyramidal and Other Effects Induced by Neuroleptic Agents," *International Series of Neuropsychiatry,* 3 (1967):131.

(29) Harrison, T., *et al.:* *Principles of Internal Medicine,* ed. 6 (New York: McGraw-Hill Book Company, 1970), p. 643.

(30) Harthorne, J., *et al.:* "Management of Massive Imipramine Overdosage with Mannitol and Artificial Dialysis," *New England Journal of Medicine,* 268 (1963):33.

(31) Henderson, L., and Merrill, J.: "Treatment of Barbiturate Intoxication," *Annals of Internal Medicine,* 64 (1966): 876.

(32) Hollister, L.: "Overdoses of Psychotherapeutic Drugs," *Clinical Pharmacology and Therapeutics,* 7 (1966):142.

(33) Innes, I., and Nickerson, M.: "Drugs Inhibiting the Action of Acetylcholine on Structures Innervated by Postganglionic Parasympathetic Nerves," in L. Goodman and A. Gilman (eds.), *The Pharmacological Basis of Therapeutics,* ed. 2 (New York: The Macmillan Company, 1961).

(34) Jarvik, M. E.: "Drugs Used in the Treatment of Psychiatric Disorders," in L. Goodman and A. Gilman (eds.), *The Pharmacological Basis of Therapeutics,* ed. 3 (New York: The Macmillan Company, 1965).

(35) Koelle, G.: "Anticholinesterase Agents," in L. Goodman and A. Gilman (eds.), *The Pharmacological Basis of Therapeutics,* ed. 3 (New York: The Macmillan Company, 1965).

(36) Koenig, M. G.: "Food Poisoning," *in* P. B. Breson and W. McDermott (eds.), *Cecil-Loeb's Textbook of Medicine,* 13th ed. (Philadelphia: W. B. Saunders Company, 1971).

(37) Levy, G., and Tsuchiya, T.: "Effect of Activated Charcoal on Aspirin Absorption in Man," *Clinical Pharmacology and Therapeutics,* 13 (1972):317.

(38) Maher, J., *et al.:* "Acute Glutethimide Intoxication," *American Journal of Medicine,* 33 (1962):70.

(39) Mathew, H., and Mackintosh, T.: "Gastric Aspiration and Lavage in Acute Poisoning," *British Medical Journal,* 1 (1968):1333.

(40) Noble, J., and Matthew, H.: "Acute Poisoning by Tricyclic Antidepressants: Clinical Features and Management of 100 Patients," *Clinical Toxicology,* 2 (1969):403.

(41) Rausten, D., and Ochs, M.: "Apo-morphine-Naloxone Controlled Rapid Emesis," *Journal of the American College of Emergency Physicians,* 5 (1973):44.

(42) Rice, A. J., and Wilson, W. R.: "Rapid Identification of Drugs in Body Fluids of Comatose Patients," *Clinical Toxicology,* 6 (1973):59.

(43) *Salmonella Surveillance: Annual Survey, 1971* (Atlanta: The Center for Disease Control, 1972).

(44) Segar, W., and Holliday, M.: "Physiologic Abnormalities of Salicylate Intoxication," *New England Journal of Medicine,* 259 (1958):1491.

(45) Sturkey, H.: "Ipecac Syrup: Its Use as an Emetic in Poison Control," *Journal of Pediatrics,* 69 (1966):139.

(46) Wright, N., and Roscoe, P.: "Acute Glutethimide Poisoning," *Journal of the American Medical Association,* 214 (1970):1704.

APPENDIX D

Poisonous parts of common house and garden plants

Plant	Toxic parts	Symptoms
Flower garden plants		
(1) Autumn crocus (meadow crocus)	All parts	Vomiting, nervous excitement.
(2) Azalea	All parts	Produces nausea and vomiting, depression, difficult breathing. May be fatal.
(3) Bleeding heart (Dutchman's breeches)	Foliage, roots	May cause convulsions and difficult breathing when eaten in large quantities.
(4) Christmas rose	Rootstocks, leaves	Inflammation of skin, numbing of oral tissues, gastric distress and nervous effects.
(5) Daffodil	Bulb	Nausea, vomiting, diarrhea. May be fatal.
(6) Delphinium	Seeds, young plants	Stomach upset, nervous excitement or depression if eaten in large quantities. Toxicity decreases with age of plant.
(7) Four-o'clock	Roots, seeds	The powdered root is an irritant to the skin, nose and throat.
(8) Foxglove	Leaves, seeds	One of the sources of the drug digitalis, used to stimulate the heart. In large amounts, the active principles cause dangerously irregular heartbeat and pulse, usually digestive upset and mental confusion. May be fatal.

Source: Prepared and published by The National Association of Retail Druggists, One E. Wacker Dr., Chicago, Ill. 60601

Plant	Toxic parts	Symptoms
Flower garden plants, *cont.*		
(9) Hyacinth	Bulb	Nausea, vomiting, diarrhea. May be fatal.
(10) Iris (blue flag)	Underground stems	Severe, but not usually serious, digestive upset.
(11) Jonquil	Bulb	Nausea, vomiting, diarrhea. Convulsions and death if eaten in large quantities.
(12) Larkspur	Seeds, young plants	Digestive upset, nervous excitement, depression. May be fatal.
(13) Lily-of-the-valley	Leaves, flowers	Irregular heartbeat and pulse, usually accompanied by digestive upset and mental confusion.
(14) Monkshood	Roots, seeds, leaves	Digestive upset and nervous excitement.
(15) Morning glory	Seeds	Produce LSD-like effects but can cause death from severe mental disturbances.
(16) Narcissus	Bulb	Nausea, vomiting, diarrhea. May be fatal.
(17) Oleander	Leaves, branches	Dizziness, nausea, irregular heartbeat. May be fatal.
(18) Peony	Roots	Juice can cause paralysis.
(19) Star-of-Bethlehem	Bulb	Vomiting and nervous excitement.
(20) Violet (pansy)	Seeds	In quantity, the cathartic effects can be serious to a child.
House plants		
(1) Caladium	Leaves, roots	Irritation of mouth, tongue and throat. Difficult breathing, nausea, vomiting and diarrhea.
(2) Castor bean	Seeds	Burning of mouth and throat, excessive thirst, convulsions. One or 2 seeds are near the lethal dose for adults.
(3) Dumbcane (dieffenbachia)	All parts	Intense burning and irritation of the mouth and tongue. Death can occur if base of tongue swells enough to block the air passage of the throat.
(4) Elephant ear philodendron	All parts	Intense burning and irritation of mouth and tongue. Death can occur if base of tongue swells enough to block the air passage of the throat.
(5) Jequirity bean	Seeds	Stomach pains, irregular pulse, cold sweat. May be fatal.
(6) Mistletoe	Berries	Acute stomach and intestinal irritation with diarrhea and slow pulse. May be fatal.
(7) Mother-in-law	Leaves	Enzyme that produces swelling of tongue.
(8) Poinsettia	Leaves	Severe irritation to mouth, throat and stomach. May be fatal.
(9) Rosary pea	Seeds	Stomach pains, irregular pulse, cold sweat. May be fatal.
Ornamental plants		
(1) Daphne	Berries, bark, leaves	Upset stomach, abdominal pain, vomiting, bloody diarrhea, weakness, convulsions and kidney damage.
(2) Golden chain	Bean-like capsules in which seeds are suspended	Severe poisoning. Excitement, staggering, convulsions, nausea and coma. May be fatal.

Plant	Toxic parts	Symptoms
Ornamental plants, *cont.*		
(3) Lantana (red sage, wild sage)	Green berries	Affects lungs, kidneys, heart and nervous system. (Grows in southern U.S. and in moderate climates.) May be fatal.
(4) Magnolia	Flower	Headache and depression.
(5) Rhododendron (western azalea)	All parts	Nausea, vomiting, depression, difficult breathing, prostration and coma. May be fatal.
(6) Wisteria	Seeds, pods	Mild to severe digestive upset.
(7) Yellow jessamine	Berries	Digestive disturbance and nervous symptoms. May be fatal.
(8) Yew	All parts, except fleshy red pulp of fruit	Foliage more toxic than berries. Convulsions with rapid death.
Trees and shrubs		
(1) Apple	Seeds	In quantity (50 or more), cyanide poisoning. May be fatal.
(2) Black locust	Bark, sprouts, foliage, seeds	Children have suffered nausea, weakness and depression after chewing the bark and seeds.
(3) Cherry	Leaves, twigs, seeds	Contains a compound that releases cyanide when eaten. Difficult breathing, excitement, paralysis of voice and prostration. May be fatal.
(4) Elderberry	All parts, especially roots	Nausea and digestive upset.
(5) Oak	Foliage, acorns	Affects kidneys gradually. Symptoms appear only after several days or weeks. Takes a large amount for poisoning.
(6) Peach	Leaves, twigs, seeds	Contains a compound that releases cyanide when eaten. Difficult breathing, excitement, paralysis of voice and prostration. May be fatal.
Vegetable garden plants		
(1) Potato	All green parts	Cardiac depression. May be fatal.
(2) Rhubarb	Leaf blade	Kidney damage. Large amounts of raw or cooked leaves can cause convulsions, coma, followed rapidly by death.
(3) Tomato	Green parts	Cardiac depression. May be fatal.
Wild plants		
(1) Baneberry	All parts	Stomach and intestinal irritation, spasms.
(2) Buttercup	All parts	Irritant juices may severely injure the digestive system.
(3) Jack-in-the-pulpit	All parts	Intense irritation and burning of mouth and tongue.
(4) Jimson weed (thorn apple)	All parts	Abnormal thirst, distorted sight, delirium, incoherence and coma. May be fatal.
(5) Marsh marigold (cowslip)	All parts	Irritation of oral tissues, digestive upset, diarrhea, respiratory depression and convulsions.
(6) Moonseed	Berries	(Blue-purple color, resembling wild grapes.) Severe digestive upset and abdominal pain.

Poisonous parts of common house and garden plants, *cont.*

Plant	Toxic parts	Symptoms
Wild plants, *cont.*		
(7) Mushrooms (fly agaric and amanita)	All parts	Stomach cramps, thirst, difficult breathing. Fatal. AVOID ALL WILD MUSHROOMS UNLESS POSITIVE OF THEIR IDENTITY.
(8) Nightshade	All parts	Intense digestive disturbances and nervous symptoms. May be fatal.
(9) Poison hemlock	All parts	Digestive disturbances. May be fatal.
(10) Poison ivy, oak, sumac	All parts	Itching, burning, redness.
(11) Skunk cabbage	Leaves, rhizomes	Burning and swelling of mouth, tongue and throat. Large quantities may cause stomach and intestinal irritation.
(12) Water hemlock (cowbane)	All parts	Diarrhea, convulsions. May be fatal.

13

Respiratory emergencies

JAMES H. COSGRIFF, JR.

Patients with acute respiratory problems are commonly seen in the emergency department and represent the highest priority of care. Compromise of respiration may result from a variety of causes, including trauma, infections, degenerative disease, neoplasms and foreign bodies. Some patients may present to the emergency department with a primary complaint of respiratory impairment, while others, particularly those in coma or with thoracic injury, may develop airway difficulties during the interval they are being treated in the emergency department.

It is important for the emergency nurse to be able to assess patients with respiratory distress and to determine what measures are necessary to correct their problems. To achieve this, the nurse must be familiar with respiratory physiology and the mechanics of respiration. This chapter will include a discussion of the anatomy and physiology of the respiratory tract, methods of airway maintenance and management of specific types of acute respiratory insufficiency.

ANATOMY AND PHYSIOLOGY

Respiration may be broadly defined as the gaseous interchange which occurs between an organism and its environment. Humans depend on oxygen to maintain normal cellular activity. Respiration depends on the transfer of oxygen and carbon dioxide between inspired air and the pulmonary capillaries, frequently called external respiration, and between the blood and tissues cells, called internal respiration. This transfer of gases occurs by diffusion, which depends on the partial pressure of each of the gases in both the air and the body tissues. Table 13–1 shows the partial pressures of oxygen and carbon dioxide in the atmosphere, alveoli and blood.

Anatomically, the chest wall is composed of a bony cage, the ribs, with supporting soft tissue structures, primarily the intercostal muscles. The lungs are paired organs lying within the chest cavity and consisting of millions of small air-containing structures called alveoli. It is in these alveoli that external respiration takes place. The lungs are covered by a thin cellular layer called the visceral pleura, which is reflected onto the chest wall as its inner lining and called the parietal pleura. Each lung is contained within its pleural cavity on either side of the mediastinum. The inferior border of the pleural cavity is the diaphragm, which separates the thoracic and abdominal cavities. The upper limit is the apex of the pleura, which extends

TABLE 13–1 PARTIAL PRESSURES OF OXYGEN AND CARBON DIOXIDE IN ATMOSPHERE, ALVEOLAR AIR AND BLOOD (AT SEA LEVEL, 760 MM. HG)

Gas	Atmosphere (mm. Hg)	Alveolar air (mm. Hg)	Venous blood (mm. Hg)	Arterial blood (mm. Hg)
Oxygen	157	100	40	93
Carbon dioxide	0.3	40	46	40
%Oxygen saturation of hemoglobin			75	97
Plasma pH			7.35	7.38

Source: Modified from pp. 6–5 and 6–6 of Charles H. Best and Norman B. Taylor, *Physiological Basis of Medical Practice*, ed. 9, ed. by John R. Brobeck. © 1973 The Williams & Wilkins Company, Baltimore.

above the level of the clavicles to the supra-clavicular space. Laterally is the rib cage, and medially is the mediastinum.

The entrance to the respiratory tract is the upper airway, including the mouth, the nasal cavity and the pharynx, which communicates at the glottis (vocal cords) with the trachea, a tubular structure extending from the level of the thyroid cartilage to approximately the second intercostal space. At this point, it divides into two main bronchi. Each bronchus leads into a lung and subsequently divides into smaller and smaller passageways within the lung until the alveoli are reached. The alveoli are thin-walled structures in which the air exchange takes place. The pulmonary capillaries are located within the alveolar walls. It is in this area that the capillary blood is separated from the alveolar air by 2 very thin membranes, through which the oxygen and carbon dioxide transfer occurs.

Unique to the pleural space (the chest cavity external to the lungs) is that intra-pleural pressure is subatmospheric, in other words, negative, in relation to environmental air and thus to the air in the alveoli. This negative intrapleural pressure is approximately −2.5 cm. of water. It is this negative pressure which assists in keeping the lungs expanded. Inspiration occurs by contraction of the intercostal muscles, which raises the ribs and expands the chest wall. The dia-phragm descends, acting as a bellows; thus air is drawn into the lungs until full expansion occurs. At the end of inspiration, the negative

intrapleural pressure rises to −7 to −8 cm. of water.

Expiration at rest is a passive action, in which the contraction of the intercostal mus-cles stops and the elastic recoil of the lungs occurs, causing the air to be expelled. The amount of air which is taken in during an ordi-nary inspiration averages 500 cc. in an adult and is called the *tidal air* or *tidal volume*. It can be easily measured by a respirometer and is one measure of respiratory activity.

As the air enters the alveoli with inspiration, the difference in partial pressure of gases in the alveolar air and the pulmonary capillary (venous) blood results in a free interchange of oxygen and carbon dioxide within the lungs. This blood, now arterialized, goes back into the left heart via the pulmonary circulation and is subsequently pumped into the systemic circulation. (See Figure 13–1.) As this blood reaches the arterial capillaries in the body, there is a diffusion of oxygen and carbon dioxide between the capillaries and adjacent tissues. The venous capillary blood leaving the tissues in the area contains a lower amount of oxygen and a relatively higher concen-tration of carbon dioxide and is returned to the right heart and lung for reoxygenation.

PULMONARY ASSESSMENT

Pulmonary function studies are rarely required in an emergency setting. More impor-tant to the emergency patient is the deter-mination of blood gases, which is a good

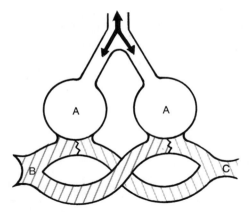

Figure 13-1 Diagrammatic illustration of the normal process of respiration. Air enters the pulmonary alveoli (A). Pulmonary venous blood (B) is oxygenated through the alveolocapillary membrane, thus producing arterial blood (C), which is then returned to the left side of the heart.

measure of pulmonary function. These tests are done on arterial blood, and the results are expressed as the partial pressures of oxygen (pO_2) and carbon dioxide (pCO_2), the oxygen saturation and the pH of arterial blood. Table 13-2 gives normal values for arterial blood gases. Such studies are essential to any emergency department patient and should be available on a 24-hour basis. Baseline arterial blood gas values should be secured on any patient with severe injury, shock or respiratory embarrassment.

History and examination

The extent of assessment will depend on the condition of the patient. Assessment of the patient with respiratory embarrassment should

TABLE 13-2 NORMAL VALUES FOR ARTERIAL BLOOD GASES

Gas	Value
pH	7.4 ± 0.3
pCO_2	40 ± 4 mm. Hg
pO_2	80–100 mm. Hg
Standard bicarbonate	24 ± 2 mEq./1
Base excess	0 ± 2.5 mEq./1
Buffer base	46 ± 1 mEq./1
Oxygenation saturation	95–97%

include a history of the onset of symptoms, i.e., whether abrupt or over a period of days or weeks. This should also note if the respiratory symptoms develop while at rest or with exertion. The nurse-assessor inquires whether the chest pain is aggravated by respiration and if there has been any cough, fever, chills, or associated injury. Another important sign is whether any sputum was raised. If so, the patient should describe the color: white, yellow, bloody. The patient should also be asked to estimate, if possible, the amount of sputum: teaspoon, tablespoon. The nurse should also inquire about any preexisting condition known to the patient, such as heart disease, hypertension, emphysema, bronchitis, asthma. Knowing whether the patient is a smoker is also important. Pulmonary problems are more common with cigarette smoking than with cigar or pipe smoking, since the latter 2 are rarely inhaled.

Physical evaluation should begin with a rapid assessment of airway patency. Excessive secretions, foreign bodies or dentures should be removed from the mouth or pharynx. If there is evidence of a mechanical obstruction in the upper airway, either it must be removed or measures must be initiated to bypass it. Once the airway is established, assessment may proceed. Vital signs are recorded. The nurse should also note any cyanosis of the lips, earlobes or nailbeds and the character of respiration. Normal respiratory movements occur by expansion of the chest through active elevation of the rib cage and depression of the diaphragm. Dyspneic patients may have an apprehensive look and utilize the accessory muscles of respiration. In such patients, supraclavicular tugging, manifested by retraction of the supraclavicular space, is common. The nares may flare with inspiration.

In patients with emphysema, the chest is typically increased in its antero-posterior diameter—the so-called barrel chest. During expiration, such a patient may be seen to expire between pursed lips. This is a mechanism which increases the expiratory pressure in the airway and allows better movement of air. Rate and depth of respiration and whether there is a labored effort to breathe, including any evidence of "splinting" of the chest wall should be noted. Splinting is quite common in patients suffering from pleurisy or chest wall injuries; because of the accompanying pain, movements of the chest wall are diminished on the involved side. In acute pulmonary edema frothy sputum may be found in the mouth or nose. It may or may not be blood-tinged. Patients with asthmatic conditions may be wheezing audibly. Auscultatory examination is done to assess the movement of air in and out of the lungs.

Following this physical examination, the remainder of the assessment should be completed.

Adjunct studies

Adjunct studies, depending primarily on the etiology of the condition, include routine blood work, chest x-ray, arterial blood gases and, rarely, pulmonary function tests. X-ray examination of the chest is probably the most helpful adjunct study in the patient with respiratory distress. Mass lesions, such as tumors, infectious processes, pneumonia, atelectasis, pneumothorax, pulmonary edema, chronic bronchitis and emphysema are among the conditions that may be identified with a routine chest x-ray. Rib fractures can also be seen.

Leukocytosis frequently accompanies infectious processes, while eosinophilia is noted in many patients with asthma of allergic origin. Tests to affirm these conditions will help in assessment.

Arterial blood gas studies are the single most important method to assess cardiopulmonary functions in the emergency department. Any condition which might affect the diffusion of gases across the alveolopulmonary capillary membrane may cause an aberration in the arterial gases (Figure 13–2). At the same time, variations in pulmonary tissue perfusion due to changes in blood flow within the lungs because of the develop-

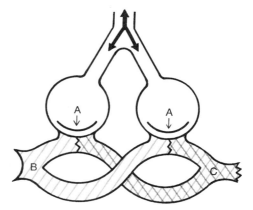

Figure 13–2 Impaired diffusion of gases. Thickening of the alveolocapillary membrane (A) impairs diffusion of gases. Pulmonary venous blood (B) is incompletely oxygenated on return to the left side of the heart via the pulmonary veins (C).

ment of precapillary shunts, may result in adequate gas exchange in some segments of the lungs and inadequate exchange in others. The result is a mixing of oxygenated blood with blood which is insufficiently oxygenated (Figure 13–3). The mixture thus produced may be less than adequate in total oxygen

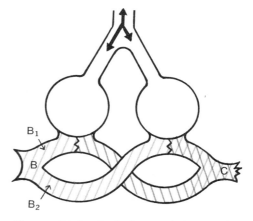

Figure 13–3 Perfusion variations due to selective shunting. Diminished perfusion of the alveoli by selective shunting within the lung causes incomplete oxygenation of the venous blood. The above diagram illustrates normal flow through one pulmonary venous channel (B₁) and diminished flow through another (B₂). The end result is incomplete oxygenation of blood in the pulmonary vein (C).

content, depending upon the percentage of lung area inadequately perfused in the shunting process. Normal arterial blood gas values are found in Table 13–2.

Another cause of abnormal blood gas levels is lowered tissue perfusion. In patients with circulatory embarrassment due to hypotension or myocardial failure, slowing of the circulation may result in lowered blood oxygen tension and elevated carbon dioxide levels (lactic acidosis).

PROVIDING AN AIRWAY

Establishing and maintaining a patent airway is of the highest priority. The ideal method used depends on the condition of the patient and the cause of the airway compromise.

Secretions should be aspirated from the mouth and pharynx when present. The oral cavity and throat are then checked for the presence of any solid foreign bodies or food particles, including ingested material and dentures. These may be removed with a finger, taking care not to be bitten by a struggling patient. If the patient's teeth are clenched tightly, the index finger may be inserted alongside the teeth in the bucco-gingival groove, reaching the pharynx behind the last molar. This safely loosens a foreign body. A device

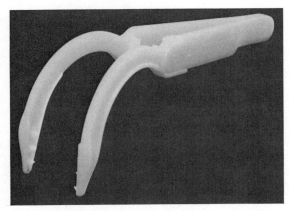

Figure 13–4 The Choke-Saver. The "teeth" at the tip of this device grasp the foreign body. A solid block at the interior neck of the device prevents its closure when in use (see inner right jaw).

often used in rescue vehicles is the Choke-Saver (see Figure 13–4). It has a protective device, which prevents tight closure of its jaws and damage to tissue.

In a critical situation involving a patient choking on a bolus of food, a technique described by Heimlich may be useful in freeing the trapped food and thus opening the airway. The rescuer stands behind the victim and extends his arms around him just below the ribs, allowing the upper body to hang forward. The rescuer, grasping his own wrists, exerts a sudden pressure on the abdomen, forcing the diaphragm upward and ejecting the obstructing bolus.[7] Since Heimlich's original report in 1974, a number of successful rescues have been reported.

In an unconscious or depressed patient, the airway may be occluded by relaxation of the jaw, which causes the mandible, tongue and floor of the mouth to collapse posteriorly into the pharynx. This situation may be corrected by pulling the tongue forward with a sponge forceps or by elevating the angles of the mandible and extending the neck (Figure 13–5). Keep in mind that in an unconscious patient, cervical spine injury must be ruled out before effecting this maneuver. To maintain this position, a rubber or plastic oropharyngeal airway (Figure 13–6) should be emplaced or a soft rubber nasopharyngeal airway inserted. If the obstruction is not relieved, endotracheal intubation is necessary.

Every emergency department should be equipped with a laryngoscope and varying size blades (Figure 13–7) and a variety of endotracheal tubes from infant to adult sizes (Figure 13–8). If the patient is vomiting, a cuffed tube should be inserted to lessen the probability of aspiration. Caution must be taken not to insert the tube too far, since it can be passed into the right main bronchus and thus occlude the left main bronchus. Should these measures fail, an esophageal obturator airway may be inserted into the esophagus and ventilatory assist added by use of a properly fitting mask. (See Figure 13–9.)

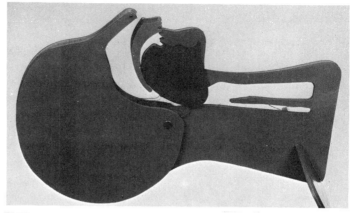

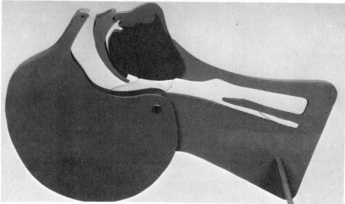

Figure 13–5 Airway occlusion and opening. Top: Model illustrates upper airway obstruction caused by a lax jaw, with the tongue collapsing into the pharynx. Bottom: Elevating the jaw and extending the neck raises the tongue from the pharynx and opens the airway.

Cricothyrotomy can be done with relative ease by inserting a large bore needle into the trachea percutaneously through the crico-thyroid membrane, which may be palpated in the midline of the neck. (The cricoid cartilage, the first tracheal ring, is usually easily felt just inferior to the thyroid cartilage. Between the 2, a diamond-shaped defect may be pal-pated. This is the cricothyroid membrane.) A number 13 needle is used. Care must be taken not to perforate the posterior wall of the trachea and the esophagus. This procedure is rarely performed in the emergency depart-ment and should be done only when other measures fail or when personnel qualified to perform a tracheostomy are not available.

Tracheostomy should be done when simpler measures fail or when better control of the airway is required to remove secretions and/or

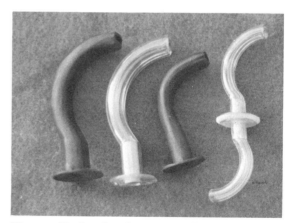

Figure 13–6 Oropharyngeal airways. Various sizes of oropharyngeal airways may be used to maintain patency of the patient's airway. The device on the right may also be used to apply mouth-to-mouth resuscitation.

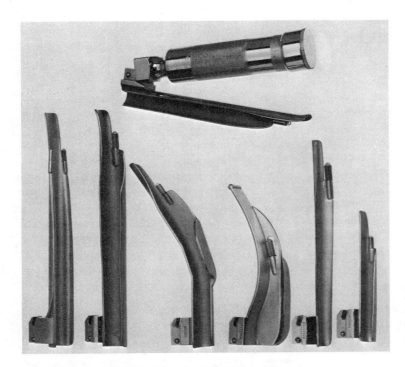

Figure 13–7 Laryngoscope and blades. Laryngoscope handle and varying sizes of lighted blades are shown, used to visualize the glottis when inserting an endotracheal tube.

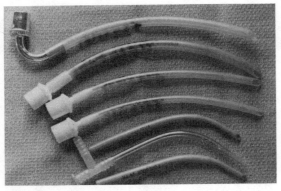

Figure 13–8 An assortment of endotracheal tubes. Endotracheal tubes are available in graduated sizes. The tubes shown do not have an inflatable cuff. Those tubes with an external diameter of 6 mm. or more can be fitted with a cuff. Most of these tubes are of the disposable type and can be purchased in individual sterile packages. The tubes in the photograph are fitted with various types of adapters, which are necessary for connection to standard resuscitation equipment.

assist with ventilation. It is *not* a simple surgical procedure and can be fraught with complications. The tracheostomized patient requires close attention. A variety of tracheos-

tomy tubes are in current use. The most common are of plastic material and contain an inflatable cuff.

SPECIFIC CAUSES OF ACUTE RESPIRATORY DISTRESS

There are many types and causes of acute respiratory distress. However, the patients who present to the emergency department with this problem, for the most part, fall into one of 3 categories:

(1) Acute pulmonary edema.
(2) Acute exacerbation or complication of chronic lung disease.
(3) Obstructive processes.

Acute pulmonary edema

Acute pulmonary edema, as the name implies, has a rather abrupt onset and is accompanied by development of fluid in the alveoli. This causes a widening of the alveolopulmonary capillary membrane. It may result from a number of factors, including inhalation of noxious fumes, pulmonary embolism,

Figure 13–9 The esophageal obturator airway. The tube has a closed end, which is inserted into the esophagus after adequate lubrication. The cuff at the lower end of the tube is inflated to occlude the esophagus, and the mask is applied tightly over the patient's mouth and nose to form a closed system. Air is then introduced into the open end of the tube either by a bag-valve device or mouth-to-tube insufflation. The air passes out of the perforations seen in the upper half of the tube and inflates the lungs.

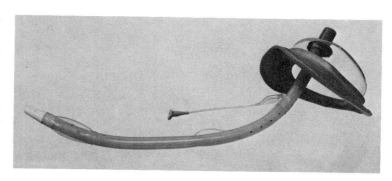

mitral stenosis, pulmonary infection and heroin overdose. But perhaps the most common cause is acute left ventricular heart failure precipitated by acute myocardial infarction or severe hypertension. Although the mechanism may vary, the physiological alteration that occurs is an increase in permeability of the alveolocapillary membrane with passage of fluid across this barrier from the capillaries into the alveoli. As a result, gas exchange is diminished, resulting in hypoxemia (lessened oxygen tension in the blood) and later in hypercarbia (increased carbon dioxide tension in the blood). The patient becomes dyspneic, tachypneic and apprehensive. This, in turn, increases the cardiac rate and may lead to further cardiac decompensation and further outpouring of fluid into the alveoli. The history of cardiac disease may be obtained, but in many patients, the initial episode may be the first evidence of cardiac abnormality. In others, exposure to fumes or drugs may be noted as causative factors.

Physical assessment will reveal an apprehensive, breathless patient. Cyanosis of the lips, earlobes and nailbeds is often present. The patient is usually unable to lie flat, and frequently frothy white or pink-tinged sputum may be flowing from the mouth or nose. Vital signs will reveal a tachypnea and tachycardia. The blood pressure may be normotensive, hypertensive or hypotensive, depending on the underlying etiology. In cardiac disease, dysrhythmias may be noted, especially auricular fibrillation. The superficial neck veins will be distended as a result of an increase in venous pressure. Auscultation of the chest reveals rales throughout with impaired breath sounds. Peripheral edema may be noted.

Important adjunct studies include complete blood count and electrolyte and arterial blood gas determinations. The latter may reveal a decrease in oxygen tension and an increase in carbon dioxide. Central venous pressure is elevated in edema of cardiac origin. Arm-to-lung and arm-to-tongue circulation time will be lengthened. Electrocardiograms may demonstrate an arrhythmia or findings indicative of acute coronary artery disease. Chest x-ray characteristically shows some increase in bronchovascular markings and commonly a hydrothorax, but these findings are not present in every patient.

Management is directed toward generally improving ventilation but more specifically toward correcting the etiology of the problem. Medication should be given by the intravenous route only, particularly in cardiac patients or when blood pressure is at hypotensive levels. Morphine sulfate in a dose of 0.008 or 0.010 gm. may be given to allay apprehension and slow the respiratory rate. An intravenous line should be placed with a large-bore needle to give medication, draw blood samples and, if indicated, perform a phlebotomy for reducing circulating blood volume.

In acute pulmonary edema of cardiac origin, specific treatment consists of oxygen by mask (40 to 60 percent O_2) or oxygen bubbled through 50 percent ethyl alcohol with intermittent positive pressure breathing. The alcohol lowers surface tension in the lungs and acts as a sedative. Cardiotonic drugs (to strengthen contractility) and diuretic agents are given as indicated. The cardiac drugs include digoxin, and ouabain. The most effective diuretics are furosemide or ethacrynic acid. Cardiac arrhythmias are managed as indicated. Severe hypertension may be managed with trimethaphan camphorsulfonate (Arfonad), given by intravenous drip. It must be monitored carefully, since it may decrease coronary artery perfusion. The patient should be transferred to the coronary care unit as soon as possible.

Patients with acute edema due to pulmonary thromboemboli frequently will have some predisposing causes, such as thrombosed leg veins or chronic heart failure. This diagnosis may be difficult to make, but the emergency nurse must have a high index of suspicion concerning patients with obvious respiratory embarrassment. It should also be kept in mind with young women who are on oral contraceptives and complain of the onset of dyspnea with chest pain. With emboli, pleuritic pain may be present, accompanied by blood-tinged sputum. Vital signs are variable. Complete assessment is mandatory. Chest x-ray may be helpful; however, a high precentage of positive diagnosis may be made by a pulmonary scan. Even more helpful is pulmonary angiography, which may demonstrate the specific vessel occluded.

Management is directed toward stabilization of vital signs and giving oxygen by mask and cardiotonic drugs or diuretics as needed. Perhaps the single most important medication and the keystone to therapy is heparin, given intravenously and repeated at regular intervals. The partial thromboplastin time or the clotting time may be used to control therapeutic levels.

The causative factor, when known, should be treated as the patient's condition permits. Varicose veins require surgical removal. Oral contraceptives should be discontinued. In massive pulmonary thromboembolism, when the patient survives the acute insult, successful emergency pulmonary embolectomy has been performed.

Asthma

Asthma (reversible airways obstruction) is a condition of the bronchial tree associated with *spasm* and increased secretion. (See Figure 13–10.) It may be due to an allergy, cardiac failure (cardiac asthma) or psychosomatic disorders. Allergic causes have received the most attention, possibly because they provide a good basis for therapy.

The end result of the process is a narrowing of the bronchial passageways due to a contraction of the muscles of the wall and retained secretions. Normally, the bronchial passages widen during inspiration and narrow somewhat in expiration. During an asthmatic episode, the spasm is associated with mucosal edema which functionally closes the lumen during expiration. Thus, expiration is interfered with and pulmonary ventilation considerably altered. Mucosal edema and spasm may affect pulmonary capillary flow and alter the permeability of the alveolocapillary membrane. Clinically, the spasm causes wheezing which frequently is audible with-

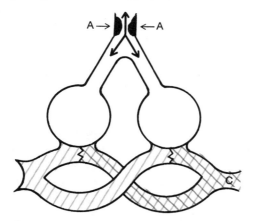

Figure 13–10 Bronchial asthma. Spasm of the bronchial tree, combined with an increase in secretions (A), causes a decrease in airflow and, thus, inadequate oxygenation of pulmonary arterial blood (C).

out the aid of a stethoscope. The asthmatic episode may be acute and of short duration, or it may last for longer periods of time extending to hours or even days. When severe and unrelieved by treatment (status asthmaticus), a fatal result may ensue.

In patients known to have asthma, an acute attack may be triggered by exposure to an allergenic agent, a superimposed pulmonary infection, extremes of temperature, nonspecific dusts or fumes or an emotional upset. The physical signs are quite characteristic and include labored respiration, particularly in the expiratory phase, associated with audible wheezing. The patient exerts a considerable effort to expire air. On auscultation, the expiratory phase is markedly prolonged and is accompanied by wheezing or rales. In mild episodes, vital signs are normal, and chest x-ray may reveal no specific change. The white blood count also may be within normal limits, while in the allergic type of asthma, an eosinophilia may be found on differential counts. Sputum samples should be obtained for smear, culture and sensitivity studies.

Management is directed toward relief of the small airways obstruction. Most patients may already be on some medication for asthma and report to the emergency department only when a complication occurs, such as a superimposed infection or an episode which is unresponsive to drugs. The most frequently used medications are epinephrine and aminophylline. Epinephrine is given subcutaneously in doses of 0.2 to 0.3 cc. of 1:1,000 solution. If no relief is achieved within 15 to 20 minutes, it may be repeated. Epinephrine may also be given as an aerosol preparation, although isoproterenol (Isuprel) and isoetharine are in more common use. Repeated observations of pulse rate and blood pressure should be made, since these particular preparations may cause tachycardia or hypertension.

Aminophylline may be given intravenously in a dose of 0.50 gm. This should be injected slowly over a 10 to 15 minute period or diluted to 250 cc. with 5 percent dextrose in distilled water, to infuse in one to 2 hours. It has a prompt action. Aminophylline suppositories may be effective but require a longer time to produce the desired effective bronchodilatation. Isoproterenol may also be used sublingually.

If an infectious process is present, specific antibiotics may be indicated. Adequate hydration is helpful in thinning the sputum, so that it may be raised more easily. Sedatives can be given to relieve apprehension. Positive pressure breathing is rarely needed.

Status asthmaticus is diagnosed when the asthmatic episode is not responsive to the usual medication. It is a serious condition accompanied by cyanosis and marked respiratory difficulty and can terminate fatally. An intravenous line should be started and aminophylline given by continuous drip; hydrocortisone may be added. Oxygen-helium mixtures in a 20:80 percent ratio, given intermittently rather than continuously, assist in better pulmonary air diffusion and may relieve the symptoms of hypoxia.

Chronic obstructive pulmonary disease

Many clinicians include chronic bronchitis and emphysema in this category. Chronic bronchitis is a disease that is characterized by chronic cough and expectoration, associated with recurrent acute infections of the lower respiratory tract. Emphysema refers to a generalized obstructive condition of the lungs, characterized clinically by dyspnea with signs of long-standing airway obstruction and hyperinflation of the lungs in which the air cannot be expelled. The abnormality occurs primarily in the alveolar portion of the lungs which are overdistended and lose elasticity. The cause of emphysema is not known, but it is seen more commonly in older patients and in association with chronic bronchitis of long-standing duration.

Emphysema patients are chronically ill with gradually increasing dyspnea without orthopnea, ease of fatigability and loss of weight and appetite. The dyspnea may increase as the disease is more prolonged. The anteroposterior diameter of the chest may equal or exceed the transverse diameter (barrel chest). Breathing is labored; respiratory movements are restricted. Typically the patient expires through pursed lips. Respiratory infections, inhalation of noxious fumes and pollution in the air may complicate emphysema and precipitate an episode of acute respiratory embarrassment.

On admission to the emergency department, the patient with acute respiratory embarrassment will exhibit apprehension and extreme shortness of breath. Cyanosis and tachycardia are usually present. Breathing is characterized by the use of the accessory muscles of respiration and by a prolonged expiratory phase. Wheezes and rales may be heard. The cough may sound as though it is loose and productive, but more often than not, the patient is unable to produce any sputum. Severe bronchospasm may accompany the attack. Arterial blood gases typically reveal hypoxemia and hypercarbia, with a lowered blood pH.

Management is directed toward relief of the bronchospasm by use of intravenous aminophylline. Expectorants may thin the sputum to enable the patient to cough more effectively. An oxygen-helium mixture given by mask may relieve the respiratory distress and allow better oxygenation of the blood. One hundred percent oxygen should be avoided, except when pneumonia is a complication. Specimens of the sputum should be obtained for cultures and sensitivity studies. A broad spectrum antibiotic may be started when an infectious process is suspected and a specific antibiotic begun after the culture and sensitivity studies have been obtained.

In the patient with severe impairment of respiratory activity and significant decrease in blood oxygen and elevation of blood CO_2, a tracheostomy with assist by a volume ventilator may be required. The patient should be placed in an intensive care unit as soon as possible. Ventilatory functions may be improved by use of positive end expiratory pressure (PEEP), which maintains better filling of the alveoli and thus may enhance diffusion.

NEAR-DROWNING

In general, the number of patients seen in any emergency department for the treatment of nonfatal submersion (near-drowning) is not great. However, with the increasing interest in water sports of all types, swimming, scuba activities, sailing and boating, the incidence of drowning and near-drowning may reasonably be expected to rise. Furthermore, with the greater public awareness of the principles of cardiopulmonary resuscitation, it can be expected that prompt initiation of resuscitative measures at the scene may result in more rescued drowning victims being seen in the hospital emergency department. It is estimated that drowning accounts for 7,000 deaths a year in the U.S. The number of near-drownings may not be accurately assessed.

Pathophysiology

The sequence of events that may occur in drowning starts with an initial phase of panic. As water enters the upper respiratory tract, laryngospasm occurs. Continued laryngospasm without aspiration causes asphyxia, hypoxemia and cardiac irregularity, with death. It is estimated that 10 percent of drowning fatalities occur by this mechanism. The process can be reversed by early rescue and control of the laryngospasm.

If the victim cannot escape or be taken from the water and laryngospasm persists, large quantities of water will be swallowed and subsequently vomited with aspiration into the tracheobronchial tree. If this chain of events is allowed to continue, it will invariably terminate fatally. Death is due to the persistent hypoxemia. Aspiration of fresh or sea water may produce changes in blood volume and alteration in serum electrolyte patterns. Other factors may play a part, especially lowered water temperature. Extreme degrees of hypothermia may limit survival time to a few minutes. Another factor which may influence the prognosis is loss of consciousness.

Upon arrival at the hospital emergency department, the victim of near-drowning may present a classic example of asphyxia, with or without congestive heart failure. Depending upon the degree of pulmonary involvement, the patient may or may not be cyanotic. Frothy sputum may be evident. Tachypnea and tachycardia with or without hypotension are noted. If asphyxia has been prolonged, the patient may be unconscious, his pupils dilated and nonreactive. The lungs may be clear on auscultation or reveal findings consistent with pulmonary edema. Clinically, there may be little distinction between near-drowning due to fresh or salt water.

Assessment and management

Venous blood samples should be taken soon after the victim's arrival in the emergency department for blood and electrolyte counts. Arterial blood gases must also be drawn to assess the magnitude of the problem. Serious alterations in blood gases may be present. Chest x-ray will give some indication of the pulmonary status and may reveal evidence of pulmonary edema, pneumonitis or atelectasis, all of which may follow asphyxia and aspiration. An electrocardiogram should be taken to detect any arrhythmia or myocardial damage.

The airway must be established immediately. If necessary, cardiopulmonary resuscitation is initiated. If cyanosis is present or the blood gas studies reveal hypoxemia, oxygen should be given by nasal catheter or mask using 40 to 60 percent O_2. If hypoxia persists, endotracheal intubation or tracheostomy is needed, and the patient should be placed on a volume ventilator. Lower concentrations of O_2 may be used with this technique, usually 25 to 40 percent. Positive pressure ventilation may reduce pulmonary edema. Since there may be portions of the lung which are incompletely aerated and arteriovenous shunts opened, positive end expiratory pressure (PEEP) may be helpful in opening these unaerated portions of the lung.

A nasogastric tube should be emplaced early during the patient's stay in the emergency department to empty the stomach contents and prevent further emesis and aspiration. When aspiration pneumonitis is considered, steroid and antibiotics are begun. Sputum cultures and sensitivity studies are initiated. A broad-spectrum antibiotic such as penicillin may be started and later changed as culture studies indicate. Furosemide (Lasix) may be helpful in lessening pulmonary edema.

Complete assessment must be done to determine other injury. This is especially true in the unconscious victim. Careful examination is needed to rule out an injury to the cervical spine, particularly when a diving injury is suspected. Close observation is needed during the patient's stay in the emergency department, with repeat assessment of vital signs at regular intervals and periodic evaluation of arterial blood gases. Blood gas evaluations and chest x-rays are the 2 most useful parameters in assessing the impact of the therapy.

BIBLIOGRAPHY

(1) Ashbaugh, D. G., and Petty, T. L.: "Sepsis Complicating the Acute Respiratory Distress Syndrome," *Surgery, Gynecology and Obstetrics,* 135 (1972): 865.

(2) Ashbaugh, D. G.; Petty, T. L.; Bigelow, D. B., and Harris, T. M.: "Continuous Positive Pressure Breathing (CPPB) in Adult Respiratory Distress Syndrome," *Journal of Thoracic and Cardiovascular Surgery,* 57 (1969):31.

(3) Cahill, J. M.: "Drowning: The Problems of Nonfatal Submersion and the Unconscious Patient," *Surgical Clinics of North America,* 48 (1969):429.

(4) Comroe, J. H.; Forster, R. E., II; Dubois, A. B.; Briscoe, W. A., and Carlsen, E.: *The Lung, Clinical Physiology and Pulmonary Function Tests,* 2nd ed. (Chicago, Ill.: Year Book Medical Publishers, 1968).

(5) Fuhs, M.; Riser, M., and Brisbon, D.: "Nursing in a Respiratory Intensive Care Unit," *Chest,* 62 (1972):14S.

(6) Giammona, S. T., and Modell, J. H.: "Drowning by Total Immersion," *American Journal of Diseases of Children,* 114 (1967):612.

(7) Heimlich, H. J.: "Pop Goes the Café Coronary," *Emergency Medicine,* 6 (1974):154.

(8) Hinshaw, H. C.: *Diseases of the Chest,* 3rd ed. (Philadelphia: W. B. Saunders Company, 1969).

(9) Levine, B. E.; Kravetz, H. M.; Spotnitz, M., and Westfall, R. E.: "The Roles of the Community Hospital in Acute Respiratory Failure Management," *Chest,* 62 (1972):10S.

(10) Moser, R. H.: "Drowning: A Seasonal Disease," *Journal of the American Medical Association,* 229 (1974):563.

(11) Nett, L. M.; Riutort, A., and Tietsort, J.: "Specialized Nurses and Therapists in Respiratory Care," *Chest,* 62 (1972): 19S.

(12) Preston, F. S.: "Water Hazards on How to Avoid a Watery Grave," *Practitioners,* 211 (1973):209.

(13) Schloerb, P. R.; Junt, P. T.; Plummer, J. A., and Gage, G. K.: "Pulmonary Edema After Replacement of Blood Loss by Electrolyte Solutions," *Surgery, Gynecology, and Obstetrics,* 135 (1972): 893.

(14) Schwar, T. G.: "Drowning: Its Chemical Diagnosis; a Review," *Forensic Science,* 1 (1972):411.

(15) Sugarman, H. J.; Rogers, R. M., and Miller, L. D.: "Positive End-Expiratory Pressure (PEEP); Indications and Physiologic Considerations," *Chest,* 62 (1972):86S.

14

Cardiac emergencies

BETTY N. LAWSON
DONNA DUELL

Cardiac emergencies have an ever-growing effect on the population of the United States. Not only does cardiovascular disease claim more American lives than all other causes of death combined, but the loss of man-days of production due to cardiac disease number 52,000,000 per year.[6] Over 675,000 lives are lost annually to myocardial infarction, which gives credence to the need for nurses to know and understand early symptoms of heart disease, as well as how to treat cardiac emergencies.

The function provided by the cardiovascular system is that of transportation. The heart is the pumping mechanism for the system, which transports nutrients, gases, electrolytes and hormones that are vital for cell metabolism. Mechanical and electrical stimuli provide the mechanism for the heart's action. The electrical stimulus originates at the cellular level and causes the conduction system of the heart to initiate and coordinate the heart action. The mechanical stimulus resulting from the electrochemical forces initiates the pumping action of the heart. The proper coordination of cardiovascular function is dependent upon: (1) the heart's effectiveness as a pumping agent, (2) neurohormonal control, (3) adequate blood volume, (4) correct acid-base balance and (5) an adequate vascular bed.

A cardiac emergency is any factor that interferes with normal pulmonary or cardiovascular function. The pulmonary system is as vital as the cardiovascular system, due to the anatomical relationship and interrelatedness of function. When one system fails to function properly, the other system also may become involved. This helps explain why patients suffering from respiratory conditions often are treated as though they were having an acute myocardial infarction until the correct diagnosis is established.

The pulmonary system is the agent for gaseous exchange to maintain cellular existence. When either the cardiovascular or pulmonary system fails to function properly, a cardiac emergency may result. Inadequate oxygenation and tissue perfusion results, and, if not reversed, cellular death occurs. Therefore, it becomes imperative that medical treatment begin immediately. Mobile coronary care units are used in many areas to serve this purpose.

THE MOBILE CORONARY CARE UNIT

More than half of all heart attack victims die within 2 hours of initial symptoms. This statistic has led to increasing use of the mobile coronary care unit. Depending on locale, these units are manned either by trained medical personnel (nurses, attendants, physicians) or by specially trained paraprofessionals.

Any time symptoms described by a person suggest a possible cardiac condition, the mobile coronary unit should be dispatched. The most frequent symptom described by the cardiac patient is persistent chest pain, usually felt behind the sternum. It can be described either as a crushing pain, which may or may not radiate across the left shoulder and down the arm, or just a tightness or pressure on the chest. The patient generally experiences diaphoresis, nausea, palpitations, fatigue and emesis. Many patients with a myocardial infarction describe their only symptom as an attack of indigestion. Others feel the pain radiating to the arms, neck or jaw. Some patients have described a feeling of impending disaster during an attack.

In order to effectively use a mobile unit, it becomes necessary to establish an emergency medical communications system in the community. A system of this type should provide for coordinated dispatching of all emergency vehicles, including fire, police, ambulance and mobile coronary unit. It is ideal to have 2-way voice communication between the rescuer and medical personnel as well as the capability to transmit the electrocardiogram by telemetry. (See Figures 14–1 and 14–2.) This is of particular importance when the mobile units are manned solely by emergency medical technicians. The type of immediate care given to the patient may profoundly influence his total outcome. It becomes essential to stabilize the patient's respiratory, metabolic and hemodynamic status early, to prevent further complications. Following the initial emergency care, it is important to provide continuity of care until diagnosis is established and the patient has been placed in a coronary care unit. (See Figures 14–3 and 14–4.)

THE EMERGENCY DEPARTMENT

Ideally, when a patient with a cardiac problem is brought to the emergency department by a medical transport team or by private vehicle, he should be placed immediately in either a Life Support Unit or an area where he can be viewed constantly as well as electronically monitored. A Life Support Unit is a self-contained unit which provides a "bed" for the patient, monitors the electrocardiogram, provides for artificial ventilation, has its own oxygen supply, and contains defibrillating equipment. (See Figure 14–5.) It should

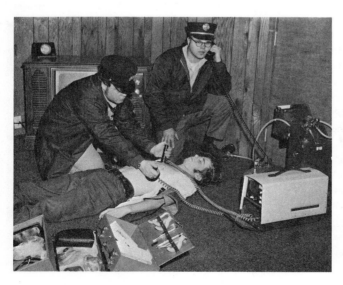

Figure 14–1 Advanced emergency medical technicians (EMT II) with cardiac patient. Equipment includes a portable monitor-defibrillator unit, with the paddles applied to the patient's chest. The paddles serve as electrodes, so that the ECG pattern can be seen on the oscilloscope. The monitor-defibrillator unit contains a radio pack, which allows the EMT II to have voice communication with the hospital and to telemeter the ECG signal to the hospital.
Source: Photo courtesy of Mennen-Greatbatch Electronics, Inc.

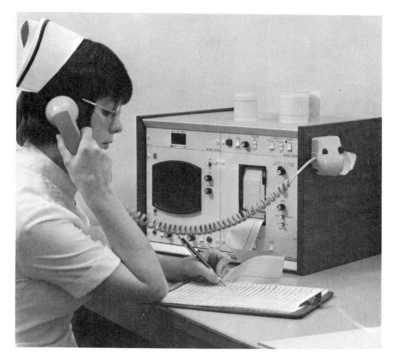

Figure 14–2 Transceiver unit in the hospital. The nurse has direct voice communication with the EMT II at the scene of the incident. This small unit receives the ECG signal on the oscilloscope and prints out a rhythm strip, which can be attached to the patient's record.
Source: Photo courtesy of Mennen-Greatbatch Electronics, Inc.

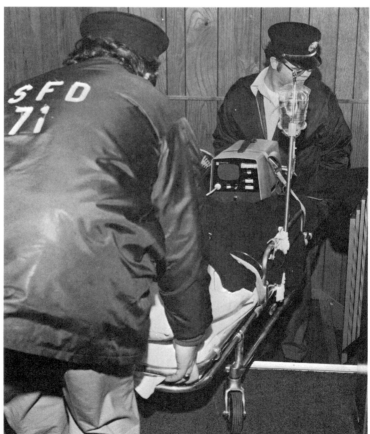

Figure 14–3 Monitoring during transportation. Patient is being transferred to the ambulance. Continuous monitoring of cardiac rhythm should be done, using fixed electrodes (rather than paddles), attached to the patient, and the portable monitor-defibrillator unit.
Source: Photo courtesy of Mennen-Greatbatch Electronics, Inc.

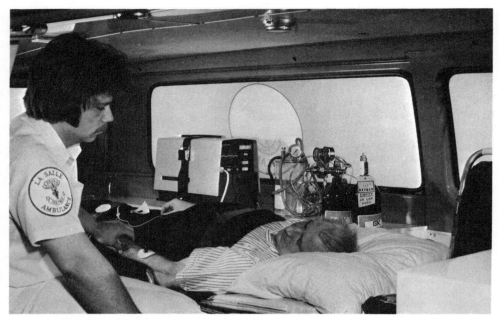

Figure 14-4 Monitoring during transportation in ambulance. The EMT II continues to monitor the ECG during the patient's transit to the hospital by ambulance.
Source: Photo courtesy of Mennen-Greatbatch Electronics, Inc.

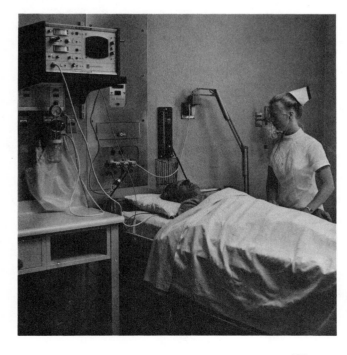

Figure 14-5 The Life Support Unit. This photo demonstrates the essential equipment included in a hospital's Life Support Unit.
Source: Photo courtesy of Mennen-Greatbatch Electronics, Inc.

also be supplied with emergency medications and intravenous equipment and fluids, in addition to cut-down and tracheostomy trays.

Emergency departments should be equipped appropriately for the management of acute cardiac patients. Standard equipment, such as monitors with ECG write-outs, cardiovertor-defibrillator units, back boards for CPR, emergency treatment and drug cart and a battery-powered portable defibrillator are essential adjunctive needs. Equipment in acute care areas, such as the ICU, CCU, post-anesthesia rooms and the emergency department, should be of the same manufacturer. This tends to eliminate most of the confusion among the professional staff in the correct operational use of life-saving equipment within the same agency. Sometimes, numerous brand names, types, direct-current and battery-powered pieces of equipment are found in each separate acute care area. Standardization of equipment aids everyone and certainly lessens the delay in caring for the patient in emergency situations. Tantamount to all else, well-prepared nursing staff is an absolute prerequisite to patient care management.

It is very important that the family be kept informed of the patient's condition. As soon as a physician is available, the family should be seated in a secluded area or quiet room, where they can have privacy to discuss the patient's status with the physician. It is not always practical to have someone stay with the family, but it is essential that someone be assigned to make periodic reports to them. Some emergency departments have secluded areas for families; if not available, the nurse might suggest using the chapel or a quiet area where family members can have privacy.

Admissions policies must be based on reasonable decisions regarding the agency's realistic capability of delivering specialized care to the acutely ill. Access and entry into the care system must be a smooth and easy operation for both the patient and his family. Senseless delays in procuring aid by the patient or his family during a cardiac emergency is a matter of better public education in recognizing the early warning signs of acute myocardial infarction; but delays and confusion within the care delivery system itself are inexcusable.

The role the nurse takes in the emergency department varies from institution to institution, depending on the availability of the medical staff as well as on the specific training the nurse has received. The most important function remains the same, however—that of assessing the patient's condition. A rapid assessment must confirm or rule out an acute myocardial infarction (MI). If the patient does indeed have an infarct, he should be transported to a coronary care unit, if one is available, as quickly as possible (Figure 14–6). If the symptoms prove to indicate some other problem, such as a pulmonary embolism or even an acute cholecystitis (the symptoms many times are confused with those of an MI),

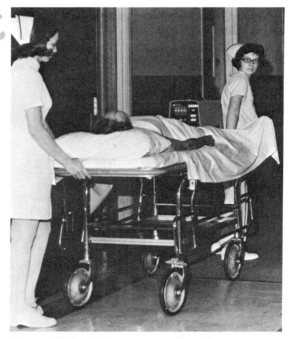

Figure 14–6 Patient en route from the emergency department to the coronary care unit. The portable monitor-defibrillator should accompany the patient during his transfer within the hospital to provide continuous monitoring of the ECG for detection of arrhythmias.
Source: Photo courtesy of St. John's Hospital, Springfield, Missouri.

the patient would then be transferred to the appropriate unit following an initial evaluation in the emergency department.

If the symptoms do suggest a cardiac condition, it is important to begin treatment for the condition even if the diagnosis is proven incorrect subsequently. Wasting time during a crucial period of establishing a diagnosis may prove fatal to the patient. It is far better to be cautious than sorry.

PATIENT ASSESSMENT

Cardiac monitoring

The initial step in treating any patient complaining of chest pain is to place him on a

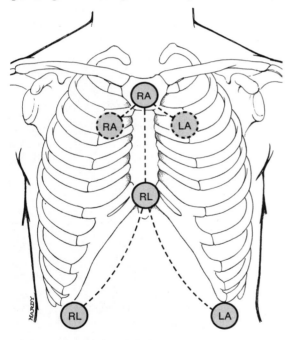

Figure 14–7 Positioning electrodes. Electrodes are placed as follows: RA: On the mid-line of the chest, just above the sternomanubrial junction. The dotted circles on either side represent electrode placement in the second intercostal space, approximately mid-way between the mid-line of the sternum and the mid-clavicular line. "RA" signifies right arm. RL: In the upper right quadrant of the abdomen, just below the costal margin in the mid-clavicular line. "RL" signifies right leg. LA: In the upper left quadrant of the abdomen, just below the costal margin in the mid-clavicular line. "LA" refers to left arm.

cardiac monitor via electrodes and observe for any cardiac arrhythmias.

An electrode may be described as a "voltage sensor." It is utilized in picking up the body's electrical impulse currents. When placing electrodes of any variety on the body surface with the intent to monitor the heart muscle, it is essential that the skin be cleansed thoroughly of dirt and oil. Body hair may be shaved in areas where electrode placement is anticipated. Figures 14–7 and 14–8 show proper positioning of electrodes. Slight abrasive rubbing is desired to improve the signal pick up; do not injure the skin by rubbing too vigorously. The electrodes are good conductors, usually of a silver–silver chloride base. Conduction is better on a moist body surface than on a dry one; therefore, conducting jellies and pastes are placed on the electrodes prior to attachment to the prepared skin areas. The internal electricity is picked up by the electrodes on the skin and transmitted via a hard-wire cable to a monitor, where an amplified wave configuration of the impulse being sensed is projected for viewing on the oscilloscope. A variety of commercial monitors are available for emergency department use. It is wise to have one with "read-out" potential. The "read-out," sometimes referred to as a "rhythm strip," is a recording of the electrical impulses seen on the oscilloscope. This strip can be used for further examination by the physician, and it provides a permanent record of the patient's initial heart pattern on admission. This may become invaluable for comparison with serial tracings during the hospitalization. The rhythm strip, however, does not preclude taking a full 12-lead electrocardiogram (ECG) when time permits.

All monitoring equipment should include: (1) skin electrodes, which are attached to the patient and transmit electrical impulses through an amplifier to an oscilloscope; (2) a heart rate meter, which indicates the heart beats per minute; (3) and an alarm system which is set with high and low limits and emits a signal when the heart rate varies outside the preset limits. In addition, monitoring of blood pressure and respiratory rate is also often provided.

If any abnormal arrhythmias are noted, a "stat" 12-lead electrocardiogram should be obtained. Arrhythmias are the most common of the 4 major complications which may result in death, the other 3 being left ventricular failure, thromboembolism and left ventricular rupture. An arrhythmia is defined as a disturbance in the rhythm, rate or conduction of the electrical impulses of the heart.

A large percentage, as high as 80 percent, of all patients with myocardial infarctions develop some type of arrhythmia within the first few days following the attack. Some arrhythmias produce sudden death; others result in circulatory inefficiency which can eventually result in left ventricular failure; some arrhythmias are relatively harmless and can be tolerated by the patient with little consequence. The death-producing arrhythmias will be discussed in detail later in this chapter.

It is important to note that many times there will be no electrocardiographic changes immediately; changes may not become evident until some days later. It is therefore necessary to take repeated (serial) tracings for an accurate appraisal of the patient's cardiac status.

Blood studies

Blood should be drawn as soon as possible and sent to the laboratory. The results of the lab studies will aid in diagnosis. These studies should be used in conjunction with the ECG findings and the patient's history. No one of the findings alone should be the basis for diagnosis.

The lab values of most benefit in confirming diagnosis are the SGOT (serum glutamic-oxaloacetic transaminase), LDH (lactic dehydrogenase) and CPK (creatine phosphokinase). These enzymes peak in the blood at varying, measurable times after infarction and return to normal limits at varying times, also. Table 14–1 displays the relative blood levels of these enzymes.

If the patient has had a myocardial infarc-

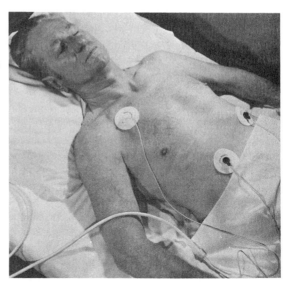

Figure 14–8 Patient monitored in bed. Fixed electrodes are attached to the patient when he is in his hospital bed, for continuous monitoring. Source: Photo courtesy of Mennen-Greatbatch Electronics, Inc.

tion, the enzymes normally found in the heart muscle escape in the blood stream and are reported at an elevated level by the lab. As myocardial cells are destroyed, the blood values increase accordingly.

INTERPRETING ASSESSMENT

Pain

A cardiac arrhythmia is one of the 2 most common signs of a possible cardiac emergency. The second is severe, persistent chest pain, unrelieved by nitroglycerine. Both findings require immediate treatment to prevent further physiological damage, which could lead to cardiac arrest.

TABLE 14–1 ENZYME BLOOD LEVELS FOLLOWING MI

Enzymes	Blood level peaks	Return to normal
(1) SGOT	1–2 days	4–6 days
(2) LDH	2–3 days	7–10 days
(3) CPK	6–24 hours	2–3 days

The nurse must elicit from the patient or his family a specific description of what type of pain was experienced during the attack. The type of pain may be diagnostically important, as it can help distinguish true myocardial infarction from transient forms of myocardial ischemia, such as angina pectoris. (Anginal pain is usually relieved by the use of nitroglycerine tablets, sublingually.) Myocardial pain becomes evident as the tissue is being damaged by anoxia and usually subsides when the damage is complete. Pain occurs when there is a discrepancy between myocardial demand for oxygen and the actual supply of oxygen provided by the coronary circulation.

Myocardial infarction is usually the result of progressive narrowing of the coronary arteries by atherosclerotic plaques, which have developed over the years. Sudden complete occlusion occurs when a thrombus forming on the rough surface of a plaque or from bleeding below it causes the plaque to dislodge and occlude the artery. The actual occlusion of the vessel does not cause sudden death; the complications which occur from the occlusion (arrhythmias, left ventricular failure) may.

As the oxygen demand needed by the myocardium is not met, hypoxia occurs, with altered cellular metabolism and a release of lactic acid. With myocardial ischemia and increased lactic acid levels, the blood pressure and heart rate increase and the myocardium becomes irritable. This compensatory mechanism to increase blood flow and oxygen may also further increase myocardial demands, which may lead to premature ventricular contractions and ventricular tachycardia. Hypoxia can also induce parasympathetic stimulation resulting in a decreased heart rate, which may lead to cardiac asystole.[7]

Rapid relief of severe chest pain is essential in order to decrease the patient's anxiety level and thus lessen subsequent release of catecholamines. Morphine sulfate is the narcotic of choice and has proven to be effective not only in decreasing pain and anxiety but also in lowering the respiratory rate, which helps to reduce the myocardial demand for oxygen.

The following 3 clinical situations will give the nurse an overview of what additional signs and symptoms the patient with a cardiac problem might present upon admission to the emergency department.

The patient seemingly not in acute distress

The clinical picture may be deceptive; the patient may appear ill but not dramatically critical or distressed. There may be only slight diaphoresis, but skin moist and cool to touch. There may be only slight cyanosis of the fingernail beds, earlobes or lips, appearing more light-bluish in hue than the red-purple color seen commonly in acute congestive heart failure or in cor pulmonale. The patient may complain of pain or pressure in the retrosternal area. Pain descriptions elicited from the patient, however, may be too vague to be of much help in diagnosing either the condition or the urgency of the situation. He may eructate "tasteless gas," with some regurgitation of a "watery fluid" and complain of nausea.

Vital signs may not be alarming to the nurse, especially when she has no idea of the patient's usual heart rate or blood pressure. What the nurse does not know is more crucial than what she can ascertain through her assessment of the patient. For example, it is not uncommon to see patients with acute myocardial infarctions in emergency departments with blood pressures of 120/70 to 140/90 upon admission who normally have been hypertensive with blood pressures ranging from 160/100 to 180/110. Thus, a blood pressure reading of 120/70 may be a highly significant drop, even though the patient's outward appearance is not that of shock.

Although the pulse may reveal irregularities in rhythm, the nurse may not have the experience to diagnose by palpation those arrhythmias which signal impending danger. The monitoring device is useful in this case, as it will provide a record of the particular arrhythmia and enable the physician to reach a diagnosis and begin treatment.

If there is no physician available in the emergency department, the patient's private physician should be contacted as soon as the patient is admitted with chest pain. Often in the busy emergency area, the acute cardiac patient who does not survive is the one whose heart history is unknown and who appeared clinically stable and not in acute distress.

The patient in acute distress

The patient with a coronary occlusion resulting in acute myocardial infarction may be dramatically ill in appearance. He may exhibit severe diaphoresis and cyanosis. How deep the cyanosis is will depend both upon the time interval from onset of symptoms and the extent of myocardial damage. Respiratory activity may vary from severe dyspnea to shallow, semi-labored breathing patterns. The patient appears apprehensive, acutely ill and fearful. The pain is classically retrosternal, often with radiation down the inner aspects of either or both arms and possibly to the shoulder or scapulae or jaw. The character of the pain is described as "severe," "crushing," "squeezing," "heavy" or "vise-like" in nature.

When the patient is a poor clinical historian, the nurse should not waste valuable time struggling to elicit difficult-to-obtain information; rather, she should rely upon her abilities to assess the clinical manifestations, such as facial expressions, physical signs and verbal or nonverbal cues, given by the patient.

The vital signs of the patient with a myocardial infarction and in shock are important. The pulse may manifest rapid or slow irregular rhythms but may be intermittent and difficult to feel. The cardiac monitor may show the infarction by deep Q waves or the current of injury by elevated S-T segments. (See Figure 14–9, following.) The normal rhythm may be disturbed by unifocal or multifocal premature beats; by intermittently or regularly blocked ventricular response, with twice as many atrial complexes (a 2:1 or 3:1 A-V block); or by complete A-V block (complete heart block), with a regular slow ventricular response and the atrium firing at its own rate. The bradyarrhythmias may lead to low blood pressure, which is a dangerous threat to life and makes stabilizing the patient difficult. These arrhythmias will be discussed in more depth later in this chapter.

Monitoring as many aspects as possible is essential, including central venous pressure, urinary output, intravenous fluid therapy and electrolyte values. The need for a possible pacemaker catheter installation, as well as assisted circulatory and ventilatory mechanisms, should be anticipated and prepared for by the nurse.

The central venous pressure (CVP) is the most important value in monitoring the true physiological status of the acute cardiac patient in shock. The most important contribution of CVP readings in the patient with shock is to provide data pertinent to the adequacy of the circulating volume of blood. This information, in conjunction with arterial blood pressure and renal output, aids the physician in his attempts to improve the function of the failing cardiac pump by minimizing the burden placed on an already inefficient muscle damaged by severe infarction.

Treatment includes oxygen therapy, drug administration for cardiac arrhythmia control and management of the hypotensive state and the electrolyte imbalances of frank or impending cardiogenic shock. The nurse must watch the infusion rate of any medications diligently and relay to the physician any changes in the CVP, blood pressure, urinary output, pulse and other observable factors, such as skin color and temperature.

The fatally stricken patient

The fatally stricken patient is one who dies suddenly, often outside an acute care facility and without the benefit of any physiological warnings. One minute he is laughing and talking to his family or friends and the next minute collapses in cardiac arrest, with no detectable blood pressure, palpable pulse or respirations. His pupils dilate, and his color is ashen-gray.

The intolerable frustration of not being able to prevent electrical death of a heart which is otherwise too healthy to die torments emergency teams, nurses and physicians alike. Most sudden deaths following acute myocardial infarction are due to electrical derangement of the heart rhythm. The electrical derangement is referred to as a "dysrhythmia." The chance of a dysrhythmia is usually greatest immediately following the attack and for several hours following myocardial ischemia.[12] Rhythm changes can occur suddenly, but death-producing arrhythmias usually give warning signs which should be observed on the oscilloscope. The two basic mechanisms involved in cardiac arrest are ventricular fibrillation and asystole.

Sudden clinical death may not be biological death; that is, there is a margin of effectiveness for life-support actions, even though the arrest usually does not conveniently happen in a hospital cardiac care unit or emergency department. Recognition of cardiac arrest by lay people who are trained in special life-saving techniques may prove to be the most important external force that can preserve life. Through mouth-to-mouth breathing, coordinated with external cardiac compression, circulation of blood, especially to the brain, may be maintained.

Cardiopulmonary resuscitation (CPR), within the usual safe margin of 4 to 6 minutes, may keep the patient biologically alive and in a retrievable state. This life-support measure, when properly performed, will maintain cerebral oxygenation to prevent brain cell death and keep the cardiac muscle "pink" enough to respond to specific therapy later. Thus, it is not as important to immediately ascertain the mechanism of cardiac arrest as it is to quickly recognize the signs and symptoms of sudden cardiac death, so that there is no delay in initiating CPR.

CARDIOPULMONARY RESUSCITATION

The newest method of CPR approved by the American Heart Association includes the use of the precordial thump, if the patient collapses and this is witnessed. It is used only if no carotid pulse is palpated. The thump may stimulate the heart to begin beating or reverse certain dysrhythmias if given within the first minute following arrest.[12]

The precordial thump consists of striking the midsternum with a closed hand. In delivering the precordial thump, these rules should be observed:

(1) Deliver a sharp, quick, single blow over the midportion of the sternum, hitting with the bottom, fleshy portion (ulnar side) of the hand from 8 to 12 inches above the chest.
(2) Deliver the thump within the first minute after cardiac arrest.
(3) If there is no immediate response, begin basic life support (CPR) at once.

The blow generates a small electrical stimulus in the heart that is reactive. The thump may be effective in restoring cardiac activity in cases of ventricular asystole due to heart block and in reversing ventricular tachycardia or ventricular fibrillation of recent onset. The precordial thump is not useful for anoxic asystole and probably won't reverse an *established* ventricular fibrillation. It is not useful in cases where electromechanical dissociation occurs.

The thump should not be used if the patient has an adequate circulation, even though ventricular tachycardia is present. It is a good idea to check the femoral pulses to ascertain if the heart is circulating an adequate blood volume. If the thump is used in cases where the heart is anoxic and still beating, the stimulus of the low voltage may be detrimental, causing ventricular fibrillation. The precordial thump is not recommended for use on children until further research is completed on its effects.

If the patient is being monitored and sudden onset ventricular fibrillation, asystole or ventricular tachycardia without a pulse is noted, give a single precordial thump. If the monitor shows that the situation is not reversed, do not waste time by continuing to use the precordial thump. Instead, countershock the patient by use of the defibrillator.

In all cases, begin CPR after the initial precordial thump. After the thump is given, again check for the carotid pulse. If the pulse is absent, begin both artificial ventilation and external cardiac massage. If there is a discernible carotid pulse, start only artificial ventilation. In all instances where you have not seen the patient collapse but have found him unconscious, check to see if there is a patent airway by going inside the patient's mouth with the fingers and feeling for foreign objects. Begin CPR by giving 4 quick breaths and then feel again for the carotid pulse. If it is absent, proceed with the external cardiac massage and artificial ventilation.

The rate of administering CPR and the exact method depends on whether it is a one- or 2-person rescue effort and whether the victim is an adult or child. Various methods will be described briefly here; however, the joint American Heart Association—American Medical Association publication on this subject provides in-depth explanations of the procedure.[5]

Administering CPR

When only one person is performing CPR on an adult, the first step is to check for a carotid pulse; if absent, begin the procedure by tilting the head back and giving 4 quick breaths by mouth-to-mouth technique while holding the nose shut. Then initiate cardiac compression by placing the palm of one hand directly on the back of the other and exerting firm, rhythmic pressure over the lower half of the sternum. Compress the sternum 15 times and then give 2 breaths. Repeat this procedure for at least 5 minutes before checking for a carotid pulse. When external cardiac massage is performed properly, it can produce systolic blood pressure peaks of over 100 mm. Hg.[1]

Effective external cardiac compression requires sufficient pressure to depress the lower sternum $1\frac{1}{2}$ to 2 inches. It is most effective if the patient is on a hard surface. A pressure of 80 to 120 pounds is required to produce the correct depression.[1] The compressions need to be firm, regular, smooth and exerted in a vertical manner. Under no circumstances should the compressions be interrupted for more than 5 seconds, as this drops the circulating blood pressure back down to zero.

This ratio of cardiac compression to ventilation (15:2) should be done at an effective rate of 80 per minute in order to achieve the goal of at least 60 artificial beats per minute. Rates below 60 beats per minute are not beneficial.

When 2 rescuers are available to administer CPR, there is a much better chance of providing optimum ventilation and circulation. The optimal ratio of cardiac compression to ventilation is 5:1. When the person doing the external cardiac massage becomes tired, the 2 can easily change places without losing rhythm.

For a discussion of CPR in children, see Chapter 18.

Evaluating CPR effectiveness

During CPR, frequent evaluation of the pupils and carotid or femoral pulses should be made to check for the effectiveness of the technique. If there is inadequate oxygenation and decreased blood flow to the brain, the pupils will remain widely dilated and will not react to light. This is an indication of serious brain damage, and continuation of the technique is questionable.

The decision to discontinue CPR, if it is apparently not effective, depends on an assessment of the cerebral and cardiovascular status.[1] Deep unconsciousness, absence of spontaneous respiration and fixed, dilated pupils for 15 to 20 minutes are indicative of cerebral death. Cardiac death is assumed when there is no return of electrocardiographic activity after one hour of continuous cardiopulmonary support. The decision to discontinue the technique is usually made by the physician who is overseeing the CPR. The resuscitation effort in children is usually continued for a longer period of time than in adults, as recovery has occurred after prolonged periods of unconsciousness. The longer the CPR is necessary, the less likely the chances of recovery.

If CPR is done correctly, there should be no complications. However, if done improperly, several severe complications can occur. If the compression is done over the xiphoid process, the bony prominence extending from the lower end of the sternum, pressure here can cause a laceration of the liver. Fractured ribs can result if the hands are placed improperly and allowed to exert pressure on the ribs. If there is air trapped in the stomach, pressure should not be exerted on it at the same time the chest is being compressed.

PATHOPHYSIOLOGY OF CARDIAC EMERGENCIES

Atrioventricular conduction defects

There are numerous grades of conduction pathway defects, ranging from a simple prolongation of the P-R interval (beyond 0.20 second) to complete atrioventricular (A.V.) dissociation.

The simple delay in impulse conduction from the sino-atrial node to the junctional area is called "first-degree A-V heart block" and is sometimes noted in normal adults. Third-degree A-V block is complete heart block. Any grade of A-V heart block in acute myocardial infarction is either watched judiciously or treated with anticipation of possible complete A-V heart block developing. The patient may proceed rapidly into higher grades of A-V heart block during the acute phase of illness, which would require immediate pacing capabilities. Therefore, if atropine fails to correct it, a temporary transvenous pacing catheter may be inserted via the brachial vein * to the superior vena cava, passed into the right atrium across the tricuspid valve and into the right ventricle,

* Other venous approaches may be utilized, e.g., the cephalic or basilic veins.

where it is embedded into the septal wall. The temporary artificial pacemaker would probably be set to fire on demand (i.e., if the rate slows too much), depending completely upon the needs of the individual patient.

The nurse should be aware of the cardiac alerts which signal the need for possible insertion of a transvenous pacemaker. Patients who are likely candidates exhibit:

(1) Bradycardias, especially associated with frequent ventricular ectopic phenomena.
(2) An anterior wall infarction and first-degree A-V block. (Posterior wall infarcts with A-V block are more likely to respond to atropine.)
(3) Serious bundle branch block involvement (right bundle branch block with left axis deviation or with anteroseptal infarction).
(4) Any evidence of progressive A-V block.
(5) Complete A-V dissociation, with atrial and ventricular pacemakers firing regularly and independently of each other.

Cardiac dysrhythmias

Cardiac dysrhythmias or abnormal rhythms are generated from several factors, including myocardial ischemia, acid-base imbalance, digitalis intoxication, mechanical interference with cardiac tissue or, in general, a disturbance in the impulse conduction system. Cardiac dysrhythmias are classified as tachycardias, bradycardias or irregular rhythms. The rhythms may occur along with either a normal or abnormal heart rate.

Tachycardias present a problem in interference with normal cardiac output due to decreased ventricular filling time. The arrhythmias included in this classification are: (1) sinus tachycardia, (2) atrial fibrillation-flutter, (3) paroxysmal atrial tachycardia, (4) ventricular tachycardia and (5) ventricular fibrillation.

Bradycardias interfere with normal cardiac

output because of a decreased rate of ventricular ejection. The arrhythmias included in this classification are: (1) sinus bradycardia, (2) partial heart block and (3) complete heart block.

Irregular heart rhythms may indicate myocardial irritability. They may not necessarily interfere with normal cardiac output, so they do not usually cause any immediate concern. They include: (1) the partial heart blocks, (2) dissociation and (3) premature ventricular contractions.

Of concern to the emergency nurse are those dysrhythmias requiring immediate intervention to prevent rapid death. They include: (1) ventricular tachycardia, (2) ventricular fibrillation, (3) third-degree (complete) heart block and (4) asystole.

Every professional nurse, whether in an acute care facility or not, needs to know and recognize basic electrocardiographic patterns and be especially astute in detecting the warning signs of possible or impending cardiac disasters. Thus, the nurse must know what is

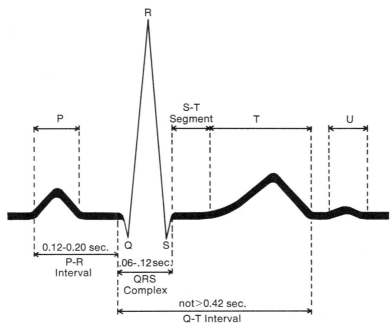

Figure 14–9 The anatomy of one heart beat.
P Wave: Represents atrial systole as a result of electrical excitation (depolarization) of the atrium arising from the sinoatrial (S-A) node.
P–R Interval: (including the P–R segment) Represents time span from S-A impulse origin, spread through atria, atrial systole, conduction of the impulse across the atrioventricular (A-V) junction, bundle of His and bundle branches to the ventricular musculature.
QRS Complex: Represents ventricular systole as a result of impulse conduction through ventricular muscle (depolarization).
T Wave: Represents ventricular repolarization.
S–T Segment: Represents time span from the end of the QRS complex to the beginning of the T wave.
Q–T Interval: Represents complete depolarization and repolarization from the beginning of the QRS to the end of the T wave.
U Wave: Cause not clear; some experts believe it is the result of residual repolarization of the ventricle while it is relaxing. (The T occurs during ventricular contraction.) It is any wave seen after the T wave but before the next P wave.

meant by the P-QRS-T-(U) * wave components that make up the electrical accompaniment of one heart contraction or one cardiac cycle. Figure 14–9 diagrams and describes the various aspects of the cardiac contraction.

Normally, the P-QRS-T waves are repetitive phenomena occurring from 60 to 100 beats per minute in a regular rhythm in the normal adult. The arbitrarily selected letters of the alphabet represent separate events within the single innervation and contraction of the heart. Distinguishing features of common arrhythmias are outlined in Table 14–2.

It is important to develop the habit of examining every rhythm strip in a uniform and systematic way:

(1) Is the rhythm regular?
   (a) QRS to QRS?
   (b) P to P wave?
   (c) T to T wave?
(2) Ascertain the rate.
   (a) Is it normal for the subject?
   (b) Is it slow?
   (c) Is it fast?
(3) Does the atrial rate differ from the ventricular rate? Calculate the rates.
(4) Is there a P wave present before each QRS complex? After each QRS?
(5) Look at the P-R interval.
   (a) Is it reasonable in relation to the QRS?
   (b) Is it unreasonable?
(6) If the QRS rhythm is irregular, is there a noticeable pattern or is it haphazard?
(7) If P waves are absent, are they hidden or buried in the QRS complexes? Or is the QRS ectopic in origin?
(8) Have the P waves been replaced by "F" or "f" waves of atrial flutter or atrial fibrillation? †

* U waves are not always apparent in all normal adults on ECG.
† "F wave" or "flutter wave" is the term used to describe the regular sawtooth P waves in the electrocardiogram of a patient with atrial flutter. In impure flut-

The answers to these questions will aid the nurse in sifting out pertinent information leading to rhythm identification. However, the lethal arrhythmias, such as ventricular fibrillation and flutter, are not mysteries of electrocardiographic interpretations. Their appearance in conjunction with patient assessment and the presenting picture leaves little doubt that life is in peril.

Electric countershock

The term "electric countershock" includes the therapies of cardioversion and defibrillation. The techniques employ the use of controlled high-energy electric current in order to interrupt unacceptable cardiac rhythms. The rationale for this approach is to stop chaotic, lethal arrhythmias and to convert both dangerous tachyarrhythmias and atrial problems which are difficult to manage and which compromise the cardiac output. These disorders of the heart beat may include atrial fibrillation (especially when control by drugs has not been satisfactory), ventricular tachycardia in acute myocardial infarction and ventricular flutter and fibrillation.

The major distinguishing element between the 2 countershock therapies is that defibrillation is employed as a life-saving measure in cardiac arrest and cardioversion is employed as a therapeutic approach in controlling certain cardiac rhythm disturbances not being controlled adequately by drugs. Comparative differences of these 2 therapies are outlined in Table 14–3.

Defibrillation produces a simultaneous depolarization of the heart muscle. If the myocardium is oxygenated and not acidotic, the spontaneous heart beat may resume. Defibrillation is used most often in patients with ventricular fibrillation. It has not been effective with the heart in ventricular asystole,

ter (when the atrial rate is above 350 to 400 per minute), the "F" wave may vary in contour.
"f wave" or "fibrillary wave" is used to describe the irregular atrial oscillation wave in atrial fibrillation. The "f" wave replaces the P wave. The configuration of the "f" waves may vary, depending on the time they occur in the cardiac cycle.

TABLE 14-2 A SUMMARY OF ARRHYTHMIAS

Rhythm	P wave	P-R interval	QRS rate & rhythm	Comment
(1) Sinus	Before each QRS	0.12 to 0.20	60–100; regular	
(2) Sinus arrhythmia	Before each QRS	0.12 to 0.20	60–100; phasic variation with respiration	
(3) Sinus bradycardia	Before each QRS	0.12 to 0.20	Less than 60; regular	Not often below 40
(4) Sinus tachycardia	Before each QRS	0.12 to 0.20	Greater than 100; regular, but may vary a little	Usually 100–160, may be higher in children
(5) Atrial premature beat	Premature P may have different configuration	May be less than 0.12 or more than 0.20	If the APC is conducted; a premature QRS will be present	No compensatory pause-USUALLY
(6) Atrial tachycardia	Before each QRS, may be hidden	May be less than 0.12 or more than 0.20	140–200; absolutely regular, USUALLY	QRS normal, USUALLY; abrupt onset and termination. Carotid pressure may terminate attack
(7) Atrial flutter	200–360, sawtooth baseline ("F" waves)	Constant or variable	75–250, depending on amount of A-V block; regular or irregular	Carotid pressure produces temporary slowing, if any
(8) Atrial fibrillation	300 or more, irregular, undulant baseline ("f" waves)	Variable	50–250, depending on degree of A-V block; irregular	"f" waves may be shown better in V2 than lead II
(9) Ventricular premature contraction	None preceding the premature QRS			Compensatory pause, USUALLY; QRS configuration different, more than 0.10, USUALLY
(10) Ventricular tachycardia	Usually not seen; if present, are not related to QRS	Variable	150–250, USUALLY; regular or nearly regular	QRS broad, different, more than 0.10, USUALLY
(11) Ventricular fibrillation	None		No well-defined QRS complexes	No palpable pulse and no audible tones
(12) 1st-degree A-V block	Before each QRS	0.21 or more	Regular	May be a warning that 2nd- or 3rd-degree block will follow
(13) 2nd-degree A-V block	Each QRS preceded by a P wave, but some P waves not conducted	Normal or long	Rate often slow, regular, with occasional "dropped" beat	May be a warning that complete A-V block will follow
(14) 3rd-degree A-V block (complete heart block)	Occur regularly but without relationship to QRS	Variable	Below 60-USUALLY; regular-USUALLY	Spells of syncope common (Adams-Stokes attacks); pacemaker is in the ventricles (idioventricular rhythm)

Source: Harold A. Braun and Gerald A. Diettert, "A Programmed Text in Electrocardiography," part I of *Coronary Care Unit Nursing* (Missoula, Mt.: The Mountain Press, 1968), p. 59.

TABLE 14–3 COMPARATIVE DIFFERENCES BETWEEN DEFIBRILLATION AND CARDIOVERSION

Defibrillation	Cardioversion
(1) Life-saving, first aid measure.	(1) Elective measure.
(2) Patient is in a lethal arrhythmia or clinically dead.	(2) Patient is alive, sedated or anesthetized for the procedure, done in the hospital.
(3) Unsynchronized shock; *defibrillator* will fire when triggers are pushed.	(3) Synchronized shock; *cardiovertor* will fire only when switches are pushed and an "R" wave is sensed.
(4) In *adult* emergencies, a dead victim after CPR may be "shocked" with 400 watt-seconds.	(4) The "countershock" energy administered by the physician is selected. It may vary with size of patient and any knowledge of past successes utilized with his patient and cardioversion therapy.
(5) It may save the life; and probably will do no serious damage.	(5) May or may not convert the undesirable rhythm. Patient will be managed on drug therapy. Life not in peril.
(6) Paddles must be well lubricated with electrically conductive jelly. It is essential to avoid contact with other monitoring electrodes, wires, metals, etc., during defibrillation.	(6) Paddles must be well lubricated with electrically conductive jelly. In cardioversion it is essential to avoid contact with monitoring electrodes, wires, etc. Metal neck chains have usually been removed.

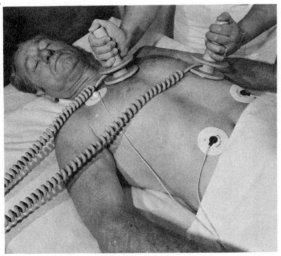

Figure 14–10 Proper positioning of defibrillator paddles. Note that the patient also has fixed electrodes in place.
Source: Photo courtesy of Mennen-Greatbatch Electronics, Inc.

but it is used when the heart is in ventricular tachycardia without a peripheral pulse.

When defibrillating a patient, one paddle should be to the right of the upper sternum below the clavicle and the other to the left of the cardiac apex (or left nipple line) (see Figure 14–10). The paddles need to be lubricated with electrically conductive jelly to provide for good conduction. While the shock is administered, be sure all other people are away from the bed.

In emergency situations, it is customary to deliver a shock of 400 watt-seconds for adults with ventricular fibrillation. The amount of myocardial damage is proportionate to the amount of energy used; therefore, some physicians elect to initiate the defibrillation at a lower setting and work up the scale until it is effective. This protocol is more applicable to slender patients with small frames. *Never start defibrillation at less than 200 watt-seconds* unless for a child.

A description of a typical portable defibrillator suitable for an emergency department is given in Table 14–4.

TABLE 14–4 DESCRIPTION OF A TYPICAL DEFIBRILLATOR/MONITOR

The defibrillator and ECG monitor should be combined in a single self-contained, portable unit. It should operate from 115 volts AC line power, as well as from a self-contained battery to permit instant operation without first locating an AC wall outlet. An internal battery charger should be included to keep the battery fully charged when the unit is plugged into a wall outlet. Typical detailed specifications are as follows:

Characteristic	Description
Defibrillator section	
(1) Energy	Stored—400 watt-seconds.
	Delivered—At least 300 watt-seconds into 50 ohm load.
(2) Waveform	Lown or Edmark (proven efficacy).
(3) Charging time	15 seconds maximum.
ECG monitor section	
(1) Display	Nonfading type, for easy visibility under all lighting conditions.
(2) Sweep speed	25 millimeters per second.
(3) ECG patient connection	3-lead patient cable or defibrillator paddles in the event of acute emergency.
(4) Isolation	The ECG input shall be isolated to allow not more than .04 microamps per volt to pass through the patient cable even when the defibrillator/monitor is connected to an AC wall outlet or to another piece of equipment.
(5) Frequency response	1 to 35 Hz. This typical "monitor" bandwidth is necessary to provide rapid recovery of the display after a defibrillation discharge and to minimize artifact and noise pickup during emergency resuscitation.
(6) Common mode rejection	High common mode rejection (typically greater than 120 dB) is very important for low artifact ECG pickup.
(7) Battery life	The unit should supply at least 4 hours of continuous monitoring and at least 40 maximum energy pulse discharges or before recharging of the battery.
Mechanical details	
(1) Construction	Rugged to withstand rough handling.
(2) Size	Shape should permit easy handling and mounting on hospital carts with the patient, to permit continuous monitoring when transporting a coronary patient from the ED to the CCU.

Source: Adapted from Mennen-Greatbatch Electronics, Inc.

DEATH-PRODUCING ARRYTHMIAS

Ventricular arrythmias

Ventricular fibrillation

The pattern of ventricular fibrillation is very distinctive and will not be mistaken for another arrhythmia (see Figure 14–11). It is impossible to detect any of the P, Q, R, S or T waves. The ventricle is unable to pump blood effectively; therefore, circulation ceases and death occurs quickly. Death can be prevented by the use of electric shock or defibrillation. It will be most effective if administered

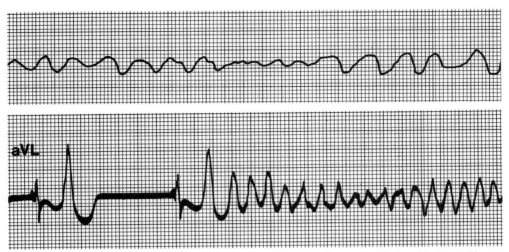

Figure 14–11 Ventricular fibrillation. Top: Common ventricular fibrillation. Bottom: Shows the sudden onset of ventricular fibrillation by a ventricular ectopic beat.
Source: Bottom strip is from p. 550 of *Learning Electrocardiography,* by J. Constant. Copyright 1973, by Little, Brown & Company.

within a 2-minute period and only if the ventricular fibrillation has developed spontaneously, not caused by some underlying problem, such as shock.

The effectiveness of the defibrillation can be increased by use of adrenalin or calcium chloride. Sodium bicarbonate should be administered to combat metabolic acidosis. The usual initial dose is one mEq. per kilogram of body weight. It can be given either in a continuous infusion over a 10-minute period or by a bolus injection.

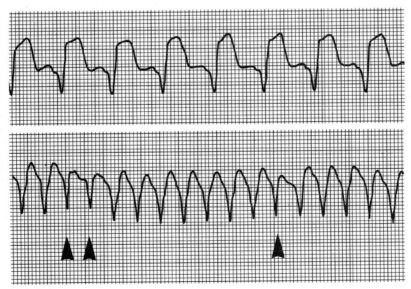

Figure 14–12 Ventricular tachycardia. Top: Common ventricular tachycardia. Bottom: Arrows indicate the occurrence of fusion beats.
Source: Bottom strip is from p. 547 of *Learning Electrocardiography,* by J. Constant. Copyright 1973, by Little, Brown & Company.

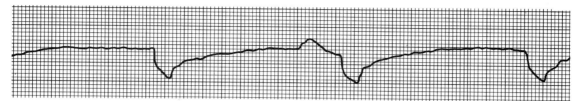

Figure 14-13 Ventricular standstill. Note the very slow heart rate.

Ventricular tachycardia

Ventricular tachycardia can lead to decreased cardiac output. If it is not reversed, it can lead to ventricular fibrillation. As seen in the rhythm strip (Figure 14–12), the ventricular rate is 150 to 250 beats per minute. A bolus of 50 mg. of lidocaine should be given immediately, and if the arrhythmia persists, a continuous lidocaine infusion should be started to prevent fibrillation. Electrical countershock may be needed to convert the arrhythmia to normal sinus rhythm.

Ventricular standstill

Before the patient experiences ventricular standstill, there is usually a warning in the form of an ECG pattern depicting second- or third-degree heart block.* If these are not treated, ventricular standstill or complete heart block may result. (Figure 14–13 shows a rhythm strip for ventricular standstill.) The heart rate will be as low as 30 beats per minute. Usually the impulses travel from the sinoatrial node to the atrioventricular node; however, in complete heart block, the impulses are totally interrupted, leaving the ventricle on its own. This results in a heart

beat so low there is great reduction in the cardiac output, leading to left ventricular heart failure—one of the complications of arrhythmias. The severe bradycardia with lowered cardiac output also causes a decrease in cerebral circulation, which may lead to syncope (Stokes-Adams attack).

The most effective method of treating heart block is by electrical pacing of the heart. This can be done on an emergency basis by means of a transvenous pacemaker (see Figure 14–14). If the heart block becomes a

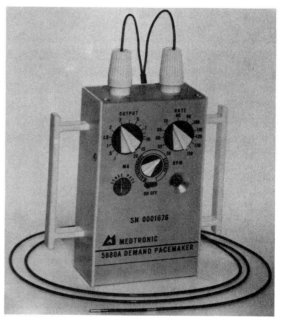

Figure 14-14 Transvenous pacemaker. The external demand pacemaker (pulse generator) is shown with a bipolar endocardial lead attached. The lead may be passed percutaneously through a peripheral vein, such as the femoral or antecubital. It is used only as a temporary pacemaker.
Source: Photo courtesy of Medtronic, Inc., Minneapolis, Minnesota.

* First-degree heart block is characterized by a prolongation of the P-R interval in excess of 0.21 second. Every atrial impulse reaches the ventricle, and a QRS complex is seen on the ECG.

Second-degree heart block is present when some of the atrial impulses do not reach the ventricles. Thus, a P wave will be found, but the following QRS complex will be absent. In second-degree block, the blocked P wave may occur in a ratio of 2:1, 3:1, 4:1, 5:1, etc.

Third-degree heart block (complete heart block) indicates that none of the atrial impulses reach the ventricles. Thus, atrial and ventricular activity are independent of each other, resulting in A-V dissociation. In complete heart block, the ventricular rhythm originating in the ventricle is called an idioventricular rhythm.

continuous phenomenon, a permanent pacemaker can be inserted at a later time. If the heart block is not immediately assessed and treated, the result is that of asystole or ventricular standstill. If the condition is not reversed by cardiopulmonary resuscitation within 4 minutes, irreversible cellular damage results.

Sodium bicarbonate is used to reverse acidosis. Drugs should be started by an intravenous route immediately. Epinephrine (Adrenalin), levarterenol (Levophed) and calcium chloride increase tissue perfusion and aid in stimulating the contractility of the myocardium.

The treatment of choice in treating asystole is cardiac pacing by electrical means. Until a pacemaker can be obtained, the use of an isoproterenol (Isuprel) drip may improve atrioventricular conduction and, thus, increase the cardiac output. The usual dose is one mg. of Isuprel to 250 or 500 ml. of intravenous fluid, administered at a rate of 30 to 60 microdrops per minute.

Premature ventricular contractions (PVCs)

The PVC is usually the warning signal that the myocardium is irritable and that the chance of ventricular fibrillation is increasing. Figure 14–15 presents 3 PVC rhythm strips. It is not always a sign of impending danger; however, if PVCs occur in excess of 6 per minute, treatment is indicated. If there are multiple foci (originating from more than one area of the ventricle) or if every other beat is a PVC, treatment is also needed. A lidocaine bolus of 50 to 100 mg. should be administered immediately. If this does not stop the PVCs, a lidocaine drip should be started, to deliver one to 3 mg. per minute.

If the lidocaine does not decrease the PVCs, the nurse should check the patient's potassium level to be sure it is within normal range; if cellular potassium is low, myocardial irritability results. Many times, the replacement of potassium will decrease PVCs.

Atrial arrhythmias

Atrial arrhythmias are not generally considered as immediate death-producing arrhythmias, but they should not be ignored, as they are indications that all is not well. Atrial arrhythmias are a result of tissue ischemia due to irritability of the muscle walls. These arrhythmias can decrease the effectiveness of the heart's pumping action by increasing the ventricular rate. Drug therapy or precordial shock are the treatments of choice for correcting the atrial arrhythmias.

Premature atrial contractions

Premature atrial contractions (PACs) originate from an ectopic focus in the atrium, which is a reflection of muscle irritability. PACs alone are of little significance; however, they present a forewarning of impending serious atrial arrhythmias (i.e., atrial fibrillation). PACs have varying contours, and the P wave may even be buried in the preceding T wave. The PAC may be conducted with a normal or prolonged P-R interval, or it may be completely blocked. (See Figure 14–16, a rhythm strip of PACs.)

Drug therapy should be instituted to control the ectopic beats when they increase to 6 or more per minute. The antiarrhythmic drugs currently being used are digitalis, quinidine and procainamide.

Paroxysmal atrial tachycardia

In a patient with coronary disease, this arrhythmia can cause cerebrovascular insufficiency, congestive heart failure or hypotension. Paroxysmal atrial tachycardia (PAT) can occur suddenly with no warning or can be preceded by PACs. It usually ends as abruptly as it begins, even without treatment. PAT does not lead to immediate death; however, the increased rate does increase the oxygen demand and consumption of the myocardium, which can lead to myocardial damage.

The rhythm is regular, but generally at a rate of 150 to 240 beats per minute. The

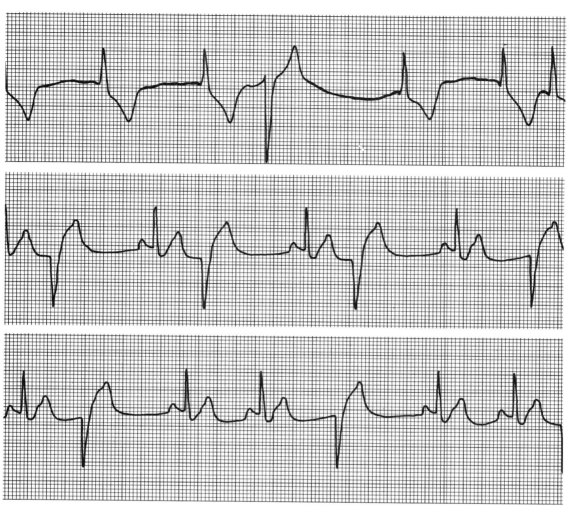

Figure 14–15 Premature ventricular contractions (PVCs) Top: Unifocal PVCs. Center: Bigeminy PVCs. Bottom: Trigeminy PVCs.

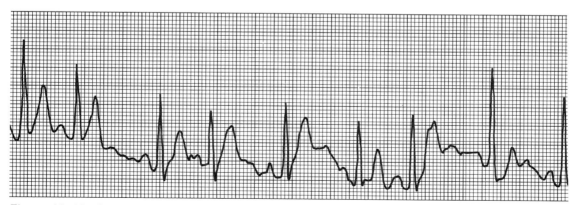

Figure 14–16 Premature atrial contractions. PAC patterns like this warn of atrial fibrillation.

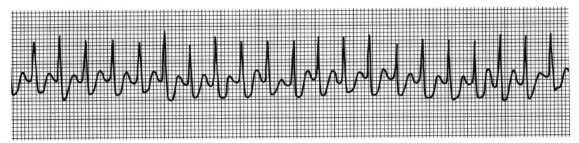

Figure 14–17 Paroxysmal atrial tachycardia. Note the regular rhythm and rapid heart rate.

ventricle is able to respond to each atrial impulse; therefore, there is no difference in the ventricular and atrial rate. (See Figure 14–17 for a rhythm strip for paroxysmal atrial tachycardia.)

The treatment of PAT consists of the use of carotid sinus massage to terminate the arrhythmia by reflex vagal stimulation. If this procedure is unsuccessful, precordial shock should be used immediately. If PAT tends to occur frequently, digitalis (the rapid-acting Cedilanid or ouabain) given intravenously will be effective in preventing recurrence.

Atrial flutter

In atrial flutter, a characteristic sawtooth (F wave or flutter wave) configuration is present on the rhythm strip (see Figure 14–18). The atrial rhythm is regular, yet there is a discrepancy between the atrial and ventricular rate, depending on how many atrial impulses pass through the A-V node. Only one half, one third or one fourth of the atrial impulses are conducted through the A.V. node and reach the ventricle. This difference

in atrial and ventricular rates is usually described as "atrial flutter," with 2:1, 3:1 or 4:1 block. With a rapid ventricular rate, the cardiac output is usually decreased, and the myocardial oxygen consumption is increased. This, then, predisposes to left ventricular failure and further myocardial ischemia.

Precordial shock (at 50 watt-seconds or less) is the treatment of choice, particularly when the ventricular rate is rapid. Digitalis (Cedilanid) administered intravenously can be effective in terminating atrial flutter, as well as in preventing its recurrence, particularly when the ventricular rate is not considered rapid.

Atrial fibrillation

Atrial fibrillation represents totally disorganized atrial electrical activity. P waves are absent; "f" waves may be noted especially in the esophageal lead; and there is an apparent grossly irregular ventricular rhythm. (See Figure 14–19.) The atrial rate is generally 350 to 600 beats per minute, with a ventricular rate of 100 to 160 beats per minute.

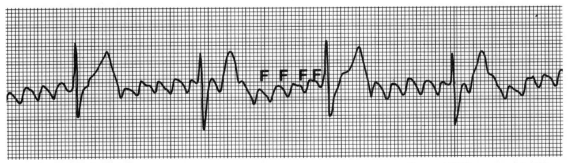

Figure 14–18 Atrial flutter. Notice the "sawtoothed" appearance of the flutter ("F") wave.

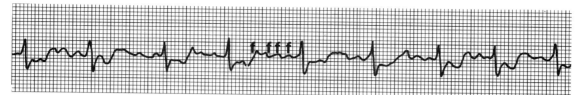

Figure 14–19 Atrial fibrillation. Notice the "wavy baseline" of fibrillatory "f" waves. P–R interval is irregular.

Atrial fibrillation can be seen in patients with acute myocardial infarction. Systemic or pulmonary emboli can result, as there is a propensity for clot formation when the atrium is in a noncontracting state. The major problem associated with atrial fibrillation is decreased cardiac output, resulting from both a rapid ventricular rate and loss of atrial contractions. This can then lead to ventricular failure and further myocardial damage.

Digitalis is used to decrease the rapid ventricular rate by increasing the degree of block at the A-V node. Digitalis does not necessarily restore the heart to a normal rhythm. The use of quinidine may be needed to convert atrial fibrillation to a normal sinus rhythm. When the patient displays evidence of left ventricular heart failure, the use of precordial shock is necessary, as drug therapy alone is much too slow.

Atrial standstill

Atrial standstill usually is indicative of death due to advanced left ventricular failure. This arrhythmia is a result of extensive myocardial damage, with progressive tissue ischemia. A warning of impending atrial standstill can be seen on the ECG monitor as a sudden decrease in shape or amplitude of the P wave or the complete disappearance of the P wave. See Figure 14–20, for a rhythm strip of atrial standstill.

Atrial standstill is usually a result of failure of the S-A node and atria to function. This leaves the less dependable A-V node and ventricles to carry out the function of pacemaker. Atrial standstill can also be a result of digitalis toxicity. Potassium or propranolol are administered to reverse the effects of digitalis.

The only treatment available is transve-

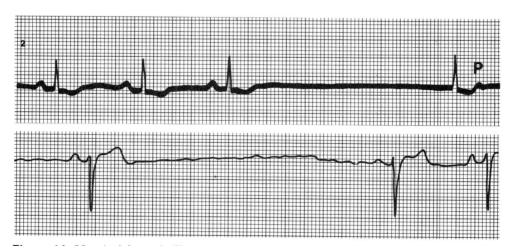

Figure 14–20 Atrial standstill. Such configurations are indicative of extensive myocardial damage.
Source: Top strip is from p. 464 of *Learning Electrocardiography,* by J. Constant. Copyright 1973, by Little, Brown & Company.

TABLE 14–5 THE RULE OF HUNDREDS

Atrial rate/minute	Tachycardia
(1) 400 ± 50 beats/minute	Atrial fibrillation
(2) 300 ± 50 beats/minute	Atrial flutter
(3) 200 ± 50 beats/minute	Atrial tachycardia

nous pacing, which is accomplished by the insertion of a transvenous pacemaker.

Defining arrhythmias

The nurse should commit to memory the above simple table (Table 14–5) on "the rule of hundreds," which will aid her about 90 percent of the time in tachycardia recognition. This rule applies only to *atrial* rates.

Cardiac ectopic pacemaker rates also aid the nurse in identifying certain arrhythmias. Table 14–6 shows the inherent rates of ectopic potential pacer sites when they are not abnormally stimulated to produce an ectopic tachycardia.

DRUG THERAPY

Drug therapy plays an essential role in the management of patients with cardiac problems. It is imperative that an intravenous line be inserted early to permit intermittent or continuous rapid administration of drugs and fluids necessary to support a stable cardiac rhythm and adequate circulation. Any one of several intravenous solutions can be used as the vehicle to transmit the drugs. The most common solutions are 5 percent dextrose in water and 5 percent dextrose and 0.2 percent normal saline or Ringer's lactate. A "cut-down" or "long line" (usually a large intracath) should not be established as the initial intravenous route, as it usually takes longer to insert; yet, a line of this type should

TABLE 14–6 INHERENT RATES OF ECTOPIC PACER SITES

Ectopic pacer site	Inherent rate
(1) A-V junction	40–60 beats/minute
(2) Ventricles [a]	20–40 beats/minute

[a] Ventricular pacers become increasingly *slower,* the more distant their location from the S-A node.

be used as soon as feasible for maintaining an open line for further drug therapy. It is important to note that the CVP line, when inserted, should not be used for drug administration as well, since it will not lend itself to a continuous accurate inflow of drug while taking frequent CVP readings.

Close monitoring of the patient's cardiac status, blood electrolytes and arterial blood gases is essential to determine appropriate drugs and dosages. Table 14–7 presents a list of drugs which should be available in any cardiac emergency situation.

Following emergency drug therapy, most patients will require the continued use of drugs in either antiarrhythmia, adrenergic vasopressor (Levophed or Aramine), or corticosteroid categories. These drugs are not discussed in this text, as the particular drugs used vary from facility to facility and physician to physician. It is recommended that the nurse become familiar with the drugs provided on the emergency cardiac cart in the facility where she is employed. Actions, side effects and normal dosages should become a part of her orientation to the usual drugs prescribed in cardiac emergencies. Table 14–8 summarizes the drugs most commonly used in cardiac emergencies, along with their recommended adult dosages. For child doses, see Chapter 18, Table 18–1.

Sodium bicarbonate

Sodium bicarbonate is used to combat metabolic acidosis or reverse acidosis caused by anoxia. An acidotic heart cannot be resuscitated; therefore, it becomes imperative that an intravenous infusion of sodium bicarbonate (one mEq./kg. of body weight) be given every 5 minutes until blood gas results are available in the absence of cardiac and respiratory activity. Ventilation must accompany sodium bicarbonate administration to remove the carbon dioxide from arterial blood. After spontaneous circulation is restored, the use of sodium bicarbonate is not indicated and may be harmful, as it could cause metabolic alkalosis.

TABLE 14-7 BASIC DRUGS FOR EMERGENCY CARDIAC CARE

Generic drug name	Trade drug name
Essential drugs	
(1) Sodium bicarbonate (prefilled syringes, 50 ml. ampules, or 500 ml. 5% bottles)	
(2) Epinephrine (prefilled syringes)	
(3) Atropine sulfate (prefilled syringes)	
(4) Lidocaine (prefilled syringe)	Xylocaine
(5) Morphine sulfate	
(6) Calcium chloride	
Useful drugs	
(1) Aminophylline	
(2) Dexamethasone	Decadron
(3) Dextrose 50%	Ion-o-trate Dextrose 50%
(4) Digoxin	Lanoxin
(5) Diphenhydramine hydrochloride	Benadryl
(6) Ethacrynic acid	
(7) Furosemide	Lasix
(8) Isoproterenol (hydrochloride)	Isuprel
(9) Lanatoside C	Cedilanid
(10) Meperidine (hydrochloride)	Demerol
(11) Metaraminol bitartrate	Aramine
(12) Methylprednisolone sodium succinate	Solu-Medrol
(13) Nalorphine (n-allylnormorphine) hydrochloride	
(14) Levarterenol (bitartrate)	Levophed
(15) Phenylephrine (hydrochloride)	Neo-synephrine
(16) Potassium chloride	
(17) Propranolol hydrochloride	Inderal
(18) Procainamide hydrochloride	Pronestyl
(19) Quinidine	
(20) Succinylcholine chloride	
(21) Tubocurarine chloride	

Source: Taken from "Standards for Cardiopulmonary Resuscitation and Emergency Cardiac Care," *Journal of the American Medical Association*, 227 (February 18, 1974):862. Reprinted with the permission of the American Heart Association.

The administration of sodium bicarbonate should be titrated in accordance with arterial blood gas results. It should not be given alone in cases of cardiac standstill or in persistent ventricular fibrillation, even following defibrillation. Cardiopulmonary resuscitation accompanied by sodium bicarbonate and adrenalin or calcium chloride should increase the effectiveness of the countershock as well as improve the status of the myocardium.

When setting up a cardiac emergency cart, it is best to supply the sodium bicarbonate in commercially prepared, prefilled syringes, as it makes the administration of the drug easier and quicker. Figure 14-21 shows 2 views of a typical cardiac emergency cart; see Chapter 2 for further information.

Epinephrine

Epinephrine (Adrenalin) is either given intravenously or injected directly into the heart through an intracardiac needle if an intravenous route is unavailable. Used intracardially, it may overcome asystole and stimulate spontaneous beating if the myocardium is simultaneously massaged to force the epinephrine through the coronary circulation.

TABLE 14–8   DRUGS USED IN CARDIAC EMERGENCIES

Drug	Suggested dose and route of administration	Remarks
(1) Sodium bicarbonate	I.V. bolus or continuous infusion. Initial dose, 1 mEq./kg. Repeat, then monitor according to blood gases.	Repeat dose following blood pH results if base deficit.
(2) Calcium chloride (10%)	I.V. bolus, 2.5–5 cc. every 10 minutes.	If digitalized, watch carefully following administration.
		Check calcium blood levels frequently, as high levels are detrimental. Don't mix with sodium bicarbonate.
(3) Epinephrine (Adrenalin)	I.V. bolus, 0.5 cc. of 1:1,000 solution diluted to 10 cc.	Note dilution. (Dilution for child is 1:10,000.)
(4) Lidocaine (Xylocaine)	I.V. bolus, 50–100 mg., may repeat. I.V. drip, 1–3 mg./minute. Mix I.V. bottle 500 mg./500 cc. D5W (yields 1 mg./cc.).	Do not exceed 100 mg./hour in children or 4 mg./minute in adults.
(5) Atropine	I.V. bolus, 0.5 mg. Repeat every 5 minutes until pulse is greater than 60.	Adult: Total dose not to exceed 2 mg. (except in 3rd-degree block).
(6) Levarterenol (Levophed)	I.V. bolus, 2–5 mg. every 5–10 minutes. I.V. drip, 0.4 mg./ml. in D5W.	Don't use in endotoxic shock or renal shutdown. Titrate for desired blood pressure.
(7) Metaraminol (Aramine)	I.V. drip, 0.5 mg. in 500 cc. D5W.	Titrate for desired blood pressure.
(8) Isoproterenol (Isuprel)	I.V. drip, 1 mg. in 500 cc. D5W.	Titrate for desired effect.

Epinephrine is used to (1) increase contractility of the myocardium, (2) increase coronary blood flow, (3) increase cardiac rate, (4) elevate perfusion pressure and (5) lower defibrillation threshold. It is important to note that epinephrine can produce ventricular fibrillation; however, this can usually be converted by defibrillation. It should be administered every 5 minutes during cardiopulmonary resuscitation. The usual dosage is 0.5 ml. of a 1:1,000 solution diluted to 10 ml.

Atropine sulfate

Atropine sulfate is used to counteract arrhythmias caused by excessive vagal action on the sinoatrial (S-A) and atrioventricular (A-V) nodes. It results in an increase in heart rate, making it a very useful drug in counteracting bradycardia. Atropine sulfate prevents cardiac arrest in profound bradycardia secondary to myocardial infarction, particularly where hypotension is also present. It is necessary to increase the heart rate to 60 to 80 beats per minute to improve the cardiac output and reduce the incidence of premature ventricular contractions and ventricular fibrillation.

Atropine is administered intravenously as a bolus of 0.5 mg. and repeated at 5-minute intervals until the heart rate is greater than 60 beats per minute in cases of sinus

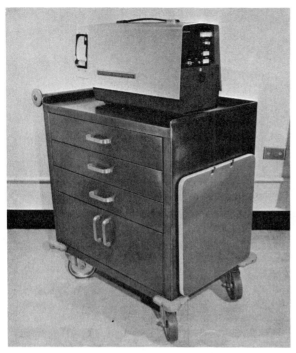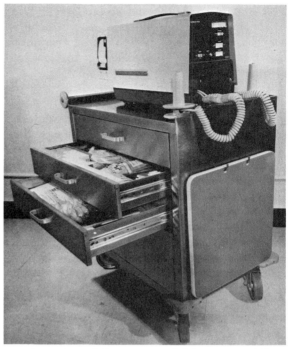

Figure 14–21 Two views of a cardiac emergency cart. A number of these are available commercially, but many hospitals modify existing equipment to fit individual needs. The cart should be easily movable and have space to contain all necessary resuscitation equipment. (See Chapter 2 for further details.) Source: Photos courtesy of Mennen-Greatbatch Electronics, Inc.

bradycardia, accompanied by premature ventricular contractions or a systolic blood pressure of less than 90 mm. Hg. Atropine is useless in ventricular ectopic bradycardia in the absence of atrial activity and in cardiac bradycardias caused by hypoxia or acid-base and electrolyte imbalances. The total dose of atropine sulfate should not exceed 2 mg. except in cases of third-degree atrioventricular block.

Lidocaine

Lidocaine (Xylocaine) stabilizes the cell membrane of the heart muscle and nerve fibers. The arterial blood pressure is not affected. It also reduces cardiac excitability and conductivity; therefore, it is useful in the treatment of acute multifocal ventricular arrhythmias and episodes of ventricular tachycardia. It is not useful in asystole.

A bolus of 50 to 100 mg. is administered intravenously, or the drug can be continuously infused, slowly, at a rate of one to 3 mg. per minute. Lidocaine should not be given in excess of 4 mg. per minute. If it is to be administered over a period of time, it is useful to mix a solution of 500 mg. lidocaine to 500 cc. 5 percent dextrose in water, which provides a one mg. per ml. solution.

Calcium chloride

Calcium chloride increases myocardial contractility, prolongs systole and enhances ventricular excitability. Sudden death can result following rapid intravenous injection, particularly if the patient is fully digitalized. Calcium chloride is used in profound cardiovascular collapse.

The usual dose is 2.5 to 5.0 ml. of a 10 percent solution. It should be given as a bolus at intervals of 10 minutes. It is important to monitor blood levels of calcium, as repeated large doses may elevate the calcium level of the blood and have negative effects.

Calcium cannot be mixed in the same I.V. or given through the same tubing as sodium bicarbonate, since they precipitate. If calcium gluconate is used, the dose should be increased to 10 mls. of a 10 percent solution, as it provides less ionizable calcium per unit volume.

Morphine sulfate

Morphine sulfate is not used in cardiac arrest, but it is a very important and essential drug in the treatment of patients with myocardial infarction. It is used to tranquilize the patient as well as relieve apprehension. It can produce periods of restful sleep.

Morphine in 3 to 4.5 mg. doses, I.V., may be needed as often as every 5 to 30 minutes for relief of pain.* The use of frequent small doses of the drug has proven more effective in reducing pain as well as avoiding respiratory distress than less frequent larger doses.

SUMMARY

The emergency nurse's diligence in detecting and caring for patients with cardiac problems has two-fold importance. Not only is cardiac disease capable of striking fatally with little warning, it is the leading killer of Americans today. The nurse's role of assessing cardiac emergencies is thus crucial.

BIBLIOGRAPHY

(1) "Cardiopulmonary Resuscitation," *Journal of the American Medical Association,* 198 (October 1966):138.

(2) Carson, P.: *Cardiac Diagnosis* (New York: McGraw-Hill Book Company, 1969).

(3) Constant, J.: *Bedside Cardiology* (Boston: Little, Brown & Company, 1969).

(4) ———: *Learning Electrocardiography* (Boston: Little, Brown & Company, 1973).

(5) *Emergency Measures in Cardiopulmonary Resuscitation,* revised (New York: American Heart Association, September 1969).

(6) *Heart Facts* (New York: American Heart Association, 1974).

(7) Houser, D.: "Emergency Cardiac Care," *Nursing Clinics of North America,* 8 (1973):401.

(8) Meltzer, L.; Abdellah, F., and Kitchell, J.: *Concepts and Practices of Intensive Care for Nurse Specialists* (Philadelphia: Charles Press, 1969).

(9) Phibbs, B., and Ewy, G.: *The Cardiac Arrhythmias* (Saint Louis: C. V. Mosby Company, 1973).

(10) Pinneo, R.: "Cardiac Monitoring," *Nursing Clinics of North America,* 7 (1972):457.

(11) Pinneo, R.: "Symposium on Concepts in Cardiac Nursing," *Nursing Clinics of North America,* 7 (1972):411.

(12) "Standards for Cardiopulmonary Resuscitation and Emergency Cardiac Care," *Journal of the American Medical Association,* 227 (February 18, 1974): 837.

---

* One ml. (15 mg.) of morphine sulfate may be diluted to 5 ml., so that one ml. of this solution contains 3 mg. of the drug. Then 3 to 4.5 mg. (one to 1.5 ml.) of the drug can be given every 5 to 30 minutes, as indicated.

15

Vascular emergencies

JAMES H. COSGRIFF, JR.
DIANN ANDERSON

The number of patients with urgent vascular problems seen in a hospital emergency department has increased in the past 2 decades. In part, this is due to increased mechanization, high-speed travel and an alarming rise in acts of violence. On the other hand, as the lifespan of the average American has lengthened into the eighth decade, the frequency of acute processes related to degenerative disease of the cardiovascular system has also increased. Less commonly, there has been a significant number of acute vascular problems arising from exposure to cold and in young women using birth control pills, the latter usually occurring in the veins.

Where 20 years ago, the prognosis for the majority of patients with vascular disease and/or injury was poor, today the outlook is considerably better. Advances in diagnostic and surgical techniques, combined with refinements gleaned by surgeons in the armed forces from battlefield experience, have resulted in better methods of evaluating patients with suspected vascular injuries, in higher rates of limb salvage and in lower morbidity and mortality. Those problems involving the extremities, though frequently serious, are usually more of a threat to limb than to life. But effective and appropriate

management of such patients in the emergency department is oftentimes essential to forestall a fatal termination.

When caring for patients with vascular problems, the nurse must be able to assess the nature of the problem, the cause and extent of the injury and, particularly in the instance of occlusive disease, whether the condition is acute or chronic. In instances of hemorrhage, she must possess the knowledge and skills to institute measures to control bleeding and support life.

Vascular emergencies can be considered under the following categories:

(1) Vascular injuries secondary to trauma.
(2) Vascular problems secondary to degenerative disease of the vessels.
(3) Vascular problems of venous origin.
(4) Vascular damage associated with cold injuries or decreased circulation and actual injury to the cells due to lower temperatures causing tissue damage.

VASCULAR INJURIES CAUSED BY TRAUMA

In patients with vascular injury due to trauma, depending upon the wounding agent, the nurse must be aware of the possibility of multiple organ injury and be familiar with established priorities of management in such instances. These patients are usually in the younger age group, and the problem will often relate to the injuries alone. Rarely is there accompanying systemic disease.

These injuries result from violence, such as stabbing or gunshot wounds or, less commonly, from automobile accidents and falls. An artery, vein or both may be damaged. Since the arterial tree is a high-pressure system, when damaged it can cause significant blood loss. While the majority of such injuries are obvious, in a small percentage of patients, presence of vascular damage may not be apparent. This is particularly true in blood vessel injury secondary to fractures and/or dislocations, in which blood loss occurs into a closed compartment of the limb as a result of partial or incomplete disruption of the vessel.

The method of injury may be important in relation to blood loss. Sharp, incised wounds of an artery may bleed massively without clotting, while blunt transection of an artery with torn, irregular edges will often clot due to deposition of platelet thrombi at the torn ends of the vessel and retraction of the vessel into the surrounding soft tissue.

The patient with vascular injury, especially when it is massive, requires immediate care by the emergency department team. Consideration of the following actions must be given:

(1) Assessing the need for life-support measures.
(2) Maintaining an adequate airway.
(3) Establishing a lifeline.
(4) Controlling hemorrhage.
(5) Obtaining a history of injury from the patient, if possible, or from a relative or friend. Time of injury, mechanism, weapon involved and the like are all important facts to substantiate.
(6) Assessing the patient for other injuries.
(7) Establishing priorities of management when multiple system injuries are present.
(8) Preparing the patient and family for anticipated surgical procedures.

It is obvious from the above list that when a patient with a vascular emergency is brought to the emergency department, the first thing the nurse must do is get help. Assessment, initiation of life-support measures and management of the injury must proceed concurrently.

Initial assessment

Prompt evaluation of the patient includes observation of the vital signs, level of consciousness, skin color and temperature, in order to obtain and record baseline data and determine if circulatory collapse has occurred. The wound should be identified and examined carefully to ascertain the presence of bleeding. Venous blood is drawn for routine studies, type and crossmatch. Arterial blood gas determinations are most helpful in evaluating ventilatory exchange and tissue perfusion, particularly in hypotensive patients. These should be obtained early in the emergency phase of care to provide baseline information and repeated as indicated.

Since various degrees of anxiety are quite common in these patients, it is important that they be kept quiet and given strong reassurance during initial assessment. Sedatives or narcotics are best *not* administered until complete evaluation of the extent of the injuries and the patient's general condition has been accomplished.

Life-support measures

Life-support measures are complex and best managed by the team approach. An adequate airway must be established and maintained and a lifeline inserted to restore circulating blood volume and maintain competency of the cardiovascular system. External hemorrhage must be controlled to prevent further depletion of circulating blood volume.

The airway

If the patient is conscious, airway patency may present no problem. In an unconscious patient or in one whose ventilation may be impaired as the result of the injury, prompt attention must be given to establishing and maintaining an adequate airway. Support to the angles of the jaw with slight extension of the neck will prevent the tongue from collapsing into the pharynx. An oropharyngeal airway may then be inserted to maintain the tongue in a more normal position. Should these prove insufficient, orotracheal or nasotracheal intubation or, on occasion, tracheostomy is required.

The lifeline

Patients with vascular injuries will suffer varying amounts of blood loss. The exact amount may be difficult to determine. The presence of hypotension and/or tachycardia should alert the nurse that significant depletion of blood volume has occurred. A large-bore needle or, preferably, a plastic catheter should be placed in a large vein in at least one or 2 extremities. After blood samples have been drawn and before type-specific blood is available, replacement of blood volume should be initiated using Ringer's lactate. Speed of infusion will depend upon the patient's circulatory status and will be determined by the physician. In a patient with a severe blood volume deficit, one liter of Ringer's lactate may be infused in a matter of minutes, if needed.

Precautions in selecting the extremities for fluid replacement are important. The fluid should not be replaced through the injured limb. In patients suspected of having injuries involving the major abdominal vessels, especially when the location of the wound might lead the nurse to suspect the inferior vena cava may be damaged, the lower limbs should not be used for the infusion. Rapid replacement via the legs in such an instance would only lead to an outpouring of the fluid directly into the abdominal cavity or retroperitoneal space. Similarly, when damage to the major vessels of the neck is suspected, the upper limbs should not be used.

Compatible, type-specific whole blood is the fluid of choice to replace lost circulating volume. Only in extremely critical situations, universal donor blood, type O Rh negative,

may be used for initial blood replacement, with the usual precautions in female patients.

Administration of blood

Transfusing blood requires special precautions, namely:

(1) Take vital signs prior to administration for baseline information and recheck the vital signs regularly throughout administration. When rapid infusion is necessary, one should monitor the central venous pressure as well as observe for clinical evidence of pulmonary overload. A doctor should be available at these times, since adverse reactions can occur rapidly.

(2) When the blood is available, 2 people should always check for donor type and number, patient's name, type of blood and expiration date.

(3) The blood should be at or near room temperature. Usually, removing the blood from refrigeration 10 to 15 minutes prior to use is sufficient. If a warming coil is used, the water in which the blood is immersed should be *tepid;* hot water will destroy cells.

(4) Flush the intravenous tubing with normal saline or lactated Ringer's solution before and after administration. The tubing should *not* be flushed with a 5 percent dextrose in water, since this solution can cause hemolysis and clotting in the tubing. A filter is used to remove any particulate matter which may have formed during storage.

(5) Take precautions in the administration of intravenous medications. Intravenous medications should never be given in the infusing blood itself. It is preferable to use a separate I.V. line. If the medications are to be given in the line infusing blood, the tubing must first be flushed with saline, the medication given and then the transfusion resumed. The "Y" tubing used for administration of blood facilitates this process, since one end is connected to saline and the other to the blood.

(6) Gently and thoroughly mix blood at intervals during the infusion. This is done by removing the blood container from the stand and inverting it 2 or 3 times.

(7) Watch the patient closely for adverse

reactions from the administration of blood. In brief, these are:

(a) *Hyperkalemia,* resulting from transfusing blood which is 2 to 3 days old and is caused by the breakdown of donor red blood cells, with subsequent release of potassium. Thus, the administration of fresh blood becomes important in patients with renal or cardiac disease. This problem usually does not arise unless a larger volume of blood is replaced.

(b) *Hypocalcemia,* occurring when a patient requires replacement of a large quantity of blood. The donor blood contains sodium citrate, which acts as an anticoagulant by removing ionized calcium in the donor blood. When large volumes of blood are replaced, the patient's circulating volume may consist wholly of donor blood.

(c) *Hemolytic reactions,* resulting from group incompatibility, such as A-B-O and Rh. Reactions usually occur during or shortly after the transfusion has been completed. It is a serious, sometimes fatal, complication, producing acute renal tubular necrosis.

(d) *Febrile reactions,* which can result when donor leukocytes are transfused into a recipient having antileukocyte antibodies. Multitransfused and multiparous recipients have increased antibodies and so are more susceptible. Usually, onset of symptoms occurs during the transfusion.

(e) *Circulatory overload,* occurring when blood is given too rapidly or in too large amounts. Patients with cardiorespiratory or renal problems and those with reduced body mass, such as amputees, are especially susceptible.

(f) *Hypothermia* may occur when the patient is rapidly infused with cold blood. The main danger here is cardiac arrest.

(g) *Anaphylaxis* is the antigen-antibody reaction of the recipient to allergens (antigens) in the donor's blood.

(h) *Infectious contamination* may result from the accidental introduction of bacteria during storage or handling or from pathogens present in the donor's blood. Hepatitis, malaria and syphilis can be transmitted in blood from asymptomatic carriers.

Close observation for changes in vital signs or clinical state is essential. Fever, chills, decreased urinary output (below 30 cc. per hour), leg or lumbar pain, cardiac or respiratory embarrassment, urticaria, nasal stuffiness, headache or unexplained parasthesia, paralysis, tingling or hyperreflexia may forewarn of further complications. When any of these occur, the blood should be discontinued immediately, the line kept open with saline or Ringer's lactate and the physician notified. The donor blood should be returned to the blood bank immediately for further testing.

In only extremely critical situations should universal donor blood, type O RH negative, be used for blood replacement. However, once O negative blood is given, it must be continued throughout the period of time the patient is in danger.

Controlling hemorrhage

The most appropriate means available to control hemorrhage are (1) pressure, (2) elevation of the part and (3) use of a tourniquet. The method selected will depend on the location and the type of vessel injured, as well as the extent of wounding. In general, exploration of the wound to clamp a major vessel is contraindicated, since a clot may be dislodged and further damage to the vessel may result, causing additional blood loss.

Pressure method

In a limb, pressure directly over the bleeding site or over the major arteries supplying the limb may diminish or completely control blood loss. When the pressure is applied over the major artery to the limb, oftentimes the collateral circulation is sufficient to preclude complete control of the blood loss.

The simplest means is to place several layers of sterile gauze over the wound and apply direct pressure with the fingers or heel of the hand. Pressure dressings may function very well in certain sites on the limbs, scalp or face. The pressure may be maintained with an outer, circular elastic bandage. In the presence of a fracture, it may be difficult to maintain adequate pressure using this method.

The most frequently used pressure points are the brachial artery in the arm and the femoral artery in the leg. Some advocate pressure over the superficial temporal artery, which lies just anterior to the ear, to control hemorrhage from scalp lacerations. Its benefit is doubtful; however, it is more advantageous than pressure applied to the carotid artery.

The brachial artery may be felt midway along the upper arm on its medial aspect. The pulse can be readily palpated by compressing the soft tissue against the medial aspect of the humerus. The lower end of the brachial artery overlies the medial half of the antecubital space and can also be used as a site of pressure. In the lower limb, the femoral artery is palpable in the mid-portion of the inguinal crease. Since the blood in both of these vessels is under arterial pressure, it may be difficult to maintain direct finger pressure for any period of time. (Figure 15–1, which illustrates locations of pulse points, may also be helpful in locating pressure points of the major arteries.)

Elevation

Elevation of an extremity with a vascular injury will lessen the pressure in the vessels. This is particularly true in injuries to the venous side, which is a low-flow, low-pressure system. Associated injuries in the limb, especially fractures, may preclude use of this technique, however.

Tourniquet

A tourniquet may be an extremely useful method of controlling blood loss from an extremity when pressure and elevation are ineffective. Much discussion has developed over the years concerning use of a tourniquet. Negative results from tourniquets are more often than not a result of improper use of the device. When applied properly, it can successfully control hemorrhage until definitive measures are instituted. The points to be stressed in the proper use of a tourniquet are these.

(1) It should be of the inflatable (pneumatic) variety so that the desired pressure may be uniformly applied and maintained.

(2) The tourniquet should exert pressure over a wide area of the skin to avoid localized pressure on the limb, which can be transmitted directly to an artery, causing damage to the vessel wall, as well as to surrounding tissue. A good example of a proper tourniquet is a blood pressure cuff, found in every emergency department. An example of an improper, potentially harmful tourniquet is the rubber tubing commonly used in obtaining blood samples.

(3) The tourniquet must be inflated above the level of systolic blood pressure. Insufficient pressure will allow for continued arterial inflow into the limb and yet cause venous outflow occlusion, which will produce an increase in pressure in the veins leading to further blood loss.

(4) To be effective, the tourniquet must be applied on the limb between the site of injury and the heart, in a position where it can exert adequate pressure on the major artery. In the arm, this level is between the elbow and the shoulder, and in the leg, between the hip and the knee. In these locations, the artery can be successfully compressed against the humerus and the femur, respectively. In the distal portion of the limbs, the arteries are positioned between the bones so

that adequate pressure cannot be applied.

(5) The time of application of the tourniquet should be noted. This is best done by placing a piece of tape on the tourniquet and recording the time.

(6) The tourniquet, when applied for control of bleeding, should not be deflated except under the supervision of the physician.

Further assessment

History

Once life-saving measures have been instituted and the patient's condition has been stabilized, a more complete assessment by history and examination is needed. As much information as possible is collected from the patient, witnesses, relatives, ambulance attendants or police officers.

When a weapon is involved, details of the type of weapon are helpful. The firearms responsible for most civilian injuries are of a relatively low-muzzle velocity and cause considerably less internal tissue damage than a high-velocity, military-type weapon. Instruments used in stabbings vary greatly in blade size and length. Details surrounding the incident and the weapon may be useful in determining the extent of injury. Whenever possible, a history of past illness, associated disease, allergies, metabolic disorders and current medical therapy should be collected as part of the complete history.

Physical assessment

Careful physical assessment is needed to ascertain both the extent of the primary injury and the presence of other injuries. It should be done with a minimum of movement of the patient. In penetrating injuries, examination of the wounds of entrance and exit may give some indication of the structures lying in between which may be injured. In limb injuries, the damaged limb should be compared to its opposite for any alteration in color and temperature.

Since the vascular structures lie immediately adjacent to nerves, which may be damaged, sensation and motor power of the limbs must be tested to rule out nerve injury. The patient may complain of sensations varying from paresthesias or numbness to partial or total paralysis of the limb. Sensory function can be tested by the pin-prick method. Motor activity can be evaluated by asking the patient to wiggle his digits or flex the ankle or wrist. Recording of these initial findings is part of the permanent emergency department record and will provide important baseline data.

The arterial pulses in each limb should be carefully palpated to evaluate the circulation to the extremities. Figure 15–1 displays their positions. It is particularly important to evaluate the pulses distal to the site of injury. In fractures involving the long bones, massive hemorrhage may occur into the muscular compartments, particularly that of the thigh, with no evidence of external hemorrhage. Such injuries may result in blood loss in excess of 1,000 ml.

Total assessment of the patient should be completed. Periodic determination of blood pressure, pulse, respiratory rate and type of respiration are taken and recorded. Since some patients will require large amounts of fluid replacement, the urine output must be measured. This is best done by means of an indwelling urinary catheter so that ongoing evaluation of renal function can be done. The urinary output should be maintained at approximately one cc. per kilogram of body weight per hour. A central venous pressure catheter may also be inserted to help guard against circulatory overload.

Vascular injuries require specialized techniques for a complete diagnosis and definitive repair, which in turn demands the skill of a surgeon familiar with such techniques. Single injection limb arteriography may be done in most emergency department x-ray units with a minimum of equipment. (See Figure 15–2.) More sophisticated diagnostic

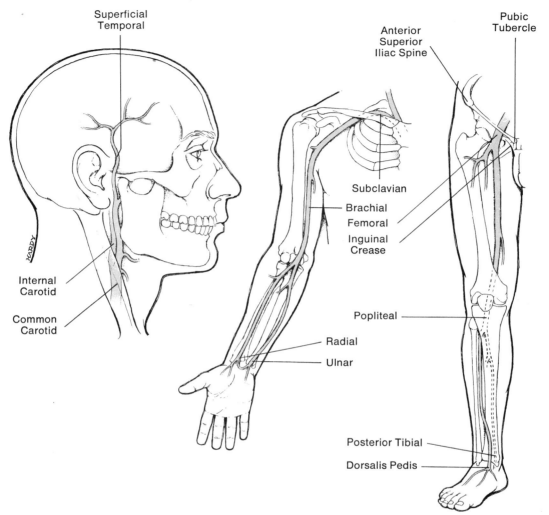

Figure 15–1 Pulse Points. The drawings indicate the points on major arteries of the head, neck and extremities where a pulse can most easily be palpated.

arteriography, when deemed necessary, may be done in the x-ray department or operating room, as conditions require.

Wound care

Primary wound care should be a minor consideration in the presence of a vascular injury. Application of a sterile dressing without any attempt at probing or examining the wound is considered adequate. Tetanus prophylaxis is given according to established recommendations (see Figure 10–11, page 133). Use of both tetanus toxoid and hyperimmune globulin may be necessary, especially when extensive soft tissue damage has occurred. Appropriate broad-spectrum antibiotic therapy may be initiated in the emergency department, depending upon the judgment of the physician.

Throughout the emergency phase of care, the nurse must be aware that the patient may need to undergo a major surgical procedure

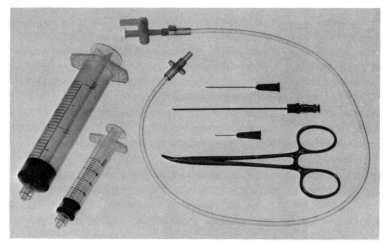

Figure 15–2 Minimum equipment for single-injection limb arteriography. Included are syringes (30 cc., 5 cc.), needles for local anesthesia (22- and 25-gauge) and for arterial puncture (19-gauge spinal), connecting tubing with 3-way stopcock, clamp. Skin prep, anesthetic solution and dye are not shown.

as soon as his condition will allow. The ultimate goal of the emergency team is to prepare the patient to withstand the anticipated surgery.

The patient and family should be advised periodically of the status of treatment and response. The nature and gravity of the problem must be expressed openly and the family prepared for unexpected eventualities. The nurse who is familiar with general information about vascular injury and repair should be able to adequately handle the needs of the family.

Occult arterial injuries

Occult arterial injuries may be the result of blunt trauma or may occur in association with fractures. They vary from contusion of a vessel wall to intimal tears and even to complete transection of a vessel. While there may be no obvious bleeding, there is invariably a decrease in circulation to the affected part which can be detected by careful assessment. Diminished arterial circulation is manifest by: (1) pain in the limb, (2) lower skin temperature, (3) pallor, (4) sensory and motor changes, (5) diminution or absence of pulses distal to the point of injury and (6) slower capillary filling.

Fractures of the long bones, such as the femur and humerus, may be associated with arterial damage. Patients exhibiting circula-

tory defects associated with fractures and/or dislocations require early reduction and immobilization. Sometimes these maneuvers correct the vascular problem. More often, diagnostic arteriography is necessary to localize the site of injury prior to starting reparative vascular surgery.

VASCULAR PROBLEMS OF DEGENERATIVE DISEASE

Patients with vascular problems secondary to degenerative disease, such as acute arterial occlusion or ruptured abdominal aneurysm, more often than not will have some associated problem of a systemic nature (diabetes) or of an organ system (arteriosclerotic heart disease, congestive heart failure or arrhythmia; chronic lung disease; renal problems). Awareness of these concomitant problems is essential to appropriate management.

Acute arterial occlusion

Sudden occlusion of the artery is accompanied by cessation of blood flow. This is found as a complication of arteriosclerosis or of a disturbance in cardiac rhythm, particularly auricular fibrillation. Primary occlusion of an artery by arteriosclerotic plaque formation is a classic example of thrombosis, while acute obstruction of arterial flow by a clot displaced from the heart and lodged in a peripheral artery exemplifies arterial embolism. In each case, the patient will demonstrate evidence of vascular compromise and lessened blood flow.

Embolic occlusion

An embolism results when a blood clot, originating in one section of the cardiovascular system (usually the heart), breaks off and enters the arterial stream until a point of narrowing is reached. The embolus then lodges there and obstructs distal flow. Typically, an embolus will lodge at the bifurcation of an artery. The most common sites are the bifurcations of the abdominal aorta and the carotid, the femoral, the popliteal and the brachial arteries (see Figure 15–3). Predisposing factors include rheumatic heart disease with mitral stenosis, auricular fibrillation or myocardial infarction. In each instance, a mural thrombus may form within the chambers of the left side of the heart. A fragment then breaks off and migrates to a peripheral artery. Less commonly, a thrombus present in an aneurysm or an arteriosclerotic plaque may fragment and migrate as well. When occlusion occurs, it is sudden. The patient is usually in the age group above 50.

The patient will usually give a history of sudden onset of pain in the affected part(s). This usually occurs in a limb, and the pain will be manifest in the limb distal to the site of the occlusion. Soon thereafter, there develops coldness, pallor, numbness and, finally, inability to move the part. When the occlusion occurs in the carotid bifurcation, the patient may appear to have had a stroke.

Physical findings will vary with the site and duration of the occlusion. Levels of physiological changes are usually detectable and will be a guide to the site of the block. The level of temperature change is some distance distal to the actual site of occlusion, because of blood flow through collateral channels which may open in an effort to allow blood to bypass the occluded site. (See Figure 15–4 for typical temperature changes.)

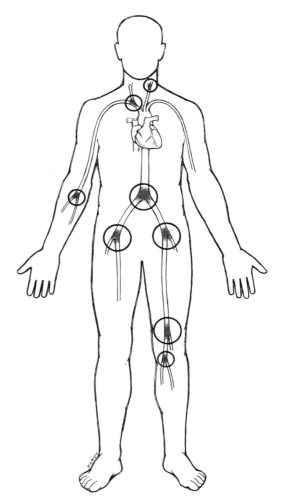

Figure 15–3 Common sites of embolic arterial occlusion. Bifurcations of major vessels are most commonly involved in occlusions.

As the period of occlusion lengthens, the pallor changes to mottled cyanosis, resulting from anoxia and decreased tissue perfusion. Motor weakness will progress to complete paralysis. Palpation will reveal absence of pulses distal to the level of occlusion. Tenderness is often elicited at the point of occlusion along the course of the artery. The veins are usually collapsed. Capillary filling is extremely slowed.

The cardinal findings of acute arterial occlusion of a limb may be summarized as: (1)

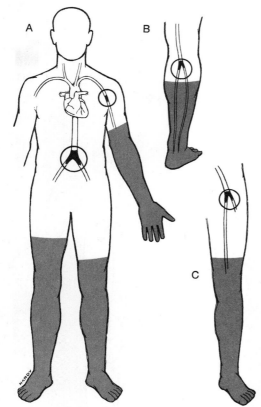

Figure 15–4 Temperature and color changes due to occlusive disease. A: In the upper limb, occlusion of the axillary artery results in a level of demarcation in the distal arm. Saddle embolus of the aorta causes change distal to mid-thigh, bilaterally. B: Occlusion of popliteal artery causes change at level of mid-calf. C: Occlusion of common femoral artery produces level of change in distal third of thigh.

pain, (2) pallor, (3) paresthesia, (4) paralysis, (5) pulselessness distal to the level of occlusion. Occlusions of the terminal aorta (saddle embolus) will result in these findings in both legs. As the interval lengthens after embolization, there may occur more extensive occlusion of the blood flow, both proximal and distal to the area where the embolus is lodged, causing further evidence of inadequate circulation and, eventually, gangrene. Patients with frank gangrene usually have a long-established occlusion and require a period of study before operative intervention. Since patients with an embolism usually have under-

lying cardiac disease, thorough assessment is indicated. Electrocardiogram and blood work, including arterial blood gases, type and cross-match, should be done. Further evaluation of the patient may include preoperative arteriography to localize the level of occlusion.

Time is a critical factor for a successful outcome in the patient with an acute occlusion. Although embolectomy has been accomplished successfully as late as 24 hours after onset, flow is more often restored in patients with shorter periods of occlusion. Definitive treatment requires urgent removal of the embolus with restoration of flow. This can usually be performed under local anesthesia, even in instances of a saddle embolus of the aorta. Long-term anticoagulant therapy is often necessary, depending on the etiology.

Thrombotic occlusion

Thrombosis is usually the result of arteriosclerotic vascular disease. As opposed to embolism, thrombosis ordinarily occurs gradually over a varying period of time and is commonly found in the lower extremities. An arteriosclerotic plaque develops on the inner lining of the artery. These plaques frequently have sharp edges and serve as a nidus for the deposition of platelets and thus development of small platelet thrombi. These gradually increase in size, narrowing the lumen of the vessel. As the blood flow lessens, the thrombus increases in size until complete occlusion occurs.

History will usually reveal that the patient had symptoms of crampy pain in the leg with exercise, or merely with walking, for some time prior to the acute episode. This is known as intermittent claudication. The patient will usually be above middle age and will present with varying complaints due to the ischemia. This problem occurs more commonly in the male than in the female. Those patients seen in the emergency setting are more often in advanced stages of the disease, with well-differentiated gangrenous changes in the limb. The majority of such patients are smokers.

Physical assessment will demonstrate those

findings resulting from gradual, progressive ischemia. The limb will be cool, with dependent rubor. When it is elevated above heart level, cadaveric pallor develops due to the restricted arterial circulation. Other characteristic signs of reduced nutrition to the part are: (1) the nails are thickened; (2) the skin of the leg is shiny, with atrophy of the skin appendages and a lack of hair; (3) pulses are unobtainable distal to the level of occlusion. Most often, the level of occlusion is the distal third of the thigh. Thus, the femoral pulse may be palpable, but the popliteal and pedal pulses are absent.

The nurse may be unable to determine the duration of the complete occlusion in the absence of frank gangrene. In many instances, patients with arteriosclerosis may provide a fairly long history suggestive of intermittent claudication, then develop sudden, total occlusion of the artery. (Figure 15–5 shows an arteriogram of such a patient.) Physician evaluation should be obtained to ascertain whether urgent treatment is necessary.

Ruptured abdominal aneurysm

Rupture of an aortic aneurysm represents a catastrophic event. An aneurysm is a local dilatation in an artery which is most often secondary to arteriosclerosis. It occurs most commonly in the abdominal aorta and is seen more frequently in males over the age of 50. The level of occurrence is commonly below or distal to the renal arteries in the terminal portion of the aorta.

Anatomically, an aneurysm may be a well-localized dilatation of the aortic wall (saccular) or one extending over a considerable length of the vessel (fusiform) (see Figure 15–6). The outpouching occurs at a point of weakness in the wall of the artery which resulted from degenerative changes in the medial layer (medial necrosis) and which accompanies arteriosclerosis. The aneurysm may be considered a single manifestation of a generalized disease process of the cardiovascular system. Once the aneurysmal dilatation occurs, it has a tendency to enlarge over a period of time, which may be measured in

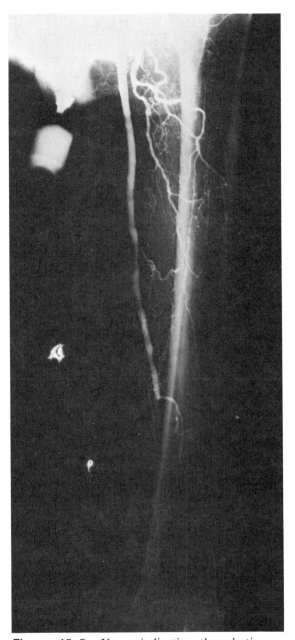

Figure 15–5 X-ray indicating thrombotic occlusion. Eighty-four-year-old female was admitted to emergency department after her left leg "collapsed" and was unable to walk thereafter. Leg was cool and pale beyond mid-calf. Arteriogram was done with emergency department x-ray. (Note notching of femoral artery, sudden termination of dye column and relative lack of collateral circulation.) At exploration, a thrombus was extracted. Diagnosis was arteriosclerotic vascular disease with acute thrombotic occlusion.

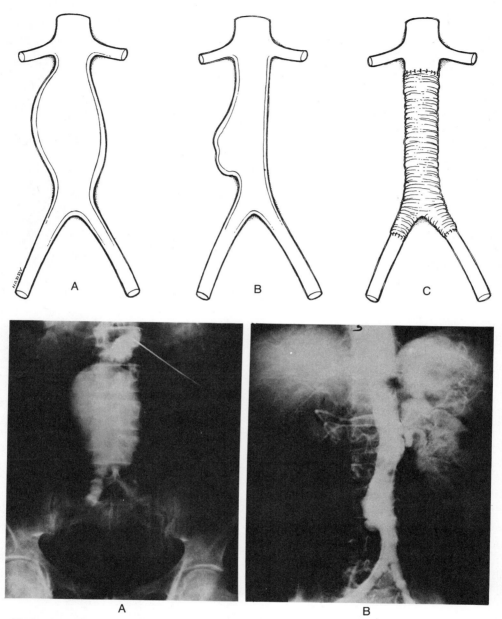

Figure 15–6 Aneurysms. A: Translumbar aortogram and diagram of fusiform aneurysm of abdominal aorta, distal to origin of renal arteries. B: Retrograde aortogram and diagram of saccular aneurysm of abdominal aorta, distal to origin of renal arteries. C: Aneurysmal segment excised and replaced by prosthetic graft.

months or years. (See Figure 15–7 for x-rays showing progressive enlargement.)

The rupture of an aneurysm may begin from a small leak with dissection into the wall of the aorta and finally through the outer wall

into the retroperitoneal space. The aneurysm usually projects to the left of the midline, and the rupture is usually to the left, which is the site of greatest weakness of the wall. In rare instances, it may rupture anteriorly into the

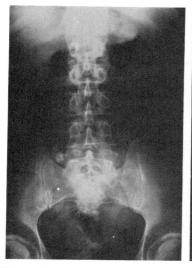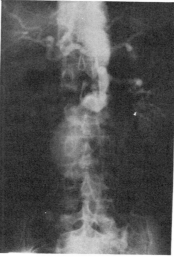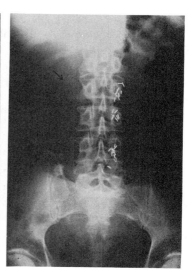

Figure 15-7 Progressive enlargement of abdominal aortic aneurysm. Left: Flat film, with rim of calcification to right of mid-line at level of second lumbar vertebra (1970). Center: Aortogram demonstrating aneurysm below renal arteries. Note rim of calcification. Aneurysm is lined with a mural thrombus. Right: Flat film 4 years later (1974). Calcification wider. Patient fainted at home. Ruptured aneurysm found at laparotomy. Aneurysm excised and replaced by Dacron graft.

peritoneal cavity or to the right. As a result of the leak, blood extravasates into the retroperitoneal space with formation of a hematoma. Since blood is an irritant to the tissues, it causes considerable pain. The loss of blood may be severe enough to produce hemorrhagic shock.

The history will vary. The patient may complain of a sudden onset of severe and unrelenting back pain associated with abdominal discomfort. As the blood loss continues with enlargement of the hematoma, vascular collapse can occur associated with weakness. Sudden onset of syncope may occur. Ordinarily, there are no symptoms suggestive of vascular insufficiency to the lower limbs.

Physical assessment will reveal an acutely ill individual, usually a male, above the age of 60. Profound shock may be present, with undetectable blood pressure in those patients with extensive blood loss. On the other hand, the patient may arrive in the hospital with blood pressure at normotensive levels or with varying degrees of hypotension. The most significant findings are in the abdomen. Careful palpation will demonstrate a pulsatile, expansile mass in the area of the umbilicus, primarily to the left of the midline. The size of the mass varies but is usually in excess of 7 cm. It is tender, though peritoneal signs are not always striking. In most patients, the femoral pulses are present. The pulses distal to the femoral region, the popliteal and pedal pulses, may be palpable or absent, depending on the degree of peripheral vascular disease.

Complete blood count and urinalysis should be obtained immediately. An indwelling bladder catheter is placed, since these patients are prone to develop significant decline in urinary output, which is most likely secondary to hypotension. Blood should be drawn for type and crossmatch. Arterial blood gases are of value in those patients in shock. An electrocardiogram is indicated, since most of these patients have arteriosclerotic heart disease. X-rays of the abdomen will often demonstrate a rim of calcification lateral to the lower lumbar vertebra. This is pathognomonic of an abdominal aneurysm and usually confirms the diagnosis when in conjunction with the other findings.

Resuscitative measures are begun immediately as indicated. Once the diagnosis is established, preparation is made to transfer the patient to the operating room. Adequate amounts of type-specific whole blood must be available for use during the surgery. As much as 2 to 3 liters of blood may be lost into the retroperitoneal space. It is not unusual for these patients to require from 8 to 12 units of blood during the surgical procedure. Fluid volume replacement may be initiated with rapid infusion of large amounts of Ringer's lactate solution. Careful attention must be given to frequent recording of vital signs. The urinary output should be maintained at approximately one cc. per kilogram per hour.

Urgent surgery is necessary. Its purpose is to obtain control of the aorta with cessation of hemorrhage, followed by resection of the aneurysmal area and replacement of the excised segment by a prosthetic graft (see Figure 15–6). Mortality varies from 30 to 50 percent.

VENOUS OCCLUSION

Occlusion in the venous system may result from thrombosis or embolism. The vast majority of problems relate to venous thrombosis, and this occurs most frequently in the leg. Anatomically, the venous system of the leg is composed of superficial and deep veins. Thrombus formation can occur in either type. Some of these thrombi may fragment and produce embolization. However, the frequency of embolization is considered more likely with deep venous thrombosis than with occlusion of the superficial veins.

Thrombosis of the superficial veins

Superficial thrombophlebitis occurs secondary to trauma, infection, birth control pills or varicose veins with stasis. The patient's symptoms may range from mild tenderness to severe pain, which may be aggravated by walking. Physical assessment will reveal a cord-like thickening of the vein at the site of occlusion, with a surrounding area of erythema and/or swelling. This swelling may be more prominent in the distal portion of the leg. There is usually no systemic reaction. Pathologically, the clot is firmly adherent to the vein wall and rarely causes embolus formation.

Management consists of analgesics for pain relief, rest and elevation of the part. Warm, moist dressings may be used to relieve discomfort and promote healing. Circumferential elastic (Ace) bandages are poorly tolerated in the acute phase, since compression of the vein may cause more pain. Anticoagulants are not necessary as a rule. Varicosities of the leg veins, when present, should be removed after the acute process has subsided, to prevent further recurrent episodes. Hospital admission is rarely necessary.

Thrombosis of the deep veins

Deep thrombophlebitis or phlebothrombosis is a serious affliction which may involve any portion of the deep venous system but particularly occurs in the leg. Various etiologic factors have been described, including stasis, trauma and inflammatory conditions. Slowing of blood flow may combine with a change in blood coagulability to produce the thrombosis.

Infectious diseases of the skin, complicated tinea infections of the foot (athlete's foot) may result in ascending involvement of perivenous lymphatic vessels which surround the vein. This, in turn, may affect a reaction in the vein wall, with subsequent clot formation. Once occlusion has occurred, the vein wall may be irreparably damaged, causing recurrent episodes to develop and eventually leading to the changes of chronic venous insufficiency and the postphlebitic syndrome.

Acute occlusion of the deep vein may be associated with slowing of blood flow above and below the thrombus and further clot formation. These clots are not usually firmly attached to the vein wall and are likely to fragment and cause embolization.

The patient will usually complain of swelling and discomfort in the limb. Bland occlusion (phlebothrombosis) may be painless, while thrombophlebitis is more often painful and associated with evidence of systemic reaction, marked by fever, tachycardia, leukocytosis.

Examination will reveal swelling of the limb. Careful palpation of the muscles of the calf or thigh elicits tenderness, especially along the course of the deep veins. The extremities should be carefully evaluated for the presence of any infectious processes, such as athlete's foot, which may be a causative factor in the occlusive process. Dorsiflexion of the foot with the knee extended causes pain in the posterior aspect of the calf (Homans's sign).

In septic conditions, the leg will appear hot, red and swollen (phlegmasia cerulea dolens). In other instances, there may be arterial spasms associated with the venous thrombosis, causing the leg to be pale, cool and swollen (phlegmasia alba dolens). Careful assessment of the peripheral pulses should be done. Enlarged tender nodes may be palpated on the involved side. It is not unusual for the venous systems of both legs to be involved.

Management is directed toward prevention of complications during resolution of the process.

The patient should be admitted for bedrest. Antibiotics are used as indicated by the presence of sepsis. Anticoagulants are given, initially heparin sodium, to bring the clotting time to therapeutic levels. Warfarin (Coumadin) should be started at the same time, and its dosage will depend on the prothrombin time. Elastic bandages are contraindicated, since they will serve only to occlude the superficial veins and drive more blood into the already occluded deep venous system, leading to further pain and aggravation of symptoms. The patient must be observed closely for any complications, the most serious being pulmonary thromboembolism.

In some areas of the country, emergency surgery is done to extract the thrombus and restore blood flow immediately. This approach is still not generally accepted, but the emergency nurse must be aware that the possibility of surgical intervention exists.

COLD INJURIES

Serious damage to tissue may occur as a result of exposure to cold. Most often the areas involved are the extremities, particularly the hands, feet, nose and ears. The problem was common in World War II and the Korean conflict, as a result of prolonged exposure to below-freezing temperatures. In civilian life, it is seen in construction workers, skiers and outdoorsmen. A combination of temperature, humidity, wind and exposure time contributes to the development of the process.

Tissue damage is thought to result from interference of circulation by sludging of blood in the smaller vessels and by actual changes within the tissue cells as a result of the lower temperature. Varieties of cold injury are frostbite, trenchfoot and chilblains. Symptoms will vary with the nature of the cold injury but generally include numbness, tingling and paresthesia in the affected area. In trenchfoot, in which the foot is immobile in damp footwear at above-freezing temperatures, there may be few symptoms until the person returns to warm environment. Then, severe burning pain is noted, with accompanying redness and swelling.

The degree of damage in cold injuries is frequently classified in a manner similar to burns. In moderate injuries, blisters may form with subsequent desquamation, as in a second-degree burn. In more serious injuries, complete necrosis of tissue can result. Varying degrees of edema may be present. Chronic alcoholic patients and derelicts who may have been exposed to cold temperatures are often not seen in the emergency department until several days after exposure, at which time frank gangrene may be present.

In the acute phase, management consists initially of thorough evaluation of the extent of the injury. Rewarming of the injured part in a tepid water bath, 103° to 107° F., should be instituted promptly until the desired effect is reached, unless frank gangrene is present. The area must be handled gently and protected from further injury. If the feet are involved, the patient should not walk. The part is dressed with a sterile bulky dressing, placing cotton or gauze sponges in the interdigital spaces to prevent maceration. Debridement of vesicles and devitalized tissues is indicated under aseptic conditions. In severe injuries, it takes a period of time to determine which tissues are permanently damaged and will require amputation. The part will often heal so that relatively little tissue is lost.

The patient who has had frostbite will often have a residual hypersensitivity to cold and should be cautioned to protect himself from exposure which may further damage the affected tissues. Such patients usually require admission to the hospital and further study of the vascular system, including arteriography, to evaluate the extent of the occlusive process. Anticoagulants may be used in selected patients.

SUMMARY

A vascular emergency may result from any one of a number of factors, including trauma, arterial or venous disease and cold injury. High-speed travel, an alarming increase in acts of violence and a longer life expectancy account in part for the increasing numbers of patients with acute vascular problems being seen in hospital emergency departments.

Improvements in diagnosis and surgical technique have resulted in lower morbidity and mortality and higher rates of limb salvage. Prompt attention to established principles of nursing management is essential to a successful outcome for these patients.

BIBLIOGRAPHY

(1) Cameron, H. S.; Laird, J. J., and Carroll: "False Aneurysms Complicate Closed Fractures," *Journal of Trauma,* 12 (1972):67.

(2) Cross, F. S., and Mowlem, A.: "Survey of the Current Status of Pulmonary Embolectomy for Massive Pulmonary Embolism," *Circulation,* 35, suppl. 1 (1967):86.

(3) Darling, R. C.: "Arterial Embolism," *Hospital Medicine,* 10 (1974):8.

(4) David, J. P.; Marks, C., and Bonneval, M.: "A Ten Year Institutional Experience with Abdominal Aneurysms," *Surgery, Gynecology, and Obstetrics,* 138 (1974):591.

(5) DeBakey, M. E., and Simeone, F. A.: "Battle Injuries of the Arteries in World War II," *Annals of Surgery,* 123 (1946): 534.

(6) DeWeese, J. A.; Blaisdell, F. W., and Foster, J. H.: "Optimal Resources for Vascular Surgery," *Circulation,* 46 (1972):A 305.

(7) Drapanas, T.; Hewitt, R. L.; Weichert, F. F., III, *et al.:* "Civilian Vascular Injuries: A Critical Appraisal," *Annals of Surgery,* 172 (1970):351.

(8) Edwards, E. A.: "Acute Peripheral Arterial Occlusion," *Journal of the American Medical Association,* 223 (1973):909.

(9) Eger, M.; Goleman, L., *et al.:* "Problems in the Management of Popliteal Artery Injuries," *Surgery, Gynecology, and Obstetrics,* 134 (1900):926.

(10) Heimbacker, R. O.; Keon, W. J., and Richards, K. U.: "Massive Pulmonary Embolism," *Archives of Surgery,* 107 (1973):740.

(11) Hermann, G.; Schechter, D. C.; Owens, J., and Starzl, T. E.: "Problems of Frostbite in Civilian Medical Practice," *Surgical Clinics of North America,* 43 (1963):519.

(12) Hewitt, R. L.: "Peripheral Vascular Injuries," *Hospital Medicine,* 9 (1973): 30.

(13) Hohf, R. P.; Epler, T.; Haskell, M., and Otto, N.: "The Threat of Thrombophlebitis," *Nursing '73,* 3 (1973):39.

(14) Hughes, C. W.: "Arterial Repair During the Korean War," *Annals of Surgery,* 147 (1958):555.

(15) Knize, D. M.; Weatherley-White,

R. C. A.; Paton, B. C., and Owens, J. C.: "Prognostic Factors in the Management of Frostbite," *Journal of Trauma,* 9 (1969):747.

(16) MacGowan, W.: "Acute Ischaemia Complicating Limb Trauma," *Journal of Bone and Joint Surgery,* 50B (1971):472.

(17) Perry, M. O.; Thal, E. R., and Shires, G. T.: "Management of Arterial Injuries," *Annals of Surgery,* 173 (1971): 403.

(18) Rich, N. M., and Hughes, C. W.: "Vietnam Vascular Registry: An Initial Report," *Surgery,* 65 (1969):218.

(19) Saletta, J., and Freeark, R.: "Injuries to the Profunda Femoris Artery," *Journal of Trauma,* 12 (1972):778.

(20) Singh, I., and Gorman, J. F.: "Vascular Injuries in Closed Fractures Near Junction of Middle and Lower Thirds of the Tibia," *Journal of Trauma,* 12 (1972): 592.

(21) Sturm, J. T.; Strate, R. G., *et al.:* "Blunt Trauma to the Subclavian Artery," *Surgery, Gynecology, and Obstetrics,* 138 (1974):915.

(22) Wright, R. S., and Edwards, W. H.: "Manifestations and Management of Acute Arterial Injuries," *Journal of Trauma,* 13 (1973):463.

16

Care of the comatose patient

JAMES H. COSGRIFF, JR.
DIANN ANDERSON

The patient in coma on arrival in the emergency department requires the highest priority of care. Such a patient represents a particular challenge to the emergency nurse, taxing her knowledge, skill and judgment to the greatest extent. In caring for the comatose patient, the nurse must base her approach on maintenance of life and, at the same time, initiate a plan of diagnostic measures which will lead to an early and correct diagnosis. Although the contents of this chapter will be presented in a step-by-step manner, it must be stressed that many of these "steps" will take place concurrently in actual practice.

The causes of coma are many, but they may be grouped into the following categories:

(1) *Metabolic* coma, due to: hyperglycemia, hypoglycemia, uremia, hepatic failure, adrenal insufficiency with addisonian crisis.
(2) *Structural* coma, due to: cerebrovascular accident, ruptured intracranial aneurysm, neoplasm, trauma, infections, seizure disorder.
(3) *Intoxication* coma, due to: drugs, alcohol, carbon monoxide.
(4) *Functional* coma, due to: psychogenic causes.

The mechanism of coma is not always fully understood. It can be said, however, that coma ensues as a result of deleterious action on the cerebral cortex and brain stem. In reality, it is a manifestation of a disease process.

HANDLING OF THE COMATOSE PATIENT

The comatose or unresponsive patient is entirely dependent for safe handling on those who provide care. In other words, it is the duty of all who come in contact with an unresponsive patient to insure that no further harm or injury results from inappropriate or improper handling.

In the emergency department, this means that the patient will not be moved from the ambulance stretcher until the vital signs are taken and a careful but rapid assessment is made to rule out any possible injury to the spine or skeletal structures. This information can be obtained by careful palpation along the spinous processes of the vertebral column and the extremities. Should there be any indication of such injury, the patient should be placed on a spine board or have the affected extremity properly splinted.

Any airway problems must be immediately corrected. The patient may then be transferred to the examining table.

The ambulance attendants should not be permitted to leave the department without providing full details of the incident from the time of their arrival on the scene until the patient entered the hospital. Similarly, any relatives, friends, co-workers or witnesses who accompanied the patient or witnessed the event should be detained until all necessary information is collected from them. Once a comatose patient has been brought into the emergency department, a staff member should remain with the patient at *all* times. The patient should be strapped to the examining cart, padded siderails in position to avert harm or aggravation of an injury.

ASSESSMENT

History

Evaluation and treatment begin at the moment the patient is brought into the emergency department. Since the patient is unable to respond to questioning, other sources must be used for the history, including family, friends, witnesses and ambulance personnel. It is helpful to know whether the patient had any condition or habit included in the 4 categories of coma which might be a prelude to the unconscious state and whether the onset of the coma was witnessed or not.

In the event there are witnesses to the onset of coma, ascertain whether the unconscious state occurred gradually, as with certain types of metabolic or structural disorders such as a neoplasm or alterations in the blood sugar level, or suddenly, such as might follow a cerebrovascular accident or a ruptured aneurysm. Was any headache noted before the onset of the coma? It occurs quite frequently in patients who suffer a ruptured aneurysm. Was there any fall or injury beforehand? Did the patient have any neurological abnormalities, such as slurred speech or motor weakness, or a seizure before becoming unconscious? Had the patient been on any drugs or prescribed medication; if so, what preparations and for what disorders? During days, weeks or months prior to the coma, had the patient any symptoms of neurological disorder?

In case of the nonwitnessed coma, the nurse should inquire as to the circumstances the victim was found in. Was there any evidence of urinary or bowel incontinence? Was there any evidence at the scene suggestive of trauma (a weapon, broken or displaced furniture)? Was any medication, drugs or drug paraphernalia found near the patient or in the household? Were any bottles of alcoholic beverages found with the patient? If in a home, garage or an enclosed area, were there any fumes noticed or any evidence of improperly vented gas heaters?

In general, every effort must be made to gather as much information as possible about the circumstances surrounding the onset of the coma state. Further information can be obtained from a careful search of the personal belongings of the patient. Look particularly for wallet cards which might contain medical information, physician's prescriptions or any material identifying an existing medical condition. Certain types of jewelry, tags or bracelets, may also be worn to identify that the person has a specific medical condition.

Physical evaluation

Probably for no other patient does the nurse rely so heavily on her senses to make a thorough assessment. A rapid, general assessment is completed prior to moving the patient onto the emergency department cart. Vital signs are taken and recorded immediately. They should be repeated at regular intervals, initially every 15 minutes during the patient's stay in the emergency department until they are stabilized. The patient must be completely disrobed once the initial assessment has revealed that no fracture is present and he is secure on the emergency cart.

The presence of any odors should be noted.

Diabetic acidosis typically creates a fruity odor on the breath, due to acetone. The person who has taken an excess of alcohol will undoubtedly have an alcoholic odor. In uremia, the breath has a faint smell of urine; and in hepatic failure, a fetid, mousey odor is detected. While noting any odors, the nurse inspects the body for evidence of trauma. She checks for blood in the ear canals, nares and corners of the mouth, and for any bruises, abrasions and bleeding or open wounds. Tongue scars or a fresh tongue wound are often found in patients with a seizure disorder.

Skin irregularities are important signs. The nurse should observe for any cyanosis which might indicate a respiratory problem. Jaundice of the skin or sclera is usually associated with hepatic failure. Look for spider angiomata of the upper trunk, sparse axillary hair in the male and a venous pattern of the periumbilical area (caput medusae) or flank regions (thoracoepigastric veins), which frequently accompany cirrhosis. Pallor of the skin may indicate bleeding. A rare condition which can be confused with cyanosis is argyria, in which the skin has a metallic, gray hue. This is found in people who have used silver preparations for a period of years as a nasal astringent; the silver gradually becomes deposited in the skin. A red, warm skin may be the result of sunburn in a patient with coma due to heat stroke. This is usually accompanied by a significant fever. A cherry-red color to the lips, along with redness of the skin, is found with carbon monoxide poisoning. Rashes, petechiae or ecchymoses might indicate a blood dyscrasia. Particularly in younger patients, who might be suspected of using drugs, look for needle marks and "tracks" along the course of a vein, on the forearm or in the antecubital space of the elbow. Also look for thrombosed veins, which frequently follow intravenous use of drugs (mainlining).

The patient's rate and depth of respirations should be observed. Cheyne-Stokes respiration is characterized by rapid, deep, labored breathing with periods of apnea. This is usually due to brain damage and heralds a poor prognosis. Kussmaul breathing accompanies diabetic acidosis or uremia and is characterized by rapid, deep respirations, often described as evidence of "air hunger." Marked hyperpnea frequently accompanies brain stem lesions. The nurse should listen for any extraneous sounds associated with respiratory activity, such as wheezes or rhonchi. The chest should be auscultated for heart and lung sounds.

In examining the heart, determination should be made of whether the apical and radial pulse rates are the same. Tachycardia is present in shock states, febrile episodes and cardiac failure. Bradycardia may be noted in patients with digitalis intoxication, myocardial infarction and heart block. The nurse counts the rate to detect any alteration in rhythm. A grossly irregular apical rhythm, accompanied by a pulse deficit in which the apical rate is more rapid than the radial pulse rate, is consistent with auricular fibrillation. Such an arrhythmia is frequently associated with thromboembolic episodes, due to the breaking off of a portion of a mural thrombus from within the heart chamber. The thrombus then enters the arterial circulation as an embolus and may lodge in the artery supplying the brain, resulting in a cerebrovascular accident.

After auscultation has been completed, the head and neck should be palpated for any swelling, wounds or depressions. The ear canals are then inspected for damage to the drums or localized bleeding, which might indicate a basilar skull fracture. Blood in the auditory canals or nares from skull fracture will not clot.

The eyes are examined next. The sclera should be searched for contact lenses, which may be used by patients of any age. Often the lens may be displaced from the cornea and found beneath the eyelid. If present, lenses should be removed (see Chapter 27) and stored for safekeeping, with identification of left and right lenses. The size and shape of the pupils are important signs, also. Under ordinary circumstances, the pupils should be round, regular and equal and reactive to light. Inequality of pupils usually results from intracranial lesion, such as a subdural hematoma. Constricted or pinpoint pupils are seen with narcotic addiction; dilated pupils accompany barbiturate intoxication or anoxia. In functional disorders, the pupils are characteristically dilated, equal and reactive. Failure of the pupils to constrict when stimulated by light may be indicative of severe brain damage. The nurse is cautioned to be alert for an ocular prosthesis (glass eye), which can be very misleading to the uninitiated.

Funduscopic examination is necessary to more completely evaluate the patient's condition. The presence of papilledema (swelling about the optic disc) results from an increased intracranial pressure and may be seen with tumor or hemorrhage. The presence of hemorrhage and exudate in association with this finding are indicative of long-standing, severe, hypertensive or diabetic retinopathy.

Estimating the depth of coma is important. A number of observations are helpful. The lid reflex can be assessed by gently touching the tips of the eyelashes. In light coma states or in those of a functional origin, the lids will blink involuntarily. Absence of the lid reflex is indicative of a deeper coma.

Spontaneous movements of the limbs are another sign. Are they unilateral or bilateral? Is there any weakness noted when comparing one side with the other? The patient's arm or leg may be raised from the cart and allowed to drop. In deep coma, the limb will drop suddenly in a limp manner; in lighter coma, it will fall gradually. Note any resistance to passive motion by the elbow or knee joints. Unilateral rigidity or flaccidity may indicate a neurological lesion. Stimulation of the limbs with a significantly painful stimulus allows an observer to note if active withdrawal occurs and if the motion is equal on both sides. (A knuckle may be pressed into the sternum or the neck pinched.) Such painful stimuli may give some evidence of the depth of coma as shown by the patient's response.

After it has been established that there is no cervical spine injury, the neck should be flexed by placing the palm of the hand behind the head. Any resistance or rigidity (nuchal rigidity) indicates meningeal irritation, which may accompany subarachnoid hemorrhage or meningitis. Deep tendon reflexes should be compared bilaterally. These include the biceps, triceps, knee and ankle jerks. A diminished, absent or hyperactive reflex on one side may indicate a lesion of the central nervous system.

Physical assessment should be completed to identify or rule out any concurrent or causative abnormality. Generally speaking, coma arising from an intracranial lesion will produce unilateral, localized neurological findings until a near terminal state is reached. On the other hand, metabolic disorders or those associated with intoxication or functional states are usually manifested by bilateral findings.

The thoracic area should be assessed for respiratory movements, noting any deformity or paradoxical motion of the chest wall, which suggests trauma. The lungs are auscultated to evaluate ventilatory exchange and to note the presence of rales, wheezes and/or rhonchi, which are seen with cardiac or pulmonary disease.

The abdomen should then be inspected for any incisional scars, which might suggest prior portacaval shunt, indicative of surgery for portal hypertension due to liver disease. In a patient who is unconscious following an automobile accident, great care must be taken to detect the presence of any internal injury. For example, any visceral enlargement is significant. Abdominal spasm or rigidity may be masked by coma. If rapid pulse or hypotension are present, particularly when coupled with the pallor of anemia, internal bleeding must be considered. Peritoneal tap or lavage may be required to detect the presence of free blood. It must be recalled that a negative tap (when no blood is recovered) does not rule out visceral damage, but false positive taps are very unusual. Therefore, the only significant finding is a positive tap.

The examination is completed with more

thorough evaluation of the limbs and skeletal structures to detect any deformity which might indicate fracture.

Adjunct studies

The number and types of adjunct studies utilized will vary with the circumstances, the tentative diagnosis and the hospital setting. Studies which may be useful in clarifying the diagnosis include blood work, urinalysis, lumbar puncture, echoencephalography and x-ray studies, which may include the skull and cervical spine, and special radiologic techniques, including brain scan and cerebral angiography.

Blood studies

As an absolute minimum, complete blood count, blood glucose and urea studies should be done on all comatose patients to uncover possible anemia, infection, hyper- or hypoglycemia or renal failure. It is appropriate also to include blood creatinine and serum electrolyte studies to better detect renal failure or severe metabolic disturbances. If the blood glucose is found to be markedly elevated, a serum acetone study is helpful. If the glucose level is low, the diagnosis of hypoglycemia is established.

In patients in whom drug overdoses are suspected, toxicology studies of the blood are routinely indicated. If the laboratory service is not available when the patient is seen, advice should be sought from the laboratory director as to proper methods of drawing and storing the blood samples until such time as the service is available.

Arterial gas studies are done when respiratory insufficiency is present or suspected. When hepatic disease is present, serum bilirubin, transaminase levels and alkaline phosphatase should be measured. The blood ammonia level should be measured, for it is frequently elevated in patients with hepatic failure. Blood cultures are indicated whenever the patient is febrile or when there is an indication of an infectious process. In patients with anemia and in patients with multiple injuries or suspected major blood loss, blood should be taken for type and cross-match.

Urinalysis

A specimen of urine obtained by catheterization is necessary in all comatose patients. Routine studies should include specific gravity, sugar, ketone bodies, protein and microscopic examination. In diabetic acidosis, the urinary sugar and ketones will both be strongly positive.

Culture and sensitivity studies of the urine are worthwhile in all comatose patients, since an indwelling urinary catheter will be necessary at least until the patient is responsive and perhaps longer. In suspected drug overdose, a urine specimen should be collected for toxicology study.

Lumbar puncture

A lumbar puncture may be helpful in further assessing the unconscious patient. It should *not* be done if there is evidence of increased intracranial pressure, particularly as manifest by papilledema. Removal of even small amounts of cerebrospinal fluid in such patients *may* cause herniation of the brain or brain stem, with serious and sometimes fatal consequences. If the physician deems the procedure safe, the cerebrospinal fluid pressure is measured and a portion of fluid removed for study. The cerebrospinal fluid pressure reflects the intracranial pressure and is normally less than 200 mm. of water.

The fluid should be observed for color. (It is normally colorless.) Grossly bloody fluid is found with fresh subarachnoid bleeding. Xanthochromic (yellow-tinged) fluid is found in patients with an old hemorrhage, such as chronic subdural hematoma. Cloudy fluid may result from infectious processes, such as meningitis. The fluid should be analyzed for the presence of blood cells, glucose, protein and serology. White blood cells indicate infection, such as meningitis, encephalitis or poliomyelitis. A decrease in sugar content occurs with infectious processes, primarily of bacterial origin, involving the central nervous system. Elevated protein levels are found particularly with neoplasms.

X-ray studies

Since x-ray studies require that the patient be moved to the radiology department, it is essential that a physician or nurse be in attendance at all times to monitor the patient and insure a patent airway.

Skull x-rays are indicated when a structural lesion is suspected, particularly due to trauma or neoplasm. Initial x-rays should include the cervical spine. It may be difficult, sometimes impossible, to diagnose a skull fracture by assessment, depending on the length and density of the hair. Anteroposterior and lateral views of the skull and cervical spine can be done with a minimum of patient movement and may provide a great deal of information.

It should be kept in mind that although a metabolic disorder or drug intoxication may have precipitated a comatose state, structural damage to the cranium and its contents may have occurred if the patient fell during or following the onset of coma. The film should be read for any evidence of fracture and pineal shift. X-rays of other body parts should be taken as clinical evaluation warrants. Children brought into the emergency department in coma and thought to be victims of abuse should have x-ray studies of the limbs, chest and clavicles, which might turn up evidence of old, healed fractures suggestive of the battered child syndrome.

Special x-ray studies, such as angiograms and brain scans, are used to localize specific intracranial lesions. These are rarely necessary in the emergency setting, with one exception—the patient suspected of having an acute extradural hemorrhage. Again, clinical evaluation may be sufficient to clarify this diagnosis. Ventriculograms and pneumoencephalograms are rarely, if ever, required as part of the emergency evaluation of a comatose patient.

Encephalography

Encephalography is of limited value in the emergency setting for suspected brain lesions. Standard electroencephalographic procedures are time-consuming. An echoencephalogram, however, can be done in a very short period of time and can provide much useful information in regard to the shift of brain structures from the midline.

MANAGEMENT

Nursing intervention for the comatose patient is directed toward provision of basic life-support measures and initiation of diagnostic procedures which will assist in identifying the cause of the coma. It is best carried out by a planned approach based on the general condition of the patient and the specific factor(s) causing the condition. By proceeding in a step-by-step fashion, the nursing therapy can be modified as more clinical and laboratory data become available. In most instances, the etiology of the comatose state will be narrowed to one of the 4 major categories discussed at the beginning of this chapter with the completion of the assessment and initial laboratory studies. (See also "Specific Causes of Coma," which follows.)

An adequate airway must be established and maintained. Support to the angles of the jaw will prevent the tongue from displacing backwards into the pharynx and occluding the airway, or an oropharyngeal airway may be inserted to maintain the tongue in position. The head should be turned to the side and secretions aspirated as indicated. If this is unsatisfactory, endotracheal intubation or tracheostomy must be used. Should the patient have shallow, ineffective respiratory movements, a mechanical ventilator may be needed.

The vital signs are taken for baseline determination. If the patient is hyperthermic, body cooling may be initiated by ice packs, alcohol towels or a hypothermia blanket. Hypotension should be treated if present. Cardiac monitoring should be reserved for those patients with a cardiac arrhythmia, to provide a continuous evaluation of the cardiac status. Tachycardia or bradycardia is managed as indicated. External bleeding should be controlled by the appropriate method.

A lifeline is inserted into a major vein, initially using Ringer's lactate solution. Since increased intracranial pressure may present a problem, the rate of infusion must be specified by the physician and closely monitored. Other fluids may be substituted as more clinical data is gathered. For example, if the initial laboratory studies reveal findings suggestive of a diabetic acidosis, the fluid may then be changed to a normal saline.

A nasogastric tube should be inserted for diagnostic and therapeutic purposes. The stomach contents are aspirated and examined for blood, fragments of capsules or pills, alcohol. If any of these are found, adequate samples should be obtained for toxicological study, and gastric lavage carried out. Gastric dilatation is common in these patients and may provoke serious consequences. Once the lavage has been completed, the tube should be placed on intermittent suction. An indwelling urinary catheter is needed to obtain a urine specimen initially, then to provide for continuous bladder drainage.

Medication is given only as required. In patients suspected of suffering a drug overdose, naloxone hydrochloride (Narcan) may be given intravenously. This is a specific antagonist to narcotics. Response is often dramatic when the comatose state resulted from narcotic use, although it may be short-lived because of the relatively longer action of the narcotic. The emergency nurse must keep a detailed record of all medications given the patient. Vital signs and neurological signs are taken and recorded at regular intervals. Antibiotics and biological vaccines are given only as the clinical condition warrants.

In patients requiring large volumes of intravenous fluids, in the elderly or in those suspected of having a compromised cardiac status, it is wise to insert a central venous pressure catheter to avoid fluid overload, which might precipitate cardiac decompensation and pulmonary edema.

Physician consultation must be available to the emergency nurse within a very short time of request.

SPECIFIC CAUSES OF COMA

Metabolic causes

The major causes of metabolic coma are hyperglycemia, hypoglycemia and uremia. Less common causes are adrenal insufficiency, lactic acidosis and hepatic failure.

Hyperglycemia

Hyperglycemia, particularly that associated with diabetic ketoacidosis, is the most common cause of metabolic coma. Diabetic ketoacidosis results from a deficiency of insulin, which leads to metabolic disturbances resulting in dehydration and in electrolyte imbalance by osmotic diuresis. It is usually seen in established diabetics, although it occurs, rarely, as an initial symptom. A history might be available from the family, or the patient may have some identification, such as a wallet card, stating he is a diabetic. Hyperglycemia most frequently results from alcoholism, infection or omission of insulin. It is important to keep in mind that coma may be induced by other causes in diabetic patients.

In diabetic ketoacidosis, the onset of coma is usually gradual. The patient appears flushed, with a fruity odor to the breath, due to ketone bodies. He frequently has the characteristic Kussmaul breathing. Dehydration is apparent. In the absence of injury, there are no localizing neurological signs.

Basic blood and urine studies will reveal elevated levels of both glucose and acetone in the urine and blood. If the patient is febrile, secondary infection must be considered, with the most likely place of origin the respiratory or urinary tracts.

Management consists of fluid replacement and administration of insulin. The amount of insulin needed depends on serial studies of blood sugar levels.

Hypoglycemia

Hypoglycemia is also seen in a diabetic as a cause of coma. The condition is usually produced by excessive insulin intake, which may have occurred as a result of administration error, skipping a meal, reducing food intake or excessive physical exertion. Oral hypoglycemic agents, with the exception of phenformin (DBI), may cause this condition, as well. The history will reveal the patient to have been sweaty, perhaps exhibiting nervousness and pallor, as the blood sugar level declined. When it reached a critical level, coma occurred.

When this diagnosis is suspected in a nondiabetic, one must consider some other cause, such as pancreatic tumors or endocrinopathies. Usually no localizing neurological signs are present.

Diagnosis is established from a blood glucose level of less than 50 mg. percent. Management consists of intravenous injection of 50 percent glucose solution, which will result in a dramatic response.

Uremia

Uremia is a less common cause of coma; coma represents the most advanced stage of central nervous system involvement in uremia. With uremia, a number of acid metabolites increase in the blood, precipitating the comatose state. If a history is available, one may detect a long-standing condition of urinary tract disease. The onset of the coma is gradual; the early phase of uremia is marked by neuromuscular and personality disorders. Seizures may occur. In any comatose patient, particularly the elderly, this cause must be considered.

Assessment may reveal dry, scaling skin (frequently described as "uremic frost"), dehydration, muscle fasciculation, typical Kussmaul respiration and, at times, a pericardial friction rub. Laboratory work will reveal an elevated blood urea nitrogen. Further studies will demonstrate an increase in creatinine and a metabolic acidosis.

Initial management consists of hydration, correction of the electrolyte imbalance and stabilization of the patient. Investigative studies are undertaken to identify the underlying cause, when the patient's condition warrants.

Structural causes

Coma due to structural causes represents serious structural change in the central nervous system. A lesion is present, which may produce localizing neurological signs.

Cerebrovascular accident

Apoplexy and stroke occur most commonly in persons over 50. They are due to compromised cerebral blood flow, with resultant damage to brain cells. The most common etiology is cerebral thrombosis; there may be symptoms of "little strokes" for a period of time. A member of the family may state the patient had a "falling out," spell or recurring episodes of momentary dizziness, loss of balance or slurred speech for varying periods of time, then was found unconscious. When due to embolus or hemorrhage, the onset is usually rapid, with little or no preexisting symptoms relating to the central nervous system.

Physical examination will usually reveal localized neurological loss, such as hemiplegia. Painful stimuli may produce a grimace by which the examiner can detect a facial palsy. The facial palsy and the extremity weakness will be on the contralateral side from the lesion in the brain. Bladder or bowel incontinence is not uncommon. Deep tendon reflexes will be diminished or absent on the side of the hemiplegia. The abdominal reflexes are usually diminished but are sometimes hyperactive. A Babinski sign will be elicited.

Initial care in the emergency department is supportive in nature. An airway must be maintained and the cardiovascular status stabilized. Further care is primarily rehabilitative in nature.

Depending on the severity of the damage to nerve cells, the coma may be short-lived. If the lesion involves the dominant side of the brain (left cerebral hemisphere in right-handed individuals, right cerebral hemisphere in left-handed persons), speech aphasia may result.

Ruptured cerebral aneurysm

A rupture of a cerebral artery aneurysm is more often found in the younger age group, those below age 40. This condition must be considered in younger adults. Such an aneurysm is congenital and may occur anywhere in the cerebral arterial tree but is most commonly seen at the bifurcation of the internal carotid artery, located at the base of the brain. Leaking or rupture causes bleeding into the subarachnoid space.

A history may reveal that the patient complained of severe headache just prior to lapsing into coma. Patients in emergency departments with severe headaches but fairly alert have been seen to lapse into coma during the course of evaluation. A frank rupture of the aneurysm has a high mortality rate.

Assessment will reveal nuchal rigidity, but localizing neurological signs are frequently absent. Vital signs may be normal, although bradycardia and high blood pressure are frequently present. With lumbar puncture, bloody fluid is recovered.

Early neurosurgical consultation is advisable, to determine whether urgent surgery is warranted. Cerebral angiography will localize the site of the lesion. Supportive measures are necessary until a decision has been made on the course of management.

Cerebral neoplasm

Neoplasms of the brain may cause coma as a late manifestation. They may be either primary or metastatic tumors. The history reveals varying periods of neurological symptoms and personality or neuromuscular disorders. It may also reveal a period of febrile illness, with gradual worsening of the victim's condition, leading to coma. Neoplasm must be considered in patients known to have malignant disease elsewhere. The most frequent malignant tumors likely to metastasize to the brain originate in the lung, gastrointestinal tract, breast and kidney.

Assessment will usually reveal unilateral localizing signs. Lateralizing neurological signs may be present. Fever, tachycardia and leukocytosis are common. Blood cultures are taken as indicated. Lumbar puncture will be helpful in clarifying the diagnosis. The cerebrospinal fluid protein content may be elevated.

Emergency department care is supportive. In the undiagnosed patient, an intensive work-up may be necessary to identify the problem. The necessary studies include meningitis, encephalitis and brain abscess, and if any of these is diagnosed, massive doses of specific antibiotics should be given early in the patient's course of treatment.

Major seizure disorder

A seizure disorder which produces coma is often referred to as a "major seizure disorder." The most common is grand mal epilepsy. It occurs more frequently in children and younger adults. Epilepsy often exists in the comatose patient seen in the emergency setting. Medication may be found in the patient's clothing.

The history will reveal that the coma was preceded by a convulsive seizure. A grand mal seizure is often heralded by an aura, in which the patient has a visual or olfactory sensation. As the seizure occurs, the uncontrollable movements are accompanied by guttural sounds. Urinary incontinence is common. The patient may have excessive salivation and fresh lacerations or scars of the tongue. The postseizure coma state is referred to as the post-ictal state and may last minutes to hours. The patient may have no recall of the event.

Neurological assessment may be unrevealing except for the presence of a Babinski reflex. Admission is not usually needed unless an injury has been incurred during the seizure. However, the importance of taking medication and avoiding excesses must be stressed to the patient. In an adult over 25, the first occurrence of a seizure is sometimes associated with a neoplasm. Therefore, a complete work-up is required in such patients to establish the cause of the disorder.

Intoxications

Alcohol

Alcohol is a potent depressor of the central nervous system. Its initial effect is the depression of certain inhibitory centers, which causes a euphoria followed by progressive loss of motor coordination, mental alacrity, judgment and discrimination. These clinical symptoms, related to elevated blood alcohol levels, render intoxicated individuals susceptible to accidents. Excessive amounts of alcohol in the blood induce narcosis. Alcohol-induced coma demands a high priority of care, since there is considerable central nervous system depression. History may be available from friends or witnesses relating to recent alcohol ingestion. One must always consider the possibility of concomitant injury, which may have resulted from a fall or altercation, and concomitant use of depressive drugs.

Complete assessment is needed. Vital signs may reveal hypothermia and hypotension. Respiratory activity may be seriously depressed. Beware the possibility of associated fractures. The patient will usually have the typical alcoholic odor to the breath, though it can be mistaken for that odor found in the diabetic. In the absence of neurological damage from associated injury, localizing signs are usually absent.

Vital signs must be closely monitored. A nasogastric tube should be inserted to prevent emesis and possible aspiration. Vasopressors and ventilatory support should be provided as needed. Acute withdrawal symptoms may be expected in the chronic alcoholic; therefore therapy should be planned to avoid this sometimes fatal complication.

Carbon monoxide

Carbon monoxide poisoning may occur under accidental circumstances or in an attempt at self-destruction. Carbon monoxide is an odorless, colorless gas which has a strong affinity for hemoglobin, estimated at 200 to 300 times that of oxygen. In carbon monoxide intoxication, the carbon monoxide-laden hemoglobin reduces the amount of oxyhemoglobin and decreases the dissociation of oxyhemoglobin. The diminished oxygen carrying capacity of the blood results in tissue anoxia, which if uncorrected will terminate fatally.

History may reveal that the patient was found in a garage or in a poorly ventilated room with a gas source present. The patient may appear cyanotic, though more typically, a cherry-red color will be present on the lips and skin. The skin is flushed; the pulse is rapid; and muscular twitching is often present. In severe cases, Cheyne-Stokes respirations are present.

Management includes supportive care. Some physicians favor inhalation of 5 to 7 percent carbon dioxide to replace the carbon monoxide on the hemoglobin and stimulate the respiratory center. The hyperbaric chamber has been demonstrated to reduce the affinity of carbon monoxide and hemoglobin by replacing the oxygen on the hemoglobin.* Chronic symptoms may arise as a result of permanent central nervous system damage.

Drugs

The current prevalence of drug use and abuse is responsible for an increasing number of visits to the emergency department for drug-related problems. The drugs that are in common abuse today include a wide variety of prescribed medications in addition to those obtained by illicit means. Coma has been one of the manifestations of the effects of these

---

* Carbon monoxide normally has a greater affinity for hemoglobin than does oxygen; thus it will displace oxygen on a hemoglobin molecule. The hyperbaric chamber, by increasing the ambient pressure, can force oxygen onto hemoglobin, thus displacing carbon monoxide.

pharmacologic agents and may occur either as a direct result of the drug, as in the case of sedative-hypnotics, or during the phase of withdrawal. Drugs which are obtained "on the street" frequently contain a high proportion of adulterants, which may cause a variety of interactions which are difficult, if not impossible, to identify.

Overuse of prescribed medication may indicate an attempt at self-destruction. This must be kept in mind when dealing with the family or friends who may appear in the emergency department with the victim. In the case of the drug addict who may have overdosed or is in the withdrawal state, friends and associates should be sought to determine what drug or drugs were being used.

In narcotic overdose, physical findings may reveal severe central nervous system depression, marked by hypotension, diminished respiratory activity and small pupils. Pulmonary edema may occur in the presence of a slower respiratory rate. It is important to rule out any coexisting injuries as a cause of the coma. Signs and symptoms of overdose from a variety of pharmacologic agents are outlined in Chapter 12.

Toxicological tests should be done to measure opiates, barbiturates, amphetamines or methadone in the urine or blood, along with the basic blood work, including electrolyte determinations. Many drug addicts suffer from diseases which are related to the manner in which they use their illicit medications. These include hepatitis, septicemia, bacterial endocarditis, tetanus, dental caries, hypoglycemia, septic emboli from injection sites and vaginitis, among others.

The management of such patients is based on the principle of treating the physiological deviations that are present. An adequate airway must be established, and maintained with proper mechanical support if necessary. Naloxone hydrochloride (Narcan) may dramatically stimulate respiratory activity and arouse the patient from his comatose state. The cardiovascular system should be supported by adequate amounts of fluid, with added vasoactive substances as needed. Gastric lavage should be instituted early in the course of emergency care to remove ingested substances remaining in the stomach.

Functional/psychogenic causes

Coma from psychogenic origin is probably least frequently seen in the emergency setting. History would usually reveal that the patient had been under psychiatric care or had exhibited personality alterations. The coma may have been preceded by a period of apprehension, overactivity and hyperpnea.

Complete laboratory studies should be done to rule out any of the other more common causes of coma. If it is psychogenic, the pupils will usually appear to be dilated and reactive. The patient may be hyperventilating. Deep tendon reflexes are often hyperactive, with no localizing neurological signs.

Management consists of close support for these patients, with care being taken to insure that there are no concomitant conditions which may have provoked or influenced the coma state.

SUMMARY

The following list outlines and summarizes the step-by-step management of a comatose patient in an emergency department.

(1) Do not move patient from ambulance stretcher until cervical spine injury has been ruled out.
(2) Establish airway.
(3) Control external bleeding.
(4) Take vital signs and record them.
(5) Place patient on emergency cart, strap in, use siderails.
(6) Obtain historical data from ambulance attendants, police, relatives, friends, witnesses present.
(7) Perform complete physical assessment.
(8) Draw venous blood for basic blood studies, and start intravenous fluids.

(9) Insert Foley catheter; obtain specimen for analysis.

(10) Repeat vital signs at intervals of 15 minutes and record them.

(11) Insert nasogastric tube; check aspirated material; perform lavage as indicated.

(12) Medication given *only as indicated; give intravenously.*

(13) Additional studies, x-rays, lumbar puncture, blood studies as indicated.

BIBLIOGRAPHY

(1) Ballantine, H. T., Jr., and Prieto, A., Jr.: "Early Recognition and Management of Neurosurgical Emergencies," *Surgical Clinics of North America,* 46 (1966):527.

(2) Bissell, G. W., and Coseglia, P. R.: "Endocrine Emergencies (Non-diabetic)," *Medical Clinics of North America,* 46 (1962):495.

(3) Canary, J. J.: "Some Complications of Diabetic Ketoacidosis," *Twenty-third Hahnemann Symposium on Emergency Room Care* (New York: Grune & Stratton, 1972), pp. 91–94.

(4) Carozza, V.: "Ketoacidotic Crisis: Mechanism and Management," *Nursing '73,* 3 (May 1973):13.

(5) Guthrie, D., and Guthrie, R.: "Coping with Diabetic Ketoacidosis," *Nursing '73,* 3 (November 1973):16.

(6) Hurwitz, D.: "Hypoglycemic and Hyperglycemic Coma," *Surgical Clinics of North America,* 48 (1968):395.

(7) Lanzoni, V.: "Drug-Induced Coma," *Surgical Clinics of North America,* 48 (1968):395.

(8) Locke, S.: "Management of the Unconscious Patient," *New England Journal of Medicine,* 274 (1966):787.

(9) Locke, S.: "The Neurological Aspects of Coma, *"Surgical Clinics of North America,* 48 (1968):251.

(10) McDermott, W. F.: "Liver Disease in the Differential Diagnosis of Coma," *Surgical Clinics of North America,* 48 (1968):327.

(11) Mancall, E. L.: "The Unconscious Patient," *Twenty-third Hahnemann Symposium on Emergency Room Care* (New York: Grune & Stratton, 1972), pp. 117–124.

(12) Pillari, C., and Naivs, J.: "Physical Effects of Heroin Addiction," *American Journal of Nursing,* 73 (1973):2105.

(13) Schumann, D.: "Coping with the Complex, Dangerous, Elusive Problem of Those Insulin-Induced Hypoglycemic Reactions," *Nursing '74,* 4 (1974):57.

(14) Singer, M. M.: "Endocrine Emergencies: Diagnosis and Intensive Care," *Medical Clinics of North America,* 55 (1971):1315.

(15) Vanamee, P., and Poppell, J. W.: "Hepatic Coma," *Medical Clinics of North America,* 44 (1960):765.

(16) Wiley, L.: "The Stigma of Epilepsy," *Nursing '74,* 4 (1974):36.

(17) Wolfson, E. A.: "Acute Drug Abuse Emergencies," *Twenty-third Hahnemann Symposium on Emergency Room Care* (New York: Grune & Stratton, 1972), pp. 257–262.

17

Care of the burned patient

FLORENCE B. DZIEKAN
GEORGE READING

Burns are a very significant emergency problem in the United States. In 1972, there were 2,000,000 burns recorded; of these, 75,000 required hospitalization. Of 12,000 deaths recorded due to burns in 1972, 6,000 occurred in the hospital, due to complications.

A burn may be defined as an injury to tissues caused by application of physical agents. This definition would include such injuries as frostbite and cold injuries, as well as chemical burns, electrical burns and injuries caused by ionizing radiation (x-ray). The most common burns, of course, are caused by heat, applied in the form of solid contact, as from a hot iron or other hot objects; by hot fluids, most commonly water or solutions such as coffee or soup; by flash, as explosion of a gas oven; and by flame, most commonly seen secondary to burning clothing.*

A burn which involves a large percentage of body surface is perhaps the most severe trauma that can occur to a living organism. The primary organ injured is the skin. In

*Most severe burns are associated with burning clothing. For this reason, the American Burn Association has instituted a program for compiling statistics on the clothes of burn victims, for use in lobbying for legislation to require that clothes be made flame-retardant.

terms of volume and weight, the skin is the largest organ of the body. The functions of the skin include: prevention of invasion of the body by microorganisms; separation of the fluid, internal environment from the dry, external environment; protection of the deeper structures from trauma; regulation of the body temperature; provision of an elastic covering for the motion of bones and joints; and, not the least, beauty or aesthetic value of the individual. All of these functions are compromised by a severe burn, and in the care of the burn, each of these functions must be considered.

Other injuries are often associated with the burn itself; of these, perhaps the most important is injury to the respiratory tract, both upper and lower, by inhalation of noxious gases (smoke), flame or heat. Burns which cover a large percentage of the total body surface are most severe, but burns of relatively small areas of the surface may be critical, if they involve specific regions. Such regions include burns of the face and neck, with the possibility of respiratory obstruction and disfigurement, and burns of the hands, feet and genitalia, with the resultant decrease in function of these structures.

FIRST AID AT THE SCENE

Very little life-saving first aid can be given a burn victim, but what can be done may be very important.

Putting out the fire by smothering it or drowning it with water is the first step in administering first aid. Smoldering garments or fragments of clothing, belts, buckles, shoes and jewelry, such as rings, should be removed completely. The victim should be separated from the burning agent as soon as possible. Persons burned with hot liquid should be covered with cold water immediately. For instance, a child who has pulled a pan of boiling water over on himself may be picked up and placed under cold water running from the kitchen tap. This is faster than removing the hot clothing.

The victim should then be assessed for other injuries, such as fractures, lacerations, head injuries or chest or abdominal injuries. Next, the wounds should be covered with the cleanest available cloth, such as a clean sheet. *No* ointments or salves should be applied. When exposed to cold weather, the victim should be covered with additional blankets or clothing over the cloth dressing, to keep him warm.

Placing the victim in a horizontal position (not the head-down position) will minimize inhalation of noxious gases. A history of smoke or noxious gas exposure is important and should be recorded promptly. Someone should reassure the victim and make him as comfortable as possible. The person is then transported by car or ambulance to a medical facility, which has been notified that a burn victim is en route.

People with critical burns should be treated at a specialized burn treatment facility, if this is at all possible. Many studies have shown markedly higher survival rates for severely burned patients treated in burn centers than for those treated in general hospitals. Moderately burned people can be treated in general hospitals, if the personnel have had experience or training, and people with minor burns can be treated as outpatients. Most burn victims, however, are first brought to a hospital emergency department, for assessment of the severity of the burn.

ASSESSMENT AT THE EMERGENCY DEPARTMENT

Initial assessment

Diagnosis of the extent and depth of the burn is necessary to determine its severity. The percentage of total body surface burned is used, along with the depth of the burn and the age of the patient, to estimate accurately the morbidity and mortality of the burn. Personnel involved in assessment, and all personnel in contact with the patient, must maintain aseptic technique. Gowns, masks and sterile gloves must be worn.

Percentage of body burned

A "critical" burn is any burn involving over 20 percent of the body surface, or smaller areas if the face and neck are involved or if the patient is under 2 or over 50 years of age. A "minor burn" involves less than 2 to 3 percent of the body surface area.

The body surface may be divided into segments, each comprising 9 percent of the body surface (see Figure 17–1), for the purpose of measuring percentage of body burned. One estimates the fraction of each area burned, figures the burn percentage in each area and adds up the percentages. The tendency is to overestimate burned area; so it is useful to estimate the unburned area as well. Children have relatively larger heads and smaller lower extremities than adults, so special charts have been devised for the estimation of burn areas in children of varying ages (Figure 17–2).

Depth of burn

A "first-degree" or "superficial" burn affects only the epidermis. It produces pain and redness, but no blistering. It is relatively easily treated and heals in 2 to 3 days. A common first-degree burn is sunburn.

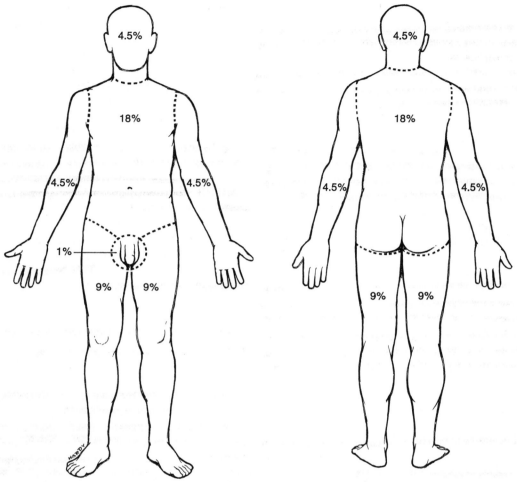

Figure 17–1 The rule of nines. The diagram of the body surface may be used to estimate the percentage of burned body area.

A "second-degree" burn or "dermal" burn destroys all of the epidermis and some portion of the dermis. There is a distinction between "intermediate" dermal burn and the "deep" dermal burn, in which all but the very deepest layers of the dermis are destroyed. In the intermediate dermal burn, there are many projections of the basal layer of the epidermal cells in the sweat glands and hair follicles of the skin, and these are available for epidermis reconstitution and growth out over the unburned dermis to produce a healed wound. In deep dermal burns, the viable projections of the basal layer are few and far between; thus, considerable time may be required for the resurfacing or reepithelization of the burn.

"Full-thickness" or "third-degree" burns denote that the dermis was entirely destroyed. If the burned areas are of significant size, skin grafting will be needed to close the wound. These burns may extend deeper than the subcutaneous tissue layer, to include fascia, muscle and bone, but this is relatively infrequent, due to the protective functions of the skin and subcutaneous tissues.

Infection can change the depth of the burn, from a burn that would ordinarily heal to a full-thickness burn that will require skin grafting. Deep dermal burns are particularly

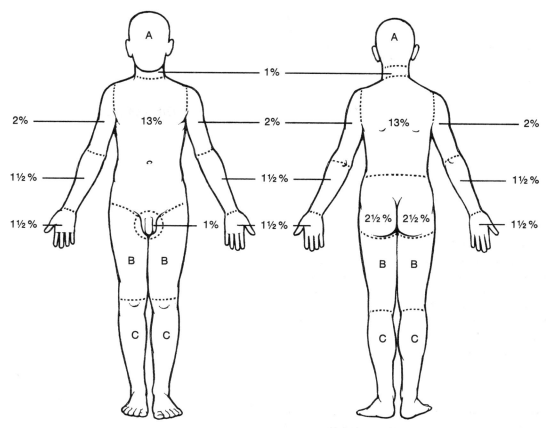

Figure 17–2 The effects of growth on the relative percentages of body surface areas. Those areas designated by numbers (reflecting percentage of body area) remain relatively stable throughout life. Those areas designated by a letter (A, B and C) represent percentages of the total body surface area which vary from birth to adult life. The table below indicates the relative percentages of these body surface areas at various stages in life.

| | Age in years | | | | | |
Area	0	1	5	10	15	Adult
A: ½ of head	9½	8½	6½	5½	4½	3½
B: ½ of one thigh	2¾	3¼	4	4½	4½	4¾
C: ½ of one lower leg	2½	2½	2¾	3	3¼	3½

susceptible to this. Dermal burns are characteristically blistered and sensitive when examined by pinprick. They are frequently caused by hot liquids and often surround the deeper burns caused by such things as burning clothing.

Accompanying conditions and injuries

Respiratory tract injuries, such as smoke inhalation, may be severe enough to cause the death of a patient in the immediate post-burn period (the first one or 2 hours). Type of exposure (e.g., burns occurring indoors in a house versus outdoors in a field), singed nasal hairs, mucosal burns of the nose and mouth, voice change, respiratory distress with wheezing and a cough with sooty sputum, all suggest respiratory complications.

Preexisting systemic diseases, diabetes and arteriosclerosis, for instance, may work towards complications and death in a patient with burns involving even a relatively small percentage of the body surface area. It must be determined whether the burn victim suffers from any disease and what effect it will have on his burn condition.

Fractures and other injuries must not be missed when attention is directed to the obvious, traumatic burn. They, also, must be assessed for treatment.

Continuing assessment

If the patient is to be given continuing care in the same institution, further assessment may be made in the emergency department. While the burn wound is being cared for, urinary output is recorded each hour, and if it is below 30 to 50 cc. an hour in adults, the rate of administration of intravenous fluids should be increased. The urine should be observed for free hemoglobin, indicated by a dark or bloody urine which suggests deep tissue involvement. This needs to be treated with immediate diuresis, usually using mannitol. Accurate measurements of fluid intake and output must be recorded in the chart.

Specimens should be taken for baseline values. These include: complete blood count, arterial blood gases, electrolytes, blood urea nitrogen and/or creatinine, urinalysis, culture of the wound and blood type and crossmatch for anticipated blood transfusions.

The amount and type of fluid administered should be calculated, using any one of a number of burn formulas. All of these formulas use 3 to 4 ml. of fluid for each percent of body burn up to 50 percent, per kilogram of body weight in the first 24 hours. The amounts of electrolyte solution, colloid solution and dextrose solution vary from formula to formula, but it is best to start with a balanced electrolyte solution, such as Ringer's lactate solution.

Vital signs (pulse, blood pressure, respiration and temperature) should be monitored hourly during the acute phase and every 4 hours, afterwards.

Tetanus immunization should be assessed and appropriate measures taken (see Chapter 10). Consideration of antibiotic therapy is made also at this time; in general, only penicillin or some other appropriate antibiotic is given in the acute phase.

INITIAL CARE

Supplies

The emergency department must be equipped with the proper supplies for care of burns. The following list summarizes these supplies; the figures in parentheses indicate the number of the specific item needed.

(1) Large scissors to cut away clothing.
(2) Sterile precaution gowns (6).
(3) Disposable masks (12).
(4) Sterile gloves (6 in various sizes).
(5) Sterile burn linen pack: sheets, gowns, pillow cases.
(6) O$_2$ (oxygen) with nebulizer, mask, cannula.
(7) Endotracheal set-up; respirator.
(8) Ambu Bag.
(9) Oral suction machine.
(10) Tracheostomy instruments.
(11) I.V. solutions, with set-ups.
(12) Cut-down instruments.
(13) Blood collecting tubes; urine specimen containers.
(14) Nasogastric tubes; gastric decompression machine.
(15) Foley catheter; catheterization tray; closed drainage system.
(16) Normal saline solution (2).
(17) Sterile water (2).
(18) Sterile hand towels.
(19) Sterile basins (2).
(20) Sterile gauze sponges, small.
(21) Sterile curved scissors (2).
(22) Sterile forceps (2).
(23) Cleansing agent, one pint.
(24) Prep razors (sterile).
(25) Wound culture tubes.
(26) ECG machine.
(27) Medications: narcotics, tetanus toxoid, antibiotics.

(28) Portable lights; extension cords.

(29) Ice and plastic containers (for blood gases).

(30) Escharotomy equipment.

(31) Topical ointments.

(32) Equipment table (Mayo stand).

(33) I.V. poles.

(34) Resuscitation cart.

Resuscitation and maintenance

Resuscitation of victims with critical burns must be started prior to transport to the burn facility or admission to the hospital. Patients with both critical and moderate burns should be started on intravenous fluids promptly. Although clinical signs of shock are rarely seen in the immediate post-burn period (one to 2 hours), intravenous fluids should be started immediately, because the loss of fluids starts at the time of burning. Shock must be prevented rather than treated after it occurs.

A urinary catheter must be emplaced, to measure urinary output; recording of urinary output by spontaneous urination is *never* satisfactory. All critical and most moderately burned patients should have a nasogastric tube emplaced to avoid acute gastric dilatation, vomiting and aspiration. If the patient is to be transferred immediately, the above treatment may be all that is necessary. Table 17-1 summarizes the steps involved in transferring a burn victim to a burn care facility.

If a specialized burn treatment facility is not available, moderate burns are best cared for in the intensive care unit. In some cases, the emergency department must initiate care. The fluid therapy is adjusted to provide for good urinary output, from 30 to 60 cc. an hour for the first 24 to 48 hours. Subsequently, as the fluid that has been sequestered in the wound is reabsorbed into the normal body fluid compartments, fluid administration should be limited to estimated fluid loss by urine, nasogastric suction and insensible loss. Insensible loss *may* be as much as 10 times normal, but the tendency, 48 hours post-burn, is to overhydrate burned patients rather than underhydrate them. Blood transfusions are seldom necessary in the first 48 hours, but may be required for a week after that period.

The respiratory status of the patient should be continuously and carefully observed. Swelling of tissues in the upper respiratory tract may take some time to become apparent. The effects of smoke inhalation may also be delayed past the period of the initial evaluation. Tracheostomy, intubation and treatment

TABLE 17-1 TRANSFER TO A BURN CARE FACILITY

Step	Explanation
(1) Communication	Call burn care facility early and get concise recommendations as to when to transfer and how much therapy to give prior to and while transferring.
(2) Airway	Check patency. Is intubation or tracheostomy needed or may it be required during transit period?
(3) Fluids	A secure veinway must be established prior to transfer and adequate electrolyte solutions started, usually Ringer's lactate. Record intake accurately.
(4) Output	An indwelling urinary catheter is essential. Record output hourly.
(5) Nasogastric intubation	Avoid acute gastric dilatation and aspiration.
(6) Burn wounds	Avoid extensive burn wound treatment. Sterile sheets and blanket are all that is needed.
(7) Transfer	A nurse or physician should accompany patient to maintain treatment and observe. Mask and gown and aseptic technique should be maintained. During transfer, resuscitation is usually optimal.

with warm humidified air may become critical. Repeated arterial blood gas determinations are required to assess ongoing respiratory function. Respiratory support with positive end expiratory pressure (PEEP) may be beneficial.

Severely burned patients rarely require strong analgesia or sedation. Deep burns are anesthetic soon after the burning, and many patients have been harmed by over-sedation prior to transfer. An attitude of quiet competence and reassurance may do more than drugs in calming and relieving a severely burned patient. Any analgesic or sedative that is given should be given in very small increments, intravenously. The effects can thus be observed immediately. It is important to avoid creating a depot of medication from intramuscular injections in unperfused tissue.

Avoiding sepsis and promoting healing

A burn provides an almost ideal environment for the growth of microorganisms. Necrotic tissue lies next to living tissue, with its fluid, warmth and low oxygen tension. It is nearly impossible to prevent bacterial growth in a burn, but the aim must be to decrease this growth so that clinical invasive sepsis does not occur.

The aim is to achieve a healed wound without infection in the soonest possible time. Several general measures are used in this effort.

(1) Cleansing and debridement are performed. Removal of the necrotic tissue is complicated by the difficulty in assessing the exact extent of the wound (how deep? how wide? where is the edge of nonviable tissue?), as well as the difficulty in assessing injury to the intact tissue (anesthesia, blood loss), which should be known before removal of necrotic tissue.

(2) Various antibacterial agents are applied topically. These include 0.5 percent silver nitrate as solution or cream, other silver compounds, mafenide (Sulfamylon), silver sulfadiazine, gentamicin and other antibiotics and povidone-iodine (Betadine).

(3) Dressings and/or isolation techniques are used to decrease contamination of the burn wound by the outside environment. However, most of the bacteria arise from the patient himself: from the deep glands of the skin and from the G.I. and respiratory tracts.

(4) Systemic measures are taken, including administration of antiobotics, nutrients, vaccinations and immune sera.

Cleansing and debridement

Gentle but thorough mechanical cleansing of the burned area should be initiated as soon as possible, using a bland soap, such as povidone-iodine (Betadine scrub), and gauze sponges. The area is well rinsed with warm, sterile saline solution. The detached epidermis is removed with sterile forceps and scissors. Blisters are usually removed by sharp dissection unless they are very firm, as on the soles or palms of the hands. Then they may be left unbroken.

Attentive nursing care must be given to burns involving the head, face and neck. The singed hair immediately surrounding or adjacent to the burned area should be removed by careful shaving and cleansing. Copious amounts of sterile saline may be used to irrigate the eyes. Gentle removal of accumulated crust and drainage from the eyes is important. Cotton-tipped sticks are appropriate here.

Particular attention to burned ears should include cleansing, careful debridement and removal of obviously necrotic tissue. Again, drainage and crusts should be removed by repeated use of saline solutions and cotton-tipped sticks. The application of a topical antibiotic ointment is useful. The mouth must also be examined for possible burns and irritation. The lips should be lubricated with an ointment, and frequent oral hygiene is soothing to the patient.

In circumferential burns of the extremities or trunk, the burned skin may act as a tourniquet, as it is unyielding to the swelling of tissues beneath it. This may result in difficulty in breathing and/or obliteration of the pulses, depending on the part involved. Should these occur, an escharotomy must be carried out. This involves cutting through the burn longitudinally on the extremities and/or chest to relieve constriction.

Full-thickness burns may require grafting to promote healing. Preparation for grafting requires removal of the dead tissue. This may be done in a number of ways.

(1) Repeated dressing changes to remove dead tissue with the dressing, along with repeated debridement at the bedside or in a Hubbard-type tank, has been used. This debridement should be carried out without pain and without bleeding.

(2) Formal excision of the burn may be carried out if it is clear which areas of the burn wound are full thickness and which are partial thickness. This debridement can include the fascia or subcutaneous tissue. However, excision through the subcutaneous tissue may not be adequate at first try, because it is very difficult to assess the viability of this tissue on immediate cutting.

(3) Tangential excision using a dermatome-type technique has been used in recent years. Usually, a small hand dermatome is used, and the excision is done under anesthesia. The excision should reach a small capillary bleeding in the viable dermis or subcutaneous tissue. This exposed area should then be immediately covered with a graft or biological dressing to prevent drying and loss of viability.

(4) Various enzymes have been used, the most recent sutlains (Travase), in attempts to remove the necrotic tissue without injuring the viable tissue adjacent or deep to it. This technique involves frequent dressing changes and is not compatible with the use of sulfamylon or other topical agents mentioned earlier.

Topical antibacterial agents

Silver nitrate, 0.5 percent solution, was introduced in the 1960s as a wet dressing for burns. It requires much nursing care for the 2 to 4 daily dressing changes. The concentration is critical; stronger solutions injure tissue, and weaker solutions are not effective in controlling bacteria. In large burns, the hypotonic solution removes salt from the patient, and extra sodium, potassium and other electrolytes must be administered. Staining is a very troublesome problem. Recently, silver nitrate 0.5 percent cream has been used with some success, employing a technique similar to that used with other creams.

Silver sulfadiazine one percent cream has been used experimentally for about 4 years and looks very promising; no major drawbacks are yet known. It has recently been released by the Food and Drug Administration (FDA) for general use. Various other silver compounds are in the testing stage.

Mafenide (Sulfamylon) 10 percent cream is effective in decreasing bacterial growth but has several important drawbacks. There is a varying degree of stinging pain produced with application. To be most effective, the cream should be removed and reapplied every 8 hours. A high percentage of patients (20 to 30 percent) develop an allergic reaction on the unburned skin after 2 to 3 weeks of treatment.

Gentamicin, neomycin, bacitracin, and other antibiotics have also been used, alone and in combinations, but in general, all topical antibiotic agents become ineffective due to the rapid development of resistant strains of bacteria. However, they may be useful for short-term therapy prior to debridement and/or grafting.

Povidone-iodine (Betadine) has recently been used, both as an ointment and as a solution, with encouraging results.

Certainly, more new agents will be developed and used in the near future, but each one will have to endure a testing period in order to determine its advantages and drawbacks. There is a relatively long delay between the beginning of clinical testing on a drug and its release for general use by the FDA.

Biological dressings

In an effort to mimic the functions of the skin that have been lost due to burning, a number of substances have been used in the treatment of burns. Homografts or skin grafts taken from cadavers are used, although obtaining them is difficult. Porcine heterografts or xenografts can be obtained in an aseptic surgical fashion from the skin of slaughtered pigs. They can be used fresh or kept at refrigerator temperature (4° C.) for up to 4 weeks and are available commercially from several firms across the country.

Frozen heterografts, as well as dry heterografts, have been used with varying success. The frozen grafts are kept at −50° C. and have an unlimited shelf life. Dried grafts are reconstituted by soaking in saline for 30 minutes prior to application. Attempts to achieve similar results with synthetic skin made of various plastic materials and foams are also being made.

Each of the above substances can be used to cover debrided or partially debrided wounds. In general, biological dressings must be changed at least every 3 to 4 days. In full-thickness burns, they aid in debridement and act as a test: if the heterograft is apparently "taking" at 3 to 4 days, the "take" of an autograft is assured.*

In partial-thickness burns, the biological dressing can be left in place for up to 2 weeks, when it peels off leaving a healed surface.

Treatment of minor burns on an outpatient basis

The burn is assessed and clothing removed. (Masks, caps and sterile gloves should be used by the personnel handling the wound.) Early cooling with cold saline or water will relieve pain, but consideration of an analgesic medication should be made at this time. General cleansing with an antiseptic soap, such as povidone-iodine (Betadine scrub), should be done, and bits of blisters and dead skin should be removed, using sterile forceps and scissors. Intact blisters over the palmar surface of the hand and the soles of the feet are left intact; all other blisters are excised.

_____

* The terms and concepts in this section are defined and developed to a greater extent in Chapter 29.

Prior to deciding that the burned patient can be treated on an outpatient basis, some evaluation of his life situation should be made. Many minor burns are small burns of the hand or face, which may interfere with the person's function at home. It is important to know if there will be someone available to care for his daily needs. Aged persons living alone, alcoholics or drug addicts are not candidates for care of burns (other than minute burns) on an outpatient basis.

Most burns cared for on an outpatient basis are best treated with a dressing technique. There is less pain and less chance of contamination from the surroundings than with an exposure technique. Any of the previously mentioned creams can be used as part of the dressing. Vaseline or nitrofurazone (Furacin) gauze may be used in one single layer next to the burn, followed by more layers of gauze and a circumferential wrap of conforming gauze (Kling). In burns of the hand, it is worthwhile to immobilize the wrist and hand with a plaster splint for 2 to 3 days.

Tetanus immunity should be evaluated and steps taken (as outlined in Chpater 10) to promote healing of minor wounds. In general, unless the burned area is known to be contaminated, antibiotics are not used in these minor wounds. Local agents containing a combination of antibiotics with or without local anesthetics (usually derivatives of benzocaine) are widely advertised and available over the counter. These medications are to be avoided because of the high incidence of local skin reactions associated with them. These small burns are usually not painful after having been dressed.

A critical part of the ambulatory care of burns is frequent follow-up. If the patient cannot be reevaluated frequently, he should not be cared for as an outpatient. One may well treat a burn for 2 to 3 weeks, then find it is necessary to admit the victim for skin grafting. Very small areas, however, may be grafted on an outpatient basis.

The patient should be seen 24 to 72 hours after the initial care for further evaluation and dressing changes. Dressing changes are effected after soaking off the intial dressing in a sterile basin with sterile saline. An evaluation as to the frequency of further dressing changes should be made, the intent being to avoid the infection which might ensue from prolonged incubation of a small amount of bacterial contamination under a dressing wet with wound exudate and dead tissue. Usually, a burn should be seen at least every 3 days until the wound is healed or grafting is obviously needed.

If there is a question of cellulitis or spreading of local infection, cultures should be obtained and antibiotics started. Usually, a penicillin or a semisynthetic penicillin effective against penicillinase-producing organisms is given prior to obtaining the culture and sensitivity reports.

In some instances, when biological dressings such as heterografts are available, they are applied to obvious partial-thickness burns and dressed into place. The dressings are changed while the heterografts are left in place until healing has occurred or until it has become apparent that the grafts are not adhering.

After the first 2 or 3 days, it is imperative that joints be routinely moved through their full ranges of motion, especially in older patients who might otherwise develop marked contractures both of small joints in the hand and of larger joints, such as elbows, knees and shoulders.

SPECIAL BURNS

Chemical burns

Chemical burns occur most often in industrial plants and laboratories. Such burns usually result from contact with strong acid or alkali solutions. The strong alkalis include sodium hydroxide, potassium hydroxide and lime. Hydrochloric, phenol, nitric and sulfuric acids are examples of strong acid solutions. Less commonly, burns may result from contact with magnesium or phosphorus. Although the skin has a protective layer of keratin and is further protected by surface oils, such strong chemical agents may penetrate or destroy the protective mechanism, with subsequent damage to tissue.

Chemical burns require immediate attention. Of first priority is irrigating the wounds with copious amounts of tap water to remove the chemical. The rinsing of the wound is effective treatment and should begin at the scene of the accident and continue at the hospital, either by showering or by submerging the patient in a tub of water. It may be necessary to continue this treatment for 24 to 48 hours to remove all of the offending agent. In general, neutralizing agents have little or no place in the management of chemical burns during the emergency phase of care, since the neutralizing agent may have a more harmful effect than the burning agent.

The wounds of chemical burns are often spotty or scattered, and the pain associated with such an injury may continue for a long period of time. After initial treatment, management is similar to that of a thermal burn.

Electrical burns

Electrical burns from household voltage (110 to 220 volts) usually do not cause severe amounts of tissue destruction but may cause death from heart or central nervous system insult.

The most common electrical burn is sustained by infants who suck on electrical apparatus, such as an extension cord. The saliva completes the circuit, and a full-thickness burn of the lips and/or tongue is sustained. These burns usually heal spontaneously but result in some degree of deformity. Most plastic surgeons feel that definitive repair is best done months after initial healing. Children with electrical burns may be treated as outpatients in homes with conscientious, well-informed parents. There is a tendency to bleed about 2 weeks post-burn, when the dead tissue separates spontaneously from viable tissue. This bleeding is usually controlled by simple, direct pressure.

High voltage may kill outright, but when it does not, the burns are often very severe and deep, involving vessels, nerves and bone, and often requiring amputations.

Tar burns

Tar burns may be treated by applying ice to the affected areas immediately. The tar will harden and may be easily removed by peeling the crusty surface away from the injured tissue. Further treatment follows that recommended for thermal burns.

SUMMARY

The following lists summarize the step-by-step care of minor and severe burns in the emergency department.

Minor burns

(1) Remove clothing, using aseptic precautions.
(2) Immediately apply cool, moist pack to burn wound for relief of pain.
(3) Gently cleanse the area with mild soap and warm normal saline.
(4) Cover the wound with sterile, non-adherent gauze dressing and wrap with conforming gauze (Kerlix) for comfort and protection from the environment.
(5) Immunize against tetanus.
(6) Administer analgesic for discomfort, if necessary.
(7) Arrange for revisit in 24 to 72 hours for redressing and evaluation of wound.

Severe burns

(1) Assure a patent airway, using oxygen, endotracheal tubes or tracheostomy, depending on indications.
(2) Perform initial veinway by inserting a plastic indwelling catheter (cutdown may be necessary).
(3) Start I.V. fluids with Ringer's lactate solution; record accurate hourly input.
(4) Communicate with attending physician.
(5) Insert indwelling Foley catheter; record accurate hourly urine output.
(6) Sedate with narcotics (intravenously, in small dose), if necessary.
(7) Immunize against tetanus.
(8) Insert nasogastric tube; attach to suction; allow nothing by mouth.
(9) Obtain complete history of burn accident and make physical assessment.
(10) Estimate percentage of body surface burned; initiate the burn diagram record.
(11) Describe depth of injury (by pinprick sensation, appearance).
(12) Obtain vital signs and record them; repeat at least hourly.
(13) Obtain laboratory studies: complete blood count, electrolytes, urinalysis, blood type and crossmatch, arterial blood gases, creatinine and blood urea nitrogen.
(14) Initiate wound care: remove or cut away burned garments and expose burn areas; gentle mechanical cleansing of burned areas with povidone-iodine (Betadine), mild scrub and warm normal saline solution; trim and remove all necrotic material with forceps and scissors; cover burns with sterile sheets and add additional blankets to keep patient warm, avoid chilling patient.

BIBLIOGRAPHY

(1) Artz, C. P.: *The Treatment of Burns,* ed. 2 (Philadelphia: W. B. Saunders, 1969).
(2) Furnas, D. W.: *A Bedside Outline of the Treatment of Burns* (Springfield, Ill.: Charles C Thomas, 1969).

(3) Laing, J. E.: *The Management and Nursing of Burns* (London: English Universities Press, Ltd., 1967).

(4) Moncrief, J. A.: "Medical Progress—Burns," *New England Journal of Medicine,* 288 (1973):444–454.

(5) Stone, N. H., and Boswick, J. A.: *Profiles of Burn Management* (Miami, Fla.: Industrial Medical Publication Company, 1938).

18

Emergency care of infants and children

SANDRA M. STEWART
THOMAS S. MORSE
DIANN ANDERSON

THE UNIQUENESS OF CHILDREN

Parents can attest to the fact that children are special—especially when the children are theirs! In terms of health care, though, parents are right; children are special in many ways. Responses to illness or injury vary among children as individuals, and among children of different age groups, both physically and emotionally.

One distinctive characteristic of illness or injury in children is that when it strikes, it does so on growing tissue. Thus, it may affect the future growth and development of the child. For example, an injury to the epiphysis of a long bone may retard or stop the growth of that bone, resulting in a shortened limb in the grown adult. Another illustration is that of hypothyroidism, which manifests as cretinism in the child and as myxedema in the adult.

While there are commonalities in identifying and treating health problems of children and adults, one cannot think of children as "little adults." Because the child's responses are influenced by so many factors (nutrition, growth and development tasks, family stabil-

ity, immunizations, previous health care), care of any one child must be based on the maturity of his body and mind, as well as on all those factors which influence their development.

The child who receives all his health care from the emergency department of a hospital requires not only treatment for his immediate problem but also assessment of nutritional, developmental and immunization status, related health screening and referral for follow-up care. Parent teaching in this situation is especially important, particularly in stressing the long-term value of preventive health care.

Care of an infant or child must also include the family, since he is dependent on and influenced by his family for many years. And parents can provide useful, detailed information about their child, information that even the most astute observer may easily overlook. Parental observations must always be seriously considered; they are usually very valid and pertinent.

In crisis situations, especially, care of the family as well as the child is essential. Listening to and supporting the family while life-support measures are being administered to the child is therapeutic as well as kind.

Helping the child cope

Methods of helping the child cope with the stress of illness or injury in the emergency department depend largely on the age of the child, his previous experiences with hospitalization and his available resources for coping. While every child's response to stress is uniquely his own, certain age group characteristics * can guide the nurse in her approach to each patient.[13]

Older infant to toddler

The older infant and toddler fears separation from his parents.[2] Most emergency department staff "bend the rules" to permit the parent to stay with the child for safety (to keep the child on the guerney †) and to reduce anxiety ("Mommy is here, so everything will be all right"). Toddlers trust their parents but not strangers. However, if their parents trust these strangers, then perhaps they will trust them, also.

The question of whether the parent should be permitted to stay with the child during treatment is one to which no inflexible rule can apply. The determination is made by considering all factors involved: the nature of the treatment, the parent's ability to tolerate the procedure being performed on the child and the child himself.

Parents need to know that it is all right to leave if they are unsure whether or not they can handle the situation. Their reassurance to the child that they are just outside the door and that they will be back as soon as the procedure is over is also important. Always, the goal is to make the emergency department experience a healthy one, to minimize the anxiety-provoking and painful experiences

and to maximize the positive, more pleasurable experiences.

Preschool to school-age children

The preschool or school-age child's major fear is that of bodily harm.[2] While the parents' presence may still be very important, his main concern is his body and what these strangers are going to do to it. The nurse can lessen the child's fears by being calm, honest, accurate and reassuring. Through these actions, she can convey that she is trustworthy.

Establishing this relationship before initiating a treatment which may be uncomfortable or painful is important, not only for gaining cooperation during the procedure, but for minimizing the negative feelings of the emergency department experience.

Older school-age children

The older school-age child fears loss of self-control;[2] he may use "delaying tactics" before an uncomfortable procedure, to give him time to regain control. He may lie still in a quiet attempt to appear brave, but he passively seeks help; he will not ask for it, but he gladly accepts it when offered. The nurse can encourage the child to verbalize his fears. Misconceptions or previous experiences with hospitalization can be explored at this time. The nurse, by asking questions which convey genuine interest, can help the child feel that there is someone who cares and will protect him or help him through this experience.

There are always some children who are absolutely terrified of anything that has to do with the hospital or its personnel. Such children are a particular challenge, especially when an uncomfortable procedure may be necessary. When all else fails and it becomes obvious that the child is going to resist, and vigorously, restraint is necessary. The nurse should have one person with her who is strong enough to help restrain the child; this is far less threatening than 3 or 4 "weak" persons. The procedure should be completed as quickly and thoroughly as possible. The child should be permitted to express his feelings about it,

---

* Care of the newborn is especially specific and unique. For that reason and since there are many excellent books dealing with neonatology, problems of the newborn will not be discussed in this chapter.

† "Guerney" is a vernacular term for a wheeled stretcher.

and afterwards the nurse might try to divert his attention to another source of interest or curiosity.

Children cooperate and respond better if allowed to handle the strange materials that will be used for their care prior to their experience with them or, if not before, after the experience.[11] Taking these materials home (the gauze or medicine cup, for example) for use in imaginative play will help the child work out his fears and, hopefully, prepare him for future visits to the hospital or doctor's office.

Family dynamics in the emergency department

For many families, the emergency department is the "family doctor"; it is their only contact with the health care system. As such, the family members receive episodic rather than comprehensive health care. They are treated for their current illness or injury but do not have the benefits of comprehensive health evaluation and preventive health care. Usually, the goals of health evaluation and preventive care cannot be accomplished while a child is ill; so the next step is to schedule or encourage the parents to schedule a follow-up appointment for a well-child visit.

A hospital may provide screening services during those hours when parents are apt to bring their children for care. These are frequently the evening hours, when the husband is home from work with the family car and the children are out of school. While the ill child receives care in the emergency department, his siblings can be screened for problems (dental, ocular, aural, nutritional, need of immunizations), then be referred to an appropriate clinic or physician for treatment.

Determining patient status

Who needs the care? In assessment, ownership of the problem is a significant question. Young parents bringing in a baby of 3 weeks with a complaint that the baby is "sick" may be more in need of assessment than the child,

especially if examination reveals a normal, healthy infant.

Circumstances leading to excessive crying may convince parents that their child is ill. If the circumstances cannot be clarified, the visit of this "well child" is indeed a waste of everyone's time. The nurse must realize that parents bring children to facilities for emergency care because they cannot deal with behaviors unrelated to illness, like crying; they also use the children as a means of requesting help for themselves.

In a facility with high volume and a great variety of problems, it is not easy to maintain the goal of assessing the key environmental variables which help define what the problem is, what it means and what can be done about it. The family seeking emergency care wants help for something; thus, assessing the family's needs must proceed concurrently with assessing the child's needs.

Communication

Because assessing the family is a part of pediatric assessment, establishing communication is likewise important. In hospitals where significant numbers of non-English-speaking families seek care, bilingual employees should be available to gather and interpret information. Families and staff share feelings of frustration and futility when they are unable to talk with one another because of the language barrier.

In addition, the staff must determine from the families their ability to comprehend the health care plan for the child and their willingness and ability to follow through with the plan at home. This demands that both staff and families listen carefully and clarify these goals with one another.

The climate of the busy emergency department is not conducive to effective health teaching. Noise, traffic and anxiety generated by unpredictable situations affect patients, families and staff, making teaching and learning difficult. Often parents don't "hear" or perceive what has been said, and written instructions are useful as supplements to the verbal teaching. A telephone number the parent can call for clarification should always be placed conspicuously on the instruction sheet.

Follow-up telephone calls may be made by nursing staff to parents of selected patients. These often reveal the inadequacy of the teaching-learning process that has occurred and provides an opportunity for clarification.

TRIAGE

Triage in pediatrics is a particular challenge. Guidelines which apply to the triage of adults don't always apply to children, especially to very young children and infants who have immature organ systems and respond globally and unpredictably to bodily stresses.

Key questions to ask early in assessment are: (1) What is the child's age? (2) How long has he been sick? (3) Is he acting very sick? (4) Does he have trouble breathing? (5) Does he have a fever? and (6) What happened that made the parent decide to bring the child to the emergency department? Using the parent's words in recording this information is helpful for the next person reviewing the record; they convey the parent's impressions rather than the triage nurse's interpretations.

Examination of the infant or child must be exacting. Vital signs should be obtained without delay; a child brought in for the chief complaint of "sick" may be moribund by the time he receives care in the emergency department if this rule is not followed.

Triage cannot be achieved without the infant unclothed and awake; young infants look deceptively well swaddled and asleep in someone's arms. Sleeping children do not exhibit enough behavior to determine if they are in a life-threatening state. They need to be awakened and engaged in developmentally appropriate activities to facilitate assessment of the problem.

Conditions requiring immediate treatment

While many basic conditions requiring immediate care are outlined in Chapter 6,

additional considerations are necessary in pediatric triage. Specific situations, often overlooked by nurses accustomed to screening adults, follow and are developed in depth later in this chapter.

(1) *Difficulty in breathing* is a first-priority emergency. Unless the triage nurse is skilled in distinguishing minor from serious respiratory problems in children, however, such conditions are often misjudged. For example, the child with "croup" is commonly misjudged, because his chest is clear, he is not breathing quickly and he is not cyanotic; but all of these criteria are late findings and are not useful in screening the "croupy" child.

(2) A child under one year of age with a *fever* should be seen by someone experienced in evaluating sickness in a child. The younger the infant, the more tenuous and critical his physiological status, and the more urgent it is that he receive prompt care. Young babies may look fairly well in spite of a high temperature. On the other hand, a very septic young infant may be afebrile. A general rule is to listen very carefully to the parent and have the infant evaluated as soon as possible.

(3) Ingestion of any possibly *toxic substance* requires immediate evaluation. Chapter 12 discusses these emergencies.

(4) A child who *"looks sick"* or *appears dehydrated* must be seen promptly before a more critical situation develops.

(5) An *alteration of consciousness* in a child may herald the onset of a serious problem requiring immediate intervention.

In general, although further evaluation may reveal a minor problem, it is always safest to triage the child as though the more serious problem existed.

ASSESSMENT

History

Information collected by interview generally follows the format outlined in Chapter 5. For the young child and infant, most information will be obtained from the parent, although the child should not be ignored during the interview; he should be talked to and played with, so that the nurse can observe his responses.

The history of a child under 2 years should include a brief survey of the pregnancy, labor, delivery, birth weight and height, early development, immunizations, previous illness, injury, hospitalizations and nutritional status, in addition to matters related to the chief complaint. One should inquire about any family history of diabetes, seizures and other conditions the child might have inherited. This information is quickly obtained and is very helpful in identifying high-risk children.

Physical examination

Examination of the infant and young child is best done with the patient unclothed, although the older child's desire for modesty needs to be respected. From observing the child without physical contact, the nurse can obtain most of the information she needs regarding respiratory status, oxygen saturation, neurological status, rashes, bruises, pain and interpersonal relationships with parents.

Vital signs and an accurate height and weight are recorded on admission to the emergency department; vital signs may need to be repeated if a significant time lapse has occurred between admission and examination.

LIFE-THREATENING EMERGENCIES

Some emergency situations that affect infants and children are obviously life-threatening, such as cardiopulmonary arrest, near-drowning and major trauma. Others may be life-threatening but may not appear so, using the criteria used for adults. The following discussions of emergency situations focus on assessment and treatment of emergencies that are not considered elsewhere in this text, or if conditions are discussed elsewhere, this chapter points out the unique features of pediatric care relating to these emergencies.

Cardiac emergencies

Cardiopulmonary arrest

Respiratory and cardiac arrest may have many causes and result in cessation of effective ventilation or circulation or both. As with the adult, the diagnosis must be rapidly made, evidenced by absence of respiration, cardiac activity and dilated, nonreactive pupils. Unlike the adult, however, events leading to cardiopulmonary arrest may be more subtle in the child,[4] and rapid, accurate appraisal becomes all the more essential. Principles of cardiopulmonary resuscitation are consistent with those outlined in Chapter 14, with some differences.

For ventilation, the head is tilted back but not hyperextended. Hyperextension of the child's neck, with its pliable structures, may cause narrowing or obstruction of the airway passages. Artificial ventilation is given through both the mouth and nose in infants and small children, using only enough air to produce good chest movement, especially of the apices. In infants, puffs from the cheeks is sufficient.

Compressions are given to the midsternum, since the ventricles of the heart lie higher in the child's chest cavity than in the adult's. The force of compression should move the sternum about one fifth of the distance from the front to the back of the chest. In infants, pressure applied with the index and middle finger is sufficient. Another method is to encircle the infant's thorax with the hands and apply pressure with the thumbs. In small children, the heel of one hand is used. As the child becomes older and approaches adult size, compressions are applied similarly, but with 2 hands.

The rate of compression depends on the age and size of the child, faster rates being used for smaller children. The compression rate should be 80 to 120 per minute and respiratory inflation quickly given after every fifth compression.

Cardiac activity may be assisted by elevating the legs, to promote venous return to the heart. The use of the precordial thump has not been sufficiently evaluated in children to endorse its use.

Gastric distention is a common problem in children and dangerous, because it promotes vomiting.[21] It may be alleviated by applying gentle pressure over the epigastrium, taking care to avoid aspiration of gastric contents; or the stomach may be decompressed by a nasogastric tube and intermittent suction.

If the infant or child has not responded to basic cardiopulmonary resuscitation, additional measures may be needed. These measures include attaching him to a cardiac monitor, providing ventilatory support until an experienced person places an endotracheal tube and establishing an intravenous route.

Equipment and medications for cardiopulmonary resuscitation must be readily available in appropriate sizes and amounts to permit their efficient and accurate use. A specific area on the resuscitation cart in the emergency department may be designated specifically for pediatric supplies. The pediatric equipment which should be accessible to the resuscitation area is listed here.

(1) Orotracheal tubes, sizes 2.5 to 8.0 (inside diameter), with adapters and stylets.
(2) Oropharyngeal airways, sizes 000 to 4.
(3) Laryngoscope and varying sizes of blades.
(4) Bronchoscope.
(5) Ambu Bag and masks for premature, newborn, infant, child.
(6) Oxygen source.
(7) Suction catheters, 5 to 14 Fr., with connectors.
(8) Suction source.
(9) Cut-down tray with pediatric instruments.
(10) Scalp vein set.
(11) Small armboards.
(12) Microdrips and metrisets.
(13) Intravenous solutions, 250 and 500 ml. bottles.
(14) Intracardiac needles, 20- and 22-guage, 6 to 8 cm.
(15) Pediatric electrodes for monitor.
(16) Pediatric defibrillator paddles.

Drug therapy is given according to body weight in kilograms. Appropriate dosages of drugs used in cardiac resuscitation are outlined in Table 18–1.

Electrical defibrillation may be necessary and should be done after the monitor is attached to the child.[18] Again, the wattage that is applied varies with the size of the child:

(1) 25 to 50 joules (watt-seconds) for infants.
(2) 100 joules (watt-seconds) for children 12 to 25 kg.
(3) 200 joules (watt-seconds) for children 25 to 50 kg.
(4) 400 joules (watt-seconds) for fully grown adolescents and adults.[9]

Near-drowning

Immediate cardiopulmonary resuscitation is the cornerstone of emergency treatment in near-drowning accidents. Resuscitation should continue for several hours, if necessary; successful resuscitations without disabling sequelae are not uncommon in children. Management follows the principles outlined in Chapter 13. Nearly drowned children are always admitted and closely monitored, since significant changes may not occur for 12 to 24 hours.

Helping the parents cope with their feelings of guilt (which are always present) is essential. Providing privacy, listening, keeping the parents informed and allowing the parents to see the child when appropriate are helpful measures in warding off a crisis situation.

Heart failure

Infants in heart failure do not have the typical signs one associates with older children and adults. Often, these children have already been identified and may be brought to the emergency department because the parents

TABLE 18–1 COMMONLY USED DRUGS FOR CPR IN INFANTS AND CHILDREN

Drug	Suggested dose	Remarks
(1) Atropine sulfate	0.01 mg./kg., I.V.	
(2) Calcium gluconate (10% solution)	0.1 to 0.2 ml./kg., I.V.	Give *slowly* and watch for bradycardia. Use with caution in digitalized children.
(3) Diphenylhydantoin (Dilantin)	2.0 to 5.0 mg./kg., I.V.	Give slowly.
(4) Epinephrine hydrochloride (Adrenalin)	0.1 ml./kg. of 1:10,000 dilution, I.V. Same, intracardiac.	Intracardiac route is used as a last resort, since coronary arteries may be damaged.[9] Note dilution.
(5) Isoproterenol hydrochloride (Isuprel)	1.0 to 5.0 mg./500 ml. of 5% dextrose/water, I.V. drip.	Titrate to desired effect.
(6) Levarterenol bitartrate (Levophed, norepinephrine)	0.1 to 1.0 μg./kg./minute, I.V. drip.	1.0 ml. of 0.2% solution diluted in 250 ml. of solution equals 4 μg/ml. Not to be used in endotoxic shock or in renal shutdown.
(7) Lidocaine, 2% (Xylocaine)	0.5 to 2.0 mg./kg., I.V.	Give slowly. Do not exceed 100 mg./hr. Excess amount may cause convulsions.
(8) Metaraminol bitartrate (Aramine)	0.3 to 2.0 mg./kg., I.V. drip.	Titrate to desired effect.
(9) Propranolol (Inderal)	0.1 to 0.2 mg./kg., I.V.	May repeat dose in 2 minutes, if necessary.
(10) Sodium bicarbonate	3.0 to 5.0 mEq./kg., I.V.	Repeat dose after pH obtained and base deficit calculated.

feel their baby has increasing distress and his pediatrician or cardiologist cannot be reached.

Early signs of heart failure in the infant are very subtle, mainly involving slight increases in respiration and pulse rates.[16] The vital signs taken during triage should be carefully compared with his baseline vitals on the hospital record. Clinical signs of late heart failure include an enlarged heart and liver, cyanosis (unless he has cyanotic heart disease) and rales, a late finding in infants but an early finding in older children and adults.

The important point is to be aware of the subtle changes in infants with heart disease so that they can be treated early and subsequent problems can be avoided.

Heart murmurs

Functional murmurs are very common in children and can be accentuated by fever and illness. When a murmur is found, reevaluation after the child recovers from his illness is in order.

Parents are often distressed when a murmur

is discovered. They need reassurance that it does not mean their child has a cardiac problem, as well as encouragement to bring the child back for reevaluation when he is well.

Respiratory emergencies

The emergency situation of near-drowning is discussed above and in Chapter 13. Respiratory obstruction is not unusual in children, known for experimenting with strange objects through their mouths. Airway obstruction from foreign objects is discussed in Chapter 26. The conditions of croup, epiglottitis, asthma and pneumonia are also frequently occurring respiratory emergencies in children.

Respiratory embarrassment

Assessment for respiratory embarrassment must be done early and carefully. The child who is sedated, poisoned, neuromuscularly impaired, acutely ill or tired may show few signs of respiratory obstruction. He may very quietly hypoventilate to hypoxemia and, possibly, to death. A shortened inspiratory phase and decreased breath sounds are significant findings, requiring early intervention. If diagnosis is unsure, the child should be reevaluated by someone experienced in pediatric assessment.

The otherwise healthy child with airway obstruction is usually restless and agitated and may show observable signs, such as retraction of accessory muscles of respiration, flaring of the lower rib margins (especially in infants), nasal flaring, grunting, tracheal tug * and the "rocking boat" † effect.[6, 16] Cyanosis is a late sign.

Stridor may occur with respirations due to upper airway obstruction between the nares and mid-trachea. In lower airway obstruction, occurring below the level of the bronchi, respirations may be very noisy, or they may be absent in areas where no ventilation oc-

curs. Grunting and nasal flaring in infants with lower airway obstruction indicates significant respiratory distress.

Croup

Laryngotracheobronchitis (croup) is an infection of the upper airway caused by several respiratory viruses and occurring in children aged 6 months to 4 years. The infection produces edema of the subglottic area, resulting in hoarseness, inspiratory whoop and a high-pitched cough ("seal bark"). As the edema increases, signs of airway obstruction (outlined earlier) begin to appear.

Treatment includes administration of steam, hydration when necessary, periodic assessment of the airway with the necessary equipment available (an appropriate size endotracheal tube and laryngoscope) and administration of corticosteroids and/or antibiotics, as deemed necessary. Children with croup should be made comfortable and kept as quiet as possible, but they should not receive sedation, which may cause respiratory depression and further compromise their respiratory status.

Epiglottitis

Children with epiglottitis may show some signs distinguishing it from "croup." Generally, these children are older (over 4 years of age); they have extreme pain on swallowing and thus drool; and they appear more toxic and feverish. Extreme care must be taken when viewing the oropharynx, since the swollen, inflamed epiglottis may suddenly obstruct the airway. Be prepared to provide an airway at any time; more than one half the children with epiglottitis require intubation or tracheostomy.[5]

Treatment consists of hydration, ampicillin, 100 mg./kg./day, chloramphenicol ‡ (Chloromycetin) 50 to 100 mg./kg./day and

---

* "Tracheal tug": The trachea descends toward the sternal notch on inspiration.

† "Rocking boat effect": The sternum retracts, and the abdomen enlarges during inspiration.

‡ Chloramphenicol is recommended for initial antibiotic coverage, pending results of culture and sensitivity tests. Strains of *H. influenzae* are developing resistance to ampicillin.

cold steam for comfort. Epiglottitis occurs much less frequently than does croup, but because the consequences can be so serious, it always deserves consideration in children with croup symptoms.

Asthma

Status asthmaticus occurs when the patient does not respond to appropriate doses of the usual asthma medication. Respiratory distress is produced by bronchoconstriction, edema and dry, sticky mucous plugs. In the young child whose chest wall is soft and pliable, bronchial obstruction may occur from the increased intrathoracic pressure that occurs with forceful expiration. Hypoxemia, hypercapnia, acidosis and dehydration are present to varying degrees. Useful indicators of the severity of the attack are the amount of aeration (not loudness of wheezes), the pulse rate and the child's appearance.

Treatment is determined by the individual child's physiological and biochemical status and may include humidified oxygen for hypoxemia, intravenous fluids for dehydration and loosening of mucous plugs and drug therapy. Taking a careful history of the child's current drug regimen and drug allergies is extremely important before administering any drug to an asthmatic individual. Some medications, especially penicillin and aspirin are potential inducers of shock in the asthmatic individual. The following drugs may be indicated:

(1) Epinephrine hydrochloride, 0.01 ml./ kg. of 1:1000 solution with a maximum total dose of 0.3 to 0.5 ml., subcutaneously.

(2) Isoproterenol hydrochloride (Isuprel) (1:200), or isoetharine (Bronchosol) 0.25 to 0.5 ml., diluted to 4 ml. with saline and given by inhalation treatment. This may be repeated in 4 hours. (Watch for cardiac or central nervous system stimulation, indicating overdosage.)

(3) Aminophylline, 3 to 4 mg./kg., in a 10 to 15 minute intravenous infusion. (The dosage may be repeated every 6

to 8 hours, but it should not exceed 12 mg./kg. in a 24-hour period, and it should not be given within 3 hours of Isuprel or Bronchosol. Watch for arrythmias and hypotension; monitor the pulse and blood pressure every 5 minutes during administration.)

Other drugs which may be indicated include corticosteroids, alkalizing agents, antibiotics and a mild sedative that will not produce respiratory depression.

After the attack has subsided and the child is stabilized, the nurse may help by working out a plan with the patient and parents for control and prevention of recurrent attacks. Identifying trigger factors, early signs and symptoms and primary methods of control is necessary. Throughout the treatment period, a calm, reassuring approach by all staff personnel is important.

Pneumonia

Pneumonia is a common problem in infants and children. As it is an example of a lower respiratory tract infection leading to obstruction, the clinical picture of pneumonia is as outlined previously. However, prior to the developing signs of lower respiratory distress, the child may present with only a fever of unknown origin; all chest findings, including x-ray, may be negative. Another early finding in the absence of respiratory symptoms may be abdominal pain, suggesting appendicitis. On examination, however, the abdomen is distended, and bowel sounds are diminished or absent, indicating an ileus secondary to the pneumonia.

In the infant, interpreting auscultation is difficult, since rales may be minimal; x-ray is invariably needed to establish the diagnosis. Respiratory grunting and nasal flaring in the infant indicates severe lower respiratory distress.

Many children with pneumonia can be treated at home if proper follow-up is available. Others are obvious candidates for admission: the child with cyanosis or severe respiratory distress, the child with pleural effusion or the child with secondary cardiac failure. The sick infant (under one year) with pneumonia may need admission until the diagnosis of staphylococcal pneumonia is excluded.

Neurological emergencies

Neurological assessment is an important aspect of the total assessment of infants and children. Much information regarding neurological status can be gathered by the nurse through making selective observations and comparing them with the known growth and development patterns for the age of the child being evaluated.

Infants

The nurse observes the infant simply by watching and holding him. She thus determines if he is alert, sleepy, fussy and whether these patterns alternate. Other observations include: good muscle tone vs. limpness and reflexes appropriate to age, such as the Moro, sucking and palmar grasp reflexes.

Deviations from the norm are important to note. Any illness can affect neurological findings, since infants respond so globally to bodily stress.

Children

In addition to the observations mentioned above, the nurse can also gather information by talking with the child or by watching the communication process between parents and the child. Thus, information about mental status, speech and perception of symptoms can be gained.

Knowledge of sophisticated techniques is not essential for a general, fairly complete neurological evaluation; rather, a practiced, keen eye and knowledge of normal growth and development patterns are the most important tools for initial evaluation.

Meningitis

Meningitis is an inflammation of the meninges, usually due to an infectious agent. The high mortality rate is related to the ease with which the infection spreads to the central nervous system tissues and to the cerebral edema which accompanies the inflammatory reaction.

Manifestations of meningitis in the very young infant may be masked, so assessment is difficult. Generally, signs in the infant may include lethargy, irritability, a high-pitched cry, a bulging fontanelle, vomiting and feeding problems or exaggerated head lag.

The child may have more specific neurological findings indicating meningeal irritation, such as positive Kernig's * and Brudzinski's † signs. In addition, he may be irritable and lethargic; have projectile vomiting, a petechial or purpuric rash; and complain of a stiff neck and severe headache. An unexplained convulsion associated with signs of infection, such as fever, must be carefully investigated to rule out meningitis.

Early, vigorous therapy is necessary, not only for treatment of the meningitis but for avoidance of life-threatening sequelae, which may also occur early in the course of the disease. These complications include septic shock, disseminated intravascular coagulation and cerebral edema, which may lead to herniation of the medulla. Assessment and treatment of these conditions are discussed in Chapters 9, 15 and 24.

Emergency department management prior to hospital admission will generally include these procedures:

(1) Obtaining specimens: cerebral spinal fluid from lumbar puncture, blood culture, throat culture, complete blood count and serum electrolytes.
(2) Starting an intravenous infusion.
(3) Administering appropriate antibiotic therapy.

---

* A positive Kernig's sign is elicited when, sitting or lying with the thigh flexed upon the abdomen, the patient is unable to completely extend his leg.

† A positive Brudzinski's sign can be elicited by 2 maneuvers: (1) flexing the neck forward results in flexion of the ankle, knee and hip, and (2) passive flexion of the lower limb on one side produces a similar movement of the opposite limb.

(4) Continuing monitoring of vital life functions and managing them as appropriate.

If the meningitis is presumed to be meningococcal in origin, the child will be placed in isolation for the first 24 hours. However, very close monitoring is essential during this time, since most of the feared sequelae develop early in the course of the disease.[5] Isolation procedures should never interfere with close observation.

Head trauma

Children, having proportionately large heads and being active and fearless, suffer their full share of head trauma. Assessment and treatment of head injury are discussed in Chapter 24.

Frequently, a parent will call the emergency department for advice as to whether he should have the child checked. It is best to advise the parents to bring the child in for evaluation, even though the injury may seem minor and signs and symptoms are minimal (nausea, vomiting, irritability and somnolence are frequent after head injury).[8] The visit will provide baseline information for subsequent evaluation and an opportunity for parent teaching.

The parent must understand the importance of periodic evaluation, what observations should be made and the need for immediate return should any develop. Instruction sheets are commonly used by emergency department personnel to reinforce this teaching when children are to be observed at home. (See Appendix E, at the end of this chapter, for an example of such an instruction sheet.)

Fever

Fever is not usually considered a life-threatening emergency in itself, since body temperature rarely becomes elevated to the point of causing brain injury.[15] Nevertheless, fever is one of the signs most commonly prompting parents to bring their child to the emergency department for care.

Parents usually equate temperature elevation with severity of illness. Thus, a calm approach to the child with fever by the nurse is a helpful educational experience for parents who need to learn that it is not the fever but associated symptoms or changes in behavior that need observation to determine seriousness.

Causes of fever are numerous, but in children, by far the most common cause of fever is an infectious process: acute tonsillitis and pharyngitis, acute gastroenteritis, otitis media, upper and lower respiratory infections, among a legion of others. While determining the cause of fever is important, measures to lower it need not wait. Such measures include undressing, sponging with tepid water (*not* cold water or alcohol), encouraging fluids, if tolerated, and administering an antipyretic, if indicated.

Antipyretic agents

Acetaminophen (Tylenol, Liquiprin) and acetylsalicylic acid (aspirin) are commonly used to reduce fever. In infants and young children, Tylenol is preferable, since it produces fewer side effects and is available in liquid form. Aspirin and Tylenol may be used simultaneously, since the combination produces slightly improved and prolonged fever reduction.[15]

The dosage for Tylenol is 5 to 10 mg./kg. every 4 to 6 hours and for aspirin, 10 to 20 mg./kg. every 4 to 6 hours. Both preparations are available in suppository form, which is useful in reducing fever in the presence of gastrointestinal upset. However, absorption is not as accurate in suppository as in oral forms and, obviously, is lessened when increased peristalsis is present.

Aspirin is not recommended for infants under 6 months of age, as infants do not metabolize aspirin as efficiently as older children and thus can be more easily overdosed. Sponging is the preferred method for reducing fever in very young patients.

Seizures

Febrile seizures most frequently occur within the first 12 to 24 hours of the fever—an important point to stress to parents, so they need not remain apprehensive through the course of the child's illness. These seizures appear as grand mal seizures, occur most frequently between the ages of 6 months to 3 years and essentially produce no sequelae.

Treatment consists of reducing the fever through sponging and administering antipyretics, determining the cause of the fever and considering the use of an anticonvulsant (usually phenobarbital, 2 to 3 mg./kg.) with the onset of fever.

Seizures in a child who has never had a seizure before is a terrifying experience for parents. Calm reassurance and instruction from the nurse regarding the therapeutic plan and preventive measures (including what to do if a seizure occurs again) are very helpful and supportive.

Dehydration

Dehydration must be assessed whenever fever or gastrointestinal fluid losses are present or whenever the child has a limited dietary intake for any reason. The nurse should observe for poor skin turgor; a sunken appearance to the eyes, with a lack of tears when crying; dry mucous membranes; and, in the infant, a depressed fontanelle.

Signs indicating severe dehydration include oliguria, tachycardia, hypotension and features of hypovolemic shock (see Chapter 9). Treatment is directed at correcting the cause for dehydration and replacing fluid and electrolyte losses by oral (if tolerated) or intravenous solutions.

Vomiting

Vomiting is a common cause of dehydration in children, especially in infants. While most episodes of vomiting are caused by an acute, nonspecific gastroenteritis, this cannot be assumed, since vomiting is a common response to systemic illness.

When the problem is identified as a nonspecific gastroenteritis, the safest and best treatment is dietary: using small amounts of clear liquids for 24 hours, with gradual progression of diet. Antiemetic drugs in sup-

pository or parenteral form may be indicated when vomiting is severe or does not respond to dietary therapy.

The aim is to prevent distention of the stomach through small, frequent and easily digested feedings and also to prevent dehydration and carbohydrate and electrolyte losses. Since vomitus is high in potassium, replacing this cation with defizzed cola and clear fruit juices is favored.

Diarrhea

As with vomiting, diarrhea is a sign that an underlying problem exists and must be identified. When the specific types of diarrhea have been ruled out and nonspecific diarrhea is the diagnosis, treatment is dietary, with selective use of antidiarrheal agents containing kaolin and pectin, such as Kaopectate. Occasionally, an antidiarrheal agent containing an antispasmotic, such as atropine (Donnagel), is useful for relief of crampy, abdominal pain.

Parents benefit from instructions regarding indications that the child's condition may be worsening and regarding appropriate foods to offer the child. Written instructions (see Appendix E) are especially helpful.

THE ABUSED CHILD

Child abuse, or the "battered child syndrome," describes the nonaccidental or deliberate physical attack on or injury of infants and children. Child neglect and deprivation is another form of child abuse, in which there is a failure to provide adequate materials (shelter, food) necessary for the child's health or a failure to nurture the child's sense of self. Both abuse and neglect demand early intervention to prevent further injury to the child and to help the abusive adult. The incidence of child abuse cannot be determined accurately, but every active emergency department encounters it.

The importance of recognizing the abused child lies in the fact that it tends to be repetitive, with each attack more savage than the one before. Many children who die or require hospitalization because of battering injuries have been treated previously, sometimes repeatedly, in an emergency department or a physician's office, for minor to moderate soft tissue injuries or fractures, which were assumed to have resulted from accidents.[14] Had the true nature of the injury been recognized at an early stage, the cycle might have been interrupted before more serious, perhaps lethal, injury occurred.

Intentional physical injury, the "battered child syndrome," is part of a spectrum of child abuse that includes intentional poisoning; physical, nutritional and emotional neglect; and all sorts of specific willful deprivation.[10] A significant proportion of children with inflicted injuries show evidence of nutritional and/or hygienic neglect, such as anemia, skin rashes or "failure to thrive." Most, but not all, of the victims are between 6 months and 2 years of age. Injuries usually occur in the home, and the perpetrator is usually a parent, most often the mother. Less frequently, siblings and babysitters are responsible.

Characteristics of abusers and the abused

Child abuse is not related to social class, income or level of education. Abusive persons have other commonalities: a lack of early mothering, themselves; feelings of worthlessness about themselves or the child; resentment or rejection of the child; expecting the child to satisfy personal or parental needs through behavior beyond that appropriate to the child's age; and a need to discipline sternly and authoritatively.

Certain reactions and attitudes of neglecting or abusive adults are also fairly characteristic. An awareness of these will guide the nurse's observations to identify the individuals who need help. Some of these characteristics are that the abusive adult:

(1) Evidences immature behavior and is preoccupied with himself.
(2) Has little perception of how a child could feel, physically or emotionally.
(3) Is critical of the child and has unrealistic expectations of him.
(4) Seldom touches or looks at the child or becomes involved in his care.
(5) Is unconcerned about the child's injury, treatment, prognosis.
(6) Gives no indication of feeling guilt or remorse regarding the child's condition; rather, may blame the child or be angry with him for becoming injured.
(7) Is concerned more about what will happen to himself and others involved in the child's injury than about the child's welfare.
(8) Often disappears from the hospital during examination or shortly after the child's admission.
(9) Asks to have the child home only when interrogation has frightened him.

Occasionally, the potentially abusive adult (usually a parent) may actively seek help, fearful that he is losing self-control and may hurt his child. Several emergency department visits within a 24-hour period may indicate a plea for help. Or, the emergency department staff may notice the parent who brings his/her child often for inconsequential symptoms. Coupled with any of the characteristics of a child abuser listed above, this behavior may suggest that the parent is becoming unable to handle an impending crisis situation.

In response to the abusive adult's behavior, the child learns to respond in ways that are also characteristic; he:

(1) Cries hopelessly during treatment or examination without any real expectation of being comforted, or he cries very little, in general.
(2) Does not look to parent (if abuser) for assurance or may actively avoid parent.
(3) Is wary of physical contact initiated by abusive parent or others.

(4) Is apprehensive when other children cry and watches them with curiosity, especially when approached by another adult.

(5) Appears constantly on the alert for danger.

(6) May constantly seek favors, food, things, services.

Early recognition of these behaviors in adults and children may be helpful to averting a crisis situation for both later.

History

The history, if taken from the abusive parent or adult, is difficult to obtain; little information is volunteered, and what is given is evasive and contradictory. Usually the history does not include a statement of abuse. If questions relative to this possibility are asked, they are generally denied.

The history of the mode of injury is often vague and may be changed if the first version does not appear to satisfy the inquirer. Often, the severity of the injury seems out of proportion to the type of accident that is said to have occurred, or the story may account for some but not all of the findings.

The most likely candidate for abuse is the infant or small child who cannot talk, who has been injured in his own home and whose wounds do not seem to fit the description of the accident. Illegitimacy, abandonment or divorce predispose to child abuse; but in at least one series, alcohol or hard drug usage was rarely a prominent factor.[14] Presumably, the abuse arises from otherwise unrelieved frustrations similar to, but more nagging and less manageable than, those felt on occasion by every parent.

It must be remembered that accidental injuries are very common in children, and health professionals lose much of their value if they become cynical and overly suspicious in dealing with parents, most of whom are struggling to deal with their own feelings of guilt over having allowed the injury to occur. When an accident is the cause of injury, the description of the incident is usually volunteered as a forthright and consistent story, which accounts in a reasonable manner for the injury which has resulted.

If the child is old enough to contribute his version of the way in which he was injured, he has lived through the age range when abuse is most frequent, but he is by no means immune. If his story is volunteered without hesitation and matches that given by a parent, child abuse is very unlikely. If he is hesitant and evasive or remains silent and terrified, the examiner may be justly suspicious.

Not all children in this latter category have been abused, however. Many simply feel guilty in the belief that wrongdoing on their part caused the accident. The older child who has been abused is particularly fearful that the parent will blame him for allowing the abuse to come to light and retaliate with further brutality. For this reason, great sympathy and tact are required to induce a child to reveal the true nature of the circumstances leading to his injury.

Physical assessment

The abused child may present with varying signs and symptoms, from the very obvious to the very subtle. The interpersonal interaction between parent and child is important to observe, as well as the physical injury.

The most common sites of physical trauma include injuries to soft tissues, bones, head and abdomen.

Soft tissue injuries

The most common injuries of early abuse are soft tissue wounds, such as multiple bruises and ecchymoses, burns such as those resulting from contact with cigarettes or other hot objects, scalds and lacerations, all of which may present in different stages of healing. Sometimes, the pattern of ecchymoses or burns suggests the shape of the instrument with which the child was attacked.

Fractures

The second most commonly inflicted injuries are fractures, and x-rays make these the easiest to document.[3, 17] Their presence may be suspected by unexplained soft tissue swelling; the child may not be aware of any problem. It is surprising how little discomfort healing fractures seem to produce in young children.

Twisting injuries result in spiral fractures of the humerus or femur or in the elevation of the periosteum by a subperiosteal hematoma, which heals with more than normal callus formation. Jerking injuries result in epiphyseal separation, with callus formation at the junction of the shaft and growth center of the bone. Rib fractures result from forceful blows or from crushing injuries.

Often, the fractures are multiple, some recent and some partially or completely healed, suggesting repetition of abuse. In the absence of metabolic bone disease, x-ray findings of multiple fractures of the long bones or ribs in varying stages of healing is pathognomonic for child abuse.

Head Injuries

Head injuries produce the highest mortality and result in the greatest amount of permanent disability.[1] Head injuries include scalp wounds, skull fractures, subdural or subgaleal hematomas and repeated concussions.

The progression of abuse appears to be from the trunk and extremities toward the head as the major target of injury, and most children with severe head injuries show evidence of earlier peripheral injuries.

Abdominal Injuries

Abdominal injuries constitute a small but serious part of the abuse syndrome. Rupture of the liver and blunt injuries to the intestine and mesentery are potentially lethal, especially if there is delay in diagnosis of an abdominal injury. A mortality of 50 percent has been reported for abdominal injuries resulting from child abuse.[12, 20]

Children who show evidence of neglect, multiple bruises or other soft tissue injuries and who complain of abdominal distress should be carefully evaluated with the possibility of abdominal injury in mind.

Management

Treatment begins with recognition that a child has possibly been abused. The nurse should inspect every child's body for evidence of injury that is more extensive or in locations other than the normal bumps and bruises a child of that age would sustain. The nurse should also always note the child/parent interactions. When these observations suggest abuse, they should be discussed with the physician and recorded on the patient's record succinctly, objectively and completely.

While the nurse need not be overly suspicious in the treatment of children with trauma, she should not deny the possibility of battering and place the child in jeopardy by sending him home. If there is any doubt, the child should be hospitalized (at that time, not sent home first) and fully evaluated medically.

Most emergency departments have protocols which guide their personnel in the handling of suspected child abuse cases. (One such protocol for a hospital in Ohio is detailed in Appendix F, at the end of this chapter.) Further, every state and territory provides a mechanism for the reporting and investigating of real and suspected child abuse cases. It is suggested that the emergency nurse familiarize herself with her hospital protocol and state reporting laws regarding suspected abuse.

In addition to careful evaluation and protection of the child, the long-term treatment plan includes counseling of the abusive parent with the ultimate goal of providing a safe environment at home for the child. The abusive adult must be helped to realize that frustration and resentment of infants and children are natural and universal and that these feelings can and must be dealt with in an appropriate manner.

If such feelings are feared, repressed and unrelieved, they are bound to surface again, sooner or later, and may result in more vicious child abuse or other socially unacceptable behavior. Punitive action against the abuser is rarely indicated. Usually the child need not be permanently removed from the home, though often a separation is needed. The child needs protection; the parent or adult needs help and counseling.[7]

An interdisciplinary team approach to treatment is desirable, recognizing that many factors contribute to child abuse and must be resolved. Treatment must be ongoing and comprehensive, and the child must be protected until his safety in the home is assured.

SUMMARY

While children may have illnesses and injuries similar to those of adults, they are not "little adults." Their responses to their health problems can be quite individual and unique and, often, unpredictable. This is especially true of the young infant from birth to 6 months of age. Careful observation of the child, attention to the parent's accounting of his behavior, knowledge of growth and development patterns are all helpful in caring for children.

The nurse can be influential in making the child's emergency department experience a positive one; often children have fearful, imagined perceptions of what will happen to them when they go to a hospital. Communicating with the child on his level and determining the meaning of the hospital experience to him may be useful in resolving his fears and reducing his anxieties.

Care of a child includes care of his family. This may take many forms, depending on child and family needs and on the nature of the care setting. Crisis assessment and intervention, patient and parent teaching, health screening and referral may all be indicated.

Implementation of the therapeutic plan requires the use of equipment and medications appropriate for the size of the infant or child. Some treatment procedures are nearly impossible without appropriately sized equipment. Since emergencies do not permit time to acquire such equipment, it should be ready at all times in the emergency department for immediate use.

The calculations of dosages appropriate for the child's weight is a special challenge to the nurse accustomed to administering medications to adults. It is always advisable to have calculations double-checked, to avoid lethal errors, and to have emergency medications available in sizes which are easily adaptable for pediatric use.

Child abuse is a special form of pediatric emergency. While much of emergency department nursing is practiced in the "caring" and "curing," of patients, with child abuse the third aspect of nursing is most important— that of "preventing." Assessing injuries and behaviors which point to abuse and identifying and reporting them can activate the mechanism for protecting the child and rehabilitating the abusive adult.

BIBLIOGRAPHY

(1) Baron, M.; Bejar, R., and Sheaff, P.: "Neurologic Manifestations of the Battered Child Syndrome," *Pediatrics,* 45 (1970):1003.

(2) Bellack, J.: "Helping a Child Cope with the Stress of Injury," *American Journal of Nursing,* 74 (1974):1491.

(3) Caffey, J.: "Multiple Fractures in the Long Bones of Infants Suffering from Chronic Subdural Hematoma," *American Journal of Roentgenology,* 56 (1946):167.

(4) "CPR with a Delicate Touch," *Emergency Medicine,* 5 (1973):80.

(5) Grossman, M.: "Upper Airway Infection," *in* D. Pascoe and M. Grossman (eds.), *Quick Reference to Pediatric Emergencies* (Philadelphia: J. B. Lippincott Company, 1973).

(6) Guy, E.: "Airway Obstruction," *in* D. Pascoe and M. Grossman (eds.), *Quick*

Reference to Pediatric Emergencies (Philadelphia: J. B. Lippincott Company, 1973).

(7) Helfer, R., and Kempe, C.: "The Child's Need for Early Recognition, Immediate Care and Protection," *in* R. Helfer and C. Kempe (eds.), *Helping the Battered Child and His Family* (Philadelphia: J. B. Lippincott Company, 1972).

(8) Hoff, J., and Wilson, C.: "Head Injury," *in* D. Pascoe and M. Grossman (eds.), *Quick Reference to Pediatric Emergencies* (Philadelphia: J. B. Lippincott Company, 1973).

(9) Hoffman, J., and Gregory, G.: "Cardiopulmonary Arrest," *in* D. Pascoe and M. Grossman (eds.), *Quick Reference to Pediatric Emergencies* (Philadelphia: J. B. Lippincott Company, 1973).

(10) Kempe, C.; Silverman, F.; Steele, B.; Droegemueller, W., and Silver, H.: "The Battered Child Syndrome," *Journal of the American Medical Association,* 181 (1962):1.

(11) Luciano, K., and Shumsky, C.: "Pediatric Procedures," *Nursing '75,* 5 (1975):49.

(12) McCort, J., and Vaudagna, J.: "Visceral Injuries in Battered Children," *Radiology,* 82 (1964):424.

(13) McFarland, J.: "Pediatric Assessment and Intervention," *Nursing '74,* 4 (1974): 66.

(14) O'Neill, J., Jr.; Meacham, W.; Griffin, P., and Sawyers, J.: "Patterns of Injury in the Battered Child Syndrome," *Journal of Trauma,* 13 (1973):332.

(15) Pascoe, D.: "Fever," *in* D. Pascoe and M. Grossman (eds.), *Quick Reference to Pediatric Emergencies* (Philadelphia: J. B. Lippincott Company, 1973).

(16) Posey, R.: "Creative Nursing Care of Babies with Heart Disease," *Nursing '74,* 4 (1974):40.

(17) Silverman, R.: "The Roentgen Manifestations of Unrecognized Skeletal Trauma in Infants," *American Journal of Roentgenology,* 69 (1953):413.

(18) "Standards for Cardiopulmonary Resuscitation and Emergency Cardiac Care," *Supplement to the Journal of the American Medical Association,* 227 (1974): 837.

(19) "Tips on Leading a Rescue Party," *Emergency Medicine,* 6 (1974):27.

(20) Touloukian, R.: "Abdominal Visceral Injuries in Battered Children," *Pediatrics,* 42 (1968):642.

(21) Ungvarski, P.; Argondizzo, N., and Boos, P.: "CPR, Current Practice Revised," *American Journal of Nursing,* 75 (1975):236.

APPENDIX E

Instructions to parents

Diarrhea and/or vomiting

Your child has been seen in the Children's Hospital Emergency Department because of diarrhea and/or vomiting. It is important that your child does not lose too much water and become dried out (dehydrated). Watch for the following signs of illness or dehydration, and call the Emergency Department or your physician if they occur:

(1) Decreased frequency of urination, with dark, strong urine.
(2) Loss of weight. (More than __ ounces.)
(3) Dry and sticky tongue.
(4) Marked listlessness.
(5) Persistent fever.

CALL BACK IF THE VOMITING OR DIARRHEA LASTS MORE THAN 24 HOURS OR BECOMES MUCH WORSE.

Liquids should be given in small amounts, one half ounce at a time. The clear liquid diet suggested includes:

(1) Water.
(2) Sugar water (one tablespoon of sugar to 8 ounces of water).
(3) Tea.
(4) Kool-Aid.
(5) Jello and Jello water.
(6) Ice popsicles.
(7) Flat soda pop (ginger ale, clear sodas or colas).
(8) Broth soup.

AVOID FEEDING MILK, ORANGE JUICE OR SOLID FOODS AS LONG AS THE CHILD CONTINUES TO HAVE DIARRHEA AND/OR VOMITING.

Telephone: _____.

Head injury

Your child has recently been seen in the Children's Hospital Emergency Department because of a head injury. Although we do not feel admission to the hospital is necessary at this time, there are several things which we would request you do at home.

It is important that the child be observed closely for the next 24 hours. Call the Emergency Department or consult your family doctor immediately for any of the following:

(1) Loss of consciousness.
(2) Increasing sleepiness or variations from normal personality or behavior. (The child should be aroused several times during the night and asked to identify familiar persons or toys, etc.)
(3) Persistent vomiting, headache, or stiff neck.
(4) Persistent nosebleed or drainage of fluid from the nose or ear.
(5) Convulsion.
(6) Fever.

Further instructions: _____.
Telephone: _____.

Source: Both instruction sheets adapted from material from Children's Hospital, Columbus, Ohio.

APPENDIX F

Protocol concerning the battered and neglected child at the Children's Hospital, Columbus, Ohio

The question of child abuse is a complex and highly emotional issue. Under the statutes of the State of Ohio, *anyone* suspecting child abuse has the *duty* to report it to the authorities.* The purpose of this protocol is not to evaluate the issues—

* Ohio Revised Code, section 2515.421 (amended).

rather, to provide a mechanism by which possible abuse may be adequately evaluated without endangering the welfare of the child.

Experience at Children's Hospital indicates that a team approach is in the best interest of the child.* Generally, this team consists of a physician, nurse, and social worker, although a psychiatrist may be consulted in many cases. It is imperative that the team concept be initiated at the time any suspected abuse is reported. Consistent communication will ensure the most appropriate disposition in most cases.

In order to help you handle this difficult situation, a few concepts may be helpful.

(1) Understandably, most people are outraged and angry when dealing with a child who has been mistreated. But remember—emotionally charged statements, notes, etc., can never replace accurate documentation of the facts. Try to maintain your composure.

(2) If there is any indication of ongoing harm to a child, either physical or emotional, the most prudent course is to place the child in a controlled environment, i.e., the hospital. If you are in doubt about this, SEEK HELP. There is no reason for one person to assume total responsibility for the disposition. An admitting diagnosis of "unrecognized trauma" is succinct, acceptable, and non-judgmental.

(3) Only the courts may take the responsibility of making an ultimate disposition of a child. To do this, accurate and unbiased data is required. The etiology of physical or mental abnormalities is frequently a matter of much debate. Careful description and documentation may resolve the issue. A statement of causality is an opinion and should be recorded as such, preferably in the form of a quote, giving the identity of the person(s) making such a statement. Whenever possible, a *carefully labeled* photograph should be obtained as permanent documentation. (Permission for photography is advisable but not mandatory in cases of suspected abuse. The decision to obtain photographs against parental wishes should be made by more than one person and noted in the record.)

(4) If we are to err, let us do so on the side of over-documentation. If a fact is not in the permanent record, it does not exist.

The remainder of this protocol deals with the mechanics of handling children who are suspected of being abused.

The battered or neglected child

Bear in mind that the signs of the battered child may be physical, emotional, or both. An excellent review of these signs may be found in the references.†,‡ When the decision is made to report suspected child abuse the following steps are taken:

(1) A "Confidential Report of Suspected Physical Abuse or Neglect" form is filled out. This is done by a physician, but a nurse, social worker, parent, neighbor,

---

* Eaton, A. P.; Vastbinder, E.: The Sexually Molested Child, *Clinical Pediatrics,* 8:8, pp. 438–441 (1969).
† Helfer, R. E.; Kempe, C. H., eds.: *The Battered Child* (Chicago: University of Chicago Press, 1968).
‡ Helfer, R. E.; Kempe, C. H., eds.: *Helping the Battered Child and His Family* (Philadelphia: J. B. Lippincott Company, 1972).

etc., may initiate the report. A single copy is made initially and electrostatic copies (xerox) made for duplicate and triplicate. This will be done by social service.

Fill out the report as completely and accurately as possible. Physical abnormalities may be outlined with the notation, "complete description in physician's examination." If the cause is unknown state "unknown at present time."

(2) A consult form is filled out from the physician to social service. Social service is *immediately* notified by the physician via phone or in person. As a rule, social service will interview the family immediately if called between 8:00 A.M. and 10:00 P.M. During other hours, the social worker on call must be notified (via hospital operator) and the time of interview will be arranged. A *primary disposition* for the child will be *arranged jointly*. Usually, this will be a matter of admitting vs. placement in a temporary home. *Only under unusual and infrequent circumstances should a child be sent home.*

(3) A meticulous physical exam should be done, carefully documenting any abnormalities (size, color, consistency) with photographs if possible. If the child is to be admitted this may be done by the house officer who works up the child. No conclusions are to be drawn from the findings!

(4) Occasionally, suspicion of child abuse may not arise until a child has already been hospitalized. Should this happen, the confidential forms are to be filled out and social service is notified immediately.

(5) Social service is responsible for coordinating the disposition for each child. This may necessitate liaison with the Public Health Nurses, other Social Services, the Police, etc. The physician is responsible for notifying social service of any changes in the child's condition, and will give advance notice when the child is medically ready for discharge.

Checklist

The physician must:

(1) Fill out "Confidential Report."
(2) Immediately notify and initiate a written consultation to Social Service.
(3) Perform a meticulous physical examination of the patient.
(4) Consummate hospital admission when indicated.

Social service must:

(1) Interview the family immediately (8:00 A.M. to 10:00 P.M.) or arrange for interview (10:00 P.M. to 8:00 A.M.).
(2) Make additional copies of the "Confidential Report."
(3) Arrange jointly with the physician and coordinate the disposition of the patient.

19

Thoracic and abdominal injuries

PAUL A. KENNEDY
GORDON F. MADDING

THORACIC INJURIES

In 1971, according to the National Safety Council, trauma caused 114,000 deaths and an additional 50,000,000 injuries in the United States. Of this number, a high percentage of the major factors contributing to death were chest injuries, and in an additional large number, chest injuries were an added factor. In many instances, death was inevitable due to the extent of the injury. In some cases, however, death resulted from inadequate treatment or from delays and errors in treatment. Since chest trauma produces urgent and profound disturbances of cardiopulmonary function, every physician and nurse caring for patients with chest injuries should have a routine protocol to follow.

A patient who has received a severe chest injury should not be considered to be "doing well" until the following criteria, suggested by Scannell,[23] have been met.

(1) Resuscitation is taken to the point that significant hypotension and hypoxia have been relieved.
(2) Bleeding is identified and controlled.
(3) Severe pain is relieved.
(4) Stability of the chest wall is established so that effective cough and ventilation are possible, as well as establishment of a clear airway.
(5) Pleural cavities are free of any significant blood and air, and the possibility of continuing or recurring pneumothorax is cared for with as complete expansion as possible of both lungs.
(6) Recognition is taken of any associated visceral injury.
(7) Care of any major external wounds is completed.

Diagnosis and treatment go hand-in-hand while an estimate of the situation is being made. Immediate attention to establishing a clear airway is the first essential. Improved position, aspiration of oral and pharyngeal secretions and the use of an oropharyngeal airway may be all that is required. A cuffed endotracheal tube, however, will be frequently necessary, and when an airway is required for a longer period of time, a tracheostomy will be indicated. A poor airway may result directly from the injury itself or from aspiration of vomitus or blood and will contribute in either event to hypotension and hypoxia. Careful inspection of the chest with frequent examination of respiratory activity and recording of

276

the details is essential to good orderly care. In urgent circumstances, immediate needle aspiration will give evidence of a tension pneumothorax and may precipitate the proper course of treatment. Arterial blood gas studies will rapidly reveal the extent of compromise of respiration.

During this early period, in which "an estimate of the situation" is being made, 100 percent oxygen is given by nasal catheter. Once the immediate, emergent problems are cared for, a more detailed complete examination can be carried out, at which time careful x-rays of the chest and abdomen can be made. Depending on the extent of the injury, all parameters should be monitored, including central venous pressure, hourly urines, electrocardiogram and blood gas studies.

Normal and abnormal respiration

The primary object of respiration is to supply the alveolar air, and consequently to supply the blood and tissues with oxygen and to eliminate carbon dioxide. A clear knowledge of the normal mechanisms of respiration is essential to understanding the influence of the untoward effects of trauma.

Generally speaking, respiration is referred to as "external" (the mass movement of gases in and out of the lungs to the arterial blood) and "internal" (the gas exchange at the arteriolocapillary level and the gas utilization at the tissue level). There is an exchange of gases between the atmosphere and the alveoli because of a pressure gradient that exists between the outside atmosphere and that within the lungs. With inspiratory effort, air flows from the atmosphere to the alveoli. Contraction of the muscles of the chest wall, together with rib elevation and the flattening (descent) of the diaphragm, results in an increased amount of alveolar gas, with a lowering of its pressure. This allows the flow of air into the lungs. For the most part, expiration is a passive action which results because of the natural recoil of the lungs.

Normal airway resistance is determined by the cross-section area of the air passages and

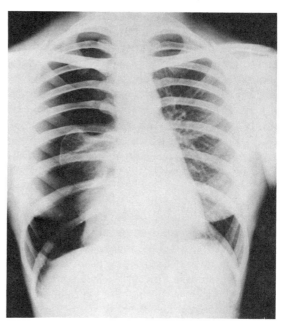

Figure 19-1 Pneumothorax. Total collapse of right lung is shown. Note the mediastinal structures shifted to the left. Patient was treated by intercostal tube drainage (closed thoracostomy), with full reexpansion.

the rate of air flow through them. Trauma by various mechanisms can interfere with exchange of atmospheric and alveolar gas and with internal respiration as well. For example, pain attendant to a simple fractured rib can limit chest wall movement and, therefore, influence ventilation unduly. Multiple fractures of ribs, producing a flail chest, can interfere greatly with exchange, depending on the extent of the paradoxical motion. Pneumothorax and tension pneumothorax may be major factors in compromising ventilation (see Figure 19-1). Injuries to the lung itself, resulting in hematomas and extensive contusions, may interfere with airflow and alveolar exchange.

Fractured ribs

The most common injury to the chest due to blunt trauma is fracture of one rib or several ribs. On occasion, severe coughing may result in fracture of a rib with resultant pain. The pain may be intense, even excruciating, and aggravated by deep breathing or motion. It causes restriction of respiratory efforts and thus limits pulmonary exchange. Careful examination of the chest by palpation will usually localize the area of the fracture. Chest x-ray with particular attention to a rib study will confirm the diagnosis. Analgesics and simple support by a chest binder, or less frequently by actual adhesive strapping, may be all that is required.

The preferable method of treating a simple uncomplicated fracture, however, is by repeated intercostal blocks. Pain is relieved, and the patient can breathe and cough without difficulty. The block is done using 0.5 percent lidocaine (Xylocaine) at a point central or proximal to the fracture. Two interspaces above and below the involved rib should also be injected. It is advisable to have an upright chest x-ray done following intercostal nerve block to be sure no pneumothorax has occurred. As respiratory excursions increase following pain relief, it is not unusual to find a delayed pneumothorax.

Limitation of cough by severe pain may result in retention of secretions, with development of atelectasis. Further immobilization of the chest by support dressings will compound the problem. In this instance, relief of pain by intercostal block together with tracheal suction will reverse the harmful process.

Usually, a simple fracture of the rib is not associated with displacement. On occasion, however, there may be some displacement, and under such circumstances, a laceration of the visceral pleura may occur by a sharp spicule of bone. This may also occur in the instance described above following intercostal block. If this happens, some degree of pneumothorax may develop. There may be evidence of crepitus (subcutaneous emphysema, air in the tissues) at the fracture site, as well as signs of pneumothorax. Chest x-ray will confirm the presence of pneumothorax.

Tension pneumothorax may result from a small wound of the lung produced by a spicule of rib fracture. Air is lost into the pleural space through the wound on inspiration and is trapped. As the amount of intrapleural air increases, the lung collapses. As this tension increases further, the mediastinum shifts to the opposite side. (See Figure 19–1.) This results in complete loss of function of the

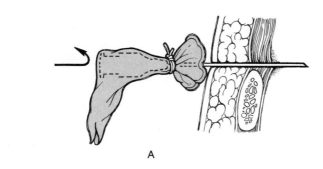

A

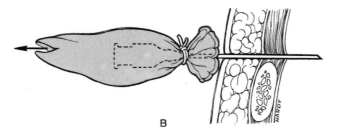

B

Figure 19–2 A simple device for emergency decompression of pneumothorax. A short bevel needle is inserted into an upper anterior intercostal space, just above the upper border of a rib. A finger cot or finger from a surgical glove with a hole in the tip is tied securely to the hub of the needle. A: On inspiration, the finger cot collapses and allows no air into the pleural cavity. B: On expiration, air is forced through the open end of the finger cot.

involved side, with severe compromise of the contralateral lung. Dyspnea quickly occurs, and the patient becomes extremely anxious. Examination of the chest reveals marked tympany over the affected side with loss of excursion.

Venous return to the heart may be adversely influenced by the shift of the mediastinal structures. Tracheal shift is easily detectable by palpation in the suprasternal notch. Under ordinary circumstances, the trachea should be in the mid-line of the suprasternal notch. Immediate treatment is called for and consists of simply inserting a needle in the second or third intercostal space anteriorly in the mid-clavicular line. If a smooth barreled glass syringe is used, the plunger will move rapidly outward as the needle enters the pleural space and the pressure is relieved. A simple flutter valve can be devised by attaching a finger cot to the needle (Figure 19–2), or an underwater trap can be established by connecting the needle with tubing to a flask containing fluid and holding the tube beneath the surface of the water.

Delay for consultation or x-rays cannot be countenanced in this emergent situation, since it may result in a fatality. Once a temporary water trap has been established as a life-saving measure, a more permanent intercostal catheter can be inserted and connected to a pleuravac or standard underwater seal (Figure 19–3). Whether or not a thoracic suction pump is needed to produce a measured amount of negative pressure will depend on the patient's response.

Fracture of one or several ribs may otherwise result in hemothorax of varying degrees (Figure 19–4). Needle aspiration in a lower intercostal space will confirm the presence of blood, which calls for evacuation of the pleural cavity, both of air and blood, until the lung is completely expanded to fill the pleural space. This can sometimes be accomplished with large-bore needles or may require intercostal drainage by means of a closed thoracostomy with underwater seal.

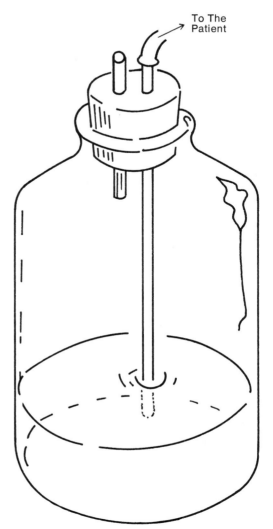

To The Patient

Figure 19–3 An underwater seal. The underwater glass tube connects via rubber tubing to the intercostal catheter. The glass tube should extend 2 to 3 cm. below the surface of the water. Air thus evacuated through this closed system will bubble into the fluid and be evacuated by means of the short glass tube vent. To maintain this closed system, the tube connected to the chest *must* remain beneath the level of the fluid.

Flail chest

A number of ribs can be fractured without incurring serious impairment of pulmonary exchange if the stability of the chest wall is not lost. At times, because of the nature of the injury and especially when a rib has been

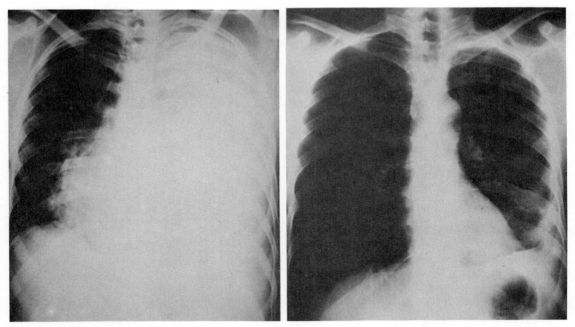

Figure 19–4 Hemothorax. Left: Hemothorax developed following a simple fracture of the eighth left rib. Right: X-ray shows improvement 3 months later, after intercostal tube drainage.

fractured in 2 places, the normal excursion of the rib is lost. Severe respiratory compromise may result, depending on the extent of the flail nature of the chest wall. This is particularly true when the injury is bilateral. Crushing injuries are more likely to lead to a flail chest.

Simple inspection will show that as the patient makes an inspiratory effort, the chest wall over the flail area will be drawn inward, and with expiration the flail area bulges outward. Therefore, the motion is said to be paradoxical. (See Figure 19–5.) Where the area of chest wall involved is small, there may be little influence on respiratory exchange. However, where the extent of the paradoxical motion is large, considerable untoward influence on respiration may result. As a result of this paradoxical motion, the underlying lung fails to draw in or expel air effectively. The respiratory compromise is in direct proportion to the extent of the flail area and to the degree of the paradoxical respiration that results. Flail chest, untreated, leads to marked dyspnea and cyanosis resulting from the hy-

percarbia and hypoxia. Unless stability of the chest wall is established, death will result from suffocation.

The simplest method of temporarily reversing instability of the chest wall is to hold it in the collapsed position by some sort of light pressure (sandbag). This will allow for increased, more effective exchange until more definitive measures can be taken. Although stability has been maintained by using external traction, the internal fixation suggested by Avery, *et al.,* is the most effective method.[2] Immediate tracheostomy will be necessary, and this in itself will reduce, to a certain extent, some of the paradoxical motion by by-passing the vocal cords and thus decreasing the dead air space and lessening respiratory effort.

Although a machine providing intermittent positive pressure may be satisfactory, a volume control respirator without a cuff on the tracheostomy tube will be considerably safer. Figure 19–6 shows the result of this treatment. Continuous monitoring by a well-informed nurse is essential. Frequent periodic

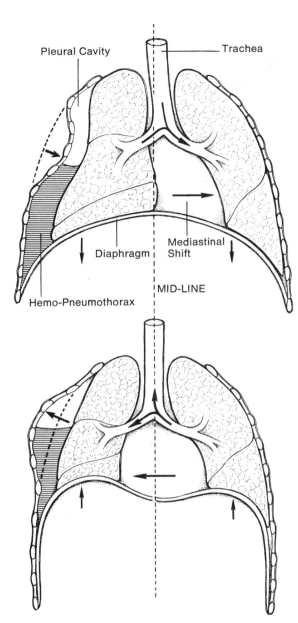

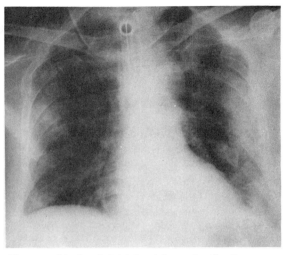

Figure 19–6 Multiple bilateral rib fractures with total flail chest. This x-ray was taken just after initiation of treatment. (Note the airway.) Patient was maintained on a volume control respirator without a tracheal cuff for 3 weeks, then gradually weaned. One year later, patient returned to light work. Pulmonary studies show continued improvement.

Figure 19–5 Respiration in a flail chest. Diagram on top shows flail area of right chest wall, which moves in with inspiration. Air moves into the left (normal) lung from the right bronchial tree as well as via normal tracheal inflow. Ventilation of the right lung is compromised. The mediastinum shifts to the uninjured side, further compromising exchange on the normal side. On expiration (bottom), air is driven out through the trachea and into the right (injured) side. This movement of air from one lung to the other is known as "pendulum movement," which leads to further deoxygenation. Hemopneumothorax further compromises oxygen exchange.

aspirations of the tracheal tube should be carried out, with care given to the sterile nature of the procedure. Ventilatory support must be continued until stabilization of the chest wall has occurred. The effectiveness of the assisted ventilation can be checked by repeated arterial blood gas analyses. It has been shown by Nealon and others that the pCO_2 is a more reliable index of when the assisted ventilation can be discontinued.[18] Intermittent use of the positive pressure breathing apparatus with frequent blood gas analyses will help to establish when the patient can be weaned from the apparatus.

Lung contusion and hematoma

Blunt trauma of the chest can produce localized injuries in pulmonary tissue or may result in a more diffuse change with varying degrees of pain and respiratory distress.[4] Chest x-ray may reveal a fairly localized area of infiltration, which in some respects might resemble a tumor. Hematoma may be well localized or generalized. The more diffuse involvement is often referred to as a "contusion." In such injury, the pulmonary alveoli in the area are filled with fluid and blood, which compromises pulmonary gas exchange.

Therapy is directed at maintaining good ventilation. Broad spectrum antibiotics may be used to prevent secondary infection, and oxygen is given as necessary. Cough is encouraged, and tracheal suction should be performed when deemed necessary. Overhydration should be guarded against; monitoring of the central venous pressure will be helpful in preventing this complication. More extensive involvement may require a tracheostomy and ventilatory assist to maintain effective exchange and a more complete and frequent pulmonary toilet.

Sternal fracture

Sternal fracture usually results from a steering wheel accident. Although the patient may be wearing the conventional seat belt, deceleration may throw him forcefully against the steering wheel, resulting in a fracture of the sternum. This may be associated with fractures of the ribs on either side of the sternum; thus there may be an element of flail chest. If so, it should be thus treated. Under some circumstances the relief of pain will be all that is necessary.

Where there is a sternal depression with an obvious paradoxical motion, external support may be adequate. In more extreme situations, tracheostomy and the use of a volume respirator are required. Under these circumstances, a consideration of myocardial injury (myocardial contusion) must be kept in mind, as must the possibility of a major vascular injury, particularly a rupture of the descending aortic arch. Serial electrocardiograms should be done to rule out a myocardial injury.

Injury to the trachea and main bronchi

Lacerations of the trachea, caused by crushing or penetrating injuries of the chest, may result in major air leaks leading to mediastinal emphysema, with extension into subcutaneous tissues of the neck. Crepitation may be palpated in the suprasternal area. Auscultation often reveals a crunching sound synchronous with the heartbeat (Hamman's sign). A tracheostomy will usually control further air loss, since with the tube in place, the tracheal pressure cannot rise much above atmospheric pressure. Also, tracheostomy prepares the patient for a thoracotomy if repair of a major tracheal laceration or bronchial fracture is indicated.

Major bronchial tears may, at times, go unnoticed, and the patient can live to develop a bronchial stenosis later. More frequently, the patient develops a pneumothorax, hemoptysis and considerable subcutaneous emphysema. Pneumothorax, with evidence of a major air leak, usually suggests the possibility of a major tracheal or bronchial tear; bronchoscopy is in order immediately. The secret to early diagnosis of this injury is a high index of suspicion.

Cardiac contusion

Blunt trauma to the heart, as seen in steering wheel injuries, occurs not infrequently and often goes unrecognized. It must always be suspected in any major contusion of the anterior chest wall. It usually is associated with a more serious injury and may be seen more frequently in already diseased hearts. The extent of cardiac damage will vary from a small, localized contusion to a more extensive injury to the cardiac muscle. It is usually manifest clinically by a tachycardia and less commonly by varying arrhythmias. Electrocardiograph findings may reveal S-T–T wave changes, which are usually temporary. Enzyme studies are elevated but are not considered helpful because of the associated soft tissue injuries which may also cause abnormal elevations of the transaminase levels.

The prognosis depends not only on the extent of the damage to the heart but also on the extent of associated injuries. In any case of suspected injury, serial tracings are in order. The patient should be monitored and kept at bedrest. Any arrhythmia that is present should be treated promptly, and major surgical operations should be avoided if at all possible under these circumstances.

Deceleration injury to the aorta

Injury to the major vessels may occur as a result of blunt or penetrating wounds. The most frequent site of a tear of the aorta is at a point just beyond the takeoff (origin) of the left subclavian artery, where there is a difference in the fixation of the aorta.[20] The usual cause is a head-on automobile accident at high speed with sudden deceleration. A fall from a height with crushing injuries may also cause a rupture of the aorta. In full-thickness tears of the aorta, death from exsanguination usually results immediately. A sizeable number of patients survive to be admitted to the hospital for immediate care.

In deceleration injuries of the aorta, the mobile, descending thoracic aorta and the more fixed portion, proximal to the ligamentous arteriosum just beyond the left subclavian artery, comprise the usual site (see Figure 19–7). The difference in the rate of deceleration in the two areas results in either a complete or partial tearing. If the adventitia (outer layer of the aorta) remains intact, the tear is partial, and a patient may survive for a period of time.

In some instances, associated chest complaints may obscure the condition. In any such injury, the diagnosis must always be considered. Pain, especially in the back of the upper chest, is a persistent complaint. Pain not influenced by respiration should suggest the diagnosis. X-ray will show a widening of the mediastinum and a retrograde aortogram will confirm the diagnosis. If a partial tear is demonstrated, exploration and repair is in order if associated injuries do not contraindicate. Unrecognized aortic tears may survive and present later as an aortic aneurysm. Compromise of the left main bronchus by the aneurysm, producing some pulmonary complaints, may also suggest the possibility of such a lesion.

Treatment consists of resection and placement of a graft. These patients may have a very unstable cardiovascular status. Frequent monitoring of vital signs and close observation is necessary. Crossmatching of

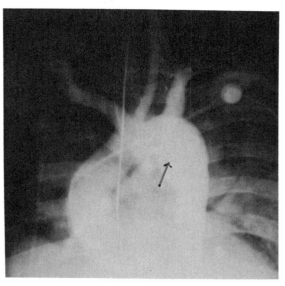

Figure 19–7 Aneurysm. Aortogram was taken because of widening mediastinum following head-on car accident. It shows traumatic aneurysm just distal to left subclavian take-off. Repair by graft was done within 12 hours after injury.

type-specific blood and initiation of volume replacement should be done soon after admission to the emergency department.

Penetrating wounds

Penetrating chest wounds may be caused by a number of agents: knives, ice picks and a variety of missiles. Some knowledge of the nature of the wounding agent is important, since it may give a clue as to the nature of the wound itself and to the extent of the involvement of the deeper structures within the chest.

Injuries caused by gunshot wounds will vary with the size and speed of the missile. High-velocity missiles will produce more damage than the wounds of exit or entrance suggest. The path of a missile is usually in a straight line, unless it is deflected by a bony structure. The wounds of entrance and exit, therefore, will usually suggest the nature of the soft tissue involvement in the bullet's path. A bizarre pathway is sometimes explained by the position of the patient at the time of wounding. In estimating the extent of the injury, all structures within the thorax and mediastinum must be considered. A line drawn from the wound of entrance to the embedded missile or the exit wound will frequently indicate the organs injured.

A persistent defect, the size of which depends on the wounding agent, may be produced in the chest wall, which allows movement of air in and out of the pleural cavity (sucking wounds of the chest). The extent to which the underlying lung collapses depends on the size of the opening in the chest wall. In some instances, the nature of the wound will allow air to flow into the chest with respiration but will prevent it from flowing outward. Air is thus trapped in the pleural cavity as in a tension pneumothorax, and with each respiratory effort the mediastinum is moved to the opposite side. This results in poor exchange between the intrapulmonary and the atmospheric air. If the mediastinal shift is severe, diminished venous return to the heart results, with accompanying hypotension.

An obvious sucking chest wound should be treated immediately. Simple closing of the wound by an occlusive dressing (usually vaseline gauze) will be adequate, temporarily. An intercostal catheter connected to a water trap will decompress the pleural space and control the situation until definitive treatment can be given. The prime indication for formal thoracotomy following a chest wound is continued bleeding into the pleural cavity (hemothorax), either from the lung or from the chest wall. When such continued bleeding is encountered, it is usually from an intercostal artery.

Hemothorax

Blood in the pleural cavity is the most common complication of a penetrating or a perforating wound of the chest. The usual finding is a combination of pneumothorax and hemothorax. Examination will reveal dullness and limited respiratory excursion, depending on the amount of blood and air in the pleural space. Treatment is by needle aspiration (a large-bore needle in a lower interspace), to remove all the blood and air and to completely expand the lung.

Most hemothoraxes are results of bleeding from the lung rather than from the chest wall. Therefore, fully reexpanding the lung will not lead to further bleeding, since the pressure in the pulmonary artery is low. Although the physical examination is important, repeated chest x-rays are more reliable in determining if bleeding is continuing and whether repeated taps are necessary. Vital signs should be recorded on admission to the emergency department and at frequent regular intervals thereafter. A falling blood pressure and a rising pulse suggest continued bleeding. When this occurs, it is usually from an intercostal artery and is a clear indication for a thoracotomy and control of the bleeding site.

When hemothorax is associated with a major air leak from the lung, adequate intercostal tube drainage is necessary. Where there may be a continuing air leak, it is safer to employ an underwater seal drainage system, with the addition of a thoracic suction pump as needed.

THORACOABDOMINAL WOUNDS

A thoracoabdominal wound is one in which both the thoracic and abdominal cavities are injured by the wounding agent. By carefully evaluating the wounds of entrance and exit, it usually can be determined whether or not one or the other or both of the 2 cavities have been involved. Where there is a single wound, with a foreign body in place, an antero-posterior and lateral x-rays of the chest and abdomen will usually give indication of the presence or absence of a thoracoabdominal wound.

The diaphragm rises to about the fourth intercostal space with expiration. This is important in considering the path of the wounding agent. The position of the diaphragm at the time of injury may determine whether or not both cavities are involved by the wound. Projecting a straight line from the wound of entrance to exit or from the wound of entrance to the missile shown on x-ray will suggest quite accurately the organs involved.

On the right side, the wound of entrance above the costal margin which exits posteriorly at the tenth rib will involve the diaphragm in 2 areas and the liver. No other intra-abdominal organs will be injured. On the left side, because of the number of organs in the left upper quadrant, a similar such wound track might involve the spleen, stomach, colon and small bowel. In thoracoabdominal wounds involving the right upper quadrant, the abdominal signs may be minimal, if bleeding from the liver is slight, or may be missing when the patient is first seen. Thoracoabdominal wounds involving the left upper quadrant are apt to present more striking abdominal signs.

Treatment of thoracoabdominal wounds first requires accurate knowledge of the missile path and the possible organs involved. Careful but complete assessment of the patient is necessary. If abdominal findings are minimal, peritoneal tap or lavage may be useful, particularly if blood is recovered. Care of the injured organs and repair of the wound of the diaphragm, with attention to pulmonary pleural toilet and complete expansion of the lung, quickly follows. Adequate amounts of type-specific blood should be given to the patient in preparation for surgery. In the emergency department, tube thoracostomy may be needed to evacuate fluid or air from the pleural space. In all instances of penetrating thoraco-abdominal wounds, surgical exploration is needed.

ABDOMINAL INJURIES

The majority of abdominal injuries in civilian life are the result of blunt trauma following high-speed automobile accidents and falls from heights; penetrating wounds of the abdomen are more common in wartime. Wounds resulting from blunt trauma are more difficult to recognize; consequently, there may be delay in diagnosis. Therefore, early recognition of intra-abdominal injury is essential to good care. The importance of ongoing re-peated assessment and evaluation of vital signs cannot be overstressed. Injury of multiple organ systems, such as the central nervous system, chest and skeletal systems, may also obscure an intra-abdominal injury, so it is important that the treatment be under the direction of one physician, usually a general surgeon, even though multiple disciplines may be involved.

Assessment

Diagnosis and treatment should occur simultaneously as an assessment of the situation is being made. An airway should be established if necessary. When spontaneous respiration is evident, all that is required is simple airway toilet. On the other hand, a comatose patient may need immediate intubation with a cuffed endotracheal tube so that assisted respiration may be given. Once ventilation is restored, an intravenous infusion line, preferably in the upper extremity, should be inserted, using an electrolyte solution such as Ringer's lactate. At the same time, an adequate sample of blood can be drawn for typing and cross-matching and for laboratory determinations, such as hemoglobin, hematocrit and arterial blood gases.

Frequently, in patients with major abdominal injuries, a central venous pressure monitoring catheter should be introduced, as it will serve as a good avenue for volume replacement. It can be inserted in the cephalic vein at the antecubital space of the elbow or directly into the subclavian vein via an infra-clavicular percutaneous approach. Sterile precautions are absolutely necessary.

An indwelling urinary catheter will give a clear picture of renal function. A urinary output of one ml./kg. per hour indicates that the kidneys are being adequately perfused. Blood in the urine will usually be present if there has been an injury of the urinary tract. A nasogastric tube should be inserted into the stomach and placed on suction and the aspirated material examined for the presence of blood. Blood on rectal examination will suggest the possibility of intestinal injury. Once respiratory and circulatory efficiency have been restored, the vital signs should be recorded at approximately 15-minute intervals. Repeated abdominal examination is important in deciding whether or not an intra-abdominal injury has occurred. Such careful observation will allow an earlier diagnosis to be made.

In the patient who is conscious, major intra-abdominal injuries are almost always accompanied by pain. Other symptoms may be present, such as nausea, vomiting, thirst and a feeling of apprehension, dependent on the extent of injury. The usual physical signs seen in visceral injuries are tenderness, spasm, diminished or absent bowel sounds and, where intraperitoneal air is present, absence of liver dullness. The extent to which these symptoms and signs are present may depend on how soon following wounding the patient is seen. When the time from injury to examination is short, the abdominal complaints and findings may be minimal. This emphasizes the importance of repeated abdominal examinations.

Peritoneal tap (abdominal paracentesis) is useful in the diagnosis of obscure intra-abdominal injuries following blunt trauma. With increasing experience, a diagnostic accuracy of 75 percent has been quoted. A positive tap, when blood has been obtained from the peritoneal cavity, is proof that there has been an intraperitoneal injury of some degree. No conclusion can be drawn, however, when the tap is negative. Aspiration of the peritoneal cavity has been advocated for years as a diagnostic aid, and its routine use has been recommended in patients where an intraperitoneal injury is suspected. Others, however, have questioned its usefulness.

The so-called 4-quadrant tap or some variation thereof, such as peritoneal saline lavage (using an indwelling catheter), will assist in making an earlier diagnosis of intra-abdominal injury in the obscure case. It must be emphasized that a negative aspiration does not exclude the presence of intraperitoneal injury; therefore, to be of any real value, the test must be positive. As with other diagnostic tests, the results must be interpreted in combination with other clinical and laboratory findings. All patients with multiple injuries who are comatose should have a routine abdominal paracentesis.

Laboratory findings at the time the patient is first seen may reveal a leukocytosis and a reduction in packed cell volume (hematocrit). In some patients with multiple system injuries, however, hemoconcentration (contraction of blood volume) may result in a normal hematocrit, which masks an underlying major blood loss. Repeated determinations of hematocrit and hemoglobin may be of considerable help in ascertaining the presence or absence of major blood loss. Serum amylase studies may indicate the possibility of pancreatic injury.

Three-way films of the abdomen (flat, upright and lateral decubitus) are helpful in a patient suspected of having an intra-abdominal injury and should be done routinely. Good films in the upright position or in the lateral decubitus will reveal the presence of free intra-abdominal air or fluid. X-ray evidence of skeletal injury, particularly to the lower ribs and the dorsal and lumbar spines, may give indirect evidence of the extent of the injury and the possibility of intraperitoneal wounding (see Figure 19–8). If hematuria has been present, whether gross or microscopic, intravenous pyelography should be done and cystograms performed, where indicated, especially if there is evidence of pelvic fractures.

Management

In management of patients with suspected thoracoabdominal injury, one should follow those principles previously enumerated, namely, establish an airway, control hemorrhage, initiate life-support measures as indicated and complete full assessment of the patient. When the history, physical findings and laboratory examinations support the presumptive diagnosis of intra-abdominal injury, the patient should be prepared for surgery. It is preferable to stabilize the patient's condition. However, if this cannot be done in a safe measure of time, the operation should not be delayed. The patient should immediately be started on parenteral antibiotics, such as a combination of penicillin and streptomycin. Tetanus prophylaxis is given as indicated (see Chapter 10). Adequate amounts of type-specific blood must be available. These patients are usually operated on under general anesthesia, since with this method, the pulmonary exchange is under complete control.

Liver injuries

The liver is the largest organ in the peritoneal cavity and the one most frequently injured in the abdomen. Being a solid viscus, damage to the liver results in blood and bile escaping into the peritoneal cavity, causing signs and symptoms of peritoneal irritation. Injury to the liver is serious, life-threatening and must be considered in any patient reporting an injury to the epigastrium, especially to the right upper quadrant.

The mechanism of injury to the liver will have a direct influence on morbidity and mortality. Penetrating wounds made by knives or low-velocity missiles frequently are associated with minimal damage, devitalization of liver tissue and continuing hemorrhage and do not present a significant problem in management. However, wounds of the liver following blunt trauma from high-velocity missiles usually result in more extensive damage to the liver parenchyma, with more resultant massive bleeding and devitalization of liver tissue. In addition, other organs are liable to be damaged. In some liver injuries from deceleration, there may be avulsion of major hepatic veins at their entrance into the vena cava, resulting in massive blood loss. The morbidity and mortality is directly related to the occurrence of multiple organ injuries.

In patients with liver trauma, the wounding may vary from a relatively minor laceration to extensive fractures. Particularly in the latter, with significant blood loss, vital signs may be unstable. Thorough assessment must be done. Details of the mechanism of injury

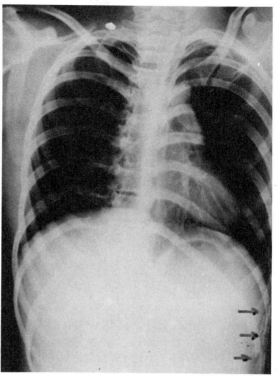

Figure 19–8 Rib fractures. The x-ray shows fractures of the left eighth, ninth and tenth ribs in a patient who struck his left chest against a gear shift lever. There also were signs of acute abdomen, and a laparotomy revealed rupture of the spleen.

may be helpful in better appraisal of the damage. Typically, there is evidence of peritoneal irritation in the upper abdomen, particularly in the right upper quadrant, with spasm and rigidity. At other times, the physical findings may be minimal. In questionable instances, peritoneal tap will be helpful. Once the diagnosis is established, it is a clear indication for operative intervention. Every effort should be made to stabilize the patient in the emergency department. Adequate amounts of type-specific blood should be available for anticipated surgery.

Whatever the nature of the liver wound, the principles of good management of liver injuries are the same: control of bleeding, removal of devitalized tissue and establishment of adequate drainage.

Wounds of the stomach and duodenum

The stomach, because of its relatively protected position behind the rib cage, is rarely injured in blunt abdominal trauma. Most wounds of the stomach and duodenum are associated with penetrating or perforating wounds, such as gunshot wounds. Invariably, these involve both the anterior and posterior walls of the stomach. In blunt injury, the diagnosis is more difficult to establish.

The duodenum, because of its relatively exposed position, is more readily injured than the stomach, both by penetrating and blunt injuries. The most frequent injury is an intramural hematoma (a blood clot within the wall of the duodenum). If left untreated, it may result in obstruction of the upper intestinal tract.

Injuries to the stomach and duodenum are difficult to diagnose for 2 reasons. First, one does not suspect this rare injury. Second, initial signs and symptoms are misleadingly absent. Physical findings may vary from none to tenderness in the epigastrium, with or without local spasm.

Management of patients with stomach or duodenum injury in the emergency department is directed primarily toward making a correct diagnosis and stabilizing the patient's condition. Repeated observation and recording of physical signs is required to properly evaluate a patient suspected of having such an injury.

Intravenous fluids and nasogastric decompression are necessary. Perforating wounds are managed by a surgical approach, while blunt injury is handled by nonoperative methods, unless a complication occurs. Complications include bleeding, upper gastrointestinal obstruction, duodenal fistula and pancreatitis. Upper gastrointestinal series is rarely used during the emergency management of such a patient but is helpful in delineating the extent of injury early in the hospital course. Patients suspected of having pancreatic injury should have serial amylase determinations on the blood and urine.

Pancreatic injuries

Wounds of the pancreas are usually associated with blunt trauma and result from severe compression across the upper abdomen. An anterior force, such as a steering wheel, compresses the pancreas against the vertebral column, resulting in a variety of injuries. There may be simple contusion, with rupture of the minor branches of the ductal system, or complete transection of the pancreas, with leakage of pancreatic juice. When injury of the pancreatic head is combined with a rupture of the duodenum, the mortality reaches as high as 73 percent, and is associated with a high incidence of serious sequelae.

Diagnosis of pancreatic injury is difficult because of the protected position of this retroperitoneal organ. Clinically, the patient may complain of epigastric pain and have localizing signs. Serum and urinary amylase studies should be made on admission, and even though normal values are obtained initially, they should be repeated in 2 to 3 hours. It has been suggested by Gambill and Mason[14] that the 2-hour collection of urine and determination of amylase is a more reliable index of pancreatic injury than the serum amylase. However, pancreatic injury may occur without serum amylase elevation. When 4-quadrant abdominal paracentesis is done in an effort to make a diagnosis of intra-abdominal injury, the fluid recovered should be studied for its amylase level.

The presence of abdominal tenderness and involuntary muscle spasm and the absence of bowel sounds indicate surgical exploration with or without elevated serum amylase.[8] Where findings are equivocal, a nonoperative course should be considered. In such instances, the treatment consists of nasogastric suction, appropriate intravenous fluids and frequent reevaluation. If there is any progression of signs or symptoms, laparotomy should be performed. A hematoma overlying the body of the pancreas may mask a pancreatic injury. Contusion of pancreatic tissue may occur without rupture of the capsule and may go unrecognized, resulting later in formation of a pancreatic pseudocyst.

The commonest major injury reported is a fracture of the pancreas at the vertebral body.[27] Complete transection results, and in this instance, a distal pancreatectomy is indicated. On rare occasions (an extensive injury involving the pancreatic head and associated structures in which salvage of the injured parts is not feasible), extensive resection is necessary for debridement of devitalized tissue. A pancreaticoduodenectomy may be the procedure of choice. The mortality in 25 reported cases has been 24 percent. It is essential, no matter what procedure is carried out, that a maximally effective drainage of the area of pancreatic injury be established. Not uncommonly, a nonoperative course is chosen. Frequent assessment, with repeated studies of serum and urinary amylase when it remains elevated, are indicative of pancreatic injury and warrant exploratory surgery.

Injuries of the spleen

Although the normal spleen, being relatively small, is well protected in the left upper quadrant, it is one of the most frequently injured organs following nonpenetrating trauma of the abdomen.[29, 30] History of a blow, fall or athletic injury involving the lower left chest or flank is frequently obtained. Abdominal tenderness and spasm in the left upper quadrant with or without evidence of rib fractures may strongly suggest the possibility of splenic injury. Systemic symptoms of acute hemorrhage, with local signs of peritoneal irritation, will suggest the diagnosis. The patient will frequently complain of pain in the upper abdomen, especially in the left upper quadrant. Enlargement of the spleen by hematoma or rupture, with blood loss under the diaphragm, may result in reflex pain being noted in the shoulder. A minor blow not readily recalled by the patient may result in splenic rupture. Because of the nature of the injury, hemorrhage may be delayed for 48 hours or longer. Although such patients may be without early symptoms, usually there are physical signs that suggest parasplenic clot or hematoma. Delay in rupture of the capsule following splenic injury may account for the latent period in the presentation of symptoms. Progressive signs of peritoneal irritation, with evidence of blood loss, is sufficient indication for laparotomy. A repeat white blood count may show a significant leukocytosis, indicating progress of the anemia.

Three-way films of the abdomen may be helpful in making the diagnosis of splenic injury by showing the presence in the splenic area of a soft tissue shadow considerably larger than a normal spleen and with medial displacement (see Figure 19–9). In some instances, selective splenic or celiac angiography may afford a more precise and adequate method of demonstrating a rupture of the spleen (Figure 19–10). Radionuclide studies may also be helpful in the study of patients who have sustained thoracoabdominal trauma and have relatively few symptoms and little or no physical findings on examination. (See Figure 19–11.) Long periods of hospitalization and observation for evidence of splenic injuries, as well as the danger of a delayed rupture with hemorrhage, may be thus avoided. In penetrating injury, damage to adjacent structures must be considered, including the stomach, pancreas and splenic flexure of the colon.

Small bowel injuries

Small bowel injuries are most commonly the result of perforating or penetrating wounds and less commonly associated with nonpenetrating trauma to the abdomen.[28] Injuries of the small bowel due to blunt trauma are the result of several mechanisms, the most common being the crushing of the bowel against the anterior lordotic curvature of the lumbosacral spine. An improperly positioned automobile seat belt may, at times, cause lacerations of the small bowel. When this occurs, it is usually in the region of the terminal ileum. Points at which the small bowel is fixed, such

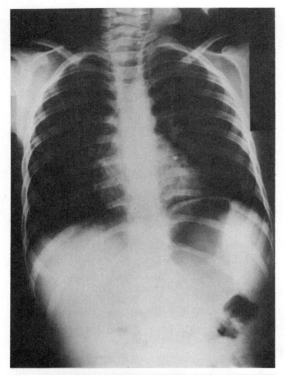

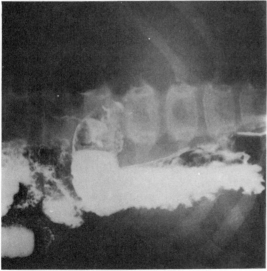

Figure 19–9 Splenic rupture. Top: Flat film of abdomen of patient who fell, striking lower left chest. Note elevation of left diaphragm and large amount of air in stomach with medial displacement of the greater curvature. Bottom: Lateral decubitus x-ray after barium swallow. Stomach displaced upward by external mass. Patient had intraparenchymal rupture of the spleen.

as the jejunum at the ligament of Treitz and the terminal ileum at the cecum, may be torn by blunt trauma. Tears and perforations may result. Fixation of the bowel by adhesions to the anterior abdominal wall or to the pelvis may also be the site of ulcerations. A bursting type injury is rare, if not unknown. Small lacerations of the mesentery of the small bowel may result from blunt trauma, and avulsion of the intestine from the mesentery over a considerable distance may occur. Major vascular injuries are rarely seen as a complication of blunt abdominal trauma.

Major wounds of the small intestine and mesentery will usually present evidence of peritoneal irritation, with spasm, rigidity and blood loss. The diagnosis can be made by careful evaluation over a period of time with such aids as abdominal tap and x-ray films. The patient should have an intravenous lifeline inserted and nasogastric suction initiated, along with crossmatch for type-specific blood. Once the diagnosis is made, operative intervention is needed. The operative management may vary from repair of mesenteric defect with control of hemorrhage to resection of irreversibly damaged bowel.

Injuries of the colon and rectum

Injuries of the colon and rectum infrequently result from blunt trauma to the abdomen, with an incidence of 3 to 5 percent. Penetrating or perforating wounds are more likely to involve the colon and rectum in a higher percentage because of the large size of these organs. The large bowel may be injured by a variety of mechanisms, such as compression against the lumbar spine, bursting effect and sudden deceleration.[9] Fractures of the pelvis account for some rectal wounds, both intra- and extraperitoneal. Penetrating and perforating wounding agents, however, account for the greatest number of rectal wounds. These include perforation by enema tip and any number of foreign bodies which might be inserted into the rectum through ordinary circumstances or in instances of erotic perversion.

There are no specific signs or symptoms to

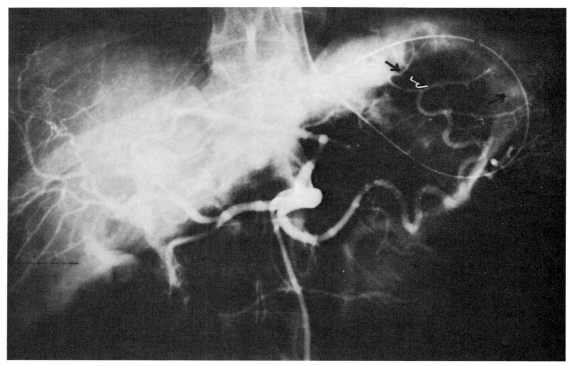

Figure 19–10 Selective celiac arteriogram. This is an x-ray of the same patient as in Figure 19–9. The arcuate appearance of splenic vessels (arrows) is abnormal and indicates hemorrhage within the spleen.

suggest a colon or rectal injury. Frequent abdominal examinations, seeking signs of peritoneal irritation are thus routine. Severe associated injuries may make recognition of colon and rectal injuries difficult.

Three-way films of the abdomen may dem-

onstrate free fluid or air in the peritoneal cavity, giving evidence of an intraperitoneal injury. Four-quadrant taps or peritoneal lavage may be of great help. The return fluid from the peritoneal lavage should be studied for blood, amylase and bacteria. Since extra-

Figure 19–11 Splenic scan. Lower arrow indicates homogenous density of normal spleen. Upper arrow indicates an area of lesser density, which is found with intraparenchymal hemorrhage of spleen. Hemorrhage was confirmed at laparotomy.

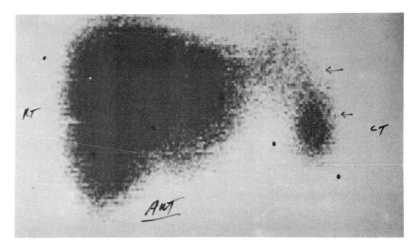

peritoneal wounds of the rectum do not reflect abdominal signs and symptoms, diagnosis is more difficult. Multiple wounds may divert attention from the anorectal region, and injuries of this area can easily be overlooked. Any wound that may possibly involve the rectum must be thoroughly examined to determine its exact extent. Digital as well as sigmoidoscopic examination is in order. The presence of blood in the rectum is strong evidence that wounding has occurred.

Intraperitoneal injuries of the colon

The management of intraperitoneal wounds of the colon will be influenced by several factors, especially by the nature of the bowel injury itself. Penetrating and perforating wounds usually are recognized more readily, and, therefore, exploration is carried out earlier, whereas injury due to blunt trauma may be recognized late, resulting in a greater degree of contamination of the peritoneal cavity. The time period from wounding to exploration will influence the severity of the problem and the procedure required. The nature of the associated injury and the general status of the patient must also be considered in planning surgical care of wounds of the colon.

Injuries to the right colon are cared for by a number of procedures, such as resection and ileotransversecolostomy to excision and creation of an end ileostomy and colostomy. The procedure will depend entirely on the particular findings in a given case. Simple closure of a wound, creating a tube cecostomy or, in some instances, colostomy, may be all that is necessary. Repair without decompression should be undertaken only in the most favorable of circumstances.

Wounds of those areas of the colon that are easily mobilized are best cared for by exteriorization, with or without the creation of a colostomy. How little or how much treatment is needed depends on the extent of the injury and the peritoneal insult. Where the wound involves a segment of colon, rectosigmoid, that cannot be exteriorized, one of several methods of surgical care can be used. Closure of the wound with completely diverting proximal colostomy may be satisfactory. Later the colostomy can be taken down and the continuity of the bowel restored. In preparing these patients for surgery, the possibility and/or probability of a colostomy (though temporary) should be discussed with the patient. If the patient's condition will not permit this, the relatives should be informed of the possibility.

Extraperitoneal wounds of the rectum

Extraperitoneal wounds of the rectum may be especially difficult to care for when the defect created is large and fractures of the pelvis are involved. A major step in the care of such wounds has been made when the diagnosis is established and the full extent of the injury is appreciated. This is often not done until the patient is in the operating room, with the abdomen opened.

Laparotomy is performed for proper assessment and care of other associated intraperitoneal injuries. Exploration of the perirectal space is carried out, and repair of the wound of the rectum is made, if at all possible. Foreign bodies, such as bone spicules, must be looked for and removed. A completely diverting proximal colostomy is usually fashioned in the sigmoid colon, for it is important that no feces spill over into the distal limb. The limbs of the colostomy should be separated. At the end of the procedure, care must be taken to empty the distal sigmoid, rectosigmoid and colon of all fecal material. Good drainage of the perirectal space through the posterior perineum alongside the coccyx is essential. Complete broad spectrum antibiotic coverage is initiated in the emergency department.

SUMMARY

Injuries to the chest contribute significantly to the number of deaths that result from trauma. A chest injury may cause major disturbances of cardiopulmonary function and, for this reason, constitutes a serious clinical problem.

The emergency nurse must be capable of

recognizing both major chest injuries and those apparently less serious but which, if not attended to promptly, could cause dire consequences. A familiarity with cardiopulmonary physiology and airway maintenance is a prerequisite for those charged with the management of patients with thoracic injuries.

A thoracoabdominal injury may be difficult to assess, particularly when it is due to blunt, nonpenetrating trauma. Priorities of care must be established in a patient with such combined injury, and diagnosis and treatment must proceed simultaneously.

BIBLIOGRAPHY

(1) Andrus, C. H., and Morton, J. H.: "Rupture of the Diaphragm After Blunt Trauma," *American Journal of Surgery,* 119 (1970):686.

(2) Avery, E. E.; Morch, E. T., and Benson, D. W.: "Critically Crushed Chests: A New Method of Treatment with Continuous Mechanical Hyperventilation to Produce Alkalotic Apnea and Internal Pneumatic Stabilization," *Journal of Thoracic Surgery,* 33 (1956):291–311.

(3) Cohen, I., Jr.; Hawthorne, H. R., and Frobese, A. S.: "Retroperitoneal Rupture of Duodenum in Nonpenetrating Abdominal Trauma," *American Journal of Surgery,* 84 (1952):293–301.

(4) Cohn, Roy: "Nonpenetrating Wounds of the Lungs and Bronchi," *Surgical Clinics of North America,* 52 (June 1972):3.

(5) Connolly, J. E.: "Practical Approach to the Diagnosis of Shock," *Hospital Medicine,* 4 (April 1968):4–13.

(6) Crandell, W. B.: "Abdominal Wound Disruption," in G. F. Madding and P. A. Kennedy (eds.), *Surgical Techniques,* 3 (San Francisco: Bancroft Whitney Company, 1970), pp. 42–55.

(7) Donovan, A. J.; Turrill, Fred, and Berne, Clarence J.: *Surgical Clinics of North America,* 52 (June 1972):3.

(8) Freeark, R. J.; Kane, J. M.; Folk, F. A., and Baker, R. J.: "Traumatic Disruption of the Head of the Pancreas," *Archives of Surgery,* 91 (1965):5.

(9) Grimes, Orville F.: "Injuries to the Chest Wall and Esophagus," *Surgical Clinics of North America,* 52 (June 1972):3.

(10) Haynes, C. D.; Gunn, C. H., and Martin, J. D.: "Colon Injuries," *Archives of Surgery,* 96 (1968):944–948.

(11) Kennedy, P. A., and Madding, G. F.: "The Incision and Wound Closure in Blunt Abdominal Trauma," *Surgical Clinics of North America,* 52 (June 1972):761.

(12) Killen, J. A.: "Injury of the Superior Mesenteric Vessels Secondary to Nonpenetrating Abdominal Trauma," *American Surgeon,* 30 (1964):306.

(13) Madding, G. F., and Kennedy, P. A.: *Trauma to the Liver, Major Problems in Clinical Surgery,* 111, ed. 2 (Philadelphia: W. B. Saunders Company, 1971).

(14) Mason, L. B.; Sidbury, J. B., and Guiang, S.: "Rupture of the Extrahepatic Biliary Ducts from Nonpenetrating Trauma," *Annals of Surgery,* 140 (1954):234.

(15) Mays, E. T.: "Observations and Management After Hepatic Artery Ligation," *Surgery, Gynecology and Obstetrics,* 124 (1967):801.

(16) Mays, E. T.: "Hepatic Lobectomy," *Archives of Surgery,* 103 (1971):216.

(17) McClelland, R.; Shires, T., and Poulos, E.: "Hepatic Resection for Massive Trauma," *Journal of Trauma,* 4 (1964):282.

(18) Nealon, Thomas F., Jr., "Trauma to the Chest," *in* J. H. Gibbon, D. C. Sabiston, Jr., and F. C. Spencer, *Surgery of the Chest,* ed. 2 (Philadelphia: W. B. Saunders Company, 1969), pp. 168–182.

(19) Nick, W. V.; Zollinger, R. W., and Pace, W. G.: "Retroperitoneal Hemorrhage after Blunt Abdominal Trauma," *Journal of Trauma,* 7 (1967):652.

(20) Rodkey, Grant V.: "The Management of Abdominal Injuries," *Surgical Clinics of North America,* 46 (June 1966):627.

(21) Roe, Benson B.: "Cardiac Trauma Including Great Vessels," *Surgical Clinics of North America,* 52 (June 1972):3.

(22) Rosoff, L.; Cohen, J. L., and Halpern, M.: "Injuries of the Spleen," *Surgical Clinics of North America,* 52 (June 1972):3.

(23) Scannell, J. Gordon: "Surgical Management of Major Chest Injury," *Surgical Clinics of North America,* 46 (June 1966):539.

(24) Shefts, L. M.: "The Initial Management of Thoracic and Thoraco-Abdominal Trauma," *American Lecture Series* (Springfield, Ill.: Charles C Thomas, 1956).

(25) Shires, G. T.: *Care of the Trauma Patient* (New York: McGraw-Hill Book Company, 1966), p. 35.

(26) Spencer, F. C.; Sharp, E. H., and Jude, J. R.: "Experiences with Wire Closure of Abdominal Incisions in 292 Selective Patients," *Surgery, Gynecology and Obstetrics,* 117 (1963):235.

(27) Thal, A. P., and Wilson, R. F.: "A Pattern of Severe Blunt Trauma to the Region of the Pancreas," *Surgery, Gynecology and Obstetrics,* 119 (1964):773.

(28) Vance, B. M.: "Traumatic Lesions of the Intestines Caused by Nonpenetrating Blunt Forces," *Archives of Surgery,* 7 (1923):197

(29) Welch, C. E., and Giddings, W. P.: "Abdominal Trauma: Clinical Study of 200 Consecutive Cases from the Massachusetts General Hospital," *American Journal of Surgery,* 79 (1950):252–258.

(30) Whitesell, F. B.: "A Clinical and Surgical Anatomic Study of Rupture of the Spleen Due to Blunt Trauma," *Surgery, Gynecology and Obstetrics,* 110 (1960): 750.

20

Care of the patient with an acute abdomen

JAMES H. COSGRIFF, JR.
DIANN ANDERSON

ANATOMY AND PHYSIOLOGY

The abdomen is the largest single body cavity. It contains a number of hollow and solid viscera and is lined by a continuous layer of tissue (parietal peritoneum), which also covers the outside of the viscera (visceral peritoneum). It is frequently referred to as the peritoneal cavity. Its boundaries are the pleural diaphragm superiorly and the pelvic diaphragm inferiorly. The innervation of the visceral peritoneum is derived from the autonomic nervous system, while the parietal portion receives its nerve supply via the peripheral nerves.

Stimulation of the visceral peritoneum results from distention of hollow viscera or traction on mesenteric attachments; the resultant pain is frequently poorly localized. Stimulation of the parietal peritoneum results from contact with an inflamed organ or irritant fluid (blood or G.I. content), and the resultant pain is localized to the point or area of irritation. Thus, in early appendicitis, the pain is usually poorly localized to the mid-abdomen and is periumbilical in location, due to distention of the appendix, a hollow organ.

As the inflammatory process spreads to involve the serosal (outer) surface, contact is made with the adjacent parietal peritoneum, and the pain is localized to the site (usually the right lower quadrant).

Innervation of the parietal peritoneum conforms to the distribution of the peripheral nerves. The umbilicus lies at the level of the tenth intercostal nerve. The innervation of the upper quadrants ranges between the sixth and tenth nerves and the lower quadrants between the tenth intercostal and second lumbar nerves. The superior border of the parietal peritoneum, which covers the undersurface of the pleural diaphragm, is innervated by branches of the phrenic nerve, which originates from the fourth, fifth and sixth cervical nerves.

Because of this distribution of nerve supply, irritation of specific areas of the peritoneal cavity may result in pain located at the site of irritation. At the same time, the stimulation of the peripheral nerve may extend along the entire length of the nerve, resulting in pain at a remote site. This is known as "referred" pain. An example of this is the frequent association of pain associated with inflammatory conditions of the gallbladder arising in the right upper quadrant and radiating along the distribution of the eighth intercostal nerve to the tip of the right scapula. Other examples will be cited in the description of specific disease conditions. As pain originating from within the abdomen may be referred elsewhere, so, too, pain arising from other areas, such as the thoracic contents, may be "referred" to the abdomen, due to cross innervation.

A knowledge of the location of the contents of the peritoneal cavity will be helpful in assessing patients with abdominal pain. Topographically, the abdomen is bounded by the costal (rib) margin above and the inguinal ligament below. The inguinal ligament attaches

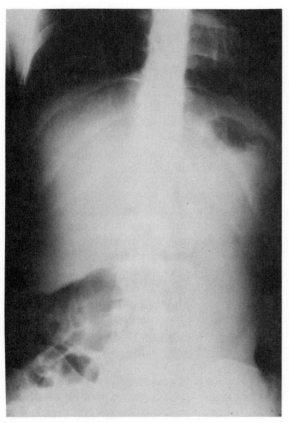

Figure 20–1 Upright film of abdomen. The liver shadow, on the left of the picture, is enlarged. Otherwise, findings are within normal limits.

to the anterior superior iliac spine of the pelvis above and laterally and to the pubic tubercle in the area of the symphysis below and medially. This ligament conforms roughly to the inguinal crease (flexion crease) at the upper end of each thigh. The lateral borders of the abdomen conform roughly to a line extending from the lateral edge of the costal margin in line with the axilla to the lateral border of the pelvis. Internally, the peritoneal cavity actually extends beyond these boundaries, as do its organs.

Pleural diaphragms will vary in position, depending on the patient's anatomical characteristics but, in general, are at the sixth intercostal space level anteriorly on the right and one lower on the left. Under ordinary circumstances, the right diaphragm lies higher than the left, being pushed up by the liver (see Figure 20–1). Although anatomical variations may occur in such instances as situs inversus (complete transposition of the organs) or incomplete or total malrotation of intestines, these conditions are quite uncommon. More often, locations of organs may vary, due to mesenteric attachments and similar minor deviations. By dropping a vertical line in the mid-line from the xiphoid cartilage to the symphysis pubis and intersecting this with a horizontal line through the umbilicus, the abdomen may be divided into 4 quadrants. (See Figure 20–2.)

The upper abdomen contains both solid and hollow viscera. Some, such as the liver, are large and extend into 2 quadrants. Organs such as the pancreas and kidneys are more properly considered retroperitoneal in location but usually produce symptoms of peritoneal irritation.

The organs found in the left upper quadrant of the abdomen are: (1) abdominal portion of the esophagus, (2) stomach, (3) spleen, (4) body and tail of the pancreas, (5) left side of the transverse colon and the splenic flexure, (6) left kidney and adrenal.

Those organs in the right upper quadrant are: (1) liver, (2) gallbladder and extrahepatic bile ducts (the cystic duct, the hepatic and common bile ducts), (3) duodenum, (4) head of the pancreas, (5) right side of the transverse colon and the hepatic flexure, (6) right kidney and adrenal.

The organs in the lower abdomen are hollow. Those in the left lower quadrant are: (1) descending and sigmoid colon and upper portion of the rectosigmoid, (2) upper portion of the small bowel, (3) left ureter. Those organs in the right lower quadrant are: (1) cecum, appendix and ascending colon, (2) lower portion of the small bowel, especially the ileum, (3) right ureter.

Lower mid-line structures include the urinary bladder and, in the female, the uterus. The ovaries, fallopian tubes and broad ligaments are paired structures in the pelvic portion of the lower abdomen, on either side of the mid-line.

ASSESSMENT OF AN ACUTE ABDOMEN

History

The history of illness is vital in assessing a patient with an acute abdominal condition. Careful attention must be given to developing the history in chronological sequence, with particular stress on the time of onset, nature and duration of the symptom(s).

If pain is one complaint, inquiry should be made to seek a description of it. The patient or family may be unable to express this adequately. The interviewer should suggest, for descriptive purposes, whether the pain is sharp, dull, aching, cramping, pressure-like. It is important to know whether it is continuous or intermittent and of constant intensity or pain that reaches a crescendo, diminishes, then increases again. The initial location of the pain along with a description of any radiation or reference should be sought.

The patient may be asked whether the pain "moves" anywhere and, if so, where; does it penetrate, "go through" or "go around" the abdomen to the back? Association with or aggravation by food intake, physical activity, increase in intra-abdominal pressure (by

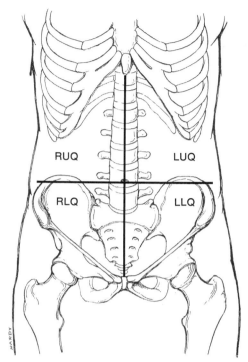

Figure 20–2 Topographical anatomy of the anterior abdominal wall, divided into quadrants. RUQ: right upper quadrant. LUQ: left upper quadrant. RLQ: right lower quadrant. LLQ: left lower quadrant.

breathing, coughing, straining, defecation) should be noted. The occurrence of related symptoms (malaise, nausea, vomiting, alteration in bowel or bladder regularity) may further aid in localizing the source of the symptoms to a specific site or organ.

In female patients, a history of menstrual activity is necessary. The nurse should establish the date the patient's last period began and whether or not it was normal. If abnormal, the nurse should seek to determine whether it was so in terms of duration, time of onset, unusual pain or associated with a smaller or larger amount of blood loss.

Not uncommonly during this opening phase of assessment, the patient may be somewhat uncooperative and ask for medication for pain relief. This is due, in part, to fear and apprehension. The interviewer must persist, however, in an effort to obtain as accurate a history as possible. Pain is an integral symptom of an acute abdomen and, as such, is discussed in Appendix G, at the end of this chapter.

Past history of prior illness, particularly of abdominal complaints or prior surgery is very important. Physical assessment must include an evaluation of the entire patient. It may be difficult to examine all areas adequately, since the patient may be immobilized by pain.

Respiratory activity and pulmonary ventilation may be lessened by the pain associated with peritoneal irritation. Splinting of the chest may cause atelectasis or collapse of the lower portions of the lung fields. Awareness of this possibility will assist in devising an appropriate plan of management.

Physical examination

Assessment directed at the abdomen is perhaps the most vital. The patient's attitude (position) should be observed. Frequently, the knees are drawn up to lessen tension on the peritoneum and decrease intra-abdominal pressure. Respiratory activity may be severely restricted.

In males, respiration is primarily abdominal, by diaphragmatic movement. With inspiration, the diaphragm descends to expand the lung, and this lessens the size of the abdominal cavity with a resultant increase in intra-abdominal pressure. As the diaphragm descends, the anterior abdominal wall protrudes and then falls as the diaphragm ascends with expiration. This motion may be sharply curtailed or totally absent with peritoneal irritation. In females, respiratory activity is effected primarily by expansion of the chest wall, using the thoracic musculature rather than the diaphragm. The most obvious sign of respiratory restriction would be splinting. Observe for any scars on the anterior abdominal wall indicating prior surgery or injury.

After inspection, auscultation is done with a stethoscope, with careful attention to peristaltic sounds. Palpation should be done only after auscultation is complete. It is preferable to begin in a quadrant "away" from the site of pain and proceed to examine the entire abdomen gently and in a manner reassuring to the patient. Children are frequently extremely difficult to examine. This may be eased by providing some distraction for the youngster.

Irritation of the parietal peritoneum causes involuntary rigidity of the muscles of the anterior abdominal wall, called "spasm." Voluntary rigidity is a result of the patient purposely splinting the abdominal musculature as a protective measure to lessen pain. Careful attention and experience will enable one to distinguish spasm from voluntary rigidity. In the former, there will be little variation in the tightness of the muscles during respiratory activity, while in the latter, muscle tone (rigidity) varies with respiration.

In the course of examining each quadrant, palpate carefully for tenderness and masses. Tenderness may be "direct" (that elicited in the area where the examining hand is) or "referred" (pressure at a remote point causes pain at another area). "Rebound" tenderness is present when pain is expressed by the patient on sudden release of the palpating hand. This invariably indicates peritoneal irritation. Pain elicited by coughing is also strong evidence of peritoneal irritation. Any palpable masses should be carefully evaluated as to size, shape, mobility by hand or respiratory activity, and whether or not it pulsates or transmits a pulsation.

Operative scars should be evaluated for sound healing or the presence of a defect or mass, which may be indicative of a hernia. Inguinal hernias are difficult to evaluate with the patient in the recumbent position, but the sites of both inguinal and femoral hernias must be evaluated for any abnormality. Pain, however, may preclude examining the patient in the upright position.

Pelvic examination in the female may be very helpful in evaluating abdominal symptoms and is necessary in a complete evaluation. Rectal examination of males and virginal females is also an important part of complete evaluation of the abdomen.

Adjunct studies

Routine blood and urine analysis should be ordered. Special biochemical tests, such as electrolyte levels, serum amylase, lipase and transaminase levels, are ordered as indicated to support a specific diagnosis. These will be discussed under each disease process.

Flat and upright x-rays of the abdomen may be helpful, especially in instances of suspected perforated viscera, intestinal obstruction or undiagnosed abdominal masses. In elderly or acutely ill patients unable to stand erect, lateral decubitus views may replace the upright film. Special studies, such as abdominal angiography or intravenous pyelography, are rarely required in the emergency department evaluation of an acute abdominal condition.

Peritoneal tap, peritoneal lavage and/or cul-de-sac aspiration may be needed to complete assessment of the patient with acute abdominal complaints.[3, 36] Equipment for these procedures should be available in the emergency department. They are all easily performed under local anesthesia. In aspirating or lavaging the peritoneal cavity, care must be taken to avoid operative scars, for laceration of the adherent bowel or omental vessels may result. Inadvertent puncture of the intestine, lying free in the abdominal cavity, is usually of no consequence.

Peritoneal tap should be done in the anterior abdominal wall, beyond the lateral borders of the rectus sheath, where large blood vessels are less liable to be encountered. A needle of sufficient length (a 4-inch spinal needle) should be used and inserted, with an obturator in place. The operator can usually identify when the peritoneum is punctured, because a small amount of resistance will be encountered and the patient may note some discomfort as the needle comes in contact with the peritoneum. With continued pressure, the needle then passes easily into the peritoneal cavity. At least a 10 cc. syringe should be attached, then gentle suction applied. If the tap is negative, it should be repeated in all quadrants. The aspirate should be examined microscopically if only a small amount is recovered. Some advocate peritoneal lavage with measured amounts of sterile saline, followed by laboratory examination of the aspirate.

Although some patients may have severe pain, narcotics should not be administered until abdominal assessment has been completed. The narcotic may mask important abdominal signs. Gentle technique and reassurance will help to allay fear until the examination is complete and appropriate medication can then be given.

Discussion of more specific details as to laboratory studies will be included with the specific disease coverage.

SPECIFIC CONDITIONS CAUSING AN ACUTE ABDOMEN

Perforated peptic ulcer

Perforation is one of the main complications of peptic ulcer and represents a most urgent indication for treatment.[13] It can occur wherever an ulcer may occur, in the esophagus, the stomach, the duodenum or at the site of a marginal ulcer, which may follow certain types of surgery for peptic ulcer.[10, 46]

Rupture of an esophageal ulcer is extremely rare and extremely difficult to diagnose. Symptoms may relate to the upper abdomen or lower retrosternal area, depending on the site of perforation.

Perforations of gastric or duodenal ulcers are much commoner, due to the higher incidence of ulcers in these locations. Most perforations occur in anterior wall ulcers and allow egress of air and gastric and intestinal content into the peritoneal cavity. The highly acid content is extremely irritating to the peritoneum and causes a "chemical" peritonitis, with outpouring of peritoneal fluid.[42] As hours pass, secondary bacterial contamination of the fluid may occur and a purulent peritonitis develop. This is an extremely serious complication, which may produce hypovolemic shock due to the outpouring of body fluid into the peritoneal cavity and subsequent diminution of circulating blood volume.[20] These patients are critically ill on admission to the emergency department, and prompt resuscitative measures are necessary.

Assessment

History and physical assessment are extremely important in diagnosis. The onset of pain is usually sudden. The pain is described as severe, sharp and constant and located in the upper abdomen. About 70 percent of patients will give a history of prior ulcer activity or use of antacids; thus 30 percent may have no previous ulcer symptoms. These statistics are important; they stress the value of assessment.

Physical assessment will often reveal restricted diaphragmatic activity. The abdomen demonstrates board-like rigidity due to spasm of the anterior abdominal muscles. The spasm is primarily in the upper abdomen, more often on the right side because of the location of the duodenum. Perforated gastric ulcers in the antral portion of the stomach may also exhibit findings in this area. Peristalsis is diminished or absent.

Vital signs should be noted and recorded, along with evaluation of the patient's general condition. Thirst and poor skin turgor indicate dehydration and a decrease in circulating blood volume. Blood samples are drawn for complete blood count and electrolyte determination. Baseline arterial blood gas levels may be helpful in future management. Flat and upright x-ray examination of the abdomen may demonstrate free air in 50 to 80 percent of cases (see Figure 20–3). In the critically ill or debilitated, lateral decubitus films taken with the patient lying on the left side will show free air, when present, above the lateral edge of the liver shadow (Figure 20–4).

Management

Intravenous fluid replacement should be instituted promptly, using glucose in saline or a balanced salt solution. Antibiotics are not required for chemical peritonitis but are necessary when bacterial contamination is suspected. A nasogastric tube is inserted and, after aspiration of gastric content, placed on intermittent suction to prevent further spillage into the peritoneal cavity. Peritoneal tap is unnecessary, except when the diagnosis is not clear.

The treatment of choice for perforated ulcer is surgery.[7, 8, 27, 43] Preliminary resuscitation in the emergency department is directed toward stabilizing the patient by restoring circulating blood volume. The most common surgical procedure is simple closure of the leaking ulcer and cleansing of the peritoneal cavity.[42] Definitive ulcer surgery may not be

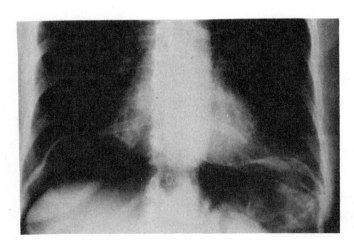

Figure 20–3 Upright film of abdomen in patient with perforated peptic ulcer. A large amount of free air is seen beneath each diaphragm.

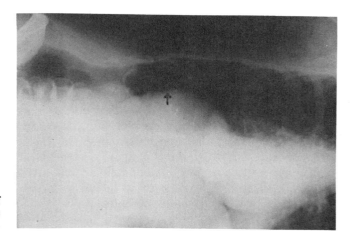

Figure 20–4 Lateral decubitus x-ray of abdomen. This x-ray demonstrates free air above the liver shadow (see arrow).

indicated until a later date, several weeks to months after simple closure. Primary gastric resection for perforated ulcer has been performed with a very acceptable morbidity and mortality rate.[24, 29, 38] However, indications for this procedure are limited by very strict criteria, including the availability of a capable surgical team.

Rupture of the spleen

Although rupture of the spleen is covered thoroughly in Chapter 19 in relation to trauma, patients with splenic rupture due to other causes may be seen in the emergency department with no history of trauma, per se.

Diseases causing splenomegaly (enlargement of the spleen) often result in rupture of this organ.[28, 34] Delayed rupture (weeks to months after initial trauma) may occur in instances of splenic injury resulting in a splenic hematoma. Internal rupture of the spleen, causing bleeding within an intact capsule, may go unrecognized until rupture of the capsule occurs, with bleeding into the free peritoneal cavity. Spontaneous rupture may also occur, frequently associated with straining or with increases in abdominal pressure.

The history will show that the patient noted a sudden onset of abdominal pain, usually in the left upper quadrant and lower left chest, posterolaterally. Pain might also be referred to the area of the left shoulder because of diaphragmatic irritation (Kehr's sign). In the patient with delayed rupture, the history may not reveal the original trauma.

Clinically, the patient will exhibit signs of pain and blood loss, pallor and tachycardia. Abdominal findings will relate to peritoneal irritation by blood, primarily including tenderness and spasm, especially in the left upper quadrant area. In the absence of a history of trauma, rupture of the spleen may not be seriously considered, but tests should be made to confirm any diagnosis.

Peritoneal tap is an easily performed and extremely helpful measure.[3, 40] Recovery of fresh blood that does not clot is pathognomonic of intraperitoneal hemorrhage and mandates surgery. Provision should be made to have an adequate amount of whole blood available for replacement and the patient prepared for surgery as soon as possible.

Acute biliary tract disease

Acute biliary tract disease includes acute diseases of the gallbladder and bile ducts, which may be difficult to distinguish. It is also important to differentiate inflammatory processes from those due to colic. Acute disease of the gallbladder may be inflammatory in nature (acute cholecystitis) or due to colic (acute biliary colic). Inflammation of bile ducts is termed acute cholangitis.

Acute cholecystitis

Acute cholecystitis is invariably associated with gallstones.[1, 14] The stones may produce a partial or complete obstruction of the outflow duct of the gallbladder (the cystic duct). This then causes an increase in intraluminal pressure and edema in the area of obstruction. As the process continues, the small veins of the gallbladder wall become obstructed, finally blocking the arterial supply. This is associated with swelling of the gallbladder wall. The process proceeds to gangrene in 10 to 15 percent of cases (see Figure 20–5) and may proceed to perforation of the gallbladder, if allowed to continue unabated.[37, 41] These are serious, sometimes fatal complications.

Gallbladder disease occurs much more commonly in women. Acute cholecystitis may occur in the absence of gallstones but is quite unusual. When it does occur, however, this form of the disease is more common in men than in women. Many texts will describe the typical gallbladder patient as "fair, fat

and forty, female and fertile." Nothing could be further from the truth.

History may be very helpful in distinguishing gallbladder disease from other problems, especially ulcer. The patient will frequently give a history of food intolerance, with varying degrees of discomfort, abdominal fullness and pain following ingestion of greasy, fried or fatty foods. The pain may last varying periods of time. A history of prior x-ray studies demonstrating abnormal gallbladder function or presence of stones may be obtained.

The pain of acute cholecystitis is typically located in the right upper quadrant, near the costal margin. As the serosal surface of the gallbladder is involved in the process, the pain may radiate around the chest to the tip of the right scapula, due to irritation of the eighth intercostal nerve. Less commonly, pain may be referred to the right shoulder, if the undersurface of the diaphragm is irritated. The pain is constant and may be aggravated by intra-abdominal pressure, coughing, straining and deep breathing.

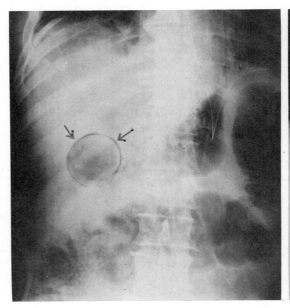 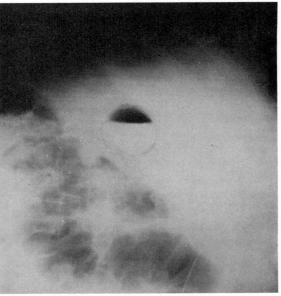

Figure 20–5   Two x-rays of a patient with gallbladder disease. Left: Abdominal x-ray, showing a "halo" around the gallbladder, characteristic of gangrenous emphysematous cholecystitis. Note also the distended intestine (ileus). Right: Lateral decubitus x-ray showing the air-fluid level in the gallbladder.

Physical assessment may reveal diminished respiratory activity, especially on the right side, with diminished breath sounds over the lower lung field. Abdominal findings are usually quite well localized to the right upper quadrant, with tenderness and spasm of the right upper rectus muscle. If the gallbladder is distended, careful palpation may reveal the pressure of a globular mass. In 25 percent of patients, the mass will be respiratory mobile (moving gently with respiration). The mass indicates complete obstruction of the gallbladder and is indicative of hydrops (benign obstruction, white bile) or empyema (purulent bile). These complications are usually accompanied by fever and leukocytosis, and in empyema, the patient may appear toxic.

To differentiate acute cholecystitis from other acute upper abdominal diseases, blood work should include a complete blood count and serum amylase. Acute cholecystitis may also be associated with mild icterus. If this is suspected, serum bilirubin and transaminase may be obtained. Serum amylase may be elevated but rarely in a significant range. Flat and upright films of the abdomen may be helpful in identifying calculi in the right upper quadrant, but this is not a frequent occurrence. Differential diagnosis includes acute pancreatitis, pyelonephritis, acute peptic ulcer and hepatitis.

Managment of patients with acute cholecystitis depends on their general condition and physical findings. Once the examination of the abdomen has been completed, appropriate doses of meperidine (Demerol) or morphine should be given for pain relief. A nasogastric tube should be inserted if the patient is vomiting and intravenous fluids begun. Urgent surgery is indicated in the presence of a palpable mass found in the right upper quadrant or if perforation of the gallbladder is suspected. Otherwise, the patient should be admitted to the hospital for further observation, study and elective surgery.

The surgical treatment of choice is complete removal of the gallbladder (cholecystectomy). In elderly, debilitated or critically ill patients, it may be too major a procedure, and simple drainage of the gallbladder with removal of stones (cholecystostomy) is indicated. If necessary, cholecystostomy may be carried out under local anesthesia. The morbidity and mortality of acute biliary tract disease is significant and, interestingly, higher for cholecystostomy than cholecystectomy. This seeming paradox may be explained by the fact that drainage procedures are used primarily in the more critically ill patients.

Acute biliary colic

Acute biliary colic also occurs in the presence of gallstones. The onset of pain is abrupt and frequently associated with emesis. It is not necessarily associated with food intake, but it may occur at anytime, even in the middle of the night, awakening the patient from sleep. The pain may persist for varying periods of time, from minutes to hours and typically stops as abruptly as it began.

A past history of biliary calculi is helpful in identifying this condition. Physical assessment may reveal surprisingly minimal findings, though tenderness may be present in the right upper quadrant. Routine blood and urine examinations should be made, as well as x-rays of the abdomen, looking for calculi.

Management usually consists of pain relief by parenteral narcotics, meperidine (Demerol) or morphine most often used. This treatment will be effective in the vast majority of cases. However, admission is frequently necessary because of the severity of pain during acute attacks. Nasogastric suction may result in more rapid dissolution of pain. Surgery is deferred until diagnosis can be definitely established by oral cholecystography. It may then be performed electively, as frequency and severity of the colic episodes are unpredictable.

Acute cholangitis

Acute cholangitis refers to an inflammation of the extrahepatic bile ducts, particularly the common bile duct. This is a serious problem, usually caused by duct obstruction with secondary infection. In most patients, obstruction is associated with the presence of stones in the common duct.[18]

Clinically, the patient is acutely ill with pain and has a systemic reaction of fever, chills, jaundice and right upper quadrant pain. Marked toxicity may be present due to severe systemic reaction. Fever is usually high, 104 to 105° F. The history confirms the above symptoms; a prior history of gallbladder disease is frequently obtained. If the inflammatory process is severe, shock and prostration may occur.

Physical assessment reveals acute tenderness in the right upper quadrant, with rigidity or spasm. The liver may be palpably enlarged and tender. Diagnostic studies should include tests for serum bilirubin, transaminases and alkaline phosphatase, all of which are elevated in acute cholangitis. Serum amylase may also be abnormal. Blood cultures should be made and sensitivity studies carried out. Invariably, these are positive, the most common organism being of the coliform group.

Massive doses of appropriate antibiotics given during intravenous fluid replacement should be started. When the patient's condition is stable, prompt surgical exploration of the biliary tract for relief of the obstruction is indicated.

Acute pancreatitis

An acute inflammatory condition of the pancreas may occur with varying degrees of severity.[25] The disease is usually associated with either biliary tract disease, alcoholism or both.[31] The conditions leading to onset of the disease process are related to duct obstruction combined with stimulation of pancreatic enzymes, resulting in autodigestion of the pancreas. Opie advanced the "common channel" theory,[34] postulating that the pancreatic duct entered the common bile duct and formed a "common channel" and that obstruction of this common channel results in regurgitation of bile into the pancreatic duct, activating the enzymes produced by the pancreas and resulting in irritation of the pancreatic tissues. Pancreatic juice comprises several enzymes which are inactive until contact has been made with bile.

The obstruction of the common channel may be due to biliary tract stones or due to overstimulation of pancreatic enzymes by alcohol. The mechanism of alcoholic pancreatitis is not clear but is thought to be associated with stimulation of gastric acid, which may activate formation of pancreatic juice, with local irritation and edema of the duodenum (duodenitis) about the entry of the duct into the bowel at the sphincter of Oddi. Less commonly, pancreatitis may be associated with acute mumps, morphinism and the effects of some other drugs.

Once the pancreatic process is established, it results in digestion of the pancreas in varying degrees of severity, then in outpouring of fluid into the retroperitoneal space and even into the abdominal (peritoneal) cavity. This outpouring of fluid, when large, may result in hypovolemia and shock, often refractory to treatment.[2, 12] Pancreatic enzymes may be found in high concentration in the peritoneal fluid. They combine with the fat tissue in the omentum and mesentery, causing saponification of the fat, seen as local areas of fat necrosis. This process, if severe enough, lowers the serum calcium to dangerous levels (less than 7 mg. percent), with resultant tetany.

Acute pancreatitis may thus develop into a mild type (acute edematous pancreatitis) or an extremely severe, highly fatal type (acute hemorrhagic pancreatitis).

Assessment

The history is usually one of severe upper abdominal pain which penetrates ("bores") directly through to the back. Less commonly, it radiates "around" one or both costal margins. The pain is constant, severe and associated with emesis. The patient may give a history of excessive alcoholic intake or dietary excess prior to the onset of symptoms. In others, symptoms compatible with biliary tract disease may be present. There may also be a history of pain associated with jaundice. Acute pancreatitis is more commonly seen in males than in females.

Physical assessment reveals the patient to be acutely ill. In more severe stages of the process, he may be febrile, toxic, in peripheral vascular collapse. The abdomen is acutely tender, especially in the upper quadrants, with spasm and/or rigidity. Rebound tenderness is present. Peristalsis may be diminished or absent. In instances of hemorrhagic pancreatitis, ecchymoses may be noted in the flanks (Grey-Turner sign). As the pathologic process continues, severe hypovolemia may develop, the patient appearing dehydrated and in shock.

Blood samples should be drawn for complete blood count, amylase content, serum bilirubin and transaminase. Serum electrolyte determinations, especially of calcium and phosphorus should be done, and if hypocalcemia is noted, replacement must be begun. Diabetes is a rare complication of pancreatitis, more often found in patients with chronic recurrent pancreatitis.

Peritoneal tap is helpful in confirming a diagnosis of acute pancreatitis. In acute edematous pancreatitis, the peritoneal fluid is opalescent and may contain fat droplets. In more severe processes, bloody fluid may be recovered. Amylase levels should be measured in the peritoneal fluid.

X-rays of the abdomen may be nondiagnostic but may exhibit signs of an ileus. Calcific densities in the area of the pancreas are strongly confirmatory of the disease. Occasionally a so-called "sentinel loop" may be visualized on x-ray. This is a loop of jejunum in the area of the pancreas which may dilate as a result of the nearby inflammatory process.

Differential diagnosis includes perforated ulcer, acute cholecystitis and mesenteric vascular occlusion.

Management

Management is directed toward resuscitation and pain relief. Choice of narcotics for pain control is important, since morphine, which is known to cause spasm of the sphincter of Oddi and pancreatitis, is usually contraindicated. Meperidine hydrochloride (Demerol), in adequate amounts, is usually sufficient. Nasogastric suction will reduce pancreatic secretion by drawing off gastric juice. Fluid replacement is instituted with Ringer's lactate, initially, and with blood, subsequently.

Urgent surgery is indicated in acute pancreatitis associated with jaundice and in acute hemorrhagic pancreatitis.[19] Surgical therapy is directed toward decompression of the biliary duct system via cholecystostomy or choledochostomy. In hemorrhagic pancreatitis, multiple incision in the retroperitoneal area may be needed to decompress the pancreas itself. Massive blood loss may occur in this instance. More commonly, the patient is treated with fluids, nasogastric suction and narcotics and admitted for further evaluation and treatment. When the acute process has subsided, thorough investigation of the biliary system is indicated. In the presence of associated biliary tract disease, definitive management is directed toward correction.

Patients with pancreatitis secondary to alcoholism are extremely difficult to cure and have a poor prognosis. Such patients may be seen time and again in the emergency department with recurring episodes of acute pancreatitis. The incidence of drug addiction in these individuals is significant, and many admittedly continue to consume large amounts of alcohol, because during that time, they may achieve some amelioration of symptoms. In general, alcoholic pancreatitis is refractory to cure.

Recurrent pancreatitis is common in patients who have not had definitive treatment. Each acute recurrent episode may produce more scarring in the pancreas, which may eventually lead to chronic pancreatitis and to pancreatic insufficiency, in which both the exocrine and endocrine functions of the pancreas may be seriously impaired, causing malabsorption, steatorrhea and diabetes.

Acute appendicitis

Acute appendicitis is the most common cause of the acute abdomen. It is regarded by many as a minor problem, but even with the advances in medicine and surgery to date, a certain number of patients will succumb to acute appendicitis and/or its complications.[44]

Appendicitis usually results from an obstructive process in the appendix. The appendix is attached to the cecum, at the lower end of the ascending colon, in the right lower quadrant. It is a hollow, long organ, its lumen ordinarily connecting with that of the cecum and its walls containing the various coats of the intestine. The obstruction may be due to a foreign body (toothpick, bone, fruit seed) or, more likely, to a fecalith or piece of inspissated feces. The obstruction blocks the lumen of the organ and initiates an inflammatory reaction characterized initially by swelling, then progressing to vascular congestion, impairment of arterial blood supply, gangrene and perforation. The perforation may be walled off and form an abscess or may occur free in the peritoneal cavity, resulting in generalized peritonitis.

Anatomically, the appendix may be in one of many positions; thus clinical findings may vary. It may lie lateral to the cecum, in the colic gutter (retrocecal appendix), or medially over the course of the ureter or the brim of the pelvis, in contact with the bladder in the male or the bladder and reproductive organs in the female (pelvic appendix). (See Figure 20–6.) As a result of these varying positions, acute inflammatory conditions of the appendix may mimic a number of other conditions causing acute abdominal pain. For example, appendicitis must be distinguished from acute gallbladder disease, perforated ulcer, acute pancreatitis, twisted or ruptured ovarian cysts and acute urinary tract disorders. The disease may occur at any age and has no predilection for sex.

Assessment

Although all textbooks record a typical history of acute appendicitis, most patients have not read these and will relate a wide variety of symptoms via history. The common denominator is pain. This may be described in a number of ways, usually initially as a vague discomfort or "belly ache" in the region of the umbilicus. At this stage, there may be a feeling of nausea and anorexia. As the inflammatory reaction involves the serosa of the appendix, the pain will shift to the area

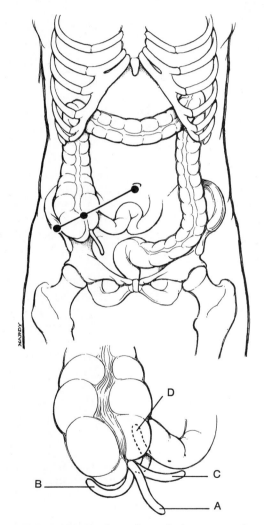

Figure 20–6 Location of the cecum in relation to McBurney's point. Appendix A is in the common location, extending from the cecum. Areas B, C and D represent other common locations of the appendix, lateral, medial, or retrocecal in position.

of irritation, usually in the right lower quadrant, commonly known as "McBurney's point."

McBurney's point is found by drawing an imaginary line from the right anterior superior iliac spine to the umbilicus; it is at the junction of the lateral and middle thirds (Figure 20–7). This anatomical point is of diagnostic value when the appendix is in juxtaposition to it. However, in retrocecal or pelvic appendicitis, the pain may be localized to the flank or iliac fossa.

The pain is constant and may radiate to the flank area, especially in the retrocecal position. It may be aggravated by walking, straining, coughing. As time passes, anorexia becomes more striking, and forced feeding may result in emesis. The inflammatory process may develop in a matter of hours and usually results in worsening of symptoms and continued pain. Occasionally, with rupture of the appendix, the patient may note lessening of the pain and feel better, only to develop more severe pain as generalized peritonitis develops.

In female patients it is particularly important to elicit a menstrual history. Pain from ruptured follicle cysts of the ovary (mittelschmerz) may be indistinguishable from pain from appendicitis.

Physical assessment must be done carefully. The patient may appear acutely ill, particularly if he is in the pediatric age group.[23] The patient will lie quite still on the examining table, reluctant to move. It is not unusual to find the right thigh flexed to lessen intra-abdominal pressure and decrease pain. Evaluation of the abdominal findings may be particularly difficult in the very young and very old.[23, 45, 47] It is not unusual for patients in these age groups to develop complications (perforation with abscess or peritonitis).

The most common findings in appendicitis are tenderness and spasm in the right lower quadrant. Referred pain may be elicited by palpation over the left colon; the pressure may be transmitted to the right side. In addition, rebound tenderness is invariably present, both local and referred. Rectal examina-

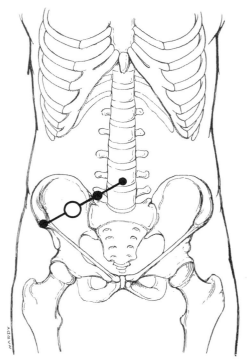

Figure 20–7   McBurney's point. The characteristic area of tenderness is in the right lower quadrant in a patient with acute appendicitis. This anatomical landmark is located at the junction of the lateral and middle thirds of an imaginary line drawn between the umbilicus and the anterior superior iliac spine.

tion in males and virginal females is helpful in localizing the site to the right lower quadrant. In females, tenderness in the area of the uterine adnexae or on motion of the cervix may indicate primary pelvic disease, although the possibility of the inflamed appendix lying in close proximity to the pelvic organs must be considered. In complicated appendicitis, a mass may be palpated in the right lower quadrant.

Complete blood count may reveal a leukocytosis with a left shift—an increase in the number of immature neutrophiles (band forms). Microscopic examination of the urine is important; usually it will be negative. However, when the inflamed appendix overlies the right ureter, a significant number of red and white cells may be found in the urine. Urinary tract symptoms of dysuria or frequency are usually absent in appendicitis, unless the organ overlies the dome of the urinary bladder. X-rays of the abdomen are usually nondiagnostic and are rarely indicated.

Differential diagnosis includes almost any intra-abdominal condition: mittelschmerz, ectopic pregnancy, gastroenteritis. In the pediatric age group, mesenteric lymphadenitis may occur, usually in conjunction with or subsequent to an acute upper respiratory infection, and the signs and symptoms may be indistinguishable from acute appendicitis.[26] Acute mesenteric lymphadenitis involves acute inflammatory changes in the lymph nodes of the mesentery of the small bowel and appendix. Careful attention to physical assessment may allow detection of more generalized abdominal tenderness (not limited to the right lower quadrant), and when the patient shifts position from side to side, a change in location of the pain may be observed.

Management

Management of acute appendicitis consists of preparing the patient for surgical removal of the appendix. In adolescent females, when it is impossible to distinguish appendicitis from ruptured follicle cysts and mesenteric adenitis, a decision must be made by weighing the possibility of complications arising from surgery in the face of an incorrect diagnosis, i.e., a delay in surgery in the face of a *possible* appendicitis. In most instances, it is much safer for the patient to elect surgery. The patient and her family should be advised both of the possibility of error in these instances and of the need for no further delay.

The patient with complicated appendicitis and long-standing symptoms may be toxic and critically ill. Fluid replacement and stabilization of his general condition may be necessary before moving the patient to the operating suite. The very old patient may be too ill to undergo surgery, and aggressive nonoperative management, consisting of fluid replacement, massive doses of antibiotics and nasogastric intubation, may be necessary.

Diverticulitis

Often referred to as "left-sided appendicitis," diverticulitis occurs in any segment of the intestine but most commonly in the colon. Similarly, diverticula and the benign, noninflammatory condition, diverticulosis, occur throughout the colon and are found most frequently in the sigmoid portion of the colon. A diverticulum is a solitary outpouching, which develops especially along the tenia of the colon. Diverticula seem to localize in groups on the area of the bowel wall where the blood vessels enter, producing an area of weakness. They are acquired and are found in the course of barium enema studies in nearly 50 percent of persons over the age of 40.[11]

Diverticulosis is a relatively asymptomatic condition; however, inflammation can occur, from inspissated feces or food content within the diverticulum. If it does not drain properly, local swelling and edema follow, and the inflammatory process continues, resulting in diverticulitis. Diverticulitis is fairly common in persons over 50. The pathologic process varies with the degree of inflammation, involving a single diverticulum or an entire segment of colon. Due to the inflammatory process, local spasm occurs, and a low-grade obstruction develops, manifested by pain. As the process continues, the complication of rupture with abscess may occur. The rupture may be walled off by omentum or an adjacent segment of bowel or, less commonly, may occur free into the peritoneal cavity. The abscess will often be walled off but may enlarge and extend into the pelvis. In cases of longer duration, abnormal communications (fistulae) may be established with the bladder (colovesical fistula) or with the vagina (colovaginal fistula).

Assessment

History may reveal some problems with constipation. The acute process is marked by the onset of pain in the area of inflammation, usually the left lower quadrant. If the inflammatory reaction is mild, the pain may be felt by the patient as a "cramp"; however, as the reaction worsens, the pain becomes more severe and constant. Local pain results from involvement of the parietal peritoneum. Without treatment, the patient will report developing fever and chills, and as the obstruction element increases, abdominal distention is coincident with constipation and lack of flatus.

The patient may also relate a prior history of chronic "bowel problems" and perhaps had a barium enema which demonstrated the condition. If fistulae to the bladder or vagina have occurred, the patient may state he or she has passed "wind" from the bladder and "wind" or stool vaginally. Rectal bleeding is uncommon in this condition.[5]

Physical findings will vary with the degree of inflammatory reaction, from mild tenderness in the left lower quadrant or iliac fossa to exquisite tenderness with spasm and rigidity, signs of peritoneal irritation. The abdomen may be distended and tympanitic to percussion. In patients with perforation and abscess, a mass may be palpable. Rectal examination may outline a cul-de-sac mass, indicative of a pelvic abscess. Complete blood count frequently demonstrates a leukocytosis with left shift. X-rays of the abdomen may be nondiagnostic, or upright films may show free air in the presence of perforation or outline a pelvic mass.

Management

Management will depend on the severity of the process. In mild cases with minimal findings, the patient may not require admission but should be placed on analgesics, stool softeners and medication to reduce the bacteria in the gut. An important part of the treatment is a low-residue diet. When the acute findings subside and the tenderness is no longer found, a barium enema may be ordered to confirm the diagnosis. These patients may be managed nonoperatively but require advice on diet.

In more complicated cases, with evidence of peritoneal irritation, obstruction or perforation, admission to the hospital is indicated, and urgent surgery may be necessary.[39] Some patients may be dehydrated, and fluid replacement is in order before surgery. Surgical management is directed toward diversion of the fecal stream by proximal colostomy and to drainage of an abscess, if present. Proximal colostomy vents the colon upstream from the level of inflammation and diverts feces from continued contamination of the involved segment. Primary resection is hazardous as an emergency procedure because of the lack of bowel sterilization. It may result in unnecessary morbidity and mortality.

Definitive surgery, removal of the diseased area, is done electively weeks to months after the colostomy, when the acute process has subsided and the surgeon may proceed safely. Following resection, the colostomy is closed to restore bowel continuity. Sigmoidoscopy is rarely necessary as an adjunct to the diagnosis of diverticulitis in the emergency setting. If it is thought necessary, caution is advised. Use of air insufflation to distend the colon is contraindicated.

Differential diagnosis includes carcinoma, urinary tract problems and appendicitis. Diverticulitis and carcinoma of the colon both occur most commonly in the sigmoid area. They may be present simultaneously and differentiation may be difficult or impossible.[30] Occasionally, in patients with acute pancreatitis, the intraperitoneal fluid may drain along the colic gutter and mimic diverticulitis.

Obstructions of the gastrointestinal tract

Mechanical obstruction

Mechanical obstruction may occur in any segment of the gastrointestinal tract. Etiologic factors include inflammatory or cicatricial scarring, as in peptic ulcer or regional enteritis, adhesion bonds, intussusception and neoplasms of the bowel.[25]

In patients with obstructive disease, severe

depletion or alteration of body fluid and electrolytes may develop. These abnormalities result from vomiting of gastric or intestinal fluids and from sequestration of electrolyte-containing fluid in the lumen of the stomach or intestine. Obstruction in the stomach or high in the small bowel causes loss of potassium and chloride ions. Obstruction lower in the small intestine may cause depletion of potassium and sodium. The degree of depletion will depend to a great extent on the duration of the obstruction.

In addition to loss of electrolytes, mild to severe fluid loss also occurs, resulting in further alterations in acid-base balance. Thus, patients with obstructions are dehydrated, may have scant urinary output and exhibit thirst and poor skin turgor. Severe contraction of circulating blood volume may result in vascular collapse.

Pyloric obstruction

Pyloric obstruction is that occurring at the lower end of the stomach or first part of the duodenum. It is most often due to the scarring of chronic active peptic ulcer, but in the older age group, especially those over 50 or 60, it may be due to carcinoma of the stomach or, less often, the pancreas. Pain is not too common, but the patient will relate a history of postprandial fullness, followed by vomiting of undigested food. As the obstruction becomes more long-standing, the stomach compensates by enlarging, and emesis may not occur until several hours after food intake. Weight loss may be noted, especially in neoplastic disease. Careful questioning may elicit a history compatible with ulcer. Prior upper gastrointestinal studies may confirm the diagnosis of preexisting ulcer disease.

Patients with pyloric obstruction usually appear chronically ill and thin. Skin turgor will be poor and eyes sunken. Physical examination may demonstrate a soft mass in the epigastric area, which is the dilated stomach. With patient observation, peristaltic waves may be seen on the anterior abdominal wall. By placing a stethoscope over the area and gently but firmly shaking the patient from side to side, a "succussion splash" may be heard, due to the splashing of gastric content back and forth within the stomach. Evidence of vascular collapse may be noted.

Electrolyte studies are mandatory, to establish baseline determinations and evaluate the degree of variation from normal. Hydrochloric acid content of the stomach should be determined. Patients with active ulcer disease ordinarily have a high gastric acidity. The most striking electrolyte deficit will be a marked lowering of the chloride and potassium ions (hypochloremic alkalosis), with an accompanied rise in serum bicarbonate or carbon dioxide ions. Patients in the seventh decade commonly have lower levels of hydrochloric acid in the stomach and may not demonstrate this severe loss of chloride ion. Loss of total fluid will cause contraction of blood volume and evidence of hemoconcentration.

The patient's general status should be evaluated. If the diagnosis is questioned, an upper gastrointestinal series will be diagnostic.

Emergency management consists of decompression of the stomach by continuous nasogastric suction and restoration of circulating blood volume and electrolyte levels to normal limits. The stomach may contain large pieces of undigested food which may plug the nasogastric tube. In such cases, gastric lavage by an Ewald tube, which can be swallowed easily through the mouth, is an effective means of cleansing the stomach.

Further management is directed toward restoring the patient's normal physiology in preparation for early surgery. Surgical treatment should be planned within 48 hours of admission to prevent further depletion of fluids and electrolytes. Nonoperative management will result in some improvement, but on discontinuance of nasogastric decompression, recurrent obstruction is common.

Small intestine obstruction

Obstruction of the small intestine may occur at any site in the small bowel. Obstruction in the proximal small bowel (duodenum or jejunum) is present more often with history of emesis, while those lower in the ileum cause distention of the obstructed bowel, with emesis occurring later in the course of the disease. The effects may be the same regardless of the level of obstruction.

Ordinarily, in a healthy individual 7,000 to 8,000 cc. of fluid, rich in electrolytes, enters the gut each 24 hour period. With obstruction, sequestration and vomiting both cause loss of fluid. As the bowel distends, fluid may be lost into the peritoneal cavity, adding to further depletion of extracellular fluid volume. As the obstructive process is allowed to continue, the intestinal wall becomes edematous, and bacteria may proliferate in the gut. This increased intraluminal pressure may then produce venous and, later, arterial obstruction, which compromise the blood supply and may lead to strangulation of the intestine. Prolongation then causes perforation and spillage of contents into the peritoneum, resulting in a severe chemical and/or bacterial peritonitis.

History will include vomiting and/or distention. Pain may be noted at the site of obstruction, crampy in nature and with crescendos occurring with peristaltic waves. Small bowel obstruction is most often due to adhesion bonds from prior surgical entry into the peritoneal cavity, but there may be other causes, such as acute appendicitis, regional enteritis, complicated hernia, intussusception or mesenteric occlusion.[21]

Assessment may reveal an incisional scar, associated with abdominal distention. Auscultation should be done carefully. Hyperactive bowel sounds may be heard, along with peristaltic rushes and borborygmi,* which are often heard without need of a stethoscope. The patient may complain of pain coincident with the peristaltic rush. Severe or generalized tenderness may indicate impairment of blood supply to the intestine (strangulation obstruction).

Serum electrolyte levels should be established on admission. X-rays of the abdomen

should be done in the flat and upright or lateral decubitus position. Multiple fluid levels and a characteristic "stepladder" pattern may be seen in the upright or decubitus film. (See Figures 20–8 and 20–9.)

Initial management relates to intestinal decompression by nasogastric or long intestinal tube (Miller-Abbott or Cantor), concomitant with aggressive fluid and electrolyte replacement. Urine output should be monitored. Of singular importance is the determination of vascular occlusion or strangulation obstruction. These conditions require emergency surgical intervention after the patient's condition has been stabilized. Their presence is heralded by physical findings of peritoneal irritation, while the ordinary "bland" mechan-

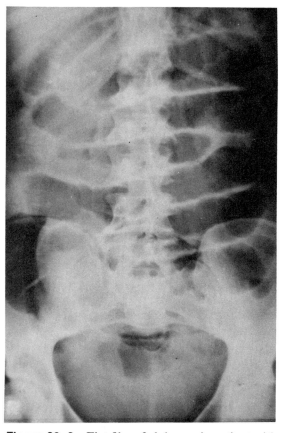

Figure 20–8 Flat film of abdomen in patient with small bowel obstruction. The small bowel is distended and in the characteristic stepladder pattern of obstruction.

* Borborygmi: Sounds of flatus in the intestines.

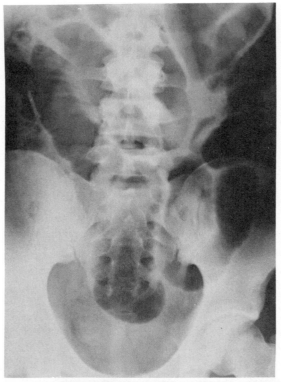

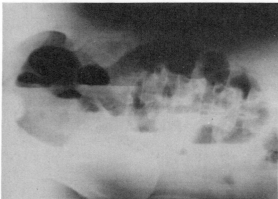

Figure 20–9 Flat and lateral decubitus x-rays of abdomen. Top: Flat film demonstrates large dilated loops of small bowel. Bottom: Lateral decubitus film shows multiple fluid levels in small bowel.

ical obstruction usually is not. Surgical care involves release of the obstruction. In patients with irreversible damage to the blood supply of the intestine, removal of the involved segment and restoration of intestinal continuity is the surgical approach of choice. Antibiotic coverage is indicated in patients with intestinal obstruction.

Certain disease states, such as pneumonia, septicemia, pyelonephritis, renal colic and hip fracture, may simulate a mechanical obstruction, called "paralytic ileus." Paralytic ileus results from interference with the autonomic nerves supplying the intestine, leading to decreased or absent peristaltic activity. It usually occurs in both the small and large bowels and has a characteristic x-ray pattern.[17] Differential diagnosis is important.

Intussusception

Intussusception occurs when a proximal segment of the bowel telescopes or invaginates into a distal segment. It may be small bowel into small bowel (ileo-ileal), small bowel into colon (ileocolic) or colon into colon (colocolic). The most frequently occurring is the ileocolic type. This condition usually occurs in the very young, in the first year of life and, less frequently, in the very old. The cause is not always apparent. Enlarged lymph follicles in the intestinal wall[32] or occasionally a polyp or Meckel's diverticulum may form the starting point for the process.

The history of intussusception in a child is readily characteristic. It is marked by sudden "spasm," with an outcry or screaming. The infant may draw its legs up and emesis may occur. The diaper may be blood-stained and contain stool of the "currant jelly" type. Physical assessment may reveal a void in the right lower quadrant and a mass along the course of the colon.

Gentle barium enema is very useful to confirm the diagnosis and is sometimes used therapeutically to reduce the intussusception. It is difficult to be certain that the reduction is complete, though, and operative intervention is usually needed to insure complete reduction. The intussusception should be reduced manually and the bowel carefully examined for compromise of blood supply. Recurrence is unusual.

Large intestine obstruction

Obstruction of the colon is usually neoplastic or inflammatory in origin. Inflammatory conditions are primarily related to complications of diverticulitis and usually occur in the left side of the colon. Malignant neoplasms causing obstruction are most often of the "napkin ring" type, which is a lesion growing circumferentially around the colon, producing a gradual and eventually complete obstruction of the bowel.[6] An infrequent cause is volvulus of the sigmoid colon due to torsion of this segment of the bowel.[16, 22]

In malignant lesions, the history will relate bowel irregularity, with alternating constipation and diarrhea, and a narrowing of stool diameter to "pencil" size. Distention will vary, depending on the duration of obstruction. Intraluminal sequestration of fluid leads to dehydration and electrolyte imbalance. Pain is not usually a significant complaint.

Physical assessment should determine the integrity of the ileocecal valve by measuring the extent of distention. If the valve is incompetent, the fecal contents will back up into the small bowel. Late in the course, fecal emesis will be noted. In x-rays of the abdomen, the colon appears enlarged (Figure 20–10).

Managment consists of nasogastric intubation and fluid replacement. X-ray evidence of distention of the colon in excess of 8 to 10 cm. in diameter is an indication for emergency surgical decompression of the colon by proximal transverse colostomy. If the patient's condition is too critical, tube cecostomy may be carried out under local anesthesia. Excessive distention can result in focal gangrenous change in the part, with perforation and massive peritoneal contamination. Delayed, elective resection of the obstructed segment is performed when the patient's condition allows, 2 to 3 weeks after the decompressive procedure and following thorough evaluation of the patient.

Volvulus can usually be reduced in the emergency department, by proctoscopy and

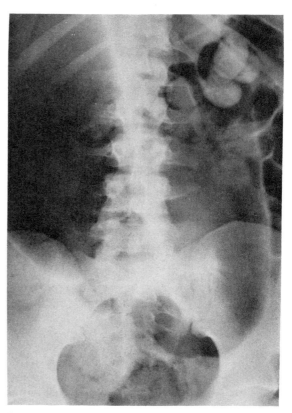

Figure 20–10 Upright film of lower colon obstruction. Note the massive enlargement of the cecum on the right side of photo.

insertion of a well-lubricated rectal tube. When reduction is impossible or evidence of infarction of the bowel is present, however, operative intervention is necessary.[22] (See Figure 20–11.)

Complicated hernias

External hernia may occur in one of several locations. The most common hernias are: (1) inguinal, (2) femoral, (3) ventral incisional and (4) spigelian. The hernia sac may contain a variety of intraperitoneal structures, such as the omentum, small bowel, colon, appendix or ovary. Hernias are not emergent conditions unless complications ensue. The 2 most common complications that may require emergency care are: (1) incarceration and (2) strangulation.

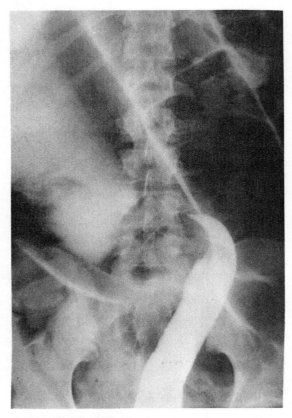

Figure 20–11 Emergency barium enema in a patient with sigmoid volvulus. Note the typical "bird beak" deformity of the rectosigmoid at the level of obstruction. Patient treated by sigmoid resection after an unsuccessful attempt to reduce by sigmoidoscopy.

In uncomplicated situations, the hernia is reducible, i.e., the protruding sac may be replaced into the peritoneal cavity when intra-abdominal pressure is decreased, as in the recumbent position with the knees flexed. With incarceration, the hernia mass cannot be reduced. Strangulation occurs when the blood supply to the bowel within the hernia sac is compromised and gangrenous change, with its attendant serious implications, develops.

Patients with a complicated hernia presenting with a complaint of pain must be carefully evaluated. Incarceration of recent origin associated with pain may or may not cause

intestinal obstruction. Reduction should be attempted by gentle manipulation of the protrusion, with the patient's knees in the flexed position, relaxing the abdominal wall. Failure to reduce such a hernia usually indicates urgent surgery.

Acute tenderness, associated with fever, leukocytosis and evidence of intestinal obstruction, is more often indicative of strangulation of the hernial contents, for which emergent surgical repair is necessary. It is possible to reduce a strangulated hernia "en masse," i.e., the entire sac and its contents may be replaced into the peritoneal cavity, but the neck of the sac may still compromise the blood supply to the hernia contents.

When it is determined that surgery is necessary, fluid replacement should be started and the patient prepared for the operating room.

Mesenteric vascular occlusion

Occlusive disease of the blood vessels of the intestine is usually found in patients over the age of 60 and associated with arteriosclerotic cardiovascular disease. Occlusion may develop in either the arterial or venous mesenteric vessels.[35] Arterial occlusion results from thrombosis or embolism. Venous occlusion follows primary thrombosis. Whether the process starts on the arterial or venous side, the end result, infarction and gangrene of the bowel, is the same.

Thrombotic occlusive disease results from buildup of atheromatous plaque in the lumen of the vessel until complete blockage occurs. In embolic occlusion, the origin of the embolus is usually a mural thrombus in the heart. The cardiac rhythm is typically auricular fibrillation, and a portion of the thrombus breaks off from the left atrium and lodges in the mesenteric artery.

The vessels involved are usually those supplying the small intestine—the superior mesenteric artery or vein. The inferior mesenteric artery, which supplies the left colon, though sometimes occluded in patients with abdominal aortic aneurysm, is much less frequently involved. If involved, it rarely results in infarction of the colon because of good collateral flow through the marginal artery.

Assessment

In acute occlusion of the mesenteric vessels, the most striking complaint is poorly localized pain. The pain is continuous but may be associated with cramps. Constipation or diarrhea may be observed as the process continues. Bleeding from the rectum develops as a result of infarction of the bowel wall. Emesis is not a common finding. The patient may give a history suggestive of mesenteric artery insufficiency or arteriosclerotic heart disease with fibrillation.

The cardiac state is carefully evaluated. Auricular fibrillation in the presence of supportive history and abdominal findings is suggestive of embolic mesenteric artery occlusion. Abdominal findings are often insignificant, especially early in the course of the disease. As the period of vascular occlusion lengthens, gangrenous changes occur in the bowel, with resultant peritonitis. Physical examination may then reveal more striking findings.

Peritoneal tap may be useful. Blood count and urinalysis are not usually abnormal, though leukocytosis can occur. X-rays of the abdomen may reveal a striking absence of gas in the intestinal tract. Arterial blood gases often reveal a significant base defect and are thus helpful in the diagnosis.

Management

Since there may be fluid loss due to peritonitis, fluid replacement is necessary. Early exploration of the abdomen is indicated. In those patients with mesenteric artery occlusion with early ischemic changes, removal of the clot with a Fogarty catheter may restore circulation. Secondary laparotomy may be done 12 to 24 hours later to check on intestinal viability and remove any bowel with impaired blood supply. In instances of frank gangrene, resection of the involved bowel is necessary. At times, massive resection involving almost the entire small bowel, may be necessary. In such cases, the prognosis is grave.

SUMMARY

Patients with acute abdominal conditions present a challenge to the knowledge, skills and ingenuity of the emergency nurse.

Familiarity with the anatomy of the abdominal organs, pain patterns and the clinical picture of the more common acute abdominal diseases will permit the nurse to make a proper diagnosis in the majority of such patients. Laboratory and x-ray studies, as indicated, are helpful in giving additional data to support the diagnosis.

The nurse should also be aware of the conditions which require urgent care. Management in the emergency department is aimed at diagnosis, initiation of measures to correct the altered physiology, control of pain and preparation of the patient for operative intervention when necessary.

BIBLIOGRAPHY

(1) Adams, R., and Stranahan, A.: "Cholecystitis and Cholelithiasis: Analytical Report of 1,104 Operative Cases," *Surgery, Gynecology and Obstetrics,* 85 (1947):776.

(2) Anderson, M. C.; Scheenfeld, F. B.; Iams, W. B., and Suwa, M.: "Circulatory Changes in Acute Pancreatitis," *Surgical Clinics of North America,* 47 (1967):127.

(3) Berne, T. V., and Shore, E. H.: "Appraisal of the Traumatized Abdomen," *Surgical Clinics of North America,* 48 (1968):1197.

(4) Brown, H.; Sass, M., and Cheng, P. Z.: "Infectious Mononucleosis and Splenic Rupture: Report of a Case," *Ohio Medical Journal,* 60 (1964):954.

(5) Byrne, J. J., and Hennessy, V. L., Jr.: "Diverticulitis of the Colon," *Surgical*

Clinics of North America, 52 (1972): 991.

(6) Carden, A. B. G.: "Acute Large-Bowel Obstruction: Aetiology and Mortality," *Medical Journal Australia,* 1 (1966):662.

(7) Carnevali, J. F., and ReMine, W. H.: "Radical Versus Conservative Surgical Managment of Acute Perforated Peptic Ulcer," *Postgraduate Medicine,* 32 (1962):119–126.

(8) Ching, E., and ReMine, W. H.: "Surgical Management of Emergency Complications of Duodenal Ulcer," *Surgical Clinics of North America,* 51 (August 1971):851–856.

(9) Clark, D. D., and Hubay, C. A.: "Tube Cecostomy: Evaluation of 161 Cases," *Annals of Surgery,* 175 (1972):55.

(10) Cleator, I. G. M.; Holubitsky, I. B., and Harrison, R. C.: "Perforated Anastomotic Ulcers," *Annals of Surgery,* 177 (1973):436–440.

(11) DeBray, C.; Hardovin, J. P.; Besancon, F., and Rainibault, J.: "Frequency of Diverticulosis of the Colon, According to Age," *Semaine des Hospiteaux de Paris,* 37 (1961):1743.

(12) Facey, F. L.; Weil, M. H., and Rosoff, L.: "Mechanism and Treatment of Shock Associated with Acute Pancreatitis," *American Journal of Surgery,* 111 (1966):374.

(13) Felix, W. R., and Stahlgren, L. H.: "Death by Undiagnosed Perforated Peptic Ulcer: Analysis of 31 Cases," *Annals of Surgery,* 177 (1973):344.

(14) Ferris, D. O., and Sterling, W. A.: "Surgery of the Biliary Tract," *Surgical Clinics of North America,* 47 (1967): 861.

(15) Floyd, C. E.; Stirling, C. T., and Cohn, I., Jr.: "Cancer of the Colon, Rectum and Anus: Review of 1687 Cases," *Annals of Surgery,* 163 (1966):829.

(16) Forward, A. D.: "Hypokalemia Associated with Sigmoid Volvulus," *Surgery, Gynecology and Obstetrics,* 123 (1966): 35.

(17) Gammill, S. L., and Nice, C. M., Jr.: "Air Fluid Levels: Their Occurrence in Normal Patients and Their Role in Analysis of Ileus," *Surgery,* 71 (1972): 771.

(18) Glenn, F., and Moody, F. C.: "Acute Obstructive Suppurative Cholangitis," *Surgery, Gynecology and Obstetrics,* 113 (1961):265.

(19) Gliedman, M. L.; Bolooki, H., and Rosen, R. G.: *Acute Pancreatitis: Current Problems in Surgery* (Chicago: Yearbook Medical Publisher, August 1970).

(20) Hardy, J.: "Mechanism of Shock in Peritonitis: Effects upon Blood Volume, Heart Action and Peripheral Vessels," *Journal of Surgical Research,* 1 (1961): 64.

(21) Harris, S., and Rudolf, L. E.: "Mechanical Small Bowel Obstruction Due to Acute Appendicitis: Review of 10 Cases," *Annals of Surgery,* 164 (1966): 157.

(22) Hines, J. R.; Geurkink, R. E., and Bass, R. T.: "Recurrence and Mortality Rates in Sigmoid Volvulus," *Surgery, Gynecology and Obstetrics,* 124 (1967):567.

(23) Holder, T. M., and Leape, L. L.: "The Acute Surgical Abdomen in Children," *New England Journal of Medicine,* 277 (1967):921.

(24) Jordan, G. L., Jr.; Angel, R. T., and DeBakey. M. E.: "Acute Gastroduodenal Perforation: Comparative Study of Treatment with Simple Closure, Subtotal Gastrectomy and Hemigastrectomy and Vagotomy," *Archives of Surgery,* 92 (1956):449.

(25) Lo, A. M.; Evans, W. E., and Carey, L. C.: "Review of Small Bowel Obstruction at Milwaukee County General Hospital," *American Journal of Surgery,* 111 (1966):884.

(26) McDonald, J. C.: "Nonspecific Mesenteric Lymphadenitis: Collective Review," *Surgery, Gynecology and Obstetrics,* 116 (1963):409.

(27) McIlrath, D. C., and Larson, R. H.: "Surgical Management of Larger Perforations of the Duodenum," *Surgical Clinics of North America,* 51 (August 1971):857–862.

(28) McIndoe, A. H.: "Delayed Hemorrhage Following Traumatic Rupture of the Spleen," *British Journal of Surgery,* 20 (1932):249.

(29) Maynard, A. deL., and Prigot, A.: "Gastroduodenal Perforation: A Report of 120 Cases over a Five and One-Half Year Period with Consideration of the Role of Primary Gastrectomy," *Annals of Surgery,* 153 (1961):261.

(30) Mayo, C. W., and Delaney, L. T.: "Colonic Diverticulitis Associated with Carcinoma," *Archives of Surgery,* 72 (1956):957.

(31) Nardi, G. L.: "Acute Pancreatitis," *Surgical Clinics of North America,* 46 (1966):619.

(32) Nissan, S., and Levy, E.: "Intussusception in Infancy Caused by Hypertrophic Peyer's Patches," *Surgery,* 59 (1966): 1108.

(33) Opie, E. L.: *Diseases of the Pancreas,* ed. 2 (Philadelphia: J. B. Lippincott Company, 1910).

(34) Orloff, M. J., and Peskin, G. W.: "Collective Review: Spontaneous Rupture of the Normal Spleen," *International Abstracts of Surgery,* 106 (1955):1.

(35) Ottinger, L. W., and Austen, W. G.: "Study of 136 Patients with Mesenteric Infarction," *Surgery, Gynecology and Obstetrics,* 124 (1967):251.

(36) Perry, J. F.; DeMeules, J. E., and Root, H. D.: "Diagnostic Peritoneal Lavage in Blunt Abdominal Trauma," *Surgery, Gynecology and Obstetrics,* 131 (1970): 742.

(37) Pines, B., and Rabinovitch, J.: "Perforation of the Gallbladder in Acute Cholecystitis," *Annals of Surgery,* 140 (1954):170.

(38) Reimer, J.: "Perforating Gastric and Duodenal Ulcers. Primary Resection Versus Suture: An Analysis of Two 15-Year Series," *Acta Chirurgica Scandinavia,* 33 (1967):38.

(39) Rodkey, G., and Welch, C. D.: "Surgical Management of Colonic Diverticulitis with Free Perforation or Abscess Formation," *American Journal of Surgery,* 117 (1969):265.

(40) Rosoff, L.; Cohen, J. L.; Telfer, N., and Halpern, M.: "Injuries of the Spleen," *Surgical Clinics of North America,* 52 (1972):667.

(41) Rosoff, L., and Meyers, H.: "Acute Emphysematous Cholecystitis: An Analysis of Ten Cases," *American Journal of Surgery,* 111 (1966):410.

(42) Schumer, W., and Burman, S. D.: "The Perforated Viscus: Diagnosis and Treatment," *Surgical Clinics of North America,* 52 (February 1972):231–237.

(43) Seeley, S. F., and Campbell, D.: "Nonoperative Treatment of Perforated Peptic Ulcer," *International Abstracts of Surgery,* 102 (1956):435–446.

(44) Talbert, J. L., and Zuidema, G. D.: "Appendicitis: A Reappraisal of an Old Problem," *Surgical Clinics of North America,* 46 (1966):1101.

(45) Thorbjarnarson, B.: "Acute Appendicitis in Patients over the Age of Sixty," *Surgery, Gynecology and Obstetrics,* 125 (1967):1277.

(46) Thoroughman, J. C.; Walker, L. G.; Graytaylor, B., and Dunn, T.: "Free Perforation of Anastomotic Ulcers," *Annals of Surgery,* 169 (1969):790.

(47) Williams, J. S., and Hale, H. W., Jr.: "Acute Appendicitis in the Elderly," *Annals of Surgery,* 162 (1965):208.

APPENDIX G

Pain and nursing care

In the emergency setting, pain is the one most frequent presenting complaint, whether it be a sore throat from an upper respiratory infection, chest pain from a hypoxic cardiac muscle or abdominal pain from the many specific causes discussed in the preceding chapter.

The emergency nurse must continually assess the nature of the patient's pain. Descriptions of site, intensity, duration and factors predisposing to pain provide useful clues in delineating the cause of the patient's pain. General observation of the patient also helps in assessing pain, noting any general or local muscle tension or rigidity, writhing, unusual postures, rubbing, restlessness, agitation, unusual quietness, withdrawal and depression. Comparing these observations with baseline information gained from the patient, his family or his hospital record is useful.

The nurse's observations aid not only in identifying the cause of pain; they also provide clues to how the patient responds to and copes with pain. His responses and coping mechanisms are as important as the diagnosis to the management of his pain.

It is not a nursing function to determine whether or not a patient does, in fact, have pain. McCaffrey's definition of pain is especially useful to nursing in this respect: "Pain is whatever the experiencing person says it is and exists wherever he says it does." * Thus, the patient knows what he feels and where he feels it; the existence of his pain is never doubted, even when a physical examination and diagnosis do not support its existence. Indeed, true pain may be felt in the absence of any physical pathology.

It *is* a nursing function, however, to assess the nature of the patient's pain, what it means to him and how he copes with it, so that measures to control his pain can be instituted. A number of factors are known to influence an individual's response to pain, such as cultural influences,† age and sex, religion, body part(s) involved, past experiences with pain, attitudes and feelings of others attending him, secondary gains from pain and his own understanding of the pain.‡ When the patient has pain, statements of the patient's response to pain should be included in a complete history.

Management of pain has traditionally been accomplished through the administration of analgesics. Further, it was thought that pain relief was best obtained if medications were repeated before the effects of the prior medication wore off and the pain became too intense. The use of analgesics has been based on the belief that pain is felt when noxious stimuli exceed the pain threshold. Analgesics were thought to alter the perception and interpretation of pain, thus controlling the pain felt by the patient.

More recent studies, however, have explained other physiological mechanisms

---

* M. McCaffery, *Nursing Management of the Patient with Pain* (Philadelphia: J. B. Lippincott Company, 1972), p. 8.

† M. Zborowski, "Cultural Components in Responses to Pain," *Journal of Social Issues,* 8 (1952):16.

‡ McCaffery, *Nursing Management;* and M. McCaffery, "Patients in Pain," *Nursing '73,* 3 (1973): 41.

for pain sensation,* which have implications for use of interventions other than medication. These studies suggest that painful sensations may be modulated or altered en route to the cerebral cortex, resulting in an altered or reduced perception. Interventions may include distraction, cutaneous stimulation (massage, use of ice or heat) and environmental control. Such measures may be used along with medication, or alone for the emergency department patient undergoing assessment, the results of which may be affected by analgesia.

Fear and anxiety are known to intensify the pain experience. In the emergency setting, where these are pervasive emotions, a calm, reassuring approach by a nurse who is truly interested in the patient and his problem may be therapeutic in itself. Being there, answering questions appropriately and dispelling the patient's fears become priority nursing measures for the patient in pain.

Surgical or medical intervention may be the only effective method of pain control in some instances, but it should be known that a number of nursing interventions are also available and that the nurse need not feel helpless without the physician's medication order. Such nursing interventions may be more time-consuming than the administration of an analgesic, but they may also be more effective and produce no side effects, as well.

* R. Melzack and P. Wall, "Pain Mechanisms: A New Theory," *Science,* 150 (1965):971.

21

Care of the patient with gastrointestinal bleeding

JAMES H. COSGRIFF, JR.
DIANN ANDERSON

Patients with gastrointestinal bleeding are frequently seen in emergency settings. Because of the usually sudden onset of symptoms and the nonvisible source, gastrointestinal bleeding can produce a frightening situation for the patient, his family and the uninitiated emergency staff.

Most episodes of gastrointestinal bleeding are minor in nature and, though potentially serious, not life-threatening. Less commonly, hemorrhage may be massive and life-threatening and require immediate action. Bleeding from any body orifice, however, presents the emergency nurse with a challenging responsibility to evaluate and diagnose the problem and institute prompt and appropriate management. The clinical picture and management will be determined by the underlying pathology, the amount of blood loss and the presence or absence of associated disease.

One concept bears repetition. Massive bleeding may be fatal and requires prompt, definitive treatment. Since the early management of the patient with G.I. bleeding may be handled by an emergency nurse, it is necessary that she be familiar with the emergency management of gastrointestinal bleeding.

EMERGENCY NURSING MANAGEMENT

The emergency management of the patient with gastrointestinal bleeding, whether massive or not, can be best achieved if the nurse meets the following objectives.

(1) Assess the patient's need for life-support measures.
(2) Institute measures to control bleeding and to restore circulating blood volume, if needed.
(3) Collect and identify pertinent data to establish both the bleeding site and a tentative diagnosis.
(4) Provide comfort and reassurance to the patient and his family.
(5) Prepare the patient and family for definitive treatment, whether surgical or nonsurgical.
(6) Evaluate the effectiveness of the nursing management.

Although each objective is important in itself, in actual practice, each measure will probably not be achieved singly. It is common in emergency nursing that several objectives are implemented simultaneously.

320

Instituting life-support measures

Assessment and management

Primary assessment consists of obtaining and recording the patient's temperature, pulse, respirations and blood pressure, bearing in mind that the position of the patient [10] and his anxiety [11] will affect the findings. Observation for other signs and symptoms of hypovolemic shock should be made. Early in the shock state, tachycardia (usually above 100 beats per minute) may be the only abnormal vital sign.

Venous blood samples should be drawn immediately and sent to the laboratory for determination of complete blood count, platelet count, prothrombin time, partial thromboplastin time, type and crossmatch. Bleeding and clotting times should also be measured to complete the "bleeding" workup and rule out hemorrhagic disorder as a cause.

When signs and symptoms of hypovolemic shock are evident, intravenous fluids should be started immediately, using the same needle by which the blood samples were obtained. Type-specific whole blood is the fluid of choice for volume replacement, but while it is being prepared, a balanced salt solution, such as Ringer's lactate, may be infused. There is little indication for the use of plasma or plasma expanders, unless whole blood is not available within a reasonable period of time.

Speed of infusion is dependent on numerous factors, such as the patient's age, the presence of cardiac and/or pulmonary disease, the volume and duration of blood loss and the response to infusion as measured by close monitoring of clinical signs. It is, therefore, the physician's responsibility to determine infusion speed.

When a large volume of blood has been lost, the patient's life may depend on volume being restored quickly. However, especially in older patients, too-rapid infusion can result in left heart failure, pulmonary congestion and edema. The use of a central venous pressure catheter, inserted via the jugular, sub-clavian or antecubital vein, provides information on the ability of the cardiovascular system to tolerate fluid replacement. Experience has demonstrated, however, that this parameter may also be misleading, for a significant rise in central venous pressure may not occur until cardiac failure is imminent. Normal pressure is in the range of 3 to 12 cm. of saline.

The amount of needed blood replacement may be estimated by figuring the difference between the initial hemoglobin and the normal value. As a rule, one unit of whole blood (500 cc.) will raise the hemoglobin level one gram. Therefore, if the patient has a hemoglobin of 10 grams on admission to the emergency facility and transfusion is deemed necessary, 4 units should be expected to raise the hemoglobin level to 14 grams in the absence of continued bleeding. Similarly, one unit of whole blood will raise the hematocrit level to 3 or 4 percent. It should be remembered that in the early hours after onset of bleeding, even when massive, hemoglobin and hematocrit may be falsely elevated or at or near normal levels. Eighteen to 24 hours may pass before hemodilution occurs and a more realistic value can be obtained.

Evaluation

During this early phase, close monitoring of vital signs and clinical state is essential to determining the effectiveness of the life-support measures. Although the vital signs are affected by numerous factors, including the patient's age and his own response to stress, it can be generally stated that additional blood replacement is needed when:

(1) The systolic blood pressure falls below 90 to 100 mm. Hg in a previously normotensive individual or is significantly lowered in a hypertensive patient.

(2) The pulse remains elevated above 100 beats per minute.

(3) There are continued signs and symptoms of hypovolemic shock, such as

322 CARE OF THE PATIENT WITH GASTROINTESTINAL BLEEDING

pallor, cold and clammy extremities, restlessness, faintness, dyspnea and thirst, apprehension.
(4) Urinary output falls below 25 to 30 cc. per hour.
(5) Blood loss continues.
(6) Hemoglobin and hematocrit are below normal levels.

The nurse should be constantly on the alert for any evidence of blood incompatibility. Prior to initiating blood infusion, she should properly identify donor blood by its laboratory number, verifying the type and a satisfactory crossmatch. While reactions due to incompatible blood may not herald a serious outcome, they may produce deleterious effects.

Among the usual reactions of incompatible blood are: (1) urticaria, (2) lumbar pain, (3) tightness in the chest and (4) a burning sensation of the face. There may be some degree of collapse, apprehension, chilling, tachycardia and fever. While body temperature readings are not routinely taken during blood transfusion, a rise in temperature often occurs before other signs and symptoms; thus, body temperature is worth observing.[2] Hematuria and anuria may also develop, indicating filtration problems in the kidneys.

Observation of any of these phenomena requires that the transfusion be stopped, the physician be notified, urine output be measured and the first specimen be saved to determine the presence of red cells. The remaining blood should be returned to the laboratory to check for type, crossmatch and bacterial contamination. The nurse should continue to observe the patient for further signs of incompatibility. Diphenhydramine (Benadryl), given parenterally, is helpful in urticarial reactions.

Further assessment

Once the life-support measures have been instituted, the nurse can collect additional information so that the bleeding site and a tentative diagnosis can be established. In order to localize the site of bleeding, the nurse should bear in mind that, for practical purposes, the gastrointestinal tract may be divided into 2 main parts by the ligament of Treitz, a ligament supporting the intestine at the junction of the duodenum and jejunum.

The upper part of the G.I. tract consists of the esophagus, stomach and duodenum. Bleeding from this portion will be manifested by vomiting blood (hematemesis) and/or passage of bloody or tarry stools (melena). In lesions of the upper tract, the vomited blood may be unaltered in appearance or resemble coffee grounds, a phenomenon caused by the action of gastric acid on hemoglobin, forming acid hematin. As little as 50 to 80 cc. of ingested blood has experimentally produced a tarry stool.[6] Blood within the gut has a tendency to stimulate peristaltic activity, which explains the presence of gross blood in the stool from lesions in the upper tract.

The lower part of the gastrointestinal tract contains the jejunum, ileum and colon, and bleeding is manifested primarily by bloody or tarry stools. In some circumstances, usually in bleeding of the small intestine, melena may be present, due to alteration of blood by gastric juices present in the intestinal tract. Gross rectal bleeding and no detection of blood in the upper tract usually places the lesion distal to the ligament of Treitz. While bleeding from the upper tract can usually be localized, it is much more difficult, sometimes impossible, to pinpoint the site of lower gastrointestinal bleeding.

The insertion of a nasogastric tube is almost always indicated, not only to provide symptomatic relief by gastric decompression, but also to assist in determining the amount, nature and site of bleeding. If coffee ground material is obtained, the content should be tested for blood by Hematest or some similar method. The presence of gross blood may indicate active bleeding and thus requires close observation of the patient.

Gastric lavage with measured amounts of iced saline may arrest active bleeding. Raising the pH of the stomach contents by irrigation with antacid solution has also successfully controlled bleeding. Gastric content is aspirated, its pH checked with nitrazine paper and antacid instilled every 15 minutes until pH reaches 7.0. Thereafter, pH is determined hourly, and adjustments are made when appropriate.

A history of the onset of the illness should be obtained, from patient or family, including careful questioning regarding ulcer disease, alcoholism and ingestion of drugs, such as phenylbutazone, aspirin or other salicylates, steroids and anticoagulants. A tarry stool may be produced by certain foods and drugs, especially iron or bismuth compounds (e.g., Pepto Bismol). A sample of stool obtained by rectal examination may be tested by the Hematest method to establish whether or not blood is indeed present. Commonly used medications which may cause gastrointestinal bleeding are listed below.

(1) Heparin sodium.
(2) Bishydroxycoumarin (Dicumarol).
(3) Warfarin (Coumadin).
(4) Phenylbutazone (Butazolidin).
(5) Salicylates (aspirin).
(6) Salicylate compounds.
(7) Steroids (prednisone, prednisolone, cortisone).

Physical assessment, in addition to observing the clinical and vital signs, as elaborated earlier, includes a careful examination for ecchymoses (they might suggest a bleeding tendency), abdominal palpation for tenderness or masses and observation for stigmata of liver disease, discussed later in this chapter. Urinalysis, including determination of glycosuria and ketone bodies and a history of allergies are important factors in planning the therapeutic program.

Emotional support of the patient and family

The sight of massive amounts of blood is a terrifying experience for the patient and his family. In gastrointestinal bleeding, the source is hidden and the event is certainly unexpected, factors which increase the fear and anxiety already present. While an episode of massive bleeding requires immediate nursing action to sustain life, emotional support to the patient and his family cannot be underestimated.

The nurse can be instrumental in providing a quiet, supportive environment for the patient and family by proceeding with emergency measures knowledgeably and calmly, explaining what is to be done for the patient and what he can do to assist in his care. Providing comfort in terms of body position, warmth and calm surroundings can be helpful in reducing further hemorrhage and shock by allaying apprehension and restlessness. When emergency surgery seems likely, the nurse should make herself available to the patient and family to listen, answer questions and offer support.

COMMON CAUSES OF GASTROINTESTINAL BLEEDING

In situations when a physician is present and available, the nurse should collect pertinent data so that a diagnosis can be established. If a physician is not present or available on the patient's admission to the emergency department, the nurse's assessment can enable her to proceed with life-saving measures and preparations for nursing and medical therapy, which can save time and reduce trauma to the patient. Understanding the symptomatology, physical findings and management of the common causes of gastrointestinal bleeding is, therefore, essential to knowledgeable and capable care.

The most common causes of upper gastrointestinal bleeding are gastritis, peptic ulcer and esophageal varices. (See Figure 21–1.) In lower tract hemorrhage, diverticular disease of the colon or small bowel is the most common source. Each of these disease entities is detailed in the following pages, with emphasis on clinical findings, as ascertained by the patient's history and physical assessment, and indicating the usual medical and/or surgical management.

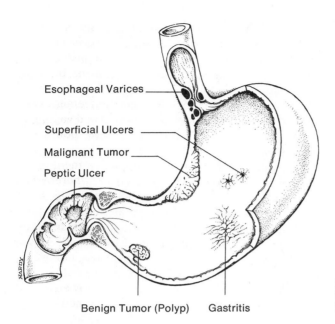

Esophageal Varices

Superficial Ulcers

Malignant Tumor

Peptic Ulcer

Benign Tumor (Polyp)   Gastritis

Figure 21–1   Upper gastrointestinal bleeding. The common sites and causes of massive bleeding are indicated.

Upper gastrointestinal bleeding

Gastritis

Gastritis is an inflammation of the mucosa of the stomach. It is the most common cause of upper gastrointestinal bleeding and is rarely massive. Gastritis is quite frequently associated with episodes of heavy alcohol intake or prolonged use of aspirin, anticoagulants, phenylbutazone, steroids or spicy foods. The symptoms are usually of short duration and not suggestive of ulcer disease. Physical assessment frequently reveals no distinctive signs. Nasogastric drainage contains fresh blood or coffee ground material.

Initial management is directed toward stabilization of the patient and preparation for diagnostic procedures, such as gastrointestinal x-rays. Should the bleeding persist or remain obscure, selective arteriography may be helpful in detecting the site of blood loss.[4, 14, 20] When the diagnosis is established, both patient and family should be advised of causative factors and properly tutored in dietary and/or medical restrictions.

Peptic ulcer

Ulcer is the most common cause of *massive* upper gastrointestinal hemorrhage. While

bleeding from peptic ulcer may occur at any age,[21] it is more commonly seen in the fifth through seventh decades. It is estimated that 20 percent of patients with ulcers bleed and that 5 percent bleed massively. The ulcer is most frequently located in the duodenum, less often in the stomach. History in ulcer patients is very important. Most will give a definite history of peptic disease or of frequent use of antacids. Nevertheless, as many as 30 percent of massive bleeders will deny prior symptoms.[21]

Physical assessment may be negative, though tenderness on palpation may be found in the area of the duodenal bulb, just above and to the right of the umbilicus. If the patient has epigastric pain which is relieved by the onset of bleeding, peptic ulcer is likely. The nasogastric aspirate may contain whole blood or coffee ground material. In some patients with bleeding duodenal ulcers, no blood may be recovered on aspiration, only gastric juice, due to the fact that the pyloric ring is closed and will not allow duodenal content to regurgitate into the stomach. For the same reason, bile will not be recovered on aspiration. The only significant symptom may be rectal bleeding.

In hemorrhage caused by an ulcer, the plan of management varies with the physician, the duration of the disease, the patient's age, the presence or absence of associated disease, the availability of type-specific blood and the capability of the surgical team. Massive bleeding from a *chronic* duodenal ulcer may be a life-threatening condition and, in a patient with coronary artery disease, may precipitate an episode of coronary insufficiency or full-blown myocardial infarction. In such patients, nasal oxygen may be needed to provide further support. Acute ulceration, secondary to medication or stress ulcers, also requires special consideration. Generally, it is treated nonsurgically.

The final decision on treatment, then, may be made from several choices. The emergency nurse should be aware of them, for, in some circumstances, this knowledge will better permit her to allay apprehension and fear of the patient and family.

In definitive ulcer care, some surgeons favor blood replacement and urgent subtotal gastric resection.[21] The general principle of transfusion and direct attack on the bleeding site is modified by the choice of the operative procedure, which may include hemigastrectomy and vagotomy, antrectomy and vagotomy or suture ligation of the bleeding point with vagotomy and pyloroplasty.

A second method of ulcer treatment is the so-called "test of transfusion," whereby the patient is managed by iced saline lavage, nasogastric decompression, transfusion and close observation. If the bleeding ceases in 24 to 48 hours, as evidenced by normal, stable vital signs and a rising hemoglobin, nonoperative management is continued. Should bleeding reoccur, the patient is treated by an urgent surgical approach, such as outlined above.

The third method of ulcer treatment consists solely of medical management by iced lavage, nasogastric decompression, blood re-

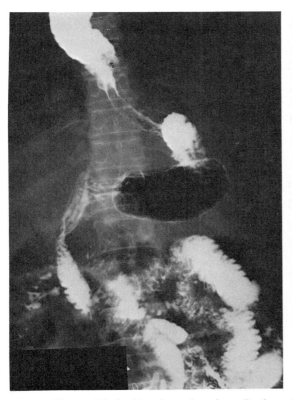 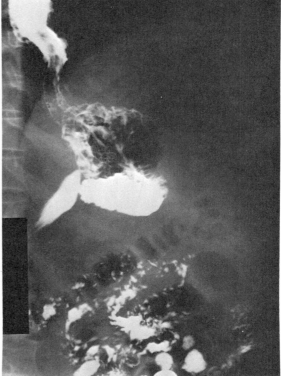

Figure 21–2   Esophageal varices. Such varices usually result from portal hypertension.

placement and feedings of milk, cream and antacids. This regimen is extremely difficult to maintain in a patient with massive bleeding or rebleeding, and surgical therapy may be required.

Esophageal varices

Esophageal varices are varicosities which develop in the portal venous system that drains the gastrointestinal tract (see Figure 21–2). Varices are most prominent in the lower portion of the esophagus and the upper stomach, resulting from portal hypertension, an increased pressure, in this system of veins. (See Figure 21–3.) Most often, portal hypertension is seen in adults, secondary to cirrhosis of the liver from chronic alcoholism (Laennec's type) or following hepatitis (postnecrotic

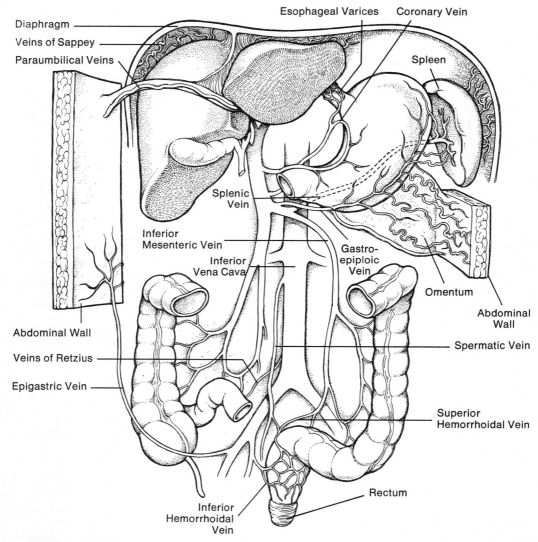

Figure 21–3 Portal hypertension. The drawing illustrates the abdominal organs and vessels which may be involved in portal hypertension.
Source: Redrawn from an article by H. K. Gray and F. B. Whitesell, Jr., in *Annals of Surgery*, 132:798–810. © 1950 by J. B. Lippincott Company.

type). Less commonly, it occurs in children in association with thrombosis of the portal vein (Banti's disease).

Bleeding from esophageal or gastroesophageal varices is usually massive. The patient may relate a history of blood "welling up" in the throat with the acute episode. A history of long-standing alcoholic intake is frequently obtained but, more importantly, physical assessment reveals one or more of the cardinal signs of chronic liver disease: jaundice, shoulder-girdle atrophy, sparse pubic hair and axillary hair, spider angiomata of the upper trunk, ascites, palmar erythema and superficial venous patterns of the trunk and abdomen (thoracoepigastric veins and caput medusa). It is also important to note that the incidence of peptic ulcer is 15 to 20 percent higher in cirrhotics than in the general population. Thus, both peptic ulcer and esophageal varices can occur concomitantly, and bleeding may then arise from either source.

When bleeding is from varices, the nasogastric aspirate is grossly bloody. If this diagnosis is suspected and bleeding continues, removal of the nasogastric tube and insertion of the triple-lumen Sengstaken-Blakemore tube is indicated, to provide esophageal tamponade. This device has 2 balloons which, when inflated, provide pressure against the lower portion of the esophagus and fundic portion of the stomach (see Figure 21–4).

Prior to passing the tube, the balloons should be inflated to detect leaks. The tube is quite bulky and at times difficult to insert. It may be lubricated with a topical anesthetic jelly, such as lidocaine, and then passed via the nose into the stomach to the 50 cc. mark. Figure 21–5 lists and depicts the equipment needed for insertion. The gastric balloon is inflated with as much as 150 to 200 cm. of air and clamped. The tube is partially withdrawn to cinch the balloon against the cardioesophageal junction, until a feeling of resistance is noted. It should then be taped to the patient's nose in this "cinched" position and the esophageal balloon inflated by means of a blood pressure cuff to 40 mm. Hg. In taping the tube

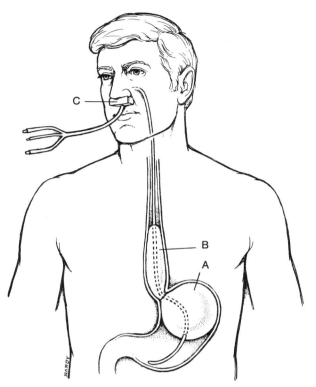

Figure 21–4 Sengstaken-Blakemore tube in place. The gastric balloon (A) and the esophageal balloon (B) are inflated. Traction is maintained by a foam sponge placed about the tube at the external nares and held by tape (C). The foam sponge also prevents ulceration of the nasal skin and cartilage. The 3 open tube ends are then connected: The one marked gastric balloon is closed with a screw clamp. The esophageal balloon is connected to a mercury or aneroid sphygmomanometer, and pressure is maintained at 40 mm. Hg. The third tube is connected to an intermittent nasogastric suction machine.

to the nose, it is advisable to use a piece of sponge to avoid undue pressure on the nasal skin and cartilage, which may lead to ulceration. The tube is then irrigated with iced saline and attached to intermittent suction.

Close observation for continued bleeding is indicated, since failure of tamponade may require emergent surgical intervention. Tamponade is usually not tolerated beyond 36 to 48 hours. At that time, the esophageal balloon should be slowly deflated and the patient observed for rebleeding. While the tube is in-

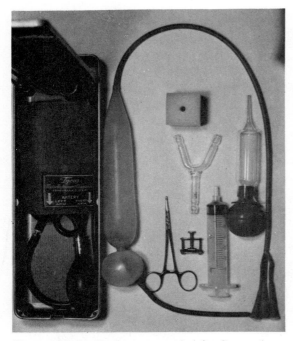

Figure 21–5 Equipment needed for Sengstaken-Blakemore tube insertion. Included are: esophageal balloon apparatus; mercury manometer for connection with a glass Y-tube; 50 cc. syringe; constant intestinal suction machine; lubricating jelly (not petroleum jelly); glass of water and straw (not shown); one Crile, Kelly or Kocher hemostat or similar clamp for rubber tubing.

flated, oral intake is restricted. When bleeding ceases, feedings may be given through the gastric lumen tube. Parenteral feedings are necessary during the entire period.

Posterior pituitary extract (Pitressin) has been effective in the emergency phase of care by reducing or controlling variceal bleeding.[7, 18] However, in addition to its therapeutic effect of reducing portal pressure by splanchnic vasoconstriction, it also causes coronary artery constriction; thus its use is contraindicated in patients with heart disease.

Further management of patients with esophageal varices will vary and depends, in part, on the parameters mentioned under the discussion of the patient with bleeding ulcer. Other considerations are the patient's liver status and whether or not the acute hemorrhage can be controlled by the esophageal tamponade and his condition stabilized with blood replacement. In all instances, venous blood samples should be drawn for the basic tests (see page 321) and baseline liver function tests should be made (SGOT, SGPT, alkaline phosphatase, bilirubin, total protein).

If there is underlying liver disease, defects in the clotting mechanism (prothrombin time) may be detected, and appropriate doses of vitamin K_1 oxide (AquaMEPHYTON) should be given intravenously. Menodione sodium diphosphate (standard vitamin K) will not be synthesized by the damaged liver and hence is of no value.

A number of operative procedures have been developed over the years to arrest the acute bleeding episode associated with varices, including transesophageal ligation and emergency decompression by portasystemic venous shunts. However, the mortality is high, and these procedures have not received general acceptance. More often than not, the Sengstaken-Blakemore tube will effectively control bleeding, allowing the patient to be stabilized and evaluated during the ensuing days or weeks until an effective surgical procedure can be accomplished. Indication for surgery is based on a firm diagnosis which can be established by x-rays of the esophagus and stomach, esophagogastroscopy and portal venography. Decompression may be effected through one of several procedures involving shunting of blood from the high-pressure portal vein to the lower pressure systemic veins (portacaval, splenorenal, mesocaval shunts).

Other causes of upper G.I. bleeding

Less common causes of gastrointestinal tract bleeding are: (1) long-standing use of aspirin or other salicylates,[1] anticoagulants or steriods, (2) acute pancreatitis with duodenitis, (3) focal areas of gastritis occurring in hiatus hernia, (4) linear tears at the gastroesophageal junction associated with vomiting and retching, usually in alcoholics (Mallory-

Weiss Syndrome) [13, 16, 24] and (5) benign or malignant neoplasms of the stomach or duodenum.

In summary, it can be said that the most frequent causes of *massive* upper gastrointestinal tract bleeding are: (1) peptic ulcer (duodenal and/or gastric), (2) gastritis (with or without hiatus hernia), (3) esophageal varices, (4) malignant and benign tumors of the stomach and (5) duodenitis with pancreatitis.

Lower gastrointestinal tract hemorrhage

As stressed earlier, one of the primary considerations in patients with rectal bleeding is determination of the source, keeping in mind the possibility it may be in the upper tract. One must first eliminate the upper tract as the source of rectal bleeding before causes of lower tract bleeding are considered.

Generally, early management of bleeding from the lower tract is similar to that of upper tract bleeding. In addition, the use of intestinal sedation (morphine) may be used cautiously to quiet the bowel. Any sedative must be administered with care in the presence of shock, since absorption of the drug may be prolonged due to peripheral vasoconstriction. Repeated injections in the presence of shock can lead to an overdose of the drug when circulation returns to normal. Hence, careful evaluation of the patient's clinical state, in relation to his need for the drug, is essential.

Diverticular disease is the commonest cause of lower gastrointestinal hemorrhage. It can be divided into 2 anatomical categories: colonic diverticula and small bowel diverticula. Other causes include hemorrhoids, fissure, proctitis, ulcerative colitis, intussusception, stercoral ulceration, benign and malignant neoplasms and the medications listed previously.

Colonic diverticula

Diverticulosis of the colon is the most frequent cause of massive lower tract bleeding, and it may occur in the absence of detectable secondary inflammation (diverticulitis). Diverticulosis is a disease common in persons over the age of 40 years and rarely seen in the younger age group. The patient may be asymptomatic prior to the bleeding or may give a history of abdominal cramps (caused by irritation of the blood in the colon). This type of hemorrhage may be life-threatening, but unlike upper tract bleeding, it is more likely to stop spontaneously.

Emergency management follows the guidelines presented early in the chapter. In addition, the equipment to perform a sigmoidoscopy should be available. This procedure may be carried out comfortably with the patient in the lateral (Sims's) position but should be undertaken only when vital signs are stable.

Urgent surgery is rarely indicated, since bleeding will usually subside and exploratory laparotomy is of little value in identifying and localizing the bleeding site, especially in the presence of an unprepared bowel. It is therefore necessary to use further diagnostic aids, especially barium studies of the colon. It is recommended that the patient be stabilized and admitted for diagnostic evaluation and elective resection of the involved colon segment when the bleeding site is found.

Small bowel diverticula

This condition is a rather uncommon cause of rectal bleeding and is frequently associated with the presence of ectopic gastric or pancreatic mucosa, a phenomenon which is thought to precipitate the hemorrhage. When bleeding does occur, it may be either massive or of the chronic low-grade variety. These lesions are outpouchings of the small intestine, and unlike the colonic diverticula which are acquired and multiple, small bowel diverticula are more frequently congenital and single in nature. The diverticulum may occur anywhere along the length of the small intestine, but the most common site is that described by Meckel in 1815 and now referred to as Meckel's diverticulum. It is found in the lower 12 to

18 inches of the small intestine in 2 to 4 percent of persons.

Bleeding from this source, if in large amounts, may be manifested by dark red or "currant jelly" stools. Typically, these lesions are found in the younger age group. When bleeding is of the chronic, low-grade variety, grossly bloody or even tarry stools may be noted. History may be important in diagnosis. Frequently, it includes crampy mid- or lower abdominal pain occurring after meals. Physical assessment may be unrevealing.

After emergency measures for stabilization, the patient is admitted for further studies. The diagnosis is frequently made by exclusion (i.e., other lesions are ruled out by barium studies of the upper and lower tracts). A new method of intestinal scanning using intravenous radioactive technetium (which may localize in a diverticulum containing gastric mucosa) has shown some promise in making the diagnosis. However, the method requires special equipment and expertise.[3, 12] Definite treatment is resection of the involved segment of bowel.

SUMMARY

Blood volume replacement, close monitoring of clinical and vital signs, collection of information to determine the bleeding site, emotional support of the patient and ongoing evaluation of nursing intervention are all responsibilities of the nurse in rendering complete care to the patient with gastrointestinal bleeding.

Setting priorities in implementing these goals depends on the individual patient's needs, as evidenced by careful assessment. In the patient with massive bleeding, for example, the need for blood volume replacement is paramount. The very anxious patient who had one episode of rectal bleeding at home before coming to the emergency facility will require emotional support first, thus reordering the priorities for nursing intervention. In the complex art of nursing, especially as it is practiced in the emergency setting, no one objective is implemented singly. Several objectives may be carried out in unison so that comprehensive quality care can be given.

BIBLIOGRAPHY

(1) Alvarez, A. S., and Sumerskill, W. H., Jr.: "Gastrointestinal Hemorrhage and Salicylates," *Lancet*, 2 (1958):920.

(2) Beland, I., and Passos, J.: *Clinical Nursing: Pathophysiological and Psychosocial Approaches,* 3rd ed. (New York: The Macmillan Company, 1975).

(3) Berquist, T. H.; Nolan, N. G.; Adson, M. A., and Schutt, A. J.: "Diagnosis of Meckel's Diverticulum by Radioisotope Scanning," *Mayo Clinic Proceedings,* 48 (1973):98.

(4) Brant, B.; Rosch, J., and Krippaehne, W. M.: "Experience with Angiography in Diagnosis and Treatment of Acute Gastrointestinal Bleeding of Various Etiologies," *Annals of Surgery,* 176 (1972):419.

(5) Child, C. G.: *The Liver and Portal Hypertension* (Philadelphia: W. B. Saunders Company, 1964).

(6) Daniel, W. A., Jr., and Egan, S.: "Quantity of Blood Required to Produce a Bloody Stool," *Journal of the American Medical Association,* 113 (1939):2232.

(7) Davis, W. D.; Gorlin, R.; Reichman, S., and Storaasli, J. P.: "Effect of Pitressin in Reducing Portal Pressure in the Human Being: Preliminary Report," *New England Journal of Medicine,* 256 (1957):108.

(8) Drapanas, T.: "Current Concepts in the Surgical Management of Portal Hypertension," *Annals of Surgery,* 159 (1964): 72.

(9) Drapanas, T.: "Interposition Mesocaval Shunt for Treatment of Portal Hypertension," *Annals of Surgery,* 176 (1972):435.

(10) Foley, M. L.: "Variations in Blood Pressure in the Lateral Recumbent Position," *Nursing Research,* 20 (1971): 64.

(11) Graham, L. E., and Conley, E. M.: "Evaluation of Anxiety and Fear in Adult Surgical Patients," *Nursing Research,* 20 (1971):113.

(12) Jewett, T. C., Jr.; Duszynski, D. O., and Allen, J. E.: "The Visualization of Meckel's Diverticulum with ggm Tc-pertechnetate," *Surgery,* 68 (1970):567.

(13) Mallory, G. K., and Weiss, S.: "Hemorrhages from Lacerations of the Cardiac Orifice of the Stomach Due to Vomiting," *American Journal of Medical Science,* 178 (1929):506.

(14) Margulis, A. R.; Heinbecker, P., and Bernard, H. R.: "Operative Mesenteric Arteriography in the Search for the Site of Bleeding in Unexplained Gastrointestinal Hemorrhage: A Preliminary Report," *Surgery,* 48 (1960):543.

(15) Menguy, R.; Desbaillets, L.; Okabe, S., and Masters, Y. F.: "Abnormal Asperin Metabolism in Patients with Cirrhosis and Its Possible Relationship to Bleeding in Cirrhotics," *Annals of Surgery,* 176 (1972):412.

(16) Miller, A. C., Jr., and Hirschowitz, B. I.: "Twenty-three Patients with Mallory-Weiss Syndrome," *Southern Medical Journal,* 63 (1970):441.

(17) Quick, A. J.: "Salicylates and Bleeding: The Aspirin Tolerance Test," *American Journal of Medical Science,* 252 (1966):265.

(18) Schwartz, S. I.; Bales, H. W.; Emerson, G. L., and Mahoney, E. B.: "The Use of Intravenous Pitressin in Treatment of Bleeding Esophageal Varices," *Surgery,* 45 (1959):72.

(19) Sengstaken, R. W., and Blakemore, A. H.: "Balloon Tamponade for Control of Hemorrhage from Esophageal Varices," *Annals of Surgery,* 131 (1950): 781.

(20) Stanley, R. J., and Wise, L.: "Arteriography in Diagnosis of Acute Gastrointestinal Tract Bleeding," *Archives of Surgery,* 107 (1973):138.

(21) Stewart, J. D.; Cosgriff, J. H., and Gray, J. G.: "Experiences with the Treatment of Acutely Massively Bleeding Peptic Ulcer by Blood Replacement and Gastric Resection," *Surgery, Gynecology and Obstetrics,* 103 (1956):409.

(22) Sugawa, C.; Werner, M. H.; Hayes, D. F., *et al.:* "Early Endoscopy: A Guide to Therapy for Acute Hemorrhage in the Upper Gastrointestinal Tract," *Archives of Surgery,* 107 (1973):133.

(23) Warren, W. D.; Zeppa, R., and Fomon, J. J.: "Selective Transplenic Decompression of Gastroesophageal Varices by Distal Splenorenal Shunt," *Annals of Surgery,* 166 (1967):437.

(24) Wychulis, A. R., and Sasso, A.: "Mallory-Weiss Syndrome," *Archives of Surgery,* 107 (1973):868.

22

Gynecological emergencies

JOHN D. BARTELS

The majority of women who present themselves to the emergency department with gynecological problems have some form of vaginal bleeding and/or abdominal pain. The causes of these symptoms vary tremendously, including aberrations of physiological menstruation, problems of pregnancy, hormonal imbalance, neoplasm, trauma, infection and postpartum or postoperative hemorrhage.

ANATOMY AND PHYSIOLOGY

The internal organs in the female pelvis include the female genital tract, consisting of the ovaries, fallopian tubes and uterus, and the urinary bladder, urethra and rectum. The external pelvic organs in the female include the vagina, the labia and the clitoris.

The uterus is a thick-walled muscular organ, lying in the mid-line between the bladder and the rectum. It is roughly pear-shaped and about 3 inches long. The upper portion is called the "corpus" or "body" of the uterus; the lower portion, the "cervix," protrudes into the vagina. It has a round, smooth surface and a central opening, the external os. The uppermost part of the body of the uterus is the "fundus," which is round and smooth. The uterus is supported by a number of ligaments.

From either side of the uterus, just below the fundus, arise the 2 fallopian tubes, which extend laterally in the uppermost portion of the broad ligament. Each tube is a hollow muscular duct which opens into the uterus medially and laterally broadens into a trumpet-shaped structure with frond-like processes, the fimbriae. The tubes transmit the ova from the ovaries to the uterus.

The 2 ovaries lie on either side of the pelvis in close relation to the fimbriated ends of the fallopian tubes. Each ovary normally measures about 1½ inches long and ½ inch in thickness. An ovary produces the ovum (egg) at ovulation in response to hormonal stimulation.

The tubes, ovaries and broad ligaments are frequently collectively referred to as the "uterine adnexae," which literally means, "lying next to the uterus."

The vagina is a fibromuscular tube, 3 to 4 inches in length, which opens on to the perineum. Its outlet is bordered by the labia and in virginal females is partially or wholly closed by the hymen. The uterine cervix protrudes into the upper part of the vagina.

The labia majora and minora are double folds of skin, connective tissue and glandular tissue on either side of the vaginal orifice. They meet in the mid-line, posterior to the vagina, to form the posterior fourchette, which lies about one inch anterior to the anus. The posterior portion of the labia contains the Bartholin glands, which are usually un-recognized except when diseased. At the anterior end of the labia minora is the clitoris. Posterior to the clitoris and just anterior to the vaginal orifice is the urethral meatus. The urethra courses upward in the anterior wall of the vagina to enter the bladder. Thus, trauma to the vaginal area and pubic bone may damage the urethra.

Blood supply to the female genitalia is derived primarily from branches of the internal iliac vessels. Innervation is through the branches of the sacral plexus.

Between the uterus and the rectum is the cul-de-sac, which is the lowermost extension of the peritoneal cavity. It comes in contact with the uppermost portion of the vagina, behind the cervix. In diseases of the female genital tract associated with internal bleeding, fluid may be recovered from the cul-de-sac by aspiration. (See Figure 22–1.) This maneuver may be very helpful in confirming a diagnosis of intraperitoneal hemorrhage, particularly when pelvic in origin.

The pelvic organs are covered by parietal peritoneum. Their sizes and locations may vary between nulliparous women and those who have borne children. Collectively, the pelvic viscera lie within the peritoneal cavity. The fimbriated ends of the fallopian tubes open into the pelvic portion of the peritoneal cavity; so blood or pus within the tube drains into the peritoneal cavity. The ovaries discharge the ova into the same area. Similarly, blood or fluid from ruptured ovarian cysts may enter the peritoneal cavity, thus accounting for abdominal symptoms in gynecological disease.

GYNECOLOGICAL ASSESSMENT

Evaluation of a female patient with suspected pelvic disease includes both careful history and physical assessment. Occasionally, particularly in bleeding complications of pregnancy, blood loss can be massive and the patient may be in shock. Naturally in such patients, initiation of resuscitative and

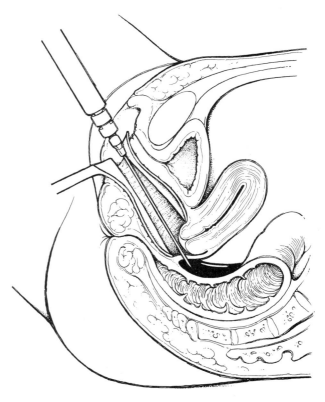

Figure 22–1 Cul-de-sac aspiration through posterior fornix of the vagina. The vagina is inspected with a speculum in place. The cervix may be grasped by a tenaculum and drawn anteriorly. A 4-inch needle attached to a syringe is inserted through the posterior fornix into the cul-de-sac for aspiration.

life-support measures take priority over complete history and physical data collection.

Whatever the complaint, be it pain, vaginal discharge or bleeding, the history must include time of onset and description of the presenting symptom (color, consistency, amount and odor of vaginal discharge, type of bleeding, presence of clots). The date of the last menstrual period and whether or not it was considered to be a normal cycle should be established. In traumatic conditions, the mechanism of injury should be determined. History data collection is particularly important in suspected rape cases.

Symptoms relating to other organs are common in many pelvic conditions. With regard to the gastrointestinal tract, nausea is common in association with pelvic disease, but anorexia and vomiting are not. Urinary symptoms are also common, particularly in inflammatory conditions of the female genital tract.

Basic instruments needed for physical evaluation of gynecological disease include sterile gloves, various sizes of vaginal specula and an adequate light source. An examining table with stirrups and clean drapes to protect the patient's modesty are essential. No pelvic examination should be performed without a female employee of the emergency department being present. Additional useful equipment include:

(1) Sponge forceps with sterile cotton and gauze squares.
(2) Uterine dressing forceps for packing.
(3) Plain or iodoform- or nitrofurazone (Furacin)-impregnated gauze packing.
(4) Uterine tenaculum for grasping the cervix.
(5) Cervical punch biopsy forceps.
(6) Endometrial aspiration biopsy forceps.

A uterine sound can also be useful at times. For cul-de-sac aspiration, to detect intraperitoneal bleeding especially when ruptured ectopic pregnancy is suspected, a 4-inch

TABLE 22–1 DRUGS USED IN GYNECOLOGICAL EMERGENCIES

Drug generic name	Drug trade name
(1) Medroxyprogesterone acetate suspension	Depo-Provera
(2) Sodium warfarin	Coumadin
(3) Heparin	
(4) Clomiphenecitrate	Clomid
(5) Hydroprogesterone caproate injection	Delalutin
(6) Penicillin	
(7) Podophyllin	
(8) Metronidazole	Flagyl
(9) Diazepam	Valium
(10) Oxytocin injection	Pitocin
(11) Probenecid	Benemid
(12) Ampicillin	
(13) Stilbestrol	

spinal needle and a 10 cc. syringe should be available.

The drugs commonly needed in treatment of gynecological emergencies are listed in Table 22–1.

Complete physical assessment is necessary, the essential points relating to evaluation of the abdomen and pelvis. In the absence of enlargement, the pelvic structures are not palpable through the anterior abdominal wall. However, bleeding or discharge from pelvic structures may cause irritation of the peritoneum, which can be detected by careful assessment of the abdomen.

Vaginal examination of the pelvic organs is one of the most important aspects of the assessment phase. It should be done gently and with a reassuring manner. In children and virginal females, particularly, a pelvic examination may be a painful and very traumatic experience. If it is the opinion of the examiner that the examination is contraindicated, limited evaluation of the pelvic structures may be carried out through the rectum.

Adequate pelvic evaluation includes speculum examination of the vagina and cervix, noting any discharge. If present, a specimen may be taken of the discharge for culture. The cervix is normally round and pink in color. In nulliparous females, the external os is round, while in parous females, the os is oblong.

Manual examination of the vagina is performed using the index and middle fingers. In females with a small introitus, examination may be carried out using one finger. A bi-

manual examination technique combines intravaginal examination with palpation of the lower abdominal wall (Figure 22–2). In this manner, the examiner attempts to outline the pelvic contents, evaluate the size of the uterus and determine whether the adnexae are enlarged. The cervix should be moved

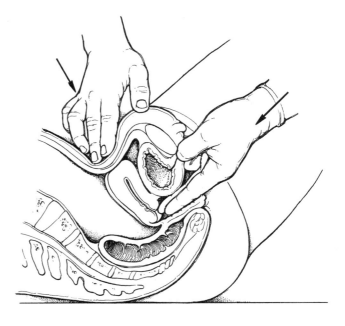

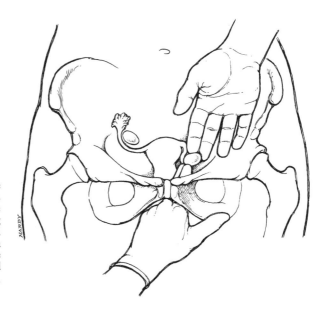

Figure 22–2 Bimanual examination of the female pelvic organs. Top: The examiner's left hand is inserted into the vagina, and the size of the uterus is evaluated by palpating the organ between the intravaginal hand and the hand on the anterior abdominal wall in the suprapubic area. Bottom: The adnexae (tubes and ovaries) should also be examined in this manner to determine any enlargement, masses. tenderness or displacement.

from side to side. In inflammatory conditions of the adnexae, particularly in salpingitis, moving the cervix to one side stretches the contralateral salpinx and will be painful.

NORMAL AND ABNORMAL MENSTRUATION

The normal menstrual cycle is a delicate mechanism involving the anterior pituitary gland, the ovaries and the uterine lining. Gonadotropic hormones from the pituitary stimulate primary follicles in the ovarian cortex to develop mature eggs and produce estrogen and progesterone. These hormones stimulate the uterine lining to develop a receptive bed for the potentially fertilized ovum.

The egg is usually released in mid-cycle. If fertilization by the male sperm does not occur within 36 to 48 hours, the egg undergoes degenerative changes, and the uterine lining is shed, about 2 weeks after ovulation. This release of the uterine lining is accompanied by arterial spasm in the uterine walls and resultant abdominal cramps, as the debris and blood are ejected. This constitutes the menstrual period.

Menstrual blood is usually nonclotting and averages 70 to 100 cc. per period. The discomfort of menstruation is related to the spasm, cramps, pelvic congestion and the smallness of the cervical os, which impedes menstrual flow. The influence of progesterone causes some water retention and the general misery associated with a young girl's periods.

The menstrual cycle varies tremendously, with a range of 20 to 46 days. Most women become fairly regular, varying only 2 to 3 days per cycle. Typically, the menstrual cycle is subject to irregularity mainly early and late in menstrual life, i.e., in the young girl and the menopausal woman. However, temporary irregularity may occur at any time, for no apparent cause.

Menstrual regularity can be affected by the action of other glands, such as the thyroid and adrenal. Emotional upsets, such as a death in the family, illness or a drastic change in environment, may cause delayed menses. However, it is important to keep in mind that a missed period in a woman of childbearing age is probably due to pregnancy until proven otherwise.

Dysmenorrhea (painful menses) may consist of abdominal pain, cramps, bloating and tension. In mild cases, analgesics may be all that is required. Diuretics and tranquilizers can be used to relieve bloating and premenstrual tension. More severe cases of dysmenorrhea respond to prevention of ovulation, which results in development of a thinner uterine lining and, therefore, less debris to be expelled. Ovulation can be prevented by large doses of estrogens, oral progestins (birth control pills) or intramuscular injections of long-acting progestins (e.g., medroxyprogesterone acetate suspension) to produce a pseudopregnancy and amenorrhea for a period of time. Smooth muscle relaxants may also give some relief. In severe dysmenorrhea, thorough evaluation is needed, and surgical treatment may be necessary, including presacral neurectomy or dilatation of the cervix to allow freer uterine flow.

In patients with abnormal bleeding, obviously, the cause must be determined before suitable treatment can be carried out. In the following pages, various types of gynecological bleeding will be discussed, along with typical symptoms and a brief outline of emergency treatment.

DYSFUNCTIONAL UTERINE BLEEDING

Premenarchal abnormalities

Vaginal bleeding in children has many causes.

Vicarious menstruation

Vicarious menstruation is seen most commonly in newborn female infants and consists of a blood-tinged mucous vaginal discharge occurring in the first 2 weeks after delivery.

This is not a pathological condition; it merely represents withdrawal bleeding from the lining of the infant uterus secondary to cessation of the estrogen which crossed the placenta from the mother's blood during pregnancy. The bleeding is of short duration and requires no treatment except reassurance to the parents bringing the child to the emergency department for assessment.

Premature menarche

The onset of menses will usually occur between the ages of 10 and 14. However, the first period may normally occur in some children as early as 8 or 9 years. It has even been reported in a girl as young as 5 years of age. However, all children with abnormally early menarche should be investigated to rule out pathological causes, such as pituitary tumors, certain types of brain tumors, ovarian tumors (such as thecal granulosa cell tumors, which are hormone-producing) or the presence of vaginal or uterine neoplasms.

Sarcoma botryoid is a rare vaginal or cervical tumor occurring in young girls or infants which may present with bleeding. It is usually a grape-like growth at the vaginal introitus. However, biopsy is necessary to prove the diagnosis. If confirmed, radical surgery is the treatment of choice.

Infection or foreign object in vagina

Many children brought to the emergency department present with a bloody, watery discharge secondary to a vaginitis. Before menarche, the vagina is very thin and easily irritated. The cells are not cornified, because there is no estrogen stimulation. Young girls, in their natural curiosity, frequently insert various items into the vaginal introitus. This may cause secondary infection, with discharge and sometimes bleeding. These self-inserted items defy description, varying from small wads of tissue to paper clips and rubber erasers. Speculum examination is difficult. However, an ear speculum, nasal

forceps or an x-ray (if the object is radio-opaque) will aid in the diagnosis. A mini-douche with saline and gentle wash often dislodges small objects.

Gonorrhea in female children may present as a vaginitis, due to the lack of protective thickening of the vagina by endogenous estrogen stimulation. This is in contradistinction to female adults, in whom cervical infection is a result of gonorrhea.

All vaginitis in children should be cultured on chochlate agar in a CO_2 environment or other suitable media to rule out gonococcus. Gram's stain smears should also be made to detect gram-negative intracellular diplococci. Treatment consists of appropriate antibiotic treatment, as well as investigation for the possible source. Once the diagnosis has been confirmed, local health authorities should be notified so that other contacts may be identified and treated.

Many females, regardless of age, in the same household will exhibit trichomonas vaginal infestation. The typical discharge is watery and yellowish and has a characteristic offensive odor. The diagnosis can be made by detection of motile trichomonads in wet drop preparations of the vaginal secretion. Treatment for a young child consists of local therapy. Nitrofurazone (Furacin) urethral suppositories inserted in the vagina are useful when the child is small and has an intact hymen. In older children and adults, there are many local preparations as well as an oral medication, metronidazole (Flagyl), which can be used.

Stilbestrol-related tumors

Recent research work has shown a significant relationship between the development of vaginal adenosis and clear cell carcinoma in female children whose mothers used diethylstilbestrol therapy during pregnancy. For a period of 10 to 15 years, beginning about 20 years ago, many high-risk pregnancy mothers were treated with stilbestrol in rather large doses to maintain the pregnancy. A very small percentage of these children have exhibited changes in the vagina and cervix which may develop into very malignant tumors.

Most of these victims will present with vaginal bleeding. Adequate examination and biopsy will confirm the diagnosis. It is recommended that all female children whose mothers took stilbestrol during pregnancy have periodic examinations and Papanicoleau (Pap) smears.

Trauma

Penetrating injuries of the vagina may cause vaginal bleeding. Careful exam is necessary. Straddle injuries, such as a fall onto a bicycle crossbar or a fence, can cause large hematomas and lacerations of the perineum. Adequate exam and x-ray studies to rule out intraperitoneal injury are necessary.

Congenital abnormalities

Imperforate hymen and obliteration of the vagina (partial or complete) may present in an emergency situation. The history is typically that a normally developed preteenage girl, with breast development, fat distribution and hair growth, has not menstruated or has only spotted. The absent or diminished menses is associated with periodic pelvic cramps, which become increasingly severe.

Inspection of the perineum shows a bulging hymen, and a bulging vagina is revealed on rectal examination. Excision of the obstruction under sterile conditions corrects the situation, usually performed in an operating suite.

Menstrual abnormalities

Menstrual abnormalities may also be due to defective hormone stimulation of the endometrial lining. It is a well-documented fact that whenever hormone stimulation of the uterine lining is suddenly stopped or fluctuates, withdrawal bleeding will occur. If complete release of the uterine lining occurs, normal menstruation results. However, if irregular shedding occurs, spotting and bleeding result and may continue over a long period of time. On occasion, prolonged estrogen stimulation results in a very thick uterine lining which bleeds readily. Mid-cycle spotting frequently occurs secondary to a slight hormone drop at the time of ovulation.

Dysfunctional uterine bleeding may be treated in one of several ways. A "D & C" (dilatation and curettage) will remove the abnormal lining and allow normal rhythmic menstrual growth to occur. Large doses of estrogen will overcome the fluctuations in physiological hormone levels and stop abnormal spotting and bleeding. Progesterone will often produce maturation of the lining, followed 5 to 10 days later by withdrawal bleeding ("medical curettage").

Recurrent dysfunctional bleeding can often be prevented by the temporary addition of estrogen and progesterone hormones to mimic a normal cycle. Oral progestins can also be used in this fashion. In most cases, a D & C is only done when the diagnosis is in doubt, where the bleeding has not responded to hormone treatment or when the problem is severe.

Dysfunctional bleeding may be associated with physiological cysts of the ovary, such as a persistent corpus luteum cyst which produces abnormal amounts of hormone and may present a clinical picture suggestive of ectopic pregnancy, appendicitis or threatened miscarriage.

Anemia in women is most commonly due to chronic blood loss associated with heavy periods over a long period of time. This is especially true in cases of marked hypothyroidism. Many authorities believe women should receive supplemental iron preparations prophylactically, to replace the body iron stores lost monthly through menstruation. Extremely heavy bleeding or clotting may respond to ergotrate preparations.

Bleeding secondary to IUDs

One of the annoying side effects of the various forms of intrauterine contraceptive devices (IUDs) is abnormal vaginal bleeding. This is commonly a menorrhagia at the time of normal menstruation or irregular bleeding in the mid-cycle, which appears to be due to local ulceration of the endometrial lining with associated endometritis. (Other complications secondary to the IUD are detailed in following pages.)

The treatment of menstrual irregularity secondary to an IUD includes Vitamin K, Vitamin C and large doses of estrogen or ergotrate preparations to cause uterine muscle contraction and reduction in menstrual flow.

Irregularity secondary to oral contraceptives

The physiological effect of oral progestins, the main component of birth control pills, is to suppress the pituitary gland by increasing hormone levels to inhibit follicle-stimulating hormone (FSH) and thus place the ovaries in a resting state similar to that seen during pregnancy. Since no ovulation occurs, no pregnancy can result. These pills are given in a cyclic fashion, usually for 20 to 21 days, then discontinued, usually for 7 days, so that withdrawal bleeding and a pseudo-period may result. These simulated periods are usually lighter in amount and are almost always painless, due to the reduced thickness of the uterine lining and the decidua-like tissue response.

Although a variety of side effects may accompany use of the pill, they are usually neither serious nor frequent in occurrence and in part depend on individual tolerance to the medication. Complications that do occur secondary to use of the birth control pill are considered later in this chapter.

If the oral progestins were given alone, there would be a marked degree of "breakthrough" bleeding. To prevent this, varying amounts of estrogen are added. British investigators have shown that it is apparently the added estrogen that is associated with the most serious complications of birth control pills, thrombophlebitis and embolic phenomena. Therefore, drug manufacturers have reduced the amount of estrogen to 50 μg. or less (or its equivalent), in order to reduce the risk.

Unfortunately, breakthrough bleeding is now more common.

Vaginal spotting can be dealt with by temporarily increasing the daily dose. Heavier bleeding may require discontinuing the pill for 7 days, even though the monthly supply has not been taken, then restarting another 21-day supply. Often, different combinations of progestins and estrogen or heavier doses will prevent the bleeding side effect.

Postmenopausal bleeding

Vaginal bleeding after 6 months of amenorrhea in a menopausal woman is always cause for concern. Gynecological malignancies reach peak incidence in the 40 to 60 age group. Postmenopausal bleeding must always be investigated to rule out a malignant cause. Cancer of the cervix or endometrium is the most common cause. Rarer tumors of the pelvis associated with vaginal bleeding include primary cancer of the vagina, ovarian tumors which may or may not produce estrogens and metastatic tumors to the vagina.

Cancer of the cervix

Carcinoma in situ may be present at any age, from 18 to 80. This is, in reality, not invasive cancer but a malignant change in the entire upper layer of the epithelium of the cervix or upper vagina. It is completely asymptomatic and can only be detected by Pap test or by use of the colposcope. Iodine solutions in the vagina will outline the abnormal areas so that punch biopsy or cone biopsy of the cervix will reveal the lesion. This type of tumor is very curable and will respond to various types of treatment.

Invasive cancer of the cervix almost always presents with vaginal bleeding as the chief complaint. A watery, serosanguineous discharge is often present. Examination will show a polypoid lesion involving the cervix or a firm cervix with an ulcer. Early cases involve the cervix only, while in more advanced disease, the vagina, broad ligament and even the bladder and rectum will be involved, sometimes with fistula formation and incontinence.

Emergency treatment in the face of hemorrhage includes transfusion, tight vaginal packing or hypogastric artery ligation. Treatment of invasive cancer of the cervix includes radical hysterectomy, radium plus cobalt radiation therapy or pelvic exenteration.

Terminal cases of cancer of the cervix usually present with uremia secondary to obstructive uropathy from tumor compression of the ureters. Distant metastasis with involvement of the lung are not uncommon.

Cancer of the endometrium

Endometrial cancer usually occurs in menopausal or postmenopausal women. The presenting symptom is almost invariably bleeding. The diagnosis is made by a D & C or endometrial biopsy. It is a very curable lesion and responds to panhysterectomy, with or without preoperative intrauterine radium. Advanced cases may respond to long-acting progestins in large doses (medroxyprogesterone acetate suspension or hydroprogesterone caproate injection).

Nonmalignant causes

(1) *Exogenous hormones* are another cause of postmenopausal bleeding. Many women receive estrogens to combat hot flashes and other menopausal symptoms, and a frequent side effect is vaginal bleeding. Endometrial biopsy or currettage is necessary, however, to rule out carcinoma.

(2) *Endometrial polyps* can also cause vaginal spotting.

(3) *Cystic glandular hyperplasia,* which is commonly seen in women undergoing waning ovarian activity, will cause postmenopausal bleeding.

(4) In some older women, bleeding may occur without evidence of abnormal lining to the uterus. Some physicians have diagnosed this as *uterine apoplexy,* that is, bleeding from a small surface artery, similar to that seen in nosebleed.

(5) *Hematometria* may also be seen in older women. This condition usually presents with some vaginal spotting plus a great deal of crampy menstrual-type pain. On pelvic exam, a large boggy uterus with a very tight or obliterated cervical os is detected. This state is often seen in endometrial cancer but may also be associated with a benign condition or a fibrotic cervix. D & C and drainage through the cervix are both diagnostic and curative.

(6) *Pyometria* (uterus full of pus) is quite similar in symptoms to hematometria, although bleeding is rare. Pyometria is usually associated with a uterine malignancy.

(7) Many older women with prolapsed uteri and cystoceles who are poor surgical risks have Gellhorn *pessaries or rings* inserted to hold their pelvic organs in place. These devices must be removed and replaced periodically to avoid tissue irritation or overgrowth of tissue, which would fix them firmly in place and make removal difficult. Some patients with pessaries will present with vaginal bleeding and discharge. Treatment consists of removal of the pessary and application of local hormone and antibacterial cream to cure the vaginitis and heal the epithelium.

(8) Some older women will present with *complete inversion of the vagina and prolapse of the uterus,* with contact ulcers of the cervix from abrasion of the organ on the underclothing. Treatment is usually surgical, but if the patient is a poor risk (and many are), a vaginal pessary may suffice.

LESIONS OF THE VULVA

Inflammatory lesions of the vulva are the type most often seen in an emergency department. Acute Bartholin's abscess is a common complaint. At one time, these were thought to be gonococcal in origin, but the vast majority encountered today are nonspecific bacterial infections due to coliform organisms.

The patient will present with an acute painful swelling in the mid-posterior aspect of the vulva, with bulging into the vaginal introitus.

Pain is aggravated by sitting or walking. There is considerable soft tissue swelling present. Emergency treatment is incision and drainage, although spontaneous rupture may often occur. The pus should be cultured for predominant organisms and gonoccocus. After drainage, antibiotics are rarely necessary. Sitz baths and analgesics will relieve the residual inflammation. Recurrences are common. A more permanent cure can be obtained by an operative procedure. The roof of the abscess wall is opened and a wedge of tissue removed. The edges of the wall are then marsupialized to create a new orifice for the Bartholin's gland.

A perirectal abscess can present as a subcutaneous abscess anywhere on the buttock or perineum. The patient will complain of a painful swelling in the area. Adequate rectal exam and the lack of bulging into the vaginal introitus can help in distinguishing this condition from Bartholin's abscess. Correct identification is important; the definitive treatment of this lesion is entirely different, since it originates within the anal crypts.

Herpes progenitalis

There has been an alarming increase in herpes progenitalis recently; it appears to have a venereal spread. The lesions are multiple small breaks in the skin and mucous membranes of the vulva and introitus. They may be single or in groups and are very painful. Enlarged, tender lymph nodes may be present in the groins. The condition is viral in origin, lasts approximately 10 days and may recur periodically.

Treatment is symptomatic, with analgesics, sitz baths and local anesthetic ointments. No satisfactory treatment other than pain relief is commonly available at this time. Antibiotics have no effect or value and should not be prescribed unless secondary bacterial infection has developed.

Syphilis

Chancre of the vulva is also being seen with increasing frequency This is a 1.0 to 1.5 cm. punched-out ulcer of the skin or mucous membrane, with a greyish, shaggy base. It is only slightly tender and appears 7 to 14 days after infectious sexual contact. A chancrous lesion is highly contagious on contact. It will disappear spontaneously in a fortnight, to be followed by the multiple mucous membrane lesions of secondary syphilis.

Blood Wasserman or other serology tests will not be positive until 10 to 14 days after the primary lesion appears. When suspected, special laboratory tests (dark field examination) on the scraping from the base of the ulcer are necessary, as well as follow-up serology in 2 to 3 weeks. Inguinal adenopathy may also be detected. Penicillin or broad-spectrum antibiotics in very large doses comprise the treatment of choice.

Syphilis is a reportable disease—once the diagnosis is confirmed, local health authorities are to be notified so that other patient contacts can be located and appropriate treatment initiated.

Condylomata acuminata

Venereal warts are now apparent in epidemic form. They are due to a virus and are usually spread by genital contact with an infected partner. They may involve the cervix and vagina but are very common on the labia, perineum and perianal areas. They occur in groups, some of which follow a linear distribution. The lesions are small, single or confluent, and may grow into very large groups.

Early lesions respond very well to 25 percent podophyllin in tincture of benzoin. This solution should be washed off in 4 hours, and abundant analgesic and local anesthetic preparations should be prescribed, because considerable local tissue reactions will occur for about 7 to 10 days. Other forms of treatment include electrocautery, surgical excision and cryosurgery. Multiple treatments are often necessary to eradicate the lesions.

Furuncles

Many sweat and sebaceous glands are present on the vulva, and infections in them are quite common. Early signs are of cellulitis, with a swollen, red area exquisitely tender to the touch. Later, the area becomes fluctuant.

In the early phase, local applications of heat or use of sitz baths and antibiotics may be indicated. However, as the area becomes fluctuant, incision and drainage under local anesthesia is the preferred treatment and will give relief. Follow-up care consists of analgesics and sitz baths. If inguinal nodes are involved, specific antibiotics effective against the predominant organism, which is usually staphylococcus, may be prescribed. In recurrent cases, skin care using a hexachlorophene soap should be used prophylactically, and blood glucose tests are in order to rule out diabetes.

VAGINITIS

Monilia vulvovaginitis

Monilia is a very common problem caused by autoinfection from an overgrowth of the yeast organism *Candida* (*Monilia*) *albicans*. The patient presents with a discharge and severe burning and itching of the vulvar and vaginal introitus areas. The tissue is reddened and weepy, and on occasion, whitish plaques can be seen. The burning is constant and is aggravated by urination.

This lesion is typical in uncontrolled diabetic patients, because the increased sugar content in the tissues and the acid environment predispose to overgrowth of the organism. To culture, the organism will grow in brownish-black colonies on Nicholson's media, which is commercially available. Wet smears or gram stains will also show the typical spores and mycelia.

Conditions which predispose to monilia infections are pregnancy, oral contraceptives, systemic antibiotic therapy which changes the normal vaginal bacterial flora (particularly penicillin) and diabetes. However, a large number of cases have no predisposing cause.

Treatment consists of local medication in the form of vaginal tablets, suppositories or ointments. The vaginal infestation must be controlled before the vulvitis will respond. Nystatin suppositories are very effective. Alkaline douches, such as 2 tablespoons of bicarbonate of soda in a quart of water, will help relieve the symptoms and restore an alkaline environment to the vagina.

Trichomonas vaginalis

Trichomonas is the second most commonly occurring vaginitis. The primary symptom is an abundant, yellowish, watery discharge with a slightly disagreeable odor. Itching and severe inflammation may be present. The condition is endemic, and many female carriers are asymptomatic, with the condition detected only on Pap smear. Trichomonas is highly contagious and can infect children; many investigators claim it is a type of venereal disease, but some cases are contacted in a nonvenereal fashion.

Diagnosis is definitive when wet saline drop preparations of the vaginal secretions are examined microscopically for the motile protozoa. Treatment consists of vaginal applications of metronidazole (Flagyl). For more persistent cases, Flagyl given by mouth will be effective most of the time. In recurrent infections, the male partner should also receive Flagyl, to prevent reinfection. Vinegar douches or commercial acid douches will also help control the condition.

Forgotten tampons

Vaginal tampons are being increasingly used by women of various ages. The neglected tampon, inadvertently left in the vagina, produces one of the most foul discharges ever encountered. Forgetting about a tampon often occurs when a new tampon is inserted before the used one is removed. The string attached to the first one will disappear, and the tampon can then be forgotten. In 3 to 4 days, a foul odor and brownish discharge occur, bringing many women to the emergency department.

Removal of the tampon will cure the condition, but during removal, the atmosphere of the treatment room will become nearly unbearable. Abundant amounts of aerosol spray are necessary. No further treatment is necessary, although sometimes antibiotic vaginal preparations may be prescribed.

OVARIAN DISEASE

In pursuit of its normal functions, both as an endocrine gland producing estrogen and progesterone and as a development site for mature ova, the human ovary during active menstrual life normally produces several types of cystic enlargements which appear and disappear. These include the graffian follicle cyst, which releases the ovum at ovulation, and the corpus luteum cyst, which replaces the graffian follicle cyst at the ovulating site on the cortex of the ovary and produces large amounts of estrogen and progesterone, which mature the endometrium to receive the fertilized egg.

Benign disease

Mittelschmerz

Ovulation pain is a common complaint and is often confused with appendicitis if it occurs on the right side. This pain may vary from vague discomfort of short duration to moderately severe pain which persists for several days. Mild pelvic and rebound tenderness may be present. The white blood count is only moderately elevated; temperature readings are 99° F. or less; and there is usually no associated anorexia. The most important sign is the expected date of the next period. This pain is almost always mid-cycle.

Cysts and tumors

(1) Hemorrhagic or ruptured corpus luteum cysts occur in the second portion of the menstrual cycle. A very tender, slightly enlarged ovary may be palpated on pelvic examination. Pain and tenderness in the lower abdomen are present. This condition must also be differentiated from appendicitis. Treatment is almost always expectant once

appendicitis and ectopic pregnancy are ruled out, merely requiring some form of pain relief and close observation.

(2) Large benign cysts of the ovary can also occur. Simple cysts are single cell layer cystic enlargements of the ovary. Unless complicated with pain or torsion, most cysts will disappear over a 3 to 4 week period. In fact, many cysts rupture asymptomatically during pelvic exam.

(3) Dermoid cysts are often found, especially in young women, as asymptomatic pelvic masses, perhaps very large. They contain hair, skin, sebaceous material and, on occasion, even teeth which can be seen on x-ray. If a dermoid cyst ruptures, it can produce a severe chemical peritonitis, but this complication is rare. Torsion of the ovarian pedicle is encountered more frequently. Women with dermoid cysts present with pelvic pain which typically is intermittent but may be constant. Treatment is surgical excision.

Other benign tumors include Brenner cell tumors, ovarian fibroids, thecomas, endometriomas, cystadenomas, pseudo-mucinous cystadenomas and many rarer types.

Malignancies

Malignant tumors of the ovary often reach extensive proportions with very few symptoms; it is an insidious disease. A large proportion of victims of malignant ovarian tumors present with abdominal ascites and palpable lower abdominal masses. Pain is seldom a presenting symptom unless torsion, hemorrhage or bowel obstruction has taken place.

Treatment consists of paracentesis, surgery, radiation treatment and chemotherapy. In the majority of cases, the prognosis is grave.

PELVIC DISEASE

Endometriosis

Pelvic endometriosis is very common, though the cause is unknown. It is due to the development of ectopic endometrial tissue, usually limited to the pelvis. This tissue, like the endometrium of the uterus, responds to the hormone cycle and bleeds internally in small amounts during menses. This causes localized blood deposits and tissue reaction. Although the tubes are usually patent and normal ovulation does occur, endometriosis is a leading cause of infertility in women.

There are two theories on causation. One posits that retrograde menstrual flow occurs through the fallopian tubes, causing random implantation of foci of viable endometrial tissue in the peritoneal cavity. The other theory is that endometrial implants occur in undifferentiated rests of embryonal tissue.

The condition may be asymptomatic. However, the typical case has marked dysmenorrhea, often with rectal pressure and backache. Common sites of endometriosis are the ovary (where rather large, chocolate-like cysts may be produced) and the posterior surface of the uterus, the uterosacral ligaments and the pelvic peritoneum (where small, tender nodules may develop).

Treatment is primarily surgical. Conservative excision is recommended in young women anxious to preserve their childbearing function. A pseudo-pregnancy can be produced by large doses of oral or intramuscular progesterone, which will cause decidual changes if carried out over long periods of time. Total removal of estrogen stimulation by removal of the ovaries will cure the most severe cases, but these patients cannot take exogenous hormones for menopausal symptoms if any abnormal tissue remains, because this will exacerbate their symptoms.

Inflammatory disease

Inflammatory pelvic disease includes all types of bacterial infections of the pelvis. The most common sites of infection are the cervix, endometrium and the fallopian tubes, although a diffuse infection of the pelvic tissues may occur (pelvic cellulitis).

(1) *Tuberculosis of the pelvis* is still seen, rarely. It is usually a silent disease, with few symptoms, and is almost invariably associated with pulmonary or renal tuberculosis. Sterility is a common result. The endometrium will grow and shed tubercular infested tissue monthly, so it may be diagnosed by D & C or endometrial biopsy. The tubes are often infected, but pain and fever are not a usual complaint. Treatment consists of prolonged antitubercular drug therapy, although, on occasion, pelvic surgery is necessary.

(2) *Cervicitis* is an infection of the cervical mucous glands. It is most commonly a low-grade infection, coliform or gonococcal in origin. The symptoms are purulent vaginal discharge and sometimes lower backache. Fever and other constitutional complaints are lacking. A large boggy, tender cervix with purulent exudate and pseudo-erosion are present. Treatment consists of suitable antibiotics followed by electrocoagulation, cryosurgery or conization of the cervix to correct the pseudo-erosion. Hospitalization is not usually required.

(3) *Endometritis* presents with pelvic pain limited to the uterus, often with lower backache and the presence of a tender, swollen uterus. The organism involved is usually *Escherichia coli* or other coliforms. It is secondary to miscarriage, D & C or intrauterine devices. Treatment consists of bedrest, antibiotics and removal of the IUD if one is present.

(4) *Salpingitis,* inflammation of the fallopian tubes, is a very common pelvic complaint. It is almost always due to gonorrhea, although it may be seen after delivery or secondary to other causes of endometritis. Women with salpingitis will present walking in a doubled-over position. Pain is prominent and usually bilateral, lower abdominal and constant, along with rebound tenderness.

The typical case of salpingitis occurs following a normal menstrual period. About the fourth or fifth day of the period, symptoms of pain develop and become progressively worse. Fever is present up to 104° F. Pelvic findings in early cases show adnexal tenderness and pain on movement of the uterus; a leukorrhea is often present. Advanced or recurrent cases may show tubo-ovarian pelvic masses or even a pelvic abscess bulging into the cul-de-sac.

Cultures should be taken from the cervix and periurethral glands for detection of gonorrhea and other organisms. Gram's stains of the exudate may show the intracellular gram-negative diplococci, even when cultures are negative. Even in typical cases, the gonococcus bacteria are not always recovered on culture, as secondary invaders, such as enterococci and other coliform bacteria, predominate cultures.

Treatment consists of bedrest, penicillin or broad-spectrum antibiotics, pain medication and drainage of pelvic abscesses, if any. If bilateral tubal masses remain after treatment, surgical removal of the tubes, ovaries and uterus should be done. If tubal enlargement persists, the tube is destroyed as an oviduct and permanent sterility occurs.

Early cases and primary infections will often completely recover with no sequelae after adequate treatment. However, peritubular adhesions, sterility and ectopic pregnancies are much more common in patients with salpingitis.

(5) *Intraperitoneal rupture of a tubo-ovarian abscess* can be a catastrophic event. Peritonitis becomes diffuse, and the patient may go into vascular collapse. Intravenous vasopressors, massive antibiotics and surgical intervention are necessary if this occurs.

Degenerating fibroids

Patients may present to the emergency department with pelvic pain secondary to uterine fibroid tumors. Pedunculated fibroids may twist on their stalks, with associated pain due to blood supply interference and tissue necrosis in the tumor. A tender fibroid tumor is found on examination. Treatment is surgical removal of the fibroid or possibly of the uterus. Large fibroids may undergo degeneration even if they are not pedunculated. The tumor, though benign, may outgrow its blood supply, causing necrosis of tissue, pain, fever or secondary infection.

Submucus fibroids can develop in the uter-

ine cavity and, by uterine contractions, deliver through the cervical os. There is usually colicky uterine pain, some bleeding and a necrotic mass presenting through the cervix. These can often be removed with a tonsil snare passed up to the stalk.

COMPLICATIONS FROM BIRTH CONTROL DEVICES

Intrauterine devices

There is an increased incidence of ectopic pregnancy in women who practice birth control by IUD. (Further discussion of ectopic pregnancies in the emergency department is presented below.) Occasionally, intrauterine pregnancy can occur despite the presence of an IUD, and such pregnancies often go to term with the IUD in situ. Salpingitis may also be seen because of infection due to the IUD, with the occasional development of tubo-ovarian or pelvic abscess. The latter conditions can render the victim sterile.

Birth control pills

Thrombophlebitis is rare, but if the deep veins are involved, it can be a serious side effect of the oral progestins. The symptoms are usually pain and swelling in one or both legs. The posterior aspect of the calf is painful on dorsiflexion of the foot, with the knee extended (Homan's sign). Sometimes a tender cord can be palpated behind the knee. Edema of the foot and lower leg may be present and in more serious cases may extend as high as the groin, with tenderness along the course of the femoral vein.

Treatment of severe cases of thrombophlebitis consists of discontinuation of "the pill" and initiation of immediate and long-term anticoagulant treatment, e.g., heparin plus warfarin sodium (Coumadin). In the face of embolic occurrences while on therapeutic doses of anticoagulants, ligation of the inferior vena cava may be necessary. Massive thromboembolism to the lungs is often fatal and may occur suddenly, without preexisting symptomatic evidence of thrombus formation in the lower extremities.

Venograms of the legs may be helpful in detecting thrombosis in the deep femoral veins which may not be clearly diagnosed on clinical examination. Acute thrombophlebitis in the superficial veins of the legs occurs more frequently, especially with preexisting varicosities. It is usually manifested by localized, red and tender areas and usually responds to elastic stockings, local heat and anti-inflammatory drugs. Although superficial thrombophlebitis has a much less grave prognosis than when deeper veins are involved, these patients should discontinue oral contraceptives and use other forms of birth control.

Other side effects of the pill are signs and symptoms of problems seen in pregnancy, which is understandable, since the 2 physiological states are quite similar. These problems include cloasma (the "mask of pregnancy," a brown discoloration of the cheeks and forehead, more prominent after ultraviolet ray exposure); nausea, especially for the first several days of the cycle; transient hypertension (rare); abnormal glucose tolerance (rare); increased ocular pressure, causing discomfort with contact lenses; an increase in occurrence of vascular headaches; and frequently, oligomenorrhea or amenorrhea.

Amenorrhea is fairly common secondary to oral contraceptives; it may be intermittent or persistent but almost invariably disappears after discontinuation of the medication. Frequently, there is a latent period before normal menstruation recurs, after the pills are discontinued, but this seldom lasts more than 6 weeks. On rare occasions, amenorrhea may persist but will usually respond to clomiphene therapy.

Vaginal monilia infections are also very common in women on the pill. Despite these side effects, however, the oral contraceptives are by far the most common type of contraceptive used today because of their great efficiency (99 percent plus effectiveness) and their lack of side effects, relative to other modes of birth control.

The "morning after" pill, though in restricted use, may be used as preventive birth control in the rape victim presenting in the emergency department. Side effects of stilbestrol, the pill's main component, are twofold. Though it must be taken daily for 5 days, it may produce severe gastrointestinal upset in the user. Secondly, if the user does not take the full dose, stilbestrol in the mother may cause future malignant tumors in a daughter if conception is not prevented. This hazard is discussed in more detail in following pages.

COMPLICATIONS OF PREGNANCY

Intrauterine pregnancy, first trimester

Nausea and vomiting

Nausea and vomiting occur often in the first 3 months of pregnancy, and in some women it may persist into the later stages. If these women become dehydrated, they may present themselves to the emergency department.

General appraisal of the patient is in order, including complete blood count, urinalysis and serum electrolyte studies. Treatment consists of fluid replacement by intravenous therapy and correction of electrolyte imbalance, as indicated. Sedation and withholding oral intake are helpful, until the symptoms are relieved. Injectable antiemetics are useful as tranquilizers. In milder cases, antiemetics given orally or by rectal suppository are adequate.

Threatened spontaneous abortion

When bleeding occurs in early pregnancy, the continuation of the pregnancy is in jeopardy. The symptoms vary from a brown or bloody spotting to bleeding as heavy as menses. The history is of one or more missed periods and an enlarged, softened uterus.

Speculum exam is always indicated, to

insure the bleeding is not from a local lesion of the cervix or vagina. As long as the cervical os is closed and no tissue has been passed, the pregnancy is presumed intact. However, such findings may also be present with a missed abortion or blighted ovum, that is, a pregnancy which has ceased and will inevitably be passed.

Treatment of threatened abortion consists primarily of bedrest. Some physicians prescribe progesterone therapy, in case the bleeding is due to inadequate corpus luteum hormone production. Additional therapy may include Vitamin C and Vitamin K preparations.

Incomplete abortion

When severe uterine cramps are associated with bleeding in the first trimester, the pregnancy will usually terminate. The passage of decidual or placental tissue is diagnostic of a miscarriage. Examination will show the cervix to be dilated, usually with tissue present in the cervical os. This tissue should be removed to slow the hemorrhage. Placental or decidual tissue has a lighter color, resembling hamburger, while blood clots more closely resemble raw liver.

Dilatation and curettage is the treatment of choice, although, on occasion, spontaneous complete expulsion of the uterine contents will occur, especially in the first 4 to 6 weeks. Further emergency treatment consists of ergot preparations or oxytocin (Pitocin) drip. Transfusion may be necessary; hence adequate blood should be available.

Hydatid mole

Hydatid mole is a rare condition which may be associated with alarming hemorrhage. Most cases are diagnosed at D & C. The passage of grape-like tissue is diagnostic. Hydatid mole is a degeneration of the placenta, causing it to overgrow and usually destroy the embryo. The uterus is often larger than expected, and spontaneous abortion most commonly occurs early in pregnancy. In rare cases, the uterus may be term-size, with huge masses of abnormal tissue present.

D & C is the treatment of choice, with close followup of gonadotropin levels, because this disease has a very real malignant potential to develop choriocarcinoma. On occasion, hypertension and toxemia may be present with hydatidform moles.

Second and third trimesters

Premature separation of placenta

All bleeding in pregnancy is due to separation of the placenta. However, it is only in the second and third trimester that the placenta has matured enough to cause alarming hemorrhage. Marginal separation may be painless, and bleeding is usually slight but may be heavy.

Abruptio or complete separation of the placenta can be catastrophic. It is almost invariably fatal to the fetus and may seriously jeopardize the mother's life. There is usually vaginal bleeding, but the separation may be occult. Severe pain, an enlarged, tense uterus and absence of fetal heart sounds will confirm the diagnosis. If the cervix is closed, immediate caesarean section is necessary

Blood specimens are drawn for complete blood count, type and crossmatch. Large veinways should be emplaced and Ringer's lactate solution begun immediately. Transfusion should be initiated as soon as type-specific blood is available. Large amounts of blood replacement may be needed.

A bleeding disorder known as afibrinogenemia may develop with any case of separation of the placenta. Thromboplastin substances may be released into the maternal circulation from the open placental sinuses. This sets up a complex reaction among the blood-clotting factors, resulting in the deposition of multiple intravascular microscopic clots. Maternal fibrinogen is also depleted, resulting in inability of the mother's blood to coagulate and uncontrolled bleeding. This is another contributing factor to the occurrence of disseminated intravascular coagulation (DIC) discussed in Chapter 9.

Afibrinogenemia should always be suspected when bleeding occurs in later pregnancy, and blood fibrinogen levels should be monitored. Samples of venous blood should be drawn and observed for times of clot development and retraction. Nonclotting blood is an ominous sign. Afibrinogenemia is treated with intravenous heparin to neutralize the circulating thromboplastin. Fibrinogen transfusions in large amounts, fresh frozen plasma therapy, blood transfusions and, most important, termination of the pregnancy should be expedited as soon as possible.

In many cases of premature separation of the placenta, labor rapidly ensues. Rupture of the membranes may control hemorrhage, by causing the uterus to contract. In fact, the sudden increase in the speed and intensity of labor should alert the nurse to the possibility of a separation, and the fetal heart tones should be monitored, especially if the bleeding increases.

Placenta praevia

If the placenta encroaches on the internal cervical os, a partial or complete placenta praevia is present. This is usually of clinical significance in the last 3 months of pregnancy. Painless bleeding is the pathognomonic sign. If bleeding is massive, transfusion and caesarean section are necessary. However, many cases will present with repeated episodes of painless bleeding.

Fortunately, many diagnostic modalities are available to pinpoint the implantation site of the placenta. These include ultrasound and isotope localization and several specialized radiologic techniques. These studies should be performed in any patient with painless vaginal bleeding in the last trimester, to avert a tragedy for mother and fetus. Vaginal examination and penetration of the cervical os should never be done in a suspected case of placenta praevia until adequate blood and operating facilities are immediately available. Treatment is usually caesarean section.

Toxemia of pregnancy

Toxemia of pregnancy is a condition typical of the last 3 months of pregnancy, characterized by this triad of symptoms: fluid retention, hypertension and albuminuria. It is a disease unique to human pregnancy, and its etiology is unknown. Most commonly, it occurs in primigravidas, multiple births and polyhydramnios. Distention of the uterus is a common factor. Other cases occur in association with preexisting hypertension, diabetes or renal disease.

If 2 of the 3 symptoms are present, the patient has pre-eclampsia. This is of no significance except to warn that many of these pregnant women will experience grand mal convulsions when the condition progresses to eclampsia. When convulsions occur, fetal loss is very high, and maternal risk is very serious. Separation of the placenta often occurs. Cerebral hemorrhage, renal shutdown or liver hemorrhage may jeopardize the life of the mother.

The pre-eclamptic mother frequently requires admission to the hospital. Treatment of pre-eclampsia consists of bedrest, diuretics, restricted salt intake, sedation and, on occasion, antihypertensive drugs. The ultimate treatment is delivery as soon as fetal maturity allows, either by medical induction or caesarean section.

The onset of convulsions requires intravenous diazepam (Valium), magnesium sulfate in large doses, antihypertensive drug therapy, sedation and delivery. The patient's treatment must be continued postpartum, because half of all eclamptics convulse after delivery. Meticulous monitoring of intake and output is necessary. Reflex activity such as clonus or a hyperactive knee jerk may indicate increasing central nervous system irritability.

Postpartum complications

Hemorrhage

Alarming hemorrhage may occur after delivery. It often happens to patients who have been discharged and sent home. They will suddenly bleed very heavily and most likely will present to the emergency department.

Postpartum hemorrhage is due to uterine relaxation, with opening of the placental sinuses. Predisposing factors include retained placental fragments or dissolution of the placental clot by saprophytic bacterial infection. The patient must be thoroughly evaluated to determine the amount of blood loss. A vaginal culture should be taken. Definitive treatment consists of blood replacement, oxytocin (Pitocin) drip (30 to 40 units/1,000 cc.) and possibly an emergency D & C, with or without uterine packing.

Infections

Salpingitis and tubo-ovarian or pelvic abscess may occur during the postpartum period. Postpartum women with infections will present with fever and abdominal pain. Assessment reveals lower abdominal and pelvic tenderness and rebound tenderness. A pelvic mass or a bulging into the vagina may be palpable on bimanual examination.

The patient should be admitted for a course of antibiotic therapy after suitable cervical, vaginal and blood cultures have been taken. Further management includes bedrest and surgical drainage of the abscess.

Ectopic pregnancy

Ectopic pregnancy is a condition commonly encountered in the emergency department. It occurs in approximately one in 100 to 120 pregnancies and develops when the fertilized ovum implants and grows outside of the uterine cavity. Tubal pregnancies are by far the most common type encountered. Less frequently, an intra-abdominal gestation may occur.

Since the fallopian tube is thin-walled, the enlarging pregnancy causes distention and eventual rupture, with subsequent intraperitoneal hemorrhage. Typically, the patient presents with a history of one missed period, lower abdominal pain and vaginal spotting. The pain is unrelenting, sharp, sudden in onset and often accompanied by weakness, dizziness or actual syncope, as a result of a blood loss. The pain may be unilateral or bilateral in the lower abdomen. Less commonly, the patient may note pain in the shoulder, due to diaphragmatic irritation (Kehr's sign). The symptoms are due to tubal rupture with varying degrees of blood loss.

Assessment reveals an acutely ill patient, who may be in shock. Blood samples are taken for complete blood count and crossmatch. Volume replacement should be instituted immediately, with Ringer's lactate and type-specific blood. As an axiom, any young woman with pelvic pain and vaginal bleeding should be considered to have an ectopic pregnancy, until proven otherwise. Temperature is usually normal or below 100° F.

Adjunct diagnostic tests include aspiration of the cul-de-sac with a spinal needle and 10 cc. syringe, laparoscopy, colpotomy or culdescope examination. Free blood in the peritoneal cavity requires surgical investigation, because by far the most common cause is tubal pregnancy. Treatment consists of blood replacement and salpingectomy.

Septic abortion

Septic abortions are less common at the present time, due in great part to the liberalized abortion laws; many septic abortions resulted from criminal attempts at interruption of pregnancy. When abortion attempt results in incomplete removal of the products of conception, the result is pelvic infection. The unfortunate victims are usually very sick, with high fever, abdominal pain and foul-smelling vaginal lochia.

Assessment will reveal an acutely ill woman with abdominal and pelvic tenderness. Bimanual examination will be painful, particularly with motion of the cervix. Blood, vaginal and tissue cultures are indicated. A high degree of clinical suspicion is necessary, as a history of attempted interruption of pregnancy is almost impossible to obtain.

Treatment consists of massive antibiotics. Since most of these infections are due to coliform bacteria, broad spectrum treatment is indicated. The uterus should be emptied of its contents as soon as adequate blood antibiotic levels are obtained. Septic shock with alarming hypotension may be present and requires vigorous treatment. Blood pressure, pulse, arterial blood gases, central venous pressure and intake and output should all be closely monitored. Vasoactive drugs may be necessary to maintain arterial pressure in order to adequately perfuse vital organs. Treatment with large doses of steroids may also be indicated. Of course, suitable blood and tissue cultures should be obtained. In this instance, also, one must maintain a high index of suspicion for disseminated intravascular coagulation, which is an ominous complication.

Trauma in pregnancy

Gunshot wounds to the abdomen during pregnancy are rare, but they do occur, often as a result of domestic altercations. They should be treated like any other gunshot wound, with the consideration that 2 humans are wounded. Adequate blood replacement and urgent laparotomy are indicated. The pregnancy should be preserved, if possible, but if penetration of the uterus has occurred, hysterotomy must be done.

Unless direct injury to the uterus occurs in an automobile accident, jeopardy to the fetus depends on the mother's condition. The fetus is well protected and will usually be uninjured unless severe force directly to the pregnant uterus causes uterine rupture or premature separation of the placenta. If prolonged hypotension to the mother occurs, the fetus will usually be lost, as intrauterine life is very sensitive. Treatment consists of adequate life-sustaining measures to the mother.

RAPE

Most victims of rape will present to the emergency department through their own volition or be brought by law enforcement officers for the purpose of obtaining evidence to sustain criminal proceedings against the suspect. This is a frightening and often humiliating experience for the woman involved; it is a situation where an understanding nurse can be invaluable.

Treatment consists of meticulous description and treatment of local and general trauma. Cultures are taken for possible gonorrhea exposure. Vaginal specimens should be obtained for wet drop preparations to discern motile sperm. Smears should be taken for permanent staining to detect the presence of sperm in the cervical mucus or vagina. In some laboratories, vaginal secretions are tested for acid phosphatase, which is present in very high concentrations in seminal fluid and usually not present in the vagina unless recent intercourse has occurred. Evidence such as seminal stains and foreign pubic hair should be described and saved for the police laboratory.

If possible pregnancy is a problem, especially when rape occurs near the fertile period, treatment with the "morning after" pill should be given. This consists of stilbestrol in high doses, 0.025 gm. twice a day for 5 days, and should be started within 72 hours of exposure to sperm. This medication will convert the endometrium to an unreceptive bed for the fertilized egg so that pregnancy will not occur. A prophylactic dose of ampicillin, 3.5 gm., and probenecid (Benemid), 1.0 gm. may be given if infection with gonorrhea or syphilis is suspected.

The "morning after" pill may cause severe gastrointestinal upset, including nausea and emesis. Thus, the patient must be advised of the importance of completing the dosage despite the upset. Incomplete treatment may result in pregnancy, and if the resulting child is female, she may have an increased susceptibility to vaginal and cervical malignancies. (See the discussion of stilbestrol-related tumors, above.)

The greatest injury to women in rape cases is usually emotional rather than physical. A number of voluntary organizations have formed to offer counsel and emotional and legal support to the rape victim. Appropriate referral to such an agency is indicated.

SUMMARY

Perhaps more than in any other emergency, the emotional and psychological support the nurse gives the patient with a gynecological problem is crucial. Many gynecological problems are nothing more than anxiety over normal variations in the menstrual cycle. Many, like rape, involve serious violation of the patient's body and mind. The emergency nurse who can assess the seriousness of the problem and respond appropriately and supportively does her patients perhaps the greatest service they will need in the emergency department.

BIBLIOGRAPHY

(1) Acker, D.; Jenson, A. B., and Tenn, G. K.: "Abdominal Pregnancy with Intrauterine Device in Situ," *Obstetrics and Gynecology,* 42 (1973):36.

(2) Acosta, A. A.; Murray, C. R., and Kaufman, R. H.: "Intrauterine Pregnancy and Coexistent Pelvic Inflammatory Disease," *Obstetrics and Gynecology,* 37 (1971):282.

(3) Bachman, F.: "The Paradoxes of Disseminated Intravascular Coagulation," *Hospital Practice,* 6 (1971):113.

(4) Barchet, S.: "A New Look at Vaginal Discharge," *Obstetrics and Gynecology,* 40 (1972):615.

(5) Beecham, J. B.; Watson, W. J., and Clapp, J. F.: "Eclampsia, Pre-eclampsia and Disseminated Intravascular Coagulation," *Obstetrics and Gynecology,* 43 (1974):576.

(6) Burgess, S. G.; Mancuso, P. G.; Kalis, P. E., *et al.:* "Clinical and Laboratory Study of Vaginitis," *New York State Journal of Medicine,* 70 (1970): 2086.

(7) Burmeister, R. E., and Gardner, H. L.: "Vaginitis: Diagnosis and Treatment," *Postgraduate Medicine,* 48 (1970): 159.

(8) Burry, V. F.: "Gonococcal Vulvovaginitis and Possible Peritonitis in Prepubertal Girls," *American Journal of Diseases of Children,* 121 (1971):536.

(9) Capraro, V. J.: "Sexual Assault of Female Children," *Annals of the N. Y. Academy of Science,* 142 (1967):817.

(10) Czernobilsky, B.; Kessler, I., and Lancet, M.: "Cervical Adenocarcinoma in Women on Long-Term Contraceptives," *Obstetrics and Gynecology,* 43 (1974):517.

(11) Davis, H. J., and Lesinski, J.: "Mechanism of Action of Intrauterine Contraceptives in Women," *Obstetrics and Gynecology,* 36 (1970):350.

(12) Dehner, L. P.: "Metastatic and Secondary Tumors of the Vulva," *Obstetrics and Gynecology,* 42 (1973):47.

(13) Dickie, E. G.: "Herpes Vulvitis," *Obstetrics and Gynecology,* 34 (1969): 434.

(14) Dwyer, J. F.: "Teenage Pregnancy," *American Journal of Obstetrics and Gynecology,* 118 (1974):373.

(15) Emmens, C. W.: "Postcoital Contraception," *British Medical Bulletin,* 26 (1970):45.

(16) Evrard, J. R.: "Rape: The Medical, Social and Legal Implications," *American Journal of Obstetrics and Gynecology,* 111 (1971):197.

(17) Harralson, J. D.; Van Nagell, J. R., Jr., and Roddick, J. W., Jr.: "Operative Management of Ruptured Tubal Pregnancy," *American Journal of Obstetrics and Gynecology,* 115 (1973):995.

(18) Holmes, K.; Counts, G., and Beaty, H.: "Disseminated Gonococcal Infections," *Annals of Internal Medicine,* 74 (1971): 979.

(19) Lang, W. R.; Fritz, M. A., and Mendecki, H.: "The Bacteriologic Diagnosis of Trichomonal, Candidal and

Combined Infections," *Obstetrics and Gynecology,* 20 (1962):788.

(20) Ledger, W. J.; Sweet, R. L., and Headington, J. T.: "Bacteroides Species as a Cause of Severe Infections in Obstetric and Gynecologic Patients," *Surgery, Gynecology and Obstetrics,* 133 (1971): 837.

(21) Massey, J. B.; Garcia, C., and Emich, J. P.: "Management of Sexually Assaulted Females," *Obstetrics and Gynecology,* 38 (1971):29.

(22) Nesbitt, R. E. L., and Rizk, P. T.: "Uterosacral Ligament Syndrome," *Obstetrics and Gynecology,* 37 (1971): 730.

(23) Nolan, G. H., and Osborne, N.: "Gonococcal Infections in the Female," *Obstetrics and Gynecology,* 42 (1973):156.

(24) Peterson, W. P.; Prevost, E. C.; Edmonds, F. T., *et al.:* "Benign Cystic Teratomas of the Ovary: A Clinicostatistical Study of 1007 Cases with a Review of the Literature," *American Journal of Obstetrics and Gynecology,* 70 (1955):368.

(25) Peyser, M. R.; Ayalon, D.; Harell, A.; *et al.:* "Stress-Induced Delay of Ovulation," *Obstetrics and Gynecology,* 42 (1973):667.

(26) Poliak, A.; Smith, J. J., and Romney, S. L.: "Clinical Evaluation of Clomiphene in Anovulatory Cycles," *Fertility and Sterility,* 24 (1973):921.

(27) Poste, G.; Hawkins, D. F., and Thomlinson, J. "Herpevirus Hominis Infections of the Female Genital Tract," *Obstetrics and Gynecology,* 40 (1972): 871.

(28) Pritchard, J. A.; Weisman, R.; Ratnoff, O. D., *et al.:* "Intravascular Hemolysis, Thrombocytopenia and Other Hematologic Abnormalities Associated with Severe Toxemia of Pregnancy," *New England Journal of Medicine,* 250 (1954):89.

(29) Sagiroglu, N., and Sagiroglu, E.: "Biologic Mode of Action of the Lippes Loop in Intrauterine Contraception," *American Journal of Obstetrics and Gynecology,* 106 (1970):506.

(30) Sharpe, N.: "The Significance of Spermatozoa in Victims of Sexual Offenses," *Canadian Medical Association Journal,* 89 (1963):513.

(31) Shore, W. B., and Winkelstein, J. A.: "Nonvenereal Transmission of Gonococcal Infections in Children," *Journal of Pediatrics,* 79 (1971):661.

(32) Smith, J. W.; Southern, P., and Lehmann, J. D.: "Bacteremia in Septic Abortions: Complication and Treatment," *Obstetrics and Gynecology,* 35 (1970):704.

(33) Spellacy, W. N.; Zaias, N., and Birk, S. A.: "Vaginal Yeast Growth and Contraception Practices," *Obstetrics and Gynecology,* 38 (1971):343.

(34) Teitze, C.: "Contraception with Intrauterine Devices," *American Journal of Obstetrics and Gynecology,* 96 (1966):1043.

(35) Teitze, C.: "Probability of Pregnancy Resulting from a Single Unprotected Coitus," *Fertility and Sterility,* 11 (1960):485.

(36) Yen, S. S. C.; Reagan, J. W., and Rosenthal, M. S.: "Herpes Simplex Infection in the Female Genital Tract," *Obstetrics and Gynecology,* 25 (1965): 479.

(37) Yen, S. S. C.; Vela, P.; Rankin, J., *et al.:* "Hormonal Relationship During the Menstrual Cycle," *Journal of the American Medical Association,* 211 (1970):1513.

23

Genitourinary emergencies

JOSEPH P. GAMBACORTA
MARY C. SAND

Patients with genitourinary problems are frequently seen for the first time in the hospital emergency department. The severe pain of renal colic, the inability to urinate or the sight of gross blood in the urine often prompts patients to seek immediate professional care. These patients deserve a thorough clinical evaluation, an accurate diagnosis and appropriate definitive treatment and care. The role of the emergency department nurse in helping to meet these objectives will be discussed in this chapter, as well as the various procedures, equipment and techniques necessary for proper management of the urological emergency.

ANATOMY AND PHYSIOLOGY

The genitourinary systems of the male and female differ considerably. In the male, the G.U. system combines the organs of urine formation and excretion with the organs of reproduction, while in the female, the lower portion of the urinary tract is closely related to the reproductive organs but entirely separate. Furthermore, in the male, the urinary tract consists of both internal organs and external genitalia (penis, testicles and scrotum). In the female, those organs that make up the urinary tract are completely within the body and in close proximity to the abdominal cavity. Common to both sexes are the components of the urinary tract: the kidneys, ureter, bladder and urethra.

The kidneys and ureters are often referred to as the upper urinary tract, the bladder and urethra as the lower urinary tract. The kidneys are paired organs, located on either side of the vertebral column, overlying the psoas muscle in the paravertebral gutter. They are extraperitoneal (outside the peritoneal cavity), in the retroperitoneal space, surrounded by loose areolar tissue, known as the perirenal fat, and a dense layer of fibrous tissue, called Gerota's fascia.

Posterior to each kidney is the lowermost rib and the transverse processes of the upper lumbar vertebrae. The angle formed by these bone structures is referred to as the costovertebral angle. Anteriorly, the kidney is in close apposition to the abdominal organs. The right kidney is slightly lower than the left, being displaced inferiorly by the liver. In a thin person, the lower pole of each kidney may be palpated by careful abdominal examination during an inspiratory movement.

The arterial blood supply to the kidneys is derived from the right and left renal arteries, which arise from the abdominal aorta. The renal veins empty into the inferior vena cava.

The 2 ureters are fibromuscular tubes which serve as conduits for urine from the kidneys to the bladder. Each extends from the pelvis of the kidney on its medial aspect, downward into the paravertebral gutter retroperitoneally. The ureter enters the brim of the pelvis as it crosses over the common iliac artery and enters the bladder at the lower posterior wall.

The bladder is roughly pyramidal in shape, with the apex inferiorly and the base superiorly. From the apex, the bladder empties through the urethra. The superior pole of the bladder is covered by peritoneum. The bladder lies behind the pubic symphysis and is not palpable through the abdomen unless distended with urine.

In the female, the urethra courses from the lower end of the bladder in close relation to the anterior wall of the vagina and reaches its external opening at the meatus just posterior to the clitoris.

In the male, the urethra is longer. Just beneath the bladder apex, the prostate surrounds it; the urethra passes through the urogenital diaphragm at the membranous portion and enters the penis. The penile urethra extends the entire length of the penis and ends at the meatus on the glans. The testicles are suspended in the scrotum, which is attached to the posterior aspect of the penis and the perineum.

ASSESSMENT

Evaluation of the patient with suspected urinary tract disease requires careful history and physical assessment. The most common symptoms are pain and some alteration in urinary habits. In traumatic injuries, urinary tract damage must be suspected in patients with penetrating wounds of the upper abdomen and in association with fractures of the pelvis.

History, symptoms and signs

Historical data to be collected include the onset, location and description of the type of pain, whether sharp, dull, aching, crampy, burning, stinging, constant or intermittent. Does voiding have any effect on the pain? Has there been any change in urination, any frequency, variation in amount of urination or nocturia? Has the patient noted any unusual color to the urine: clear, cloudy, concentrated ("strong") or containing blood? Is there any history of fever or chills?

Pain originating from the urinary tract is located at the site of the problem. Lesions of the kidney, infection or trauma will usually produce pain in the area of the costovertebral angle and the upper abdomen (epigastrium). When a ureter is involved, as in calculous disease, pain may be felt in the flank, radiating along the course of the ureter and upward into the kidney or downward and anteriorly into the lower abdomen. In obstructive disease of the lower third of the ureter, the pain may radiate into the labia or testis. Obstruction of the ureter, particularly by calculi, causes a typical colicky type of pain, which is one of the most severe experienced by humans. The pain cycle begins in a crescendic manner, with the pain reaching a peak that may last for minutes and gradually subsiding. The cyclic pain is due to the peristaltic activity of the ureter against the obstructing lesion.

Symptoms arising from the bladder are usually localized at the site of the bladder, in the lower abdomen, and are frequently associated with pain or burning on urination (dysuria). Gastrointestinal symptoms may occur secondary to urinary tract lesions.

In infectious diseases of the kidney, pyelonephritis for example, a reflex intestinal ileus may occur, with abdominal discomfort and fullness. Anorexia may be present, but nausea and vomiting are uncommon. Systemic reactions of fever and chills occur with significant frequency in urinary tract infections, especially when the kidney itself is involved.

Physical examination

Examination of the patient with complaints referable to the urinary tract should begin with the vital signs, temperature, pulse, respiration and blood pressure. Complete physical examination is advisable. The urinary tract can be evaluated to a great extent by careful examination of the abdomen. In renal disease, tenderness may be present on deep palpation in the epigastric region. The kidneys are not normally palpable through the abdomen, except in a thin person or in pathologic conditions associated with enlargement of the kidney. With the patient sitting, percussion or a light punch in the costovertebral angle will usually elicit pain. With ureteral obstruction, tenderness is often present along the course of the ureter. The physical findings are rarely consistent with the severity of the pain, in that abdominal spasm and rebound tenderness are rarely, if ever, found.

When the bladder is involved, tenderness is usually present in the suprapubic area of the abdomen. The bladder is not palpable unless enlarged because of urinary retention; then a mass may be palpable in the mid-portion of the lower abdomen. Careful percussion will reveal a dull to flattened note in the area of the enlarged bladder. Bladder enlargement can be confirmed in the female by bimanual and vaginal examination. The urethral meatus should be examined visually at all times. A urethral caruncle may be identified. This is a polypoid tumor of the urethra which is usually found at the meatus; it may be a source of bleeding.

In the male, the external genitalia should be inspected and the scrotal contents palpated to determine that the testes are completely descended. Each testis is suspended by the spermatic cord, an elastic structure which extends from the testis upward into the inguinal area and enters the abdominal wall at the level of the internal inguinal ring. The structure contains blood vessels, nerves, and vas deferens (the spermatic duct). In inflammatory conditions of the testes, cord enlargement and tenderness may be present.

Injuries of the urinary tract should be suspected in penetrating wounds of the abdomen and fractures of the pelvis. When the history of physical findings points to urinary tract involvement, a number of adjunct studies are available and should be used as needed to confirm the diagnosis.

Adjunct studies

A great number of tests are available to assist in evaluation of the patient with urinary tract symptoms or injury. The one most frequently used is simple analysis of the urine. Gross examination for color, specific gravity, sugar and protein and microscopic study for blood cells, sediment and bacteria are extremely helpful.

X-ray studies available in the emergency department includes the K.U.B. (kidneys, ureters, bladder) plate, which will aid in identifying the size and location of the renal shadows. The film should also be carefully examined for any calcification in the area of the renal shadow, along the course of the ureters, for urinary stones.

In a patient with abdominal pain suggestive of renal colic, use of an I.V.P. (intravenous pyelogram) can be most helpful in outlining the excretory ducts of the kidney to locate a stone. It can be done in the emergency department if necessary. More involved studies, such as infusion pyelograms, retrograde pyelograms and renal scintiscans and angiograms may be useful in determining renal functioning and/or damage, especially in the patient suspected of urinary tract injuries. Any patient with a renal injury that may involve removal of a whole or part of a kidney *must* have an intravenous pyelogram preoperatively to evaluate the function of both kidneys and assure the physician that both kidneys are, indeed, present.

Patients with pelvic fracture and blood in the urine must be evaluated for injury to the bladder. A simple technique, which can be carried out in the emergency department, is retrograde cystography. Sodium diatrizoate (Hypaque Sodium) is injected into the bladder through a catheter, and x-rays of the region are taken. Deformity of the bladder wall may indicate a contusion or hematoma, while extravasation of urine is pathognomonic of perforation of the bladder. Failure to recover urine may be indicative of damage to the urethra, in which instance extravasation of the dye will be apparent on x-ray study.

CALCULOUS DISEASE

Urinary calculi have plagued man from the beginning of recorded history. Despite ongoing research, stone formation is still a common problem, and cause and prevention of the majority of calculi are still unknown. Calculous disease may occur anywhere in the urinary tract, kidney, ureter, bladder or prostate. This discussion will be limited mainly to ureteral stones, since this type causes the severe colicky pain that prompts most patients to seek care in the hospital emergency department.

Ureteral calculi occur mainly in middle life; 69 percent of calculi victims are between the ages of 20 and 50 years. It is seen more often in men than women and more often in the spring and fall months. Ureteral calculi are formed in the kidneys, around a nucleus which may be composed of pus, blood, a crystal or devitalized tissue. Chemical analysis reveals that 91 percent of calculi contain calcium in some form, 8 percent are uric acid and one percent are cystine stones. Thus, some are not radio-opaque.

The known causes of urinary calculi are multiple. A urinary tract infection with a urea-splitting organism, such as staphylococcus or proteus, seems to predispose to stone formation. Immobilization, which impairs renal drainage, alters the calcium mechanism and results in skeletal decalcification, is another predisposing factor. Metabolic disorders, which result in hypercalcemia and/or hypercalciuria (such as hyperparathyroidism and hyperthyroidism), are known to cause renal stones. Other metabolic diseases which cause urinary calculi are gout and cystinuria. Some stones are formed secondary to disorders within the urinary tract.

Assessment

The symptoms produced by urinary tract stones are influenced by the presence or absence of obstruction and infection and by local irritation of the renal pelvis or ureter, resulting in edema. Renal stones cause some discomfort or a dull ache in the kidney area, which is usually not disabling. Ureteral stones more often cause an acute onset of colic without prodromal symptoms. The pain is severe and intense. It may be in the area of the costovertebral angle, generally radiates down the ureter and may be referred to the testicle or vulva. The pain may last for hours or may subside within a few minutes.

The patient with ureteral colic is often cold and clammy; his pulse is weak and rapid, and there may be a drop in blood pressure. If the kidney is obstructed and the urine is infected, he may have fever and chills. Nausea and vomiting are fairly common, and in some instances all the symptoms may mimic gastrointestinal disease. The stone may pass down the ureter, and as it nears the bladder, the patient may complain of frequency and burning on urination. In most patients with ureteral calculi, there is hematuria, either gross or, more commonly, microscopic.

A detailed history will reveal the nature of the pain, its location and radiation, as well as any previous similar episodes or any metabolic disorders, such as gout or parathyroid disease. On physical examination, tenderness can usually be elicited with deep pressure to the renal area anteriorly and gentle percussion in the costovertebral region.

To make certain a diagnosis of ureteral calculi, laboratory and x-ray studies are necessary. Routine urinalysis should be made and noted for the presence or absence of red blood cells, white blood cells and bacteria. In the female, a "clean catch" sample should be obtained. During the menstrual period, catheterization will be necessary. At this time, a culture should be submitted to the laboratory. Blood should be drawn for routine blood count and chemistry profiles, including serum protein, urea, calcium, phosphorus, chloride, CO_2, uric acid and acid phosphatase.

Perhaps the most helpful diagnostic study for ureteral calculi is x-ray of the abdomen, ordinarily referred to as a K.U.B. plate, followed by an intravenous pyelogram. In the latter, the renal shadows are outlined, the position of the stone is revealed, any obstruction is evident, the status of the opposite kidney is ascertained and the status of renal function is indicated. It should be noted that 15 percent of all renal calculi are not visible on x-ray. Admission is usually required for further workup and treatment.

Electively, a cystoscopy may be performed. If a stone has passed, it will be apparent by the edema about the ureteral orifice. Retrograde pyelograms may be necessary because of incomplete visualization of the entire length of the ureter or poor concentration of the contrast material by the kidney at the time of the I.V.P. This is done during cystoscopy by passing a fine catheter into the ureter and injecting contrast material. A complete stone workup is in order to uncover any of the organic or metabolic diseases that are manifested by urinary calculi. Helpful, in this respect, are urinary excretion studies of calcium, phosphorus, uric acid, oxalate and cystine, the phosphate reabsorption test and a parathormone assay.

Management

The treatment of ureteral calculi depends on many factors. To be considered are: (1) the size of the stone, (2) the degree of obstruction, if any, (3) the severity and duration of the symptoms, (4) the status of the opposite kidney, (5) the presence or absence of infection and (6) the occupation, age and general condition of the patient.

Generally, the patient with a small stone that is not accompanied by infection or progressive hydronephrosis and whose colic is not too frequent or disabling may be simply observed, with the hope that it will pass. Of all renal calculi, 90 percent will pass through the ureters, bladder and urethra spontaneously.

An intermediate treatment of ureteral stones is ureteral manipulation. This can be done in 2 ways. At the time of cystoscopy, a wire basket enclosed in a ureteral catheter is passed up the ureter to the stone, the basket is opened and the stone hopefully engages in the basket and is pulled into the bladder. The second method, also done at the time of cystoscopy, is passing a ureteral catheter up to the kidney and leaving it in place for a time. This will relieve any obstruction to the kidney, and it will dilate the ureter, making passage of the stone somewhat easier after the catheter is removed.

Elective surgical intervention is the treatment of choice for stones larger than 1.0 cm., when renal parenchyma is being destroyed due to obstruction and/or infection or when the symptoms are persistently severe. In all instances of ureteral calculi, individualization of patient treatment is necessary. This requires sound clinical judgment to determine whether to pursue a policy of watchful waiting or intervene surgically.

The long-range treatment of a patient with ureteral calculi depends on the chemical analysis of the stone and the presence of any contributory organic or metabolic disease. Parathyroid adenomas are treated with an appropriate surgical procedure. Gout can be treated with a low purine diet, allopurinol, alkalinization of the urine and a high fluid intake. Cystinuria can be treated to some extent with D-penicillamine. The vast majority of patients with calculous disease will pass calcium-containing stones and will have a negative workup for organic or metabolic disease. At present, the long-range regime for these patients is a diet low in calcium, a high fluid intake and, possibly, the administration of ascorbic acid to lower the urinary pH.

Nursing considerations

The most immediate problem for a patient with a ureteral stone is relief of the intense colic that it causes. The patient may be unable to remain in bed and may walk about doubled up in agony. Fairly high doses of narcotics are usually needed to control this pain, and with the administration of these drugs, precautions should be taken to prevent the patient from injuring himself. Pain must be evaluated and dealt with individually, but the usual nursing measures used in caring for a patient in pain can be applied here. (See Appendix G, which follows Chapter 20.)

The next consideration for the emergency department nurse is the proper collection of preliminary laboratory work. Special care should be given to the collection of urine for analysis and culture. Cleanly voided urine is taken unless ordered otherwise. If there is to be a significant delay in transporting it to the laboratory, the urine should be refrigerated. The results of the urinalysis may directly influence diagnosis and subsequent treatment.

Fluids should be taken liberally; 4 to 5 liters in 24 hours is an appropriate amount. This increases the urinary output and, hopefully, puts an extra "push" behind the stone. Many patients with ureteral stones have accompanying gastrointestinal symptoms, such as nausea and vomiting. If their oral intake is inadequate, the urologist may order intravenous therapy. An adequate fluid intake is especially important if the patient is febrile.

If infection is present and the patient is febrile, antibiotics are ordered. Any allergic sensitivity to these drugs must be ascertained. For a markedly elevated temperature. an antipyretic may be needed.

The next step is an x-ray of the abdomen and pelvis, which may be followed by an intravenous pyelogram. It is necessary to determine any allergenicity to iodine, since this is present in the contrast material. If the I.V.P. is done on an emergency basis, there will be no bowel preparation, as there would be for an elective procedure. It is not unusual for a quiescent patient to have another bout of ureteral colic during or just after the I.V.P. The contrast material used for this procedure is an osmotic diuretic and acts much the same as any diuretic in producing a large urinary output.

Once the diagnosis is established, the patient should be made aware of it and given a fairly detailed description of the possible ensuing events. Most patients who understand their diagnosis, their symptoms and the expected course of events are better able to tolerate their pain.

Perhaps one of the most important procedures in caring for a patient with a ureteral stone is straining the urine. This may be done with a tea strainer, several open gauze sponges or one of the commercially made strainers for urine. Every single voiding must be strained. If a stone is passed and recovered, the diagnosis is definite, and the patient may be spared further diagnostic studies. The stone can then be chemically analyzed and the patient put on an appropriate long-range program.

HEMATURIA

Hematuria may be microscopic or gross in character. Of importance is that hematuria is not a disease but a *symptom*. As such, it is essential that a complete and thorough urological investigation be undertaken. Such a program consists of urinalysis, urine culture and sensitivity, intravenous pyelogram, cystoscopy with or without retrograde studies, renal scan and selective renal angiography. With these modalities, a true diagnosis of the etiology of the hematuria can be made in almost all instances. The most common causes of hematuria are infection, benign prostatic hypertrophy, calculous disease, hydronephrosis, tumor, polycystic disease, anticoagulant therapy and injury.

When it is not possible to make an accurate diagnosis of the cause of bleeding, percutaneous needle biopsy of the kidney should be considered, to rule out medical diseases of the kidney, such as glomerulonephritis or pyelonephritis. In the Negro race, all patients with hematuria should have a sickle cell study to rule out that form of anemia. There are instances when a positive diagnosis cannot be made, even after a complete urological survey. It may then be necessary to do a complete bleeding profile study, including bone marrow studies.

Tuberculosis of the urinary tract is not an uncommon cause of hematuria. When urinary studies show a persistent pyuria in the presence of an acid urine despite adequate and prolonged urinary antibiotic treatment, a temporary diagnosis of tuberculosis should be made, and routine studies of skin testing and urine culture for acid-fast organisms should be instituted. Once the diagnosis is confirmed, a definitive plan of treatment should ensue with proper follow-up.

Nursing considerations

On admission to the emergency department of a person with hematuria, accurate measurements of vital signs, especially blood pressure and pulse, should be taken and recorded. Hematuria, unless it is unusually massive or has been allowed to continue over a long period of time, is rarely an immediate life-threatening situation. However, careful observation of the patient for signs of shock is important.

A detailed history and thorough physical examination will reveal any preexisting urinary disease, blood disorders, possible injury, recent use of anticoagulants, abnormal bleeding tendencies or any coexisting medical problems. Urinalysis and complete blood count (C.B.C.) are the first laboratory studies performed. The C.B.C. reveals if the amount of blood lost has been significant enough to affect the hemoglobin and hematocrit determinations. Blood for type and crossmatch may also be drawn at this time. The urine should be noted for color, amount and presence or absence of clots before transmittal to the laboratory. The method of urine collection, especially in female patients, is an important consideration. At times, urine obtained with a catheter will prove the true site of bleeding to be the vagina.

Generally speaking, there is no way to stop bleeding from the upper urinary tract, and at this point, there is usually no need to do so. The patient will be admitted to the hospital and undergo a thorough diagnostic evaluation and appropriate treatment.

In contrast, bleeding from the bladder can be controlled, in some instances, by an indwelling catheter and irrigation, and this procedure *will* be initiated in the emergency department. Before beginning this procedure, it is the nurse's responsibility to give the patient an adequate explanation, to assemble the necessary equipment and to position the patient. A routine catheterization tray will provide the basic sterile items, such as gloves, drapes, antiseptic prep and lubricant. Catheter size depends on the urologist's preference. Usually, a large size, such as a 22 or 24 Fr. with a 5 cc. balloon, has a lumen large enough to permit adequate drainage, irrigation and passage of clots or other debris.

Irrigating equipment should include an Asepto syringe, a Toomey syringe (a 50 cc. piston syringe with a catheter-adapted tip) and several bottles of irrigating solution, usually normal saline. Once the catheter is inserted, it becomes the responsibility of the nurse to keep it patent. Catheter irrigation should be done as frequently as necessary and under careful aseptic technique. The Asepto syringe should be used routinely and the Toomey syringe only when the catheter has become obstructed with clots. Once the bleeding is under control, the patient will be admitted to the hospital and subjected to a complete urological investigation.

Blood in the urine, as with bleeding from any body orifice, is a frightening experience for the patient. A small amount of blood in the urine will turn the entire urinary output pink or red and will seem to the patient much more severe than it actually is. Emotional support, calm reassurance and a skilled, knowledgeable performance of professional duties are vital to the patient and his family.

URINARY RETENTION

Acute urinary retention is a malady very commonly seen in the emergency department. Generally speaking, this problem is usually encountered in the age group of 60 to 80 years. The causes of retention, in order of frequency of occurrence, are:

(1) Benign prostatic hypertrophy.
(2) Urethral stricture.
(3) Adenocarcinoma of the prostate.
(4) Calculi.
(5) Neurogenic bladder.
(6) Drug-induced retention.

The patient usually gives a history of increased difficulty in voiding, manifested by hesitation, straining, voiding with a slow, weak stream and the sensation of incomplete emptying of the bladder. On examination, the patient is most usually very restless and in considerable discomfort. He may not have voided at all, or he may dribble constantly or urinate small amounts intermittently. This is usually an overflow incontinence, indicating a much greater amount of urine remaining in the bladder.

The most immediate treatment is to establish urinary drainage through urethral catheterization. Once the bladder has been decompressed, the catheter should be attached to a closed gravity drainage unit. Much has been said and written about the rate at which the bladder is decompressed. Studies have shown that while rapid decompression may cause transient hematuria, it does not generally cause hemorrhage or shock. However, experience has shown that an *atraumatic* catheterization and a rapid decompression causes the patient no ill effects whatsoever.

Once the patient is comfortable, routine laboratory and x-ray data should be obtained. After this, a complete urological workup is undertaken, including urine for culture and sensitivity, an intravenous pyelogram and a cystoscopic evaluation. Following complete medical and urological studies, a diagnosis is made, and the appropriate treatment is instituted.

Nursing considerations

On the patient's admission to the emergency department, routine laboratory samples are obtained, and the patient is prepared for catheterization. An adequate explanation of the procedure should be given the patient. A sterile catheterization tray, including gloves, drapes, lubricant and an antiseptic prep, will be needed. The size of the indwelling catheter is determined by the urologist. Generally, an 18 Fr. catheter with a 5 cc. balloon is the size of choice. It is small enough to permit easy passage and large enough to permit adequate flow of urine. Other routine supplies needed at this time are collection containers for urinalysis, culture and sensitivity studies, a closed gravity drainage unit and possibly an irrigation set. Since the vast majority of patients with retention will have a pathologic obstruction either in the urethra or at the vesicle neck, a few instruments and catheters unique to the practice of urology should be assembled, as outlined in the following paragraphs.

(1) *Urethral dilators* (filiforms, followers, LeFort and Van Buren sounds). A filiform is a small plastic catheter with a metal-threaded female tip at one end, used as a guide to bypass urethral strictures. They range in size from 3 to 6 Fr. A follower is a plastic catheter with a threaded male tip that can be screwed into the filiform. Followers of increasing sizes are passed to dilate the stricture, from 12 to 28 Fr. (See Figures 23–1 and 23–2.) LeFort sounds are rigid metal instruments with an "elbow" curve at one end and a threaded male tip. Van Buren sounds do not have the threaded tip. The curve is designed to negotiate the curve of the prostatic and bulbar urethra, as it passes under the symphysis pubis. (See Figure 23–3.)

(2) *Coudé catheters* are indwelling catheters with a curved tip, similar to Van Buren sounds. They are particularly useful for patients with bladder neck elevation due to prostatic hypertrophy. (See Figure 23–4.)

(3) *Catheter stylet* is a wire guide, inserted into a catheter to give it a curved tip and some rigidity. This is an extremely dangerous instrument and should be used only by those qualified to do so. It is possible to cause serious injury should the stylet accidently protrude from the proximal end of the catheter. (See Figure 23–4.)

The procedure of catheterization is carried out with strict aseptic technique. The patient is draped with a sterile towel, and the meatus is cleaned with generous amounts of antiseptic solution. The catheter is then well lubricated, or the urologist may prefer to inject sterile lubricant through the meatus

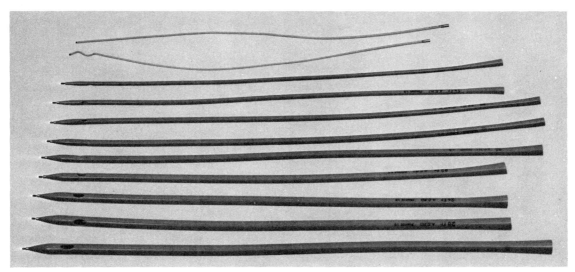

Figure 23–1 Filiforms and Philips followers. The filiforms (at the bottom of the picture) are the straight and spiral type. The followers attach to these and are passed through the urethra in graduated sizes, beginning with the smallest.

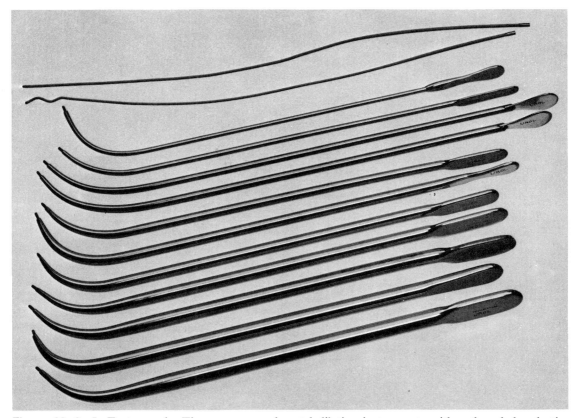

Figure 23–2 LeFort sounds. These are curved metal dilating instruments with a threaded male tip. They are used in conjunction with filiforms in the same manner as followers. The choice of followers or LeFort sounds depends on the personal preference of the urologist.

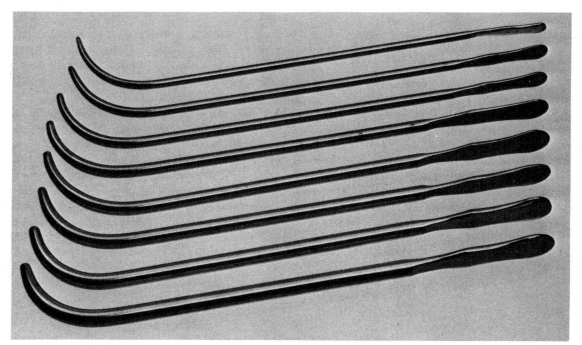

Figure 23–3 Van Buren sounds. These are smooth metal dilators, available in graduated sizes, from 16 Fr. to 30 Fr.

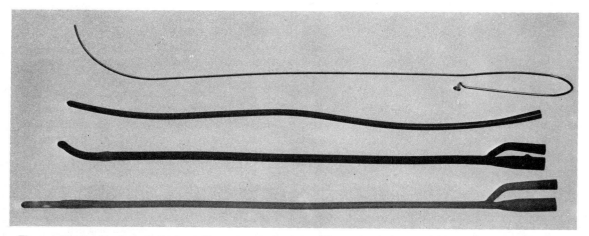

Figure 23–4 Various catheters. From top to bottom: The stylet is inserted into a catheter, giving it a degree of rigidity. The Robinson catheter is a nonretentive catheter, used for a single insertion. The coudé catheter is a retentive catheter, with a curved tip. The Foley catheter is a retentive catheter with a straight tip.

into the urethra. The catheter is passed, using constant, steady, gentle pressure. After a free flow of urine is obtained, the catheter should be connected to a closed drainage unit.

Following catheterization, the amount of residual urine should be noted. Urine is then sent to the laboratory for analysis, culture and sensitivity studies.

A chemistry profile should be drawn, including blood urea nitrogen, creatinine, sugar and electrolyte determinations. It occasionally happens that a patient has been in retention so long that it has caused some degree of renal impairment, and this may first become evident in his serum chemistries. Most patients are started on antibacterials at this time; thus, any allergenic sensitivity to these drugs should be ascertained. An adequate fluid intake is always important, but especially so to this particular patient in retention. The patient is often admitted to the hospital for a complete diagnostic workup.

VENEREAL DISEASE

Venereal disease is by far the most common of the communicable diseases of the genitourinary tract. In 1974, nationwide, there were over 900,000 reported cases of gonorrhea alone, with private physicians reporting only one out of every 9 cases of venereal disease they treated. Syphilis cases were estimated in 1974 at near 25,000. As more emergency departments become community health centers, the number of patients with venereal disease seen by emergency personnel can be expected to rise.

Patients with venereal diseases come from all ethnic backgrounds and occupations and range in age from 13 to 70 years. No parental consent is needed to treat venereal disease in a minor. Ignorance and fear still surround venereal disease, and the attitude of the nurse can help in bringing the disease and its treatment into proper perspective.

Gonorrhea

Gonorrhea, the most prevalent of the venereal diseases, is generally seen in the emergency department 2 to 9 days after sexual contact with an infected individual. The presenting symptoms are burning on urination and a thick, profuse, purulent urethral discharge. Diagnosis is made from a smear and/or culture of the exudate; the smear will show gram negative intracellular diplococci. To obtain a culture, the swab containing the exudate is inoculated on Thayer-Martin or Transgrow medium. It takes at least 24 hours before a culture report is available.

Treatment usually consists of procaine penicillin G, 4.8 million units intramuscularly divided into 2 separate doses, one injected into each buttock. Tetracycline may be used for penicillin-sensitive patients. In some areas of the country, ampicillin, 3.5 gm., and probenecid (Benemid), 1.0 gm., is given orally.

Nursing considerations

It is important that the urethral swab is obtained prior to urination, when the discharge is most concentrated. Due to the fragility of the *Neisseria gonorrheae,* the swab should be taken to the laboratory as soon as feasible. Principal precautions revolve around preventing spread of the infection to the eyes or nasopharynx of the nurse, other personnel and other patients. It is thus important to discard or wash and autoclave *anything* that comes in contact with the exudate. Careful handwashing is mandatory, since the *Neisseria gonorrheae* cannot survive soap and water. As penicillin is the treatment of choice, any history of allergy to this drug must be established. The patient should be observed carefully following penicillin injection, and emergency resuscitative equipment should be ready in the event of anaphylactic shock. Between 2 and 10 percent of all patients receiving penicillin have an allergic manifestation.

Arrangements should be made for follow-up care, either with a private physician, the hospital clinic or a community venereal disease treatment center. Victims of gonorrhea rapidly become asymptomatic and because of this may stop taking their medication and feel no need to continue under a physician's care. It should be emphasized to them that prompt diagnosis and treatment will in most cases prevent complications, such as urethral strictures, posterior urethritis, prostatis, epididymitis and cystitis.

Chapter 22 presents further information on gonorrhea in the female.

Syphilis

Syphilis, caused by the organism *Treponema pallidum,* is transmitted exclusively by sexual contact with a person harboring an open spirochete-containing lesion. After the incubation period of 10 to 90 days, the initial lesion, the chancre, appears on the genitalia.

Diagnosis is made from a positive darkfield examination of serous material obtained from a moist lesion or, more commonly, from a serological response to the infection (VDRL). Treatment consists of benzathine penicillin G, 2,400,000 units, half injected in each buttock. Tetracycline is given to patients who are allergic to penicillin.

Nursing considerations

Nursing responsibilities in caring for a patient with suspected syphilis are very much the same as caring for a patient with suspected gonorrhea. They include meticulous attention to handwashing, and proper care of supplies and equipment that come into contact with the lesion, as well as the precautions necessary when administering penicillin. Follow-up care is especially important and should be stressed to the patient. Untreated or inadequately treated primary syphilis can go on to secondary, latent and, finally, late syphilis, which ultimately may cause diseases of the heart, arteries and central nervous system.

Evaluation and treatment of *all* sexual partners of the infected individual are essential. Information regarding community resources for venereal disease should be given the patient. Often, community clinics provide treatment without cost.

TRAUMA

Foreign body in the G.U. tract

Patients with a foreign body in the genitourinary tract are occasionally treated in the emergency department. The most frequent predisposing causes for bodily use of foreign bodies, whether internal or external, are abnormal psyche, inebriation, eroticism and senility.

The bladder and urethra are the most common sites for foreign objects, with one qualification: the object must be small and firm enough to be passed up the urethra. Symptoms center around the associated infection. There may be frequency, dysuria, urethral discharge and, possibly, abdominal pain. Occasionally, the foreign body becomes a nucleus, around which a stone forms. Diagnosis can be established by urinalysis showing blood and pus, x-ray studies showing a metallic object or encrustation surrounding a nonopaque foreign body and cystopanendoscopy showing the object under direct vision. Foreign bodies in the urethra and bladder can usually be removed at the time of cystoscopy.

External foreign bodies are most often used to constrict the external genitalia, usually the penis. They can be anything, from a thread or hair to a metal ring. The penis becomes swollen and inflamed and, at times, necrotic up to the point of obstruction. Also accompanying are a purulent discharge and, in extreme cases, urinary retention.

Nursing considerations

Patients with internal foreign bodies will usually be admitted for an attempt at transurethral removal of the object. Most external foreign bodies can be removed successfully in the emergency department. A minor instrument set-up, with sterile towels, sponges, antiseptic prep, scissors and hemostat should be prepared. A sedative or tranquilizer is given before the procedure is begun; provisions should be available for administration of local anesthetic. In difficult patients, like children, it may be necessary to admit and attempt removal under a general anesthetic.

Patients presenting in the emergency department with this problem are usually guilt-ridden and embarrassed. A matter-of-fact approach by the medical and nursing staff can help allay such feelings.

Injuries to the G.U. tract

Injuries to the genitourinary tract may be divided into penetrating and nonpenetrating types. Blunt trauma (nonpenetrating) is more common and most frequently results from automobile accidents. Less often, it follows a fall, a direct blow or an athletic injury. Penetrating injuries result from guns, knives and icepicks, among other instruments.

Isolated injuries to the urinary tract are not common and rarely life-endangering. When urinary tract injuries occur in conjunction with trauma to other organ systems, total evaluation of the patient must be made, priorities of care established and principles of resuscitation followed. Thus, a patent airway must be established and maintained and the cardiovascular system must be stabilized. Initial urinary tract evaluation may be brief, and unless the problem involves major blood loss, the urinary tract may assume a lesser priority of care.

Renal injury

Injury to the kidney occurs much more commonly in the male with a ratio of approximately 3 males injured to every one female, and it is more frequently seen in those below the age of 40. Trauma to the kidney may vary from a mild contusion to complete fragmentation or avulsion from its vascular pedicle. In general, abnormal kidneys are more prone to injury than normal ones. Signs and symptoms of renal trauma are hematuria, pain, tenderness and abdominal rigidity of varying degrees. Renal injury must be considered in blunt or penetrating injury to the upper abdomen or direct blows to the costovertebral angle area.

After the patient has been assessed, the diagnosis can be confirmed by excretory urography (I.V.P.). Systolic blood pressure should be at least 60 mm. of mercury to assure adequate renal perfusion. The accuracy of diagnosis can be increased by use of an infusion technique, using 120 cc. of 50 percent sodium diatrizoate (Hypaque). Pyelogram will usually show the extent of injury and allow assessment of the uninjured side. On occasion, renal arteriography may be necessary, particularly when major vascular injury is suspected (see Figure 23–5).

Management of renal trauma is generally conservative. Rest and observation will bring recovery to 80 percent of patients. Emergency surgery is indicated if the vital signs cannot be stabilized with transfusion of whole blood or if there is an expansion of the perirenal hematoma. The options at time of surgery include drainage of the renal area, repair of the damaged kidney and a complete or partial nephrectomy.

Trauma to the bladder and urethra

Bladder trauma includes contusion, intraperitoneal rupture, extraperitoneal rupture or a combination of the latter. It is usually associated with a fractured pelvis. Pelvic fracture as evidenced by x-ray should indicate suspicion of bladder trauma. Symptoms of a ruptured bladder are pain over the pubic area, an extreme desire to void (urinary tenesmus) or extreme dysuria, hematuria, shock and evidence of blood loss.

Diagnosis is verified by means of a retrograde cystogram. Surgical treatment is usually necessary to establish suprapubic drainage and thorough drainage of the perivesical area. Immediate diagnosis and treatment is imperative in rupture of the bladder. Deaths have been reported with delayed exploration.

Rupture of the urethra almost exclusively results from an automobile accident and is associated with a fractured pelvis. As a consequence of trauma, urine extravasates into the tissue at the site of injury, setting up an intensive inflammatory reaction. Injury should be suspected in patients complaining of pain in the bladder area and experiencing urinary tenesmus but unable to void.

Diagnosis may be confirmed by insertion of a catheter. In most instances, urine will not be obtained. Injection of sodium diatrazoate (Hypaque) will confirm the extravasation of urine about the site of injury. The objectives of treatment are to drain the extravesical

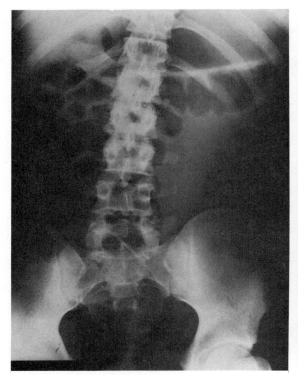
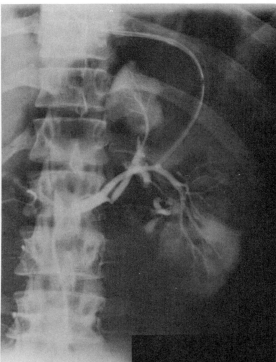

Figure 23–5 Renal injuries. Left: Flat film of abdomen of young man injured in a motorcycle accident, complaining of abdominal pain. Note gaseous content of small bowel and stomach indicative of ileus (upper right). Note also displacement of loops of bowel to the patient's right side (left side of illustration) by mass in left side of abdomen. Left psoas shadow not visualized. Right: Left renal arteriogram revealing a fracture of the kidney at the junction of its upper and middle thirds. In both fragments, there is extravasation of blood, due to damage to the major arteries. Note the sharp kink at the takeoff of the artery supplying the upper pole, indicating partial rupture. Curved radiopaque density in upper right corner of illustration is a nasogastric tube. Patient required nephrectomy.

urine, to reestablish urethral continuity and to control hemorrhage.

Injuries to the external genitalia

Genital injuries include abrasions, hematomas and minor lacerations of the penis and scrotum or vulva. Patients with fracture of the penis are occasionally seen in the emergency department. It is caused by direct blow to an erect organ and results in hemorrhage, hematoma and distortion of the organ.

Conservative management of penile fracture consists of splinting the penis, inserting an indwelling catheter and applying ice packs. Surgical evacuation of the hematoma is sometimes done.

Lacerations of the penis or vulva are managed as any similar wound elsewhere on the body. Loss of skin requires immediate coverage, usually by means of split-thickness graft.

Torsion of the testicle is a condition in which a testicle twists on its spermatic cord, disrupting its own blood supply. It may be caused by an injury but more often occurs spontaneously. Torsion causes severe scrotal pain, unrelieved by rest. There is generally a normal urinary sediment. The treatment is surgical exploration of the scrotum and bilateral fixation of both testes. It is important for the emergency nurse to understand that delay in treatment will cause the loss of the testicle; the organ must be reduced and fixed within a few hours to preserve fertility.

Nursing considerations

Patients admitted to the emergency department with genitourinary trauma will present in a variety of ways. Some will have multiple injuries and be in immediate danger of death. Others may have only one or 2 complaints and appear to be in no acute distress. The specific needs of each patient must be evaluated and dealt with individually, using the basic procedures and techniques familiar to every nurse, including the maintenance of an adequate airway, the treatment of hemorrhagic shock with fluid replacement, close monitoring of vital signs, obtaining blood and urine samples for laboratory studies, accurate intake and output and, above all, close observation of the patient.

Two points deserve special mention relative to urological procedures. An intravenous pyelogram is of no value if the patient is in shock. Renal perfusion, and thus perfusion of the contrast material, depends on blood pressure. Renal perfusion is impaired with arterial pressures under 60 mm. Hg. However, shock is no contraindication to renal arteriography. Secondly, it is important to keep a Foley catheter patent. Occasionally, anuria or oliguria can be traced to a nonfunctioning indwelling urethral catheter.

SUMMARY

Most patients with genitourinary complaints seen in the emergency department are not in an immediate life-threatening condition. They are, however, vitally concerned about their health. Some will have additional fears, such as loss of sexual potency, discovery of an incurable disease or feelings of guilt or embarassment. Patients with genitourinary problems deserve utmost privacy. They also need understanding, explanation, reassurance and, above all, the nurse's sincere interest.

BIBLIOGRAPHY

(1) Brosman, S. A., and Fay, R.: "Diagnosis and Management of Bladder Trauma," *Journal of Trauma,* 13 (1973): 687.

(2) Brown, William J.: "Acquired Syphilis," *American Journal of Nursing,* 71 (April 1971):713–715.

(3) Campbell, Meredith, and Harrison, J. Hartwell: *Urology* (Philadelphia: W. B. Saunders Company, 1970).

(4) Desautels, Robert E.: "Mismanagement of Urethral Catheterization," *Hospital Medicine,* 1 (March 1965):10.

(5) Gross, M.; Arnold, T., and Waterhouse, K.: "Fracture of the Penis: Rationale of Surgical Management," *Journal of Urology,* 106 (November 1971):708–710.

(6) Howard, John: "Tried, True, and New Ways to Treat and Prevent Kidney Stones," *Resident and Staff Physician,* 70 (December 1970):67–79.

(7) Keuhnelian, John G., and Sanders, Virginia E.: *Urologic Nursing* (London: Macmillan Company, 1970).

(8) Lauler, David P.: *Venereal Disease* (New York: Medcom Learning Systems, 1972).

(9) Mathews, Rosemary: "TLC with the Penicillin," *American Journal of Nursing,* 71 (April 1971):720–723.

(10) Morel, Alice: "Urethral Catheters—An Ancient Device," *RN,* 72 (April 1972):40–43.

(11) Parker, Richard, and Robison, Jack: "Anatomy and Diagnosis of Torsion of the Testicles," *Journal of Urology,* (August 1971):243–247.

(12) Waterhouse, Keith, and Gross, Melvin: "Trauma to the Genitourinary Tract: A 5 Year Experience with 251 cases," *Journal of Urology,* 101 (March 1969): 241–246.

(13) Winter, Chester, and Roehm, Marilyn: *Sawyer's Nursing Care of Patients with Urologic Diseases* (Saint Louis: C. V. Mosby Company, 1968).

24

Injuries of the head, neck and spine

JAMES H. COSGRIFF, JR.
DIANN ANDERSON

The area of the head and neck is most vulnerable to trauma and one of the most commonly injured body sites. A study of victims of automobile accidents revealed that over 70 percent suffered injuries to the head/neck region.[6] Other than vehicular accidents, injuries to this region may be due to falls, acceleration and deceleration, blunt and penetrating trauma and athletic trauma.

Within the head and neck is a complex variety of structures involving many different organ systems, all closely related anatomically. Injury to the head or neck may damage portions of the central and peripheral nervous systems, upper gastrointestinal tract, airway, major blood vessels and lymphatics, lungs and pleura and musculoskeletal structures. Because of the close proximity of the structures, multiple organ injury is quite common.

The spine, in its relationships to the head and neck, will be discussed throughout the chapter when appropriate and in a special section at the end of the chapter.

ANATOMY AND PHYSIOLOGY

The head

The head consists of the skull, brain and overlying scalp (see Figure 24–1). The scalp is comprised of 5 layers of soft tissue covering the skull. The innermost layer is the galea, which consists of coarse connective tissue. The skull is formed by the cranium and facial bones. Its only moveable joint is the temporomandibular joint. The cranium itself consists of 8 bones that are open during the first years of life and later fuse at suture lines.

Of the 5 special senses of the human body which provide protection from the outer world, 4 are located exclusively in the head. These include the so-called "visceral senses" of taste and smell and the "special somatic senses" of sight and hearing. The fifth sense, touch, is present in the head and neck region but is not as acute as in the fingers.

Within the bony vault of the skull is the brain, the seat of the central nervous system. It is covered by 3 layers, the meninges. The

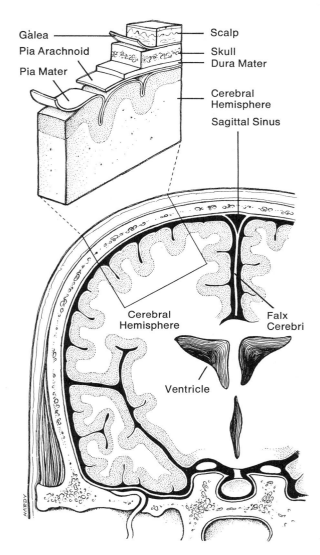

Figure 24–1 Coronal view of the head. The various levels of the scalp, the skull and the coverings of the brain are depicted.

innermost is a fine-cellular layer which conforms to the convoluted surface of the cerebral hemispheres, called the "pia mater." The medial layer is the "pia arachnoid," and the outer is the "dura mater," a dense layer attached to the interior of the skull.

The brain consists of 2 large lobes or cerebral hemispheres which attach to the brain stem and the cerebellum. The cerebral hemispheres govern human function, thought and motor and sensory activity. The cerebellum primarily controls the vestibular sense. The brain stem is the seat of vegetative activity; the cardiac and respiratory centers are located there, and the nerve pathways from the brain to the spinal cord pass through it.

The neck

The neck, or cervical region, extends from the mandibles to the clavicles, with large muscles and the cervical spine serving as the circumferential boundaries. This region contains a large number of both hollow and solid organ structures which are part of the nervous and cardiovascular systems and the gastro-intestinal and respiratory tracts. Excepting the cranial vault and the cervical spine, the protective layers of skin and muscle on the neck do little to shield its vital structures from injury. Much of the neck's protection results from the 5 special senses and the mobility of the head and neck.

Beneath the skin and subcutaneous tissue, the neck is encased in a muscular coat, the "platysma," which extends over its entire anterior and lateral aspects. This is a thin muscle located deep to the subcutaneous tissue. It serves little in the way of protective function, but in terms of wound management, it may be compared to the peritoneum. Penetration of this layer usually mandates surgical exploration of the site of injury, for serious, even mortal, wounds may result to deep-lying vital structures.

In considering the anatomy of the neck, it is helpful to divide it into 2 structural groupings, the mid-line and the lateral regions. Midline structures include: (1) trachea, (2) thyroid gland, (3) larynx and vocal cords, (4) esophagus, (5) spine and spinal cord. Lateral structures include: (1) brachial plexus, (2) carotid, subclavian and jugular vessels, (3) major lymphatic ducts, (4) sympathetic chain and ganglia, (5) apex of the lung and pleura.

Thus, cervical injuries may affect both hollow and solid organs. The site of wounding may indicate specific structural (organ) injury. In penetrating injuries, particularly those due to gunshot or stabbing, multiple organs may be damaged.

ASSESSMENT

Awareness of possibility of injury to the cervical spine and spinal cord is paramount in assessment. A good axiom, especially in an unconscious trauma patient, is that the cervical spine should be considered damaged until proven otherwise.[22] Unconscious patients are usually brought to the emergency department by ambulance; thus proper immobilization should have been initiated during the prehospital phase of care by the emergency medical technician. (Figure 24–2 illustrates use of a spine board on a patient transported by ambulance.)

When proper splinting has not been previously done, the emergency department nurse must evaluate the spinal column before moving the patient from the ambulance stretcher or other vehicle, being alert to the fact that any movement of an unstable cervical vertebra could produce spinal cord damage, with resultant quadriplegia and possibly fatal consequences. Careful palpation of the neck in the mid-line posteriorly will allow examination of the spinous processes. Any alteration in alignment should make the nurse suspicious of a spinous injury. In the conscious patient, pain will be elicited at the site of injury, allowing the nurse to distinguish, by palpation *and* patient response, bony tenderness from pain due to soft tissue injury.

If pain is elicited or a malalignment detected on spinal assessment, further evaluation should be delayed until the head and neck are immobilized. This may be done by placing sandbags on either side of the head or by strapping the head and chin to a spine board (see Figure 24–8, especially photo "A").

A serious problem may arise when a patient with suspected spinous injury also has airway difficulty. *In no case when cervical spine injury is suspected should the patient's neck be extended in the usual manner to achieve airway maintenance.* Neck extension could result in displacement of a fracture fragment or a dislocation of the spine. with resultant cord damage. Instead, the mandible is brought forward and held in that position until immobilization has been accomplished. Then an attempt may be made to pass an oropharyngeal or soft rubber nasopharyngeal airway. Should this be unsuccessful, tracheostomy is needed.

Once a patient's airway is established, control of hemorrhage is next accomplished, and life-support measures are then initiated. Vital signs should be observed and recorded for baseline information. Too often in patients

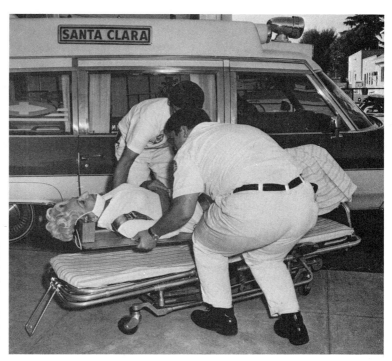

Figure 24–2 Use of a spine board. This photo illustrates the proper use of a spine board by EMTs to immobilize a patient for transportation to the emergency department.
Source: Photo courtesy of the Santa Clara County GSA, Eddie Chong, Chief Photographer.

with head injury are these basic principles of emergency care neglected.

History

The history of injury, including onset and etiology, is helpful. Knowing the mechanics of the trauma, including where the injury was received, may enable the examiner to localize the site of injury. A good many patients were under the influence of alcohol when injured, making history data collection difficult. Others may have been dazed or may have suffered a period of unconsciousness following injury, while still others are unconscious when brought to the emergency department. History must then be sought from family, witnesses, police officers or ambulance attendants, anyone who may be able to supply information about the circumstances of the incident.

Important facts include the bodily location of the injury, whether or not the patient was dazed or actually unconscious or suffered a convulsive seizure, the nature and amount of blood loss and the occurrence of any coughing, spitting or emesis of blood. The nurse should also establish any history of voice change, hoarseness, respiratory difficulty, dysphagia and motor or sensory loss, since they may indicate tracheal, esophageal or specific neurological injury. In vehicular accidents, knowledge of interior damage to the automobile, the position of the injured in the vehicle before and after impact and whether or not lap or shoulder restraints were in use may be of value, in assessment and diagnosis.

Physical examination

Thorough physical evaluation may be delayed until the patient's condition has been stabilized. Bleeding or presence of blood is an obvious sign of injury. Not uncommonly, especially with lacerations of the scalp and face (very vascular areas), blood may be splattered over a wide area from relatively minor wounds. Careful inspection and palpation for wounds should be done. The head is also examined for lacerations, swellings or depressions which might indicate a skull fracture.

The ear canals are examined with an otoscope. Presence of blood in the external auditory canal (otorrhea) of a patient with head trauma is strongly indicative of basilar skull fracture. Keep in mind, however, that bleeding may occur with simple rupture of the tympanic membrane (eardrum), and such blood will usually clot. Blood from the ear associated with skull fracture is mixed with cerebrospinal fluid and will not clot.

Similarly, bleeding from the nose may follow contusion or fracture of the nose, and the blood will clot. However, fractures of the basilar portion of the frontal bone will frequently result in cerebrospinal rhinorrhea, drainage of blood and spinal fluid from the nose, and this will not clot.

The nurse should then observe the eyes and eyelids. Ecchymoses of the lids and lateral subconjunctival hemorrhage are often associated with frontal skull fracture. Extraocular movements are to be noted, as well. Pupils should be examined for size, regularity and reaction to light. Fixed dilatation or constriction of one or both pupils, with no reactive light reflex, indicates cerebral damage in the absence of preexisting ocular disease.

Complete neurological examination of motor and sensory modalities is done to rule out damage to the central and peripheral nervous systems. In addition to pupillary reflexes, evaluation of level of consciousness, speech, sensation (pinprick, touch, painful stimuli), deep tendon reflexes, motor activity of limbs and digits must be made. Flaccidity or spasticity of muscle groups can be determined by evaluation of active and/or passive motion of each limb. Extreme rigidity (decerebrate type) is indicative of severe brain damage. Flaccidity or paralysis result from either brain or cord damage.

Opposing limbs should be compared in each test. The presence of a Babinski reflex indicates pyramidal tract damage. In the course of examining the upper extremities, the nurse should palpate the distal pulses. Differences in opposing pulses can occur secondary to vascular damage in the supraclavicular area of the involved side.

An awareness of level of consciousness is important. Stupor (when the patient does not respond intelligibly) may be an important sign of cerebral damage, either from intracranial injury or as a result of a carotid artery wound with impaired blood flow to the brain.[3]

The neck should be inspected carefully for open wounds, abrasions, contusions. The position of the head in relation to the shoulders is important. After acceleration-deceleration injuries (whiplash), the head and neck are frequently held in a rigid, protective position and moved reluctantly. Even passive motion by the examiner may be difficult. Blunt injuries, such as those caused by blows or being "clotheslined," may result in local pain, swelling and restricted motion. Dysphagia or hoarseness is often present.

Blunt injuries can prove very deceiving, since serious deep tissue damage may occur with minor superficial wounds. Similarly, some penetrating injuries may bleed very little and mask more serious, even fatal internal injury. Inspection of the wounds of entry and exit, when present, may allow determination of the path of the missile or knife.

Following visual inspection, palpation of the neck for muscle spasm, rigidity and areas of tenderness or swelling is carried out. Subcutaneous emphysema (crackling or crunching under the skin) indicates release of air into the fascial planes of the neck, as a result of damage to hollow organ structures such as the trachea, esophagus or lung. In a more serious injury of the supraclavicular space involving the lung or pleura, a sucking wound may be present.

Assessment of the entire patient should then be completed to evaluate the full extent of injury. All findings are recorded to establish baseline data. One of the most important aspects of managing patients with suspected head injury is periodic reassessment of vital signs, level of consciousness and neurological status. Pupil size and reactivity, motor and sensory loss are especially important parameters to observe and record at regular time intervals, usually every 15 to 30 minutes.

Adjunct studies

X-ray studies should not be undertaken until the patient's condition is stable and, when spine injury is suspected, only after proper immobilization has been effected. Simple anteroposterior and lateral x-rays of the skull and cervical spine will usually suffice to rule out fracture. Since most fractures of the cervical spine occur in the lower neck, one must be certain that the entire cervical spine is visualized on the films (see Figure 24–3). Upright x-rays of the neck and chest will reveal any subcutaneous emphysema and the presence of pleural complications, such as pneumothorax or hemothorax.

Every effort should be made to localize any foreign bodies which may be lodged in the deeper tissues following a penetrating injury. Not uncommonly, such missiles may be found on the side opposite the wound of entry. Radio-opaque objects will be located by x-rays.

Skull x-rays should be viewed for fracture and pineal shift. The pineal gland is a mid-line structure, lying close to the pituitary gland. In most adults, it is calcified. Under normal circumstances, it will be seen in the mid-line on an anteroposterior view. A shift from this position to one side of the mid-line indicates a tumor or mass on the opposite side.

Special x-ray studies, such as an esophogram and angiogram, will be helpful in detecting specific organ injury. These studies are rarely performed in the emergency department, however. In other specific instances, a brain scan may be useful. Lumbar puncture is done infrequently to evaluate patients with craniocerebral trauma.

Baseline laboratory studies in the emergency department phase of care should include a complete blood count, urinalysis, arterial blood gases and electrolyte levels. Type-specific blood is ordered as indicated.

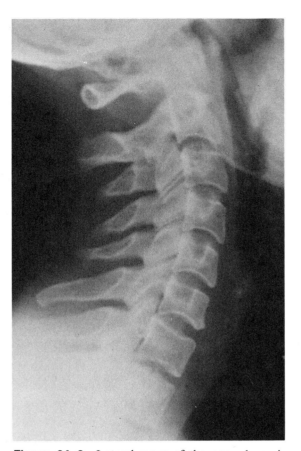

Figure 24–3 Lateral x-ray of the normal cervical spine. The entire cervical spine is well visualized and in normal alignment.

MANAGEMENT OF HEAD INJURIES

Head injury is the most frequent cause of death between the ages of one and 44 years. It accounts for death in two thirds of all fatal accidents.[26] The most serious aspect of head injury is that the brain may be damaged. It should be noted that shock is not a reliable sign of brain damage. In general, shock rarely results from intracranial injury alone; one must look to other causes.[6, 11]

Injury to the scalp and skull

Scalp wounds are very common, but each must be examined carefully for serious damage. The scalp, being very vascular, when wounded may result in blood loss significant enough to produce hemorrhagic shock, especially in children. The management of simple scalp wounds is discussed in Chapter 10. All scalp wounds should also be evaluated for possible skull fracture. If the patient was dazed or unconscious when seen, skull x-rays are indicated.

Simple skull fracture is, in itself, not a serious injury. Its serious connotation results from concomitant damage to the brain. Fractures of the skull result from external forces applied directly to it, such as from a blow or fall. The fracture may assume a variety of configurations, such as linear or stellate (radiating in a star-like fashion). Skull fractures may be present without any external open wound. Whenever a patient gives a history of a blow to the head followed by being dazed, or a loss of consciousness, skull x-rays should be taken to rule out fracture. In the absence of a neurological deficit, no specific treatment is needed.

Complicated skull fractures include the open (compound) and closed (depressed) types and require specific treatment by a physician. In the open variety, the wound must be fully cleansed, debrided and closed. In depressed fractures, the skull is actually driven centrally into the cavity of the cranium, and, depending on the depth of the depression, may press on or penetrate brain tissue. These fractures usually require elevation.

Patients with complicated skull fracture require complete assessment and a period of observation to rule out brain damage. Appropriate antibiotic therapy is required to prevent intracranial infection. Additional studies include electroencephalogram and echoencephalogram. Depressed fractures are treated by management of the soft tissue wound and elevation of the bony fragment to relieve pressure on the brain.

Brain injury

Brain injury is the most serious consequence in the patient with craniocerebral trauma. Generally, injury to the brain may result from di-

rect force, compression or anoxia. An example of direct force is a bullet entering the brain, injuring the tissue it severs. A compressive injury is caused by hemorrhage or clot formation, such as any of the hematomas discussed below.

A "contrecoup" injury is a compression injury. It is found at a site opposite to where the initial blow or injury was sustained. This type of injury occurs when the head is struck and the brain, being like gelatin, moves with the direction of the force until it strikes the rigid skull on the opposite side, resulting in trauma to the tissues involved.

Brain injury caused by anoxia occurs when the blood supply to the brain, carrying the needed oxygen and glucose, is interrupted. The metabolic needs of the brain are so high that if its blood supply is lost for 4 minutes, irreversible brain damage results.

Cerebral concussion is the most frequent and least serious type of brain injury. It has been defined as a clinical syndrome "characterized by immediate and transient impairment of neural function such as alteration of consciousness, disturbances of vision, equilibrium . . . due to mechanical factors."[6] The concussion victim may complain of headache, nausea or emesis when awake but is rarely found to have a neurological deficit. Complete assessment must be done to rule out more serious injury. The finding of neurological abnormality, more often than not, indicates an injury more serious than simple concussion. If the trauma is severe enough, contusion or bruising of the brain occurs, with subsequent neurological change depending on the site of injury.

In all concussion patients, skull x-rays should be done in the emergency department. Experience has shown that it is preferable to admit such patients to the hospital for at least 24 hours of observation. An electroencephalogram and echogram are indicated to complete minimal diagnostic studies. Repeated observation of vital signs and level of consciousness and neurological assessment should be adhered to during the observation period. Any deviation from initial findings may indicate more serious brain injury. The most common change is alteration in level of consciousness. Significant widening of pulse pressure with lowering of pulse rate is indicative of increased intracranial pressure.

Intracranial hemorrhage

Intracranial hemorrhage is a serious complication of head injury and may terminate fatally. In general, bleeding within the rigid bony skull will result in increased intracranial pressure, which may cause local or generalized pressure on the brain itself. Elevation of intracranial pressure, secondary to hemorrhage, will cause varying types of neurological deficit. Common to all is progressive loss of consciousness.

The prognosis for intracranial hemorrhage is related to the type and extent of bleeding and the period of time over which the pressure has risen. Arterial bleeding is more serious than venous bleeding, though they may occur concomitantly. As a result of the increase in intracranial pressure, small vessels supplying the brain may be occluded, with resultant death of brain tissue. By repeated observation of head injury patients, early signs of increased intracranial pressure may be detected (see Figure 24–6), so that further studies and specific therapeutic measures may be undertaken. Increased pressure may lead to herniation of the brain and the brain stem inferiorly into the foramen magnum, with fatal consequences.

Hemorrhage within the cranium is of 4 main types: (1) epidural hemorrhage or hematoma, (2) subdural hematoma, (3) subarachnoid hemorrhage and (4) intracerebral hemorrhage.

Epidural hematoma

Bleeding into the epidural space, which lies between the skull and the dura, results in epidural hematoma (see Figure 24-4). Although it may be either venous or arterial bleeding, the most serious hemorrhage is caused by laceration of the middle meningeal artery, associated with a fracture in the temporal bone.

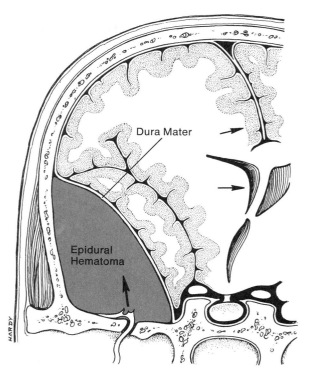

Figure 24–4 Epidural hematoma. The dark area in the lower left area of the drawing represents the hematoma. Note the broken blood vessel and the shift of mid-line structures.

The history is rather typical. The patient suffers a blow to the head, rather severe, causing momentary unconsciousness. There follows the so-called "lucid interval," which may last from minutes to several hours. This is followed by progressive loss of consciousness and deterioration of vital signs.

Assessment may reveal a dilated, nonreactive pupil on the side of damage (ipsilateral) and paralysis on the contralateral side. If the damage occurs on the dominant side of the brain (the left in right-handed individuals, the right in left-handed individuals), aphasia or speech deficit may be noted. Skull x-rays will frequently reveal the temporal fracture and pineal shift. Angiography or brain scan may reveal an abnormality, though many of these patients are diagnosed without these specialized studies.

Treatment depends on early recognition

and demands emergency evacuation of the hematoma, with control of the hemorrhage. The mortality rate approximates 50 percent.

Subdural hematoma

Subdural hematoma is caused by hemorrhage into the subdural space, between the dura and the arachnoid (see Figure 24–5) and may be either of the acute or chronic variety.

Acute subdural hematoma results from severe head trauma which causes both arterial and venous bleeding within a short time after injury. The bleeding originates from laceration of a cerebral vessel or from a cortical laceration or contusion. It may occur unilaterally or bilaterally and is often associated with an intracerebral injury.[14]

The history is usually similar to that of a severe head injury. The patient is unconscious. Lateralizing signs of an ipsilateral dilated, nonreactive pupil, with or without contralateral limb weakness or paralysis, may be noted. In bilateral or advanced cases, pupillary changes may be seen bilaterally.

Skull x-rays may or may not reveal a fracture and/or pineal shift. Bilateral carotid angiography is valuable in demonstrating and localizing the extracerebral mass lesion.[14, 23] Such procedures, however, are not usually performed in the emergency department. Lumbar puncture is rarely done.

Treatment is of an emergent nature and requires drainage of the hematoma. Although the prognosis is grave, with a mortality rate varying between 46 and 90 percent, it is favorably affected by surgical intervention soon after injury.

Chronic subdural hematoma usually becomes manifest weeks to months after injury. It occurs more commonly in infants and the aged. History of the injury, being so remote, may be almost forgotten. The mechanism of injury is usually a fall or blow to the head and may have been relatively minor. After injury, bleeding, usually venous, occurs from the surface of the brain. The hematoma expands over a period of time, causing gradual increase in intracranial pressure with resultant headache, alteration in consciousness, visual disturbances and other neurological deficits. The patient may also complain of nausea and emesis.

Skull x-rays and echogram will demonstrate a shift of mid-line structures. Angiography may confirm these findings. Lumbar puncture will reveal an increase in spinal fluid pressure. The fluid, rather than being clear, is often yellow-tinged (xanthochromic), due to absorption of breakdown products from the hematoma into the spinal fluid.

Once the diagnosis is established, the hematoma is evacuated to allow reexpansion of the brain. Contrary to acute hematoma, prognosis in the chronic type is excellent, with a 90 percent survival rate. In some patients, however, a neurological deficit may remain.

Subarachnoid hemorrhage

Subarachnoid hemorrhage is the most common type of intracranial hemorrhage due to

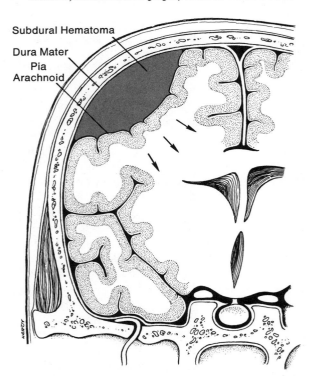

Figure 24–5 Subdural hematoma. The dark area in the upper left area of the drawing represents the hematoma. Note the shift of mid-line structures.

head trauma. History of head injury is noted, but no localizing signs may be seen on assessment. Headache is common, and bleeding into the subarachnoid space causes irritation of the meninges, which reflexly causes stiffness of the neck. Attempts to flex the neck, with the patient in the supine position, by lifting the head gently with the palm of a hand will be difficult. At times, the patient's neck is so rigid that the trunk is raised as well. This evidence, "nuchal rigidity," is strongly indicative of blood in the subarachnoid space.

Skull x-rays may be inconclusive; angiography may reveal no localizing signs. Lumbar puncture will reveal grossly bloody fluid. Management is usually nonoperative, unless a specific lesion is identified, such as cerebral artery aneurysm.

Close observation of the patient with a suspected head injury is an important nursing function. Cerebral edema, a feared sequela of head trauma, is manifest by signs and symptoms which should be familiar to the nurse and for which the patient should be observed at regular intervals.

Increased intracranial pressure

As pressure from hemorrhage or edema formation is exerted within the rigid cranial vault, a number of clinical signs are elicited. (See Figure 24–6 for one cause of increased intracranial pressure.) These signs reflect the body's ability to cope with the increased pressure (compensation). Frequent observation and recording of the patient's neurological status is necessary to initiate indicated treatment before irreversible brain damage from this pressure occurs. If the pressure continues to increase, brain damage and, possibly, death occurs. Failure of compensatory mechanisms (decompensation) may also be observed in neurological signs.

Nursing assessment of cerebral function includes observing for (1) level of consciousness, (2) motor and sensory function, (3) vital signs and (4) pupil size, reaction and movement. (Table 24–1 summarizes and compares level of consciousness, vital signs and pupil sizes for the 3 states of normalcy, compensa-

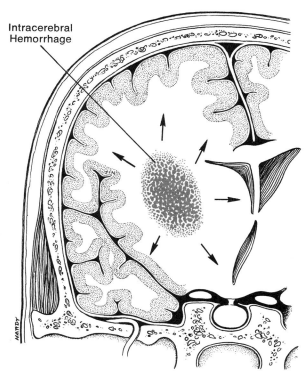

Figure 24–6 Intracerebral hemorrhage. The central large dark area represents the hemorrhage. Note the mid-line shift.

tion and decompensation.) While alterations may occur because of trauma or illness originating elsewhere in the body, it is wise to note these signs to provide baseline information for subsequent comparison and evaluation.[9]

Headache may be the first symptom of intracranial pressure, caused by tension on intracranial blood vessels.[30] While not uncommon in patients with head trauma, it does forewarn the nurse to watch closely for other neurological signs. Confusion, disorientation and delerium are seen early; later, somnolence and deepening coma ensue.

As cranial pressure rises, the systolic blood pressure rises and the diastolic pressure falls, resulting in a widened pulse pressure (the difference between the two pressures). The pulse slows and becomes full and bounding. Respirations are important in terms of rate and quality. The respiratory rate may slow as cranial pressure rises, but changes in the

TABLE 24–1 NEUROLOGICAL SIGNS OF INCREASED INTRACRANIAL PRESSURE

Sign	Normalcy	Compensation [a]	Decompensation [b]
(1) Level of consciousness	Conscious	Progressive unconsciousness	Comatose
(2) Pupils			
(3) Blood pressure 160 120 80 60			
(4) Pulse 160 120 80 60			
(5) Respiration 40 30 20 10			
(6) Temperature 106° F. 102° F. 100° F. 98.6° F.			

[a] Compensation is the period of time post-trauma when the body strives to compensate for increased intracranial pressure.

[b] Decompensation occurs when the body can no longer deal with the increased intracranial pressure.

quality of respiration may be even more significant.[16, 30] Maintaining a patent airway and providing respiratory support are important aspects of emergency care.

Temperature is not an accurate indicator of early increase in intracranial pressure, although a terminal rise may be noted in the stage of decompensation. But, temperature monitoring is important in controlling hyperthermia, so that the metabolic needs of an already compromised brain can be minimized.

Pupillary signs are a valuable indicator of cerebral status. They should be observed for size, shape, equality and response to light. Increased intracranial pressure may cause irritation of the oculomotor nerve, resulting in a fixed, dilated, ipsilateral pupil.[18] Bilateral fixed, dilated pupils indicate more generalized cerebral edema and are a grave prognostic sign. Eye movements can also provide valuable assessment data. Nystagmus, when present, should be observed for direction of movement. Other examinations such as the doll's eye maneuver and the caloric test are useful tools in evaluating intactness of the brain stem.[17]

Another important criterion of cerebral function is assessment of motor and sensory function. The patient's response to stimulation (verbal, pressure, pinprick) should be noted. Evaluating the movement as purposeful or nonpurposeful, as in spastic movement or decorticate or decerebrate posturing. also indicates the degree of cerebral function.

If the patient lost consciousness following head trauma, he is often admitted to the hospital for a 24-hour period of observation. Patients who sustained trauma to the head without loss of consciousness and without other abnormal neurological findings are usually discharged, with instructions to return or call the emergency department if signs of cerebral edema occur. Some hospitals give out instruction sheets (Table 24–2) as well as oral instructions and note on the emergency department record that these instructions were given and were understood by the patient or a responsible adult.

Cerebral edema in the inebriated patient

When a brain injury is sustained by a person whose brain is already depressed by alcohol, assessment becomes especially difficult, as the decreased level of consciousness and sensory-motor functioning can be due to either the alcohol or cerebral edema (secondary to injury). Likewise, bradycardia and vomiting may be caused by either.

In intoxicated patients, as well, the onset of cerebral edema is delayed, possibly because of the antidiuretic effect of alcohol, until the alcohol has been metabolized. But the edema may then persist for a longer period of time.[16] Hence, an inebriated patient with evidence of head trauma should be evaluated periodically for an extended period of time for alteration in his neurological status.

Prevention of cerebral edema

In patients with serious head injury, parenteral fluids should be administered with extreme caution to avoid causing or aggravating cerebral edema. The amount and rate of fluid intake should be prescribed by the physician and carefully monitored. An indwelling urethral catheter should be inserted and an accurate intake and output record maintained.

The use of urea solutions or concentrated sucrose and mannitol has been helpful in reducing the occurrence of cerebral edema.[25]

The anti-inflammatory effects of steroids have also been of value. Narcotics are generally not used, because they may mask important clinical signs. Slight sedation with a non-narcotic agent may be desirable to quiet the restless patient.

TABLE 24–2 HEAD INJURY OBSERVATION SHEET

If any of the following symptoms occur, call or return the patient to Santa Clara Valley Medical Center (telephone number: _____).

(1) Lethargy, confusion, sleepiness or inappropriate speech (Awaken injured person every 2 hours during the first 18 hours following the injury.)
(2) Vomiting
(3) Unequal pupil size (black central portion of eyes not of equal size)
(4) Blurred vision or seeing double
(5) Dizziness or unsteady gait
(6) Fever over 100°F.
(7) Slowing of pulse (less than 50 beats per minute)
(8) Marked reduction of muscular strength or inability to move arms or legs
(9) Convulsion or unconsciousness
(10) Colorless fluid coming from ears or nose

Source: Adapted from a form prepared by the hospital staff at the Santa Clara Valley Medical Center, San Jose, Cal., as a handout for observation of the head injury patient.

MANAGEMENT OF CERVICAL INJURIES

Acceleration-deceleration injury

Whiplash injury is most frequently associated with an automobile accident. The victim was probably in a vehicle stopped for a traffic signal or at an intersection when it was struck in the rear by a second vehicle. As a result, the first auto is pushed forward, and the head and neck of the victim is first extended, then flexed sharply. This extension-flexion injury results in a sprain or strain of the muscles and ligaments about the neck. Not uncommonly, but to a lesser extent, the muscles of the lower back will also be involved. Symptoms may not occur for 24 hours.

Whiplash victims enter the emergency department in varying degrees of distress. Head movements are restricted in all spheres: flexion, extension, lateral flexion and rotation. Careful palpation of the neck muscles may reveal spasm of the anterior strap muscles and the trapezius muscles. Pain is elicited on palpation, and localized tenderness may be present. There is rarely sensory loss.

The lower back should be examined similarly to determine the extent of involvement, since the strap muscles of the back on either side of the mid-line, known as the paraspinous muscles, extend the entire length of the vertebral column and can be involved, as well. X-rays of the cervical spine are indicated to rule out any bony injury. The normal lordotic curve of the neck is frequently lost due to muscle spasm.

Rarely do whiplash victims require hospitalization when that is their only injury. Treatment consists of applying a padded cervical collar for support of the neck, plus analgesics and muscle relaxants, as indicated. Correct fitting of the cervical collar produces a straight neck, with the chin tucked in, preventing cervical spine hyperextension (see Figure 24–7). Whiplash patients may be extremely apprehensive, as a result of the

injury and require strong reassurance. Diazepam (Valium) has been used effectively as a muscle relaxant/tranquilizer.

Success with an early physical therapy program in the acute phase of muscle strain has been reported. Treatment consists of massaging with ice, using a specific technique, followed by range of motion and mobilization exercises in the involved area. Other physical therapy modalities used with varying degrees of success has been diathermy, massage and ultrasound. Cervical traction may be required to overcome persistent muscle spasm, particularly when symptoms of cervical nerve root compression (paresthesias radiating into the upper limbs) are present.

Cervical spine injuries

History is very important in evaluating patients with cervical spinal injury, especially when the spinal cord may be involved. Injuries to the vertebrae that can result in damage to the cord are usually caused by acute flexion, as seen in the classic diving accident—the victim strikes his head at the bottom of a shallow depth of water. Similar injuries may result from a blocking injury in football, when the blocker, in an improper position, suffers an acute forceful flexion injury to the neck. It should be determined immediately whether any neurological deficit is present, and if so, when it occurred, whether immediately after injury or after a period of time.

The patient, when conscious, will invariably complain of neck pain and varying alteration in movement and sensation. In every instance, proper handling of the patient is mandatory. The head should be maintained in one position, by use of a sandbag on either side.

If there is suspicion of cervical spine injury, the patient should be placed on a special board designed to immobilize the spine. A variety of immobilization boards are available (see Figure 24–8), and one should be carried on the ambulance and used whenever

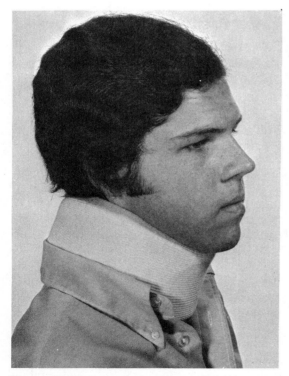

Figure 24–7 A cervical collar applied. The collar helps to immobilize the injured neck, thus protecting it from further harm.

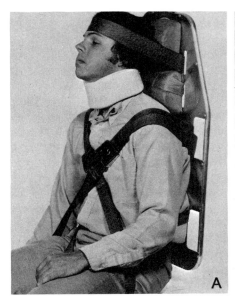

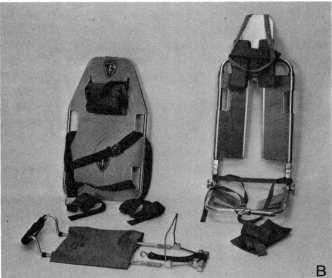

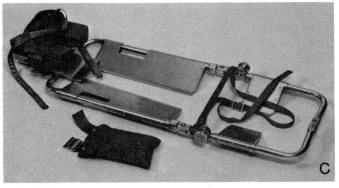

Figure 24–8 Splinting devices. A: Half-length spine board applied, along with cervical extrication collar. Note immobilization of head; when cervical collar is not needed or not applied, more padding is inserted behind the head for greater support. This board may be applied prior to extrication of a victim from a vehicle. B: Various splints for extrication and transfer of patient suspected of spine or lower limb injury. Upper left: half-spine board. Upper right: full-spine board. Foreground: Hare traction splint. C: Full-length, adjustable spine board in extension.

a back or neck injury is suspected. One such board, known as the "Prolo Board" (Figure 24–9), is in common use in some areas and is designed for immediate immobilization of the cervical spine at the accident site. Its distinct advantage to emergency department personnel is that x-rays can be taken with the device in place, and the patient can remain on this board in reasonable comfort until definitive therapy is instituted.[18]

Palpation of the cervical spinous processes by gentle examination of the posterior midline of the neck may reveal localized tenderness and, sometimes, malalignment. Diagnosis can be confirmed by anteroposterior and lateral x-rays of the cervical spine (Figure 24–10). Remember not to move the patient off the spine board. Most often, injuries occur to the lowermost portion of the cervical spine; thus, it is essential that the last cervical and first thoracic vertebrae be visible on the film.

If the spine has been damaged but no neurological injury has occurred, the patient should be kept immobile until the physician can determine the extent of injury and further management. If the injured area is unstable and neurological deficit is absent, skeletal traction may be required. Commonly used are Vinke or Crutchfield tongs or a halo traction device, which are inserted into the outer

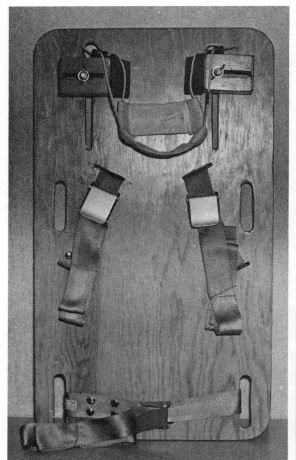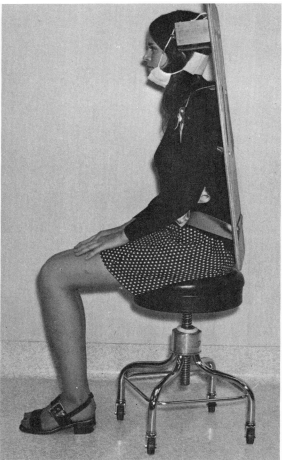

Figure 24–9 The Prolo board. In the photograph at right, the device was applied while the patient was in the sitting position. This splint can be placed on the patient before removal from a vehicle.

table of the skull under local anesthesia. This procedure can be performed in the emergency department.

All personnel must keep in mind that improper handling of a patient with cervical spinal injury could convert a simple bony injury into a complicated, possibly fatal one. Utmost caution is imperative in all actions.

Spinal cord damage

If a neurological deficit is noted, the nurse should assume the spinal cord has been damaged. Depending on the degree and level of damage, dramatic systemic alterations may result. Symptoms and findings may include sensory changes, such as numbness, tingling and altered sensation, and motor loss (weakness or total paralysis) distal to the level of injury. The cervical cord areas most frequently injured are between the fourth and fifth and between the fifth and sixth cervical vertebrae. It is in these areas that the greatest degree of flexion and extension mobility occurs.

Respiratory embarrassment results from an acute cord injury. Respiration may be shallow, with little or no movement of chest muscles but *with* movement of abdominal muscles. The muscles of normal respiration are those of the chest wall and the diaphragm.

The diaphragm is innervated by the phrenic nerve, which arises from the third, fourth and fifth cervical nerves. A cord injury at or above the level of the mid-cervical region causes severe respiratory embarrassment, which can be fatal if untreated.

Airway management may be difficult; passage of an endotracheal tube can cause further damage to the neck. The best approach is tracheostomy. A mechanical ventilator will be required to maintain or assist the patient's respirations. Arterial blood gases should be taken for baseline information.

Hypotension secondary to neurological injury is a common occurrence, due to alteration in functioning of the autonomic nervous system, with splanchnic pooling and sequestration of blood in the large bed of vessels of the abdominal viscera.

Similarly, gastric dilation is frequently noted, due to gastric atony. As a result, fluid and air collect in the stomach. If untreated, it may lead to further circulatory and respiratory embarrassment, emesis and possibly aspiration. This latter complication can be prevented or treated by insertion of a nasogastric tube soon after the patient has been stabilized, since the patient may have had fluid or solid food a short time prior to injury which could be aspirated.

Bladder control will also be affected by any spinal cord injury, and an indwelling catheter is necessary.

A complete examination of the patient is

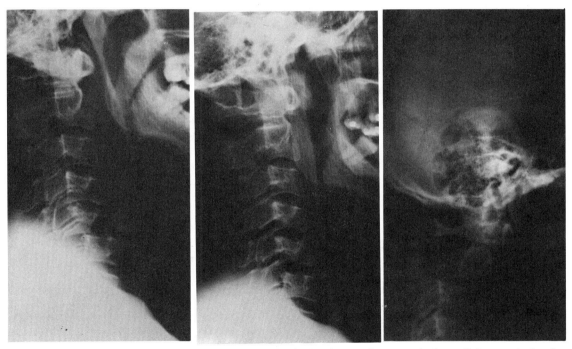

Figure 24–10 Fracture and dislocation of the cervical spine. Left: Lateral view of the cervical spine reveals a fracture dislocation of the fifth cervical segment. The lowermost vertebra is not well visualized on this film but was well seen in other studies. Patient suffered an acute flexion injury of the neck after diving into shallow water and was quadraplegic at the time of admission to the emergency department. Center: Same patient after application of Crutchfield tongs and traction is seen. Good reduction was obtained, but there was no recovery of neurological function. Right: Fracture dislocation of the second cervical vertebra can be visualized. This patient was involved in an automobile accident and ejected from the vehicle. Marked hypotension and severe respiratory embarrassment were present on entry to the emergency department. The patient expired within several hours of injury.

necessary to rule out any associated injury. Since patients with cord injuries have little. or no pain sensation below the level of injury, assessment may be difficult, and care must be taken to determine the presence of other fractures and soft tissue or visceral injury. Close observation is required. The patient should not be moved until the physician has completed his evaluation.

When a previously active, independent person sustains a spinal cord injury and is suddenly thrust into a role of dependence, it can be a very traumatic experience for patient and family. Feelings of grief, loss and helplessness are common.[12, 15] The sensitive emergency nurse can be influential in supporting the patient and his family during this acute phase of care. Reassurance that everything possible is being done and that resources are available to rehabilitate the patient to a full, productive life can be helpful during this time.

Blunt injury to the neck

Blunt trauma usually results from a blow or fall. As mentioned previously, the bone and muscles of the cervical area protect it from blunt injury posteriorly and laterally. Anteriorly, however, the strap muscles afford little protection and the neck structures are extremely vulnerable to injury.

Direct blows to the anterior neck may cause delayed airway obstruction from hematoma expanding deep to the pretracheal fascia.[2, 22] Less severe injuries to the trachea may cause dyspnea and stridor and must be evaluated to rule out more serious damage. When the trachea has been damaged sufficiently to produce a leak of air, subcutaneous emphysema is invariably present, which will be manifest by a "crackling" sensation over the area, when palpated.

If the patient is alive on entry to the emergency department, airway compromise must be dealt with swiftly. If possible, an endotracheal tube should be passed; otherwise, tracheostomy must be done. Rupture of the trachea is associated with a high mortality rate. Urgent operative treatment is necessary, with every effort made to stabilize the patient's condition prior to transfer to the surgical suite.

Sharp blows, such as karate chops, can cause varying degrees of injury to neurovascular structures in the lateral portions of the neck. Damage to the esophagus from blunt injury is rather uncommon but must be kept in mind; an esophagram may be helpful in detecting perforations of the esophagus. Similarly, injury to the apex of the lung or pleura must be considered.

As a rule, patients with blunt injuries to the neck are more difficult to assess than those with penetrating wounds.

Penetrating injury to the neck

Penetrating injuries resulting from a stabbing, gunshot wound or flying object are potentially life-threatening injuries. The nurse should not be misled by what appears to be an innocuous flesh wound. A number of series of patients with penetrating neck injuries have been reported in the medical literature with a mortality rate of 6 to 10 percent.[10, 22,26] If the principle that penetration of the platysma mandates exploration of the site of injury is followed, many fatalities may be averted. Higher survival rates are found in patients of those institutions adhering to the principle of early exploration. Most fatalities are due to vascular injury, particularly of the carotid and subclavian arteries and veins, and the remainder are due to wounds of the larynx, esophagus and trachea.[20, 21] Exploration of a hemmorhaging wound is done in the operating suite, not in the emergency department.

Assessment of the entire patient is necessary, with particular attention to vital signs and the wound itself. An adequate airway must be established and maintained. Not uncommonly, endotracheal intubation or tracheostomy must be done. The circulatory status of the limbs should be evaluated, and in patients with hemorrhagic shock, volume replacement should be started with large-bore needles, allowing rapid infusion with Ringer's lactate solution. Type-specific whole blood should be prepared and infused as soon as available. If the nurse suspects injury to a major vein in the neck, particularly the subclavian, which drains the upper extremities, the lifeline should be placed in the lower limbs. The large-bore needle or Angiocath should be inserted into the saphenous vein at the ankle percutaneously or through a cut-down.

Once the patient has been stabilized, more thorough assessment may be completed. *No penetrating wound should be ignored or underestimated.* The neck should be inspected for any swelling or mass. Careful palpation for subcutaneous emphysema or the presence of a pulsatile mass must be made. The position of the trachea is appraised. Ordinarily, the trachea should be in the mid-line in the suprasternal notch, between the medial ends of the clavicles. Deviation from the mid-line may result from pressure of a mass, such as a hematoma, against the trachea or from a hemothorax or pneumothorax.

Examination of pulses and motor and sensory modalities should be done in the upper limbs to discover any damage to the vascular or nervous system. The wound should be inspected and the path of injury identified, if possible. Upright x-rays of the neck and chest are needed to determine the presence of a pneumothorax, hemothorax or air in the tissues of the neck. The location of retained missiles may also be noted on film.

Hemorrhage from a penetrating neck wound may be controlled by pressure while resuscitative measures are instituted. *In no instance should the wound be probed in the emergency department,* lest a thrombus be dislodged and further hemorrhage result. Rather, this should be done in the operating suite.

Prior to World War II, when treatment of penetrating wounds was largely nonsurgical, most deaths from penetrating wounds were due to vascular damage and secondly to airway damage. Since that time, penetrating wounds of the neck have generally been explored surgically. This has resulted in a much lower mortality rate.

It is important to know that innocuous penetrating neck wounds are often associated with major structural damage to the neck,[10, 29] such as injuries to the major vessels, esophagus and thoracic duct. Studies have shown that even though the wound appears minor, surgical exploration for associated trauma and repair is often necessary.[7, 19]

INJURIES TO THE SPINE

Injuries to the cervical portion of the spinal column have been discussed above. They undoubtedly represent the most dramatic vertebral injury because of the rather high incidence of associated spinal cord damage and resultant neurological deficit. Damage to the thoracic (dorsal) and lumbar vertebrae occurs more frequently than cervical spine injury, involving the twelfth (or last) thoracic and the upper 2 lumbar vertebrae.

The usual mechanism of thoracic and lumbar injury is acute hyperflexion of the spinal column, resulting from a fall in which the patient landed on his feet or on his buttocks, in a sitting position. As a result of the sudden deceleration, the body weight causes acute flexion of the spine, with compression of the vertebral body. This "wedging" results in a compression-type fracture (Figure 24–11), which is more apt to occur when the fall is from a height or in a patient with demineralization of the body, as with osteoporosis. This type of injury accounts for approximately 60 percent of all spinal injuries. In more serious injuries, the vertebral body may actually fragment, and one vertebra may dislocate on the adjacent one.

In patients who have suffered a fall, as from a ladder or scaffold, especially when landing on the feet, great force is exerted on the lower leg, particularly in the region of the heel. Thus, fractures of the heel (os calcis) or lower tibia may be found in association with thoracolumbar spinal injury.

Other deceleration forces may produce vertebral fractures. Lap-type and shoulder-type restraints mandated in the modern-day

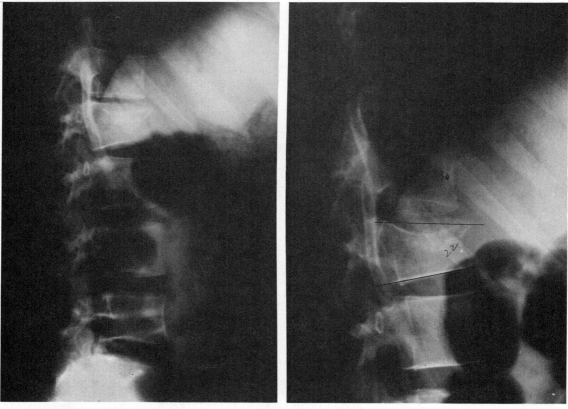

Figure 24–11 Lumbar vertebra fracture. Left: X-ray shows a compression fracture of the first lumbar vertebra in a patient who fell from a height of 3 stories, landing on his feet in soft earth. There were no other injuries. Right: In the same patient, spot film shows marked degree of wedging.

automobile may be one factor in such injury. In rapid deceleration at impact, the passenger is thrown forward while being restrained by the lap or shoulder belt. As a result, the upper body may flex sharply over the restraining device, with compression fracture resulting. Torsional injury may also occur and is more likely to be found in the area of the dorsal vertebrae. Such injuries are rarely associated with any neurological damage, however.

Anatomically, the spinal cord terminates at the level of the second lumbar vertebra; thus, it is unusual to have any serious neurological damage accompanying vertebral injury below this point. The cauda equina may be damaged, however. In patients with suspected fracture of the thoracic or lumbar vertebrae, transport within the hospital should be done carefully and the patient moved about as little as possible.

Assessment

In the absence of neurological injury, fractures of the dorsal or lumbar vertebrae are usually manifested by local pain. Rarely is a detectable deformity present. The incidence of spinal cord damage is low, being associated with fracture-dislocations or with penetrating injury, such as a gunshot or stab wound, with direct damage to the cord. The patient will relate a history of injury, such as a fall or auto accident, with acute flexion followed by pain in the back.

In extensive injury, involving several vertebrae, there may be enough damage to cause retroperitoneal bleeding, which can produce a reflex paralytic ileus involving both the intestinal tract and urinary bladder (see Figure 24–12). When thus indicated, a nasogastric tube and indwelling bladder catheter should be placed. Vital signs are determined and recorded for a baseline value upon entry and should be reassessed at periodic intervals during the patient's entire stay in the emergency department.

Physical evaluation may be negative or may demonstrate tenderness in response to palpation (pressure) or percussion over the spinous process of the involved vertebra(e). Spasm of the adjacent paraspinous musculature may also be present. Careful neurological examination is necessary to determine whether spinal cord damage has occurred. Motor and sensory function and deep tendon reflexes should be thoroughly assessed. Nerve injury may be manifest by symptoms varying from paresthesias to total paralysis below the level of injury.

If there are no findings suggestive of spinal cord injury, the patient should be moved to the x-ray department, where roentgenological examination of the entire spine is performed. Every effort must be made to move the patient as little as possible until the nature of the injury is established. If neurological injury is suspected or diagnosed, the patient should be moved in the prone position. Under no circumstances should the patient be allowed to walk or sit if a spine fracture is suspected, even though he or she may have walked into the emergency department. After the x-rays have been completed, the physician should decide on further handling of the patient.

Management

Patients with no neurological injury are admitted and maintained at bedrest until the pain has subsided. In some instances, reduction of the fracture by hyperextension, traction and application of plaster dressings may be indicated.[1] This is rarely, if ever, done in

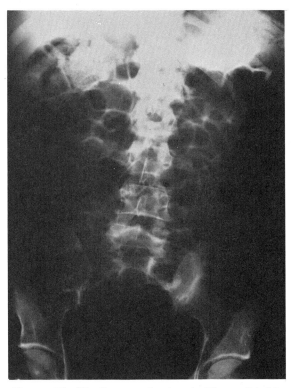

Figure 24–12 Same patient as in Figure 24–11. Note large amount of gas scattered throughout both small and large bowel, indicative of reflex ileus. The body of the first lumbar segment is narrowed, especially on the right side.

the emergency department. When spinal cord injury has occurred, neurosurgical consultation should be sought. Further diagnostic tests may be in order to establish the presence of a block in the spinal canal. One technique is to perform a lumbar puncture (spinal tap), using the Queckenstadt test. When evidence of a block within the spinal canal is found, urgent decompression of the spinal cord may be necessary.

The patient should be stabilized in preparation for anticipated surgery. Nasogastric and bladder drainage, intravenous fluid replacement and measurement of intake and output are essential to good patient care. Calm, decisive action on the part of the emergency department team will serve to allay apprehension and provide assurance to the patient.

SUMMARY

The head, neck and spine comprise a region of the body which is frequently injured in emergency trauma situations. A combination of thorough assessment, suspicion of further injury and caution on the part of the emergency nurse will help insure a positive result for the patient.

BIBLIOGRAPHY

(1) Baab, O. D.: "Fractures of the Dorsal and Lumbar Spine," *Clinical Orthopaedics and Related Research,* 49 (1966):195.

(2) Beall, A. C.; Noon, G. P., and Harris, H. H.: "Surgical Management of Tracheal Trauma," *Journal of Trauma,* 7 (1967):248.

(3) Bradley, E. L., III: "Management of Penetrating Carotid Injuries," *Journal of Trauma,* 13 (1973):248.

(4) Enker, W. E., and Simonowitz, D.: "Experience in the Operative Management of Penetrating Injuries of the Neck," *Surgical Clinics of North America,* 53 (1973):87.

(5) Grant, A. E.: "Massage with Ice (Cryokinetics) in the Treatment of Painful Conditions of the Musculoskeletal System," *Archives of Physical Medicine,* 45 (1964):233.

(6) Hekmatpanah, J.: "The Management of Head Trauma," *Surgical Clinics of North America,* 43 (1973):47.

(7) Hubay, C. A.: "Soft Tissue Injuries of the Cervical Region," *International Abstracts of Surgery,* 111 (1960):511.

(8) Jackson, R.: *The Cervical Syndrome,* 3 ed. (Springfield, Ill.: Charles C Thomas, 1966), p. 35.

(9) Johnson, M. R.: "Emergency Management of Head and Spinal Injuries," *Nursing Clinics of North America,* 8 (1973):389.

(10) Jones, R. F.; Terrell, J. C., and Salyer, K. E.: "Penetrating Wounds of the Neck: Analysis of 274 Cases," *Journal of Trauma,* 7 (1967):228.

(11) Kurze, T., and Pitts, F. W.: "Management of Closed Head Injuries," *Surgical Clinics of North America,* 48 (1968): 1271.

(12) Lee, J.: "Emotional Reactions to Trauma," *Nursing Clinics of North America,* 5 (1970):577.

(13) Maroon, J. C., and Gosling, C.: "A Head and Neck Trauma Teaching Model," *Journal of Trauma,* 13 (1973):245. (Medical Plastics Laboratory (Gatesville, Texas) Lifelike Anatomical Model.)

(14) Moiel, R. H., and Caram, P. C.: "Acute Subdural Hematomas," *Journal of Trauma,* 7 (1967):660.

(15) Murray, R.: "Principles of Nursing Intervention for the Adult Patient with Body Image Changes," *Nursing Clinics of North America,* 7 (1972):697.

(16) Parsons, L. C.: "Respiratory Changes in Head Injury," *American Journal of Nursing,* 71 (1971):2187.

(17) Plum, F., and Posner, J.: *The Diagnosis of Stupor and Coma,* ed. 2 (Philadelphia: F. A. Davis Company, 1972), pp. 44–46.

(18) Prolo, D., and Hanbery, J.: "Cervical Stabilization—Traction Board," *Journal of the American Medical Association,* 244 (1973):615.

(19) Quesenbury, J., and Lembright, P.: "Observations and Care for Patients with Head Injuries," *Nursing Clinics of North America,* 4 (1969):237.

(20) Rich, N. M.; Baugh, J. H., and Hughes, C. W.: "Acute Arterial Injuries in Vietnam: 1,000 Cases," *Journal of Trauma,* 10 (1970):359.

(21) Rich, N. M.; Hobson, R. W.; Jarstfer, B. S., and Geer, T. M.: "Subclavian Artery Trauma," *Journal of Trauma,* 13 (1973):485.

(22) Saletta, J. C.; Folk, F. A., and Freeark, R. J.: "Trauma to the Neck Region,"

Surgical Clinics of North America, 53 (1973):73.

(23) Schisano, G., and Burzaco, J.: "Acute and Chronic Subdural Hematomas," *Acta Chirugica Scandinavia,* 128 (1964):471.

(24) Schwartz, Henry G.: "Management of Acute Head Trauma," *Surgical Clinics of North America,* 38 (1958): 1475.

(25) Stein, A., and Seaward, P. D.: "Penetrating Wounds of the Neck," *Journal of Trauma,* 7 (1967):239.

(26) Walker, A. E.: *Head Injury Conference Proceedings: Univ. of Chicago, February 6–9, 1966* (Philadelphia: J. B. Lippincott Company, 1966).

(27) Watson-Jones, R.: *Fractures and Joint Injuries,* ed. 4 (Baltimore: Williams & Wilkins Company, 1955).

(28) Weitzman, G.: "Treatment of Stable Thoracolumbar Spine Compression Fractures by Early Ambulation," *Clinical Orthopaedics and Related Research,* 76 (1971):116.

(29) Yoder, R. L.: "Innocuous Appearing Stab Wounds to the Neck:" *Southern Medical Journal,* 62 (1960):113.

(30) Young, J.: "Recognition, Significance and Recording of the Signs of Intracranial Pressures," *Nursing Clinics of North America,* 4 (1969):223.

25

Injuries of bones, joints and related soft-tissue structures

JAMES M. COLE
JAMES H. COSGRIFF, JR.
KARILYN R. DUARTE
CARL T. ANDERSON

Injuries to the bones, joints and related supporting structures are commonly seen in the emergency department setting. Such injuries may occur singly or in association with other trauma. Nursing intervention is important, for often the nurse is the first trained professional to see the victim. As such, the nurse should be adequately prepared to assess the patient and initiate appropriate treatment and diagnostic studies.

ANATOMY AND PHYSIOLOGY

Bone is living tissue formed by organic materials (mostly protein), minerals, water and fatty tissue, which is located in the marrow cavity. The organic materials comprise about 30 percent of bone weight and the minerals about 45 percent, including mainly calcium, phosphorus and magnesium.

Adult bone consists of an inner fatty marrow cavity surrounded by the strong, hard, osseous tissue which comprises the main structure of the bone. The outer layer is covered by the periosteum, from which new bone cells grow. Vascular supply to bone is derived from blood vessels arising from neighboring arteries which penetrate the bone through small channels called Haversian canals. These vessels are often referred to as nutrient arteries.

The bony skeleton lends structural support to the body. Mobility of the body depends upon the joints and their supporting muscles and ligamentous structures. The skeleton is surrounded by varying amounts of soft tissue, which, in addition to muscles and ligaments, includes tendons, fascia, blood vessels and nerves. Injury to a bone involves damage to these many other tissues, which must be taken into consideration in the management of the patient suspected of having a fracture.

Fractures may assume a number of configurations and occur anywhere in the length of the bone: in the shaft, at either end or extending into the joint. Bone growth occurs in the child from ossification centers usually located near the ends of each bone, called the epiphyseal plate, or more commonly, the epiphysis. Bone growth is completed by approximately age 17. Fractures which occur in the epiphysis before full bone growth has occurred may cause a subsequent failure of growth in the affected bone.

A fracture results from stress applied to a bone or joint. The type of stress may be a direct blow, a penetrating injury (in which a high-energy missile strikes the bone) or ligamentous or muscular stresses about a joint (in which the joint is overflexed, overextended or undergoes torsion).

In joint stresses, type of injury depends on the strength of the structure involved. For example, if an individual twists his ankle stepping off a curb, the usual mechanism is to land on the lateral side of the foot so that the foot is inverted. This results in 2 types of stress. On the lateral aspect of the ankle, the ligamentous structures about the joint are stretched, and this stretching (tensile) force is exerted on the bones at the site of attachment of the ligaments. At the same time, on the medial aspect of the ankle, the bones are crushed against each other in another form of stress. The result may be a fracture on the medial side of the ankle joint and laterally a ligamentous tear or avulsion fracture. The ligamentous tear results if the stress is sufficient to pull the ligament apart (often referred to as a sprain). If a ligament holds and pulls the bone away at its site of attachment, that is an avulsion fracture.

Displacement of fracture fragments results partly from the mechanism of the causative injury but is more likely due to muscle pull. After disruption of the skeletal structure by fracture, the muscles contract and cause angulation, overlapping or other deformity of the bone at the fracture site. This assumes great importance, especially if an effort is made at securing a reduction.

Fracture healing

The healing of a fracture does not vary significantly from the healing of soft tissue wounds, from the physiological standpoint. Fracture healing occurs primarily as a local phenomenon at the site of injury. As in other wounds, proper healing depends on accurate apposition of tissue (bone ends), proper immobilization and adequate blood supply.

After a fracture is incurred, blood and tissue fluid enter the fracture site in a manner similar to granulation tissue. As healing progresses, the blood clots and areas of cartilage and calcification develop within the clot as the first stage of callus formation. The amount of callus formed varies in amount, depending on how the bone ends are anatomically approximated. Calcium cells are deposited in the callus, and true bone is then formed. As bone formation progresses, excess callus is resorbed, and periosteum covers the area of the fracture site.

The new shape of the bone after fracture healing will depend to a great extent on the initial alignment and on maintenance of position of the fracture fragments. Depending on the site of the fracture and the factors mentioned above (proper reduction, immobilization and blood supply), healing will occur in 3 weeks (for phalanges) to many months (for femur and hip).

Failure of the fracture to heal is called *non-union*. Non-union results from a number of causes, including failure to adhere to principles of fracture management, inadequate mobilization, loss of reduction, interposition of soft tissue between the bone ends, metabolic diseases and infection. In addition, aseptic necrosis of the bone may occur after fractures in which the blood supply to bone ends has been interrupted. It most commonly occurs in the head of the femur following a fracture through the anatomical neck.

TYPES OF INJURIES

The common injuries to the bones, joints and related soft tissue structures are: (1) fracture, (2) dislocation, (3) sprain and (4) strain.

Fracture

A fracture is any break in continuity of a bone. Although various types may be described (transverse, oblique, spiral, greenstick, comminuted or impacted), this is only of relative importance to the emergency nurse. The diagnosis of fracture type is made by x-ray, since the clinical appearance in many instances is the same. (See Figure 25–1.)

However, differentiation between so-called "closed" fractures and "open" fractures is of primary importance to the emergency nurse. A closed fracture denotes no direct communication between the fracture and the overlying skin. An open fracture is one where direct communication exists between the fracture and the overlying skin. At times, distinguishing the two may be difficult, as in a patient with both a laceration and an obvious fracture present, although there does not appear to be a direct communication between the two. To avoid such confusion, any patient with an obvious fracture of an extremity and with a wound in the vicinity of the bony injury should be assumed to have an open fracture until proven otherwise. The physical signs really only assist the nurse in making a proper diagnosis by x-ray investigation.

Dislocation

A "dislocation" is an injury to a joint, involving *complete* disruption of the contiguous surfaces of the two articulating bones from one another. A "subluxation" of a joint is a lesser, similar injury, in which part of the joint is still articulating.

Symptoms of a dislocation are primarily those of pain about a joint and complaints of inability to use the extremity. The most common signs of a dislocation are obvious deformity about the joint and lack of motion.

Sprain

A "sprain" is an injury to a ligament which results from incomplete tearing of the ligamentous fibers, involving no loss of continuity to the ligament. There are many degrees of sprain, manifested clinically from very mild pain and swelling about a joint to a more serious disruption of the ligamentous structure.

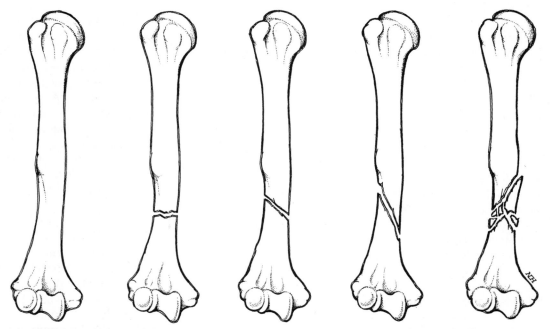

Figure 25–1 Various types of fractures. From left to right: intact bone, simple transverse fracture, simple oblique fracture, spiral fracture, comminuted fracture.

The primary symptom of a sprain is pain in the area of the joint. The most obvious physical finding is swelling. It is, many times, extremely difficult to differentiate a sprain from a fracture. The nurse should consider a painful swelling about a joint to be a fracture until x-ray examination proves otherwise.

Strain

O'Donoghue defines a "strain" as "damage of some part of the muscle, or tendonous attachment occasioned by overuse (chronic strain) or overstress (acute strain)."[20, p. 59]

The symptom of a strain is pain in the area of the muscular or tendonous attachment unit that has been traumatized. As opposed to a sprain, the pain is usually away from the joint. The physical sign of swelling is less constant in this injury. Pain in the area following trauma, along with findings of tenderness and swelling, should suggest a fracture; a fracture must be ruled out before treatment is instituted.

TRANSPORTATION

Since disturbances of normal ambulation may be one of the prime effects of bony injury, special equipment is necessary, or at least desirable, for moving these patients. This is particularly true with injuries to the back, pelvis and lower extremities. (See Chapter 24 for discussion of immobilization equipment for spinal injuries.) Simple coordination of personnel and equipment will do much to ease admission and subsequent care, and prior warning of the patient arrivals will allow preparation and assembly of equipment and personnel.

Many ambulances and fire rescue vehicles utilize stretchers to lessen patient movement and manipulation. Having a Transaver or similar device ready for transfer of the patient from the ambulance stretcher is advisable, not only in terms of patient comfort but also in decreasing the number of personnel needed for patient movement. If a scoop stretcher has been used by the ambulance attendants, the patient should preferably not be removed from it until the x-rays have been completed, if this is feasible.

All movement of the patient, particularly of the injured part(s) should be performed slowly and cautiously, eliciting the patient's voluntary help when possible. Quick movements, even with an uninvolved extremity or body part, can provoke painful muscle spasms. Slight muscle tension is desired when the patient is moving his own fractured arm. He should be encouraged to relax the involved muscles only after personnel have supported the limb with their hands or other splinting methods.

The injured part should be firmly supported above and below the fracture site. Once hands have been placed on the patient, they should not be shifted to a different position. This involves planning ahead. Rather than manipulating clothing off the patient's body, quicker access may be gained by cutting it away. Conditions allowing, there is usually no necessity to cut up the middle of a piece of clothing when a seam line cut could accomplish the same result and also salvage the garment.

TRIAGE

Whether or not a triage nurse is specifically designated as part of the organizational plan of the emergency department, it is essential that the emergency nurse be familiar with triage principles and their application in the management of patients with fractures. Triage is considered throughout the chapter, in discussing assessment and management of specific situations.

Fractures occupy a low-priority position in the overall treatment of the trauma victim—with the exception of fractures associated with vascular and/or neurological impairment, to be discussed later in this chapter. Within the limited category of fractures, a setting of priorities does exist. The elderly adult with a fractured hip and stable vital signs may be placed lower on the priority list than the young person with a comminuted fracture of the femur and in hypovolemic shock.

While life-threatening situations take precedence for treatment, the nurse must always remain vigilant for associated problems, particularly with the older adult. Falls may have been precipitated by momentary loss of consciousness, signaling underlying cardiovascular and/or neurological disorders. Visual disorders, such as glaucoma and cataracts, may have been the causative factor in the fall but were unrecognized and untreated prior to injury because of their insidious nature. A history of any recent ingestion of medications which may have caused muscle incoordination or changes in the sensorium should be brought to the doctor's attention.

HISTORY AND ASSESSMENT

It is extremely important for the nurse to recognize that a true emergency exists in the mind of the patient even if not substantiated by the presenting symptoms and subsequent assessment. Accidents are not planned; thus, the sudden onset of trauma to bones and joints often leaves the patient stunned and in varying degrees of pain. Obtaining a history of injury can be a trying situation for both nurse and patient. Emotional support is important in allaying anxiety and eliciting cooperation.

Historical data should include the mechanism of injury and the circumstances surrounding the injury. These facts are sometimes difficult to elicit in any great detail, since the fall or incident may have happened so rapidly that the patient has little recall of the event. It should be determined whether the patient had full use of the involved limb(s) after injury.

A record should be made of all of the patient's symptoms or complaints; attention must be given to every detail. It is not uncommon, when confronted with a patient with multiple injuries, for emergency personnel to attend to the major, life-threatening injuries and give little or no recognition or treatment to a minor injury, which could result in a prolonged occupational disability. Thus, it should be determined whether the symptoms are localized to one area or involve others.

Obviously, the amount of history needed will depend on the patient's complaints. For example, a young patient presenting with pain in the ankle and inability to bear weight does not require the extensive inquiry that is needed to properly evaluate the patient with multiple injuries. In the latter case, as many details as possible should be gathered. Although the victim may be accompanied to the emergency department by relatives or friends, they may not have been at the accident scene. Information should then be sought from police officers and ambulance personnel, especially when the patient is not a reliable historian.

EMERGENCY MANAGEMENT

The general principles of early emergency department management of the patient with suspected fracture includes assessment of the patient, immobilization of the injured part, to minimize pain and avoid complications, and initiation of appropriate x-ray studies as soon as the patient's condition permits. One must be suspicious of fracture in any patient complaining of pain, especially pain in a limb or about a joint, accompanied by obvious swelling, deformity or inability to use the part.

Physical assessment depends on the patient's symptomatology. Common sense, experience and good judgment will determine the extent of evaluation. In patients with multiple injuries, the emergency nurse must first insure that the airway is adequate. The cardiovascular system must also be evaluated and stabilized. Attention may then be directed to the area of suspected fracture(s), keeping priorities in mind. (See Chapter 6, on triage.) When the patient has a single injury, attention may be limited to the site of injury.

Thorough examination of the part should be done gently, looking for the presence of any open wound. The most common signs associated with fracture are: (1) local tenderness, (2) local swelling, (3) deformity, (4) diminution or total absence of active motion, (5) false motion at the fracture site and (6) crepitation (grating of the bone ends).

Injuries or fractures may occur at sites remote from the fracture site itself. For example, in certain ankle injuries involving the medial malleolus, the upper shaft of the fibula may be fractured. Likewise, in falls in which the patient landed on the feet, fracture of the heel bone, the os calcis, is common, but accompanying compression fractures of the dorsolumbar vertebrae are also frequent occurrences (see Chapter 24). These are primarily at the level of the twelfth thoracic and the upper 2 lumbar vertebrae.

Soft tissue structures about the area of injury must also be evaluated. Loss of motion may be due to major tendon damage. The most commonly injured tendons are the biceps brachii in the upper arm, the quadriceps tendon on the anterior aspect of the knee and the achilles tendon just above the heel. Rupture of these structures may occur with seemingly little stress, resulting in an inability to use the part.

The circulatory and neurological status of the limb must be evaluated, by assessing the arterial pulses and motor activity and sensation distal to the level of injury. The possibility of neurovascular damage is important to assess, for when present, it may necessitate modification of the usual mode of therapy.

The 5 Ps of vascular occlusion (pain, pallor, pulselessness, paresthesia, paralysis) serve as an excellent assessment guide. Palpate the pulse(s) distal to the fracture site, comparing the findings with the opposite, uninvolved area, if possible. Presence or absence of a pulse cannot be considered sufficient, in itself, to rule out vascular damage. Repeated evaluation at regular intervals is important.

Ischemia slows metabolic processes so that the involved areas become cooler to the touch. Temperature and color comparisons with an uninvolved area are helpful. (See

Figure 15–4, page 224.) Metabolic acidosis occurs as cellular energy sources are rapidly depleted. This may progress until capillary permeability increases, allowing edema in the soft tissue. The result is an edematous, cool and pale extremity, with poor capillary refill in the nailbeds.

The patient will experience some degree of pain as the result of a fracture and ensuing muscle spasm. Careful questioning by the nurse may better describe the quality and location of the pain. At first, the pain of anoxia is burning in nature, progressing to a deep throbbing sensation. Pain produced when the nurse passively extends the fingers or toes of the injured extremity is a reliable sign of early ischemia.

Motor paralysis can accompany or follow loss of sensory modalities, which include touch, proprioception and temperature. In testing for nerve involvement due to ischemia, it is important to remember that loss of deep pain sensory fibers, causing numbness, begins distally, with the insensitive area having a glove- or stocking-like distribution. Unlike singular nerve involvement caused by sharp transection or blunt trauma, nerve damage due to ischemia does not correspond to normal anatomical patterns of nerve supply.

Findings indicative of ischemic tissue constitute a true emergency situation.

Immobilizing injured parts

Once assessment has been completed and the patient's condition is stable, preparation should be made for x-ray studies. The injured part should be properly immobilized, if not already so, to minimize discomfort and prevent any undue motion at the fracture site.

In many instances, the victim will arrive at the emergency department with a splint in place. The type of splint may vary from several thicknesses of newspaper, to light wood, to the inflatable plastic variety (Figure 25–2), to more sophisticated types such as the Keller-Blake or Hare traction or Thomas ring-traction splint. While these splints may limit the extent of assessment of the injured part,

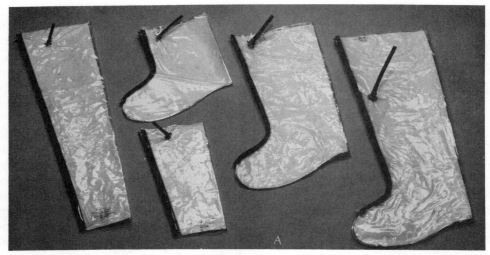

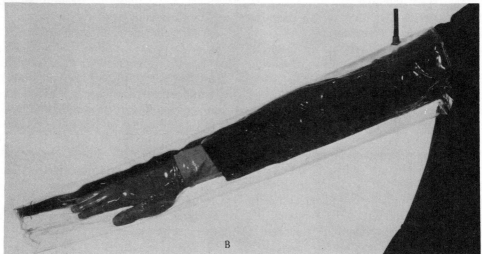

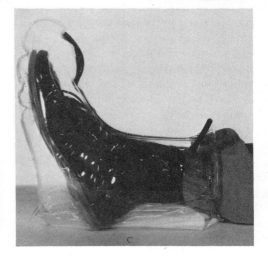

Figure 25–2 Various splints used on ambulances. A: Several sizes of plastic "air" splints. B: An air splint in place on an arm. C: An air splint in place on an ankle. Note that the splint fits over the shoe. (For illustrations of supportive and traction devices used on ambulances, see also Figure 24–8.)

it is generally preferable to leave the splint in place, providing it has been properly applied. When necessary, the splint should be removed by a physician.

Proper splinting includes the joint above and below the suspected fracture site. Most splints are held in place by circumferential wrappings. The injured limb should be evaluated to ascertain that circulation is not impaired by too tightly applied dressings. Inflatable plastic splints are commonly used by ambulance crews to immobilize an injured extremity. They are usually inflated by mouth and rarely is pressure sufficient to damage the limb. When properly inflated, the surface of the air splint should dent under the pressure

of the thumb. If this is not the case, the splint may be partially deflated until the desired pressure is attained.

If a splinting device has not been applied prior to entry into the hospital, some form of immobilization is indicated. The type used will vary from one hospital to another; it may be a padded board, a wire ladder splint, a metal gutter-type splint or one of other options (see Figure 25–3). In upper extremity fractures, the limb may be immobilized with a chest swathe arrangement, while in suspected lower limb fractures, especially of the femur, the legs may be bound together with pillows between the knees.

Removal of a splinting device is not re-

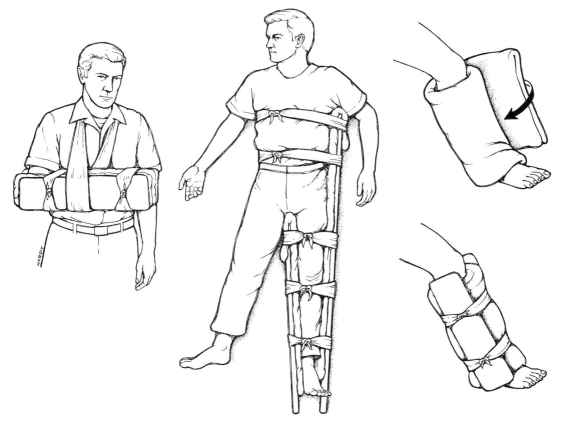

Figure 25–3 Splinting techniques using padded boards and circular conforming gauze bandage. Patients with a suspected forearm fracture should be immobilized using splints and a simple sling. A lower extremity may be immobilized using longer padded-board splints and circular conforming gauze. The ankle can be splinted by wrapping it in a towel (to keep pressure off bony prominences) and using supporting, lightly padded splints exteriorly, maintained in position by circumferential conforming gauze.

quired for routine x-ray studies and should not be done without a physician's order. Indications to remove a splint include evidence of improper application, signs of vascular impairment caused by the splint, initial x-ray studies negative for fracture or dislocation or the need for additional, special x-ray examinations. When a splint is to be removed and a fracture is present, provision should be made for use of other techniques of immobilization. Gentle traction should be applied and the limb carefully removed from the splinting device. This is best done by or under the direct supervision of a physician.

Adjunct studies

The most helpful and frequently used study of a patient with a suspected bone or joint injury is x-ray of the injured part. While multiple views are taken, it is not unusual to find the fracture evident in only one view. Most of the splinting devices in popular use today will allow complete x-ray study without removing the splint. If the patient's condition is tenuous, a nurse or physician should accompany the patient to the x-ray area, once it has been established that the study is necessary.

In patients with obvious injury to a joint area but no x-ray evidence of fracture, a ligamentous injury must be considered. If a major ligament supporting a joint has been completely disrupted, significant false mobility of the joint occurs and can be identified by taking special x-ray views of the part while the suspect ligament is stretched (stress films). This is a painful process for the patient and usually requires local anesthesia.

Other studies will be determined by the seriousness of the injury, the presence of associated trauma or disease and the mode of anticipated treatment. For example, a patient with a Colles' fracture or ankle injury which is to be reduced under local anesthesia in the emergency department is unlikely to need further tests. A patient with a fracture of the forearm requiring internal fixation under general anesthesia will need more thorough

study. When vascular damage is suspected, emergency arteriography is helpful in localizing the site and delineating the nature of the injury. Additional studies include complete blood count, urinalysis, electrocardiogram, blood chemistry tests and any other special tests which may be indicated.

Injuries to the extremities

Severity of injury to an extremity varies widely, from a simple, undisplaced fracture to a badly comminuted open fracture, to multiple injuries with the patient in a life-threatening condition. Early management of lesser injuries is directed toward immobilization of the affected part, to minimize discomfort and prevent complications until definitive treatment is given.

In patients with more serious or life-threatening injuries, attention is directed to established principles of care, based on known priorities. These include: (1) airway maintenance, (2) control of hemorrhage, (3) management of shock, (4) evaluation of neurological or vascular complications and (5) immobilization of the fractures. Then, attention must be given to *every* injury, lest one which is seemingly minor later prove to be a major source of disability.

Airway maintenance has been discussed in detail in Chapter 13.

Control of hemorrhage in the presence of a fracture may be difficult. In closed fractures of the long bones, such as the femur, or in fractures of the pelvis, significant blood loss can occur into adjacent tissues but exhibit few clinical signs except tachycardia and hypotension. It is impossible to initiate any measures aimed at control of the hemorrhage, since this is usually limited by the confines of the anatomical tissue compartment affected by the injury.

With open fractures, however, extensive blood loss may occur if a major vessel has been damaged. In this circumstance, control of bleeding is often difficult because of instability at the fracture site. The best initial treatment method is application of direct pressure to the bleeding wound. After cleansing the skin about the wound, sterile dressings are applied with an outer circumferential elastic dressing. No effort should be made to replace protruding bone ends beneath the skin. If the bleeding continues uncontrolled, a tourniquet may be used, following principles outlined in Chapter 15. Uncontrolled bleeding in association with a fracture is uncommon in the absence of major vessel injury.

Hypovolemic shock may develop following major blood loss. Replacement of circulating blood volume is often not directed toward restoration of the total lost volume; increase in blood pressure to near-normal levels could cause further hemorrhage. Maintenance of the patient's systolic blood pressure at approximately 90 mm. Hg is considered adequate to maintain urinary output until the hemorrhage can be surgically controlled. In patients normally hypertensive, adjustments must be made according to clinical signs and symptoms. Initially, circulating volume may be replaced with Ringer's lactate until type-specific whole blood is available.

While it is common for a patient to complain of pain at the fracture site, pain distal to the level of injury is uncommon, unless the blood and/or nerve supply is compromised. Comparison with the opposite, uninjured limb is helpful in confirming this diagnosis. Neurological damage may be contusion or partial or complete transection of a nerve. Physician assessment is needed to determine the extent of injury. Contusions of a nerve are usually managed by watchful waiting, while transection of a nerve may require surgical repair at the time of reduction of the fracture.

Basically, management of vascular injury is similar to that for neurological damage. Any suspicion of impaired blood flow into an injured limb mandates full assessment of the problem, including angiography. In some patients, the vessel may be trapped or angulated by bone ends at the fracture site. Proper reduction of the fracture may alleviate the problem. Transection of a major artery requires immediate surgical attention.

Amputation

Perhaps the most severe degree of soft tissue injury and bone involvement is exemplified by amputation, whether it be of a single digit or of a major portion of an extremity. Controversy still continues as to the advisability of replantation, primarily because of the long rehabilitation period, including several stages of operative procedures, and the often uncertain results. The fact remains that occasionally patients are brought to the emergency department, and the amputated part is brought with them, wrapped in anything from a clean sheet to an oily mechanic's rag.

While it is not the responsibility of the nurse to decide about replantation, the nurse does have the responsibility of preserving the integrity of the amputated part and the remainder of the extremity. The amputated part should be placed in sterile normal saline or Ringer's lactate solution, iced, if possible. Preservation of larger parts, such as an arm, can be accomplished by placing the amputated part in a large, sterile plastic bag containing the solution.

Generally, the sooner after injury the surgery can be completed, the greater the chance of survival of the limb. Maximum elapse of time has not been established, but studies indicate that when replantation has been completed within 4 to 6 hours from injury, better results are obtained.

Pain

The management of pain caused by a fracture or related soft tissue injury should be individualized. It depends on the type of fracture, the size and age of the patient, any accompanying trauma or complications, anticipated definitive treatment and the final disposition of the patient. To a great extent, pain is caused by muscle spasm; therefore, positioning the patient to reduce movement of the affected area can do much to increase comfort.

The patient with a fracture of the femoral neck or intertrochanteric region should be supported by pillows under the thigh and the lateral aspect of the leg; this reduces muscle fatigue from attempts to hold the limb, already externally rotated, in a position of least tension and pain. Individuals with fractures in this location will also tend to have their buttocks squeezed together, much as does an individual anticipating a gluteal injection. Moving the unaffected buttock slightly outward (laterally) will help relieve the tensed position. Attention to the shoulder area will assist in identifying malalignment. With fractures of the pelvis and/or lower extremities, leverage involved in voluntary movement of the upper part of the body is diminished. Assistance should be offered to the patient to move his torso a few inches to one side or the other.

Edema, occurring at the fracture site, adds to discomfort, as nerve endings are further stimulated. Applications of covered ice bags or packs during the first hours after fracture will lessen the rate of swelling and increase comfort. Unfortunately, there are patients whose fractures have occurred more than 12 to 24 hours prior to evaluation in the emergency department. Application of ice is of little value at this point. Positioning the affected part so it is at or above the level of the heart will assist in improving venous return, hopefully with reduction of local congestion. In patients with multiple injuries, positioning all affected areas to the best advantage is difficult.

Administration of analgesics should be a very selective process. The temptation is to relieve the patient's discomfort immediately with medication rather than with nursing measures. When shock is present, absorption of intramuscular analgesics is impeded and of little immediate value to the patient. Repeated administration of analgesics is also a potential hazard to the resolution of the shock. When sedation or analgesia is necessary, reduced amounts should be administered intravenously over a period of several minutes and timed to have maximum effect during a particular procedure, such as a closed reduction or manipulation of a dislocation. Local anesthesia may be used in the latter situation to afford maximum comfort.

EMERGENCY CARE OF SPECIFIC INJURIES

The upper extremities

In order to avoid confusion, management of fractures and dislocations of extremities will be considered for isolated injuries.

Fracture of the clavicle

The clavicle is one of the most commonly fractured bones, constituting between 5 and 10 percent of all fractures. The victim will usually give a history of a fall or blow to the shoulder area and subsequent pain and swelling in the region of the clavicle. On examination, swelling and deformity may be noted, and tenderness can be elicited on palpation of the fracture site.

It should be remembered that in children particularly, incomplete fracture of the clavicle may be present although swelling is minimal. The child may be very irritable. Careful palpation of the clavicle will reveal localized tenderness at the area of injury. Typically, the patient will support the affected limb with the opposite.

Following x-ray studies (Figures 25–4 and 25–5), the management of the fracture involves application of a figure-8 dressing. Figure-8 dressings are available commercially and should be applied carefully, with the patient sitting upright on an examining table and the shoulders in the "position of attention" (shoulders squared, chest out). Liberal amounts of powder or cornstarch should be placed in each axilla to prevent irritation of the skin from perspiration or rubbing.

The major vessels of the limb, the subclavian and axillary arteries, lie in close proximity to the middle third of the clavicle. Careful evaluation of distal pulses is neces-

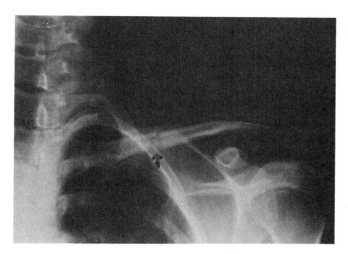

Figure 25–4 Simple fracture of the clavicle. (See arrow for fracture.) Fragments were stable and in good position in a 30-year-old female. She was treated by sling only, with good results.

sary, as well as observation for any significant hematoma of the supraclavicular area which might indicate vascular damage. Rarely is internal fixation necessary.

Acromioclavicular separation

Separation of the shoulder is a ligamentous injury at the lateral aspect of the shoulder which usually occurs from the force of a fall directly on the "point" of the shoulder. The patient will complain of pain and deformity over the point of the shoulder at the lateral end of the clavicle. Physical examination will reveal what appears to be a sagging of the injured shoulder with the clavicle appearing to ride higher, tenting the skin. Careful palpation over the distal end of the clavicle will elicit tenderness.

To establish diagnosis by x-ray a special technique involves the patient being examined in the upright position, holding weights in each hand. Due to damage to the structures supporting the joint on the injured side, there will be a widening of the acromioclavicular joint.

Management of this injury depends on the severity of ligamentous damage and the individual involved. In lesser injuries, taping of the part and application of a sling is all that is required. In more extensive injuries, internal fixation may be necessary.

Anterior dislocation of the shoulder

The shoulder is the joint most commonly injured by dislocation, accounting for 50 percent of all dislocations. It is a serious injury, in which the head of the humerus is displaced from the shallow articulating surface of the scapula and is associated with a tear in the joint capsule. The humeral head may be dislocated into a number of positions, anterior, inferior or posterior, in relation to the glenoid fossa of the scapula.

The usual mechanism of shoulder dislocation is a fall on the outstretched (abducted) arm, resulting in severe pain and inability to use the shoulder. The patient ordinarily presents holding the injured limb with its opposite. Any attempt to move the involved shoulder will cause considerable pain. Physical assessment will reveal a bulge over the anterior aspect of the shoulder, if the patient is thin enough, and a depression below the point of the shoulder. The patient will usually refuse the use of a sling and be reluctant to let go of his arm for fear of increasing the pain.

Once the diagnosis has been established, reduction should be carried out. If the patient is seen within a relatively short time after injury, muscle spasm may not be a problem, so that reduction can be achieved easily using a minimum of analgesia. Diazepam

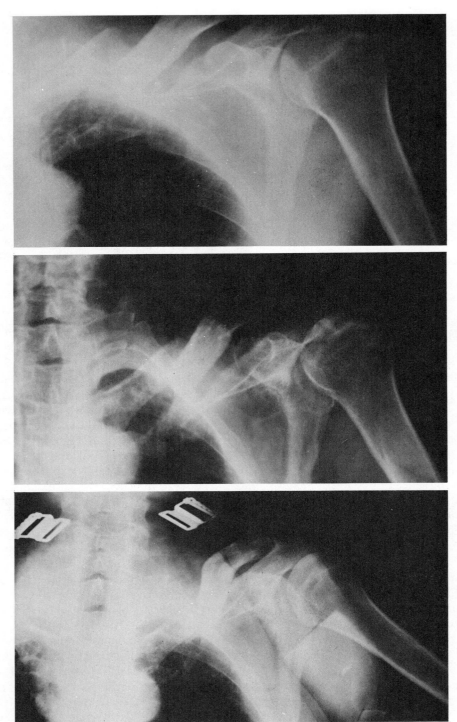

Figure 25–5 Progress of a displaced, fractured clavicle. Top: Severe displaced fracture, left clavicle, middle third. Center: Partial reduction with figure-8 dressing. Bottom: Failure to heal 3 months later. Note marked osteoporosis of disuse. Patient symptomatic, later treated by resection of medial half of clavicle, with good results.

(Valium), meperidine (Demerol) or morphine, given in appropriate doses intravenously, may be used. If the dislocation occurred many hours previously and muscle spasm is significant, general anesthesia is often necessary to reduce the dislocation.

In some patients, this injury will recur on numerous occasions, related to permanent stretching of the muscular and ligamentous structures about the shoulder joint. With each recurrence, there may also be damage to the articulating surfaces of the involved bones. In persons with recurrent dislocations, surgery may be necessary as an elective procedure, to shorten the damaged periarticular structure.

In instances where the dislocation is not confirmed by x-ray, and thus reduction is unnecessary, ligamentous damage is a likely sequela. In such a patient, immobilization of the arm in a sling at the side for at least 3 weeks is advisable, to insure sufficient ligamentous healing.

Fractures about the shoulder

Shoulder fractures usually occur as a result of falls. The victim, usually elderly, will have fallen on the outstretched hand or arm and will present complaining of pain or inability to move the shoulder. Often, such persons are not seen until several days after injury. The degree of swelling will vary but is usually present about the area of the shoulder, and in instances where the injury occurred several days previously, the swelling and ecchymosis may extend to the region of the elbow.

Most shoulder fractures involve the neck of the humerus. Careful palpation will elicit tenderness in the upper third of the arm, and x-rays will confirm the diagnosis. The fragments may be impacted or displaced. Management usually consists of application of a sling and analgesics. These patients must be observed closely and have physical therapy instituted early, to encourage active motion and prevent a "frozen" shoulder resulting from shortening and scarring of the periarticular structures.

Fracture of the shaft of the humerus

A fall or direct blow to the arm, with subsequent pain and deformity in the mid-portion of the upper limb often results in fracture of the shaft of the humerus. Assessment will reveal swelling, tenderness and false motion at the humeral area. A grating sensation may be elicited at the fracture site.

The radial artery and nerve lie in close proximity to the middle third of the humeral shaft; thus, vascular and neurological integrity must be evaluated before any care is provided. The radial pulse at the wrist should be palpated. The radial nerve can be evaluated by asking the patient to dorsiflex the wrist, and sensation may be tested on the dorsum of the hand, in the area of supply of the radial nerve. Radial nerve injury must be considered in the presence of "wrist drop" and inability to actively dorsiflex the wrist.

The patient may require a sling and swathe, which will fix the arm to the side by means of a circumferential dressing around the chest. Following x-ray confirmation of the diagnosis (Figure 25–6), management may consist of either application of a cast or open reduction and internal fixation of the fracture fragments.

Fractures of the distal end of the shaft and the supracondylar area of the humerus, just above the elbow joint, are much more serious than those involving the shaft; vascular and/or nerve damage is not uncommon in such fractures. Further, the injury will frequently involve the joint surfaces, which constitutes a major complication. Joint injury usually occurs as a result of a fall on the arm or elbow. More often than not, internal fixation is necessary.

Fractures of the forearm and wrist

Falls on the outstretched hand may cause injury to the wrist area, fracture of the navicular or radius and ulnar styloid just above

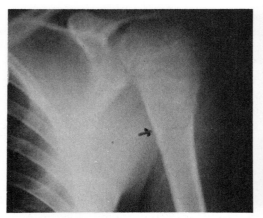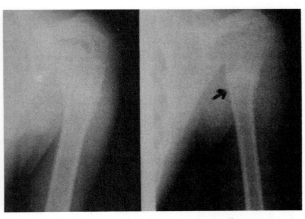

Figure 25–6 Simple fracture of the humerus. Left: Simple fracture of upper shaft of the left humerus on a 15-year-old male. Fracture was stable; treated with sling and swathe. Right: Good callus formation and partial healing, 5 weeks later.

the wrist (Colles' fracture, Figure 25–7) or to the mid-forearm or elbow area (fracture of the radial head or the humeral condyles). These are more commonly seen in children. There is a history of falling on the outstretched hand, resulting in pain and deformity. Evaluation will reveal a typical deformity of the forearm just above the wrist, called a "silver-fork deformity." This injury commonly involves both the radius and the ulnar styloid just above the wrist; the degree of deformity varies.

Other fractures about the wrist involve the carpal bones, particularly the navicular, which also results from a fall on the outstretched hand, with subsequent pain and swelling at the wrist. The typical silverfork deformity is not present, however. Careful evaluation of these patients will usually reveal local tenderness at the fracture site. In instances of suspected navicular fracture, pressure may be exerted against the tip of the extended thumb. By pushing this tip of the thumb toward the wrist area, compression of the fracture fragments will occur, and pain can be elicited.

These patients frequently have considerable pain, and a simple padded wooden splint should be applied before x-ray studies. If the films reveal no fracture of the radius or ulna, special studies of the navicular bone

should be ordered. Magnified views may be necessary to localize the site of fracture. In some patients, particularly the young, the fracture line may not be visible immediately after injury. In such instances, the patient should be advised that no fracture can be identified at that time; however, the injury should be managed as a fracture by immobilizing the part, and repeat x-ray studies should be done in approximately 10 days. At that time resorption of the bone at the site of fracture can clarify the clinical diagnosis.

Fractures of both bones of the forearm are invariably displaced and unstable. The position and degree of displacement will vary with the level of the fracture and the resultant muscle pull on the fragments, particularly the proximal fragments. This injury is severe. Closed reduction may be attempted; however, if the fragments are not able to be maintained in satisfactory alignment, open reduction and internal fixation is required. (See Figure 25–8.)

On the other hand, greenstick fractures of the mid-portion of the radius and ulna are quite stable. This injury is most common in children. During the time the patient is awaiting x-ray studies, application of a splint may add to the patient's discomfort; therefore, in this instance, a simple sling might be applied

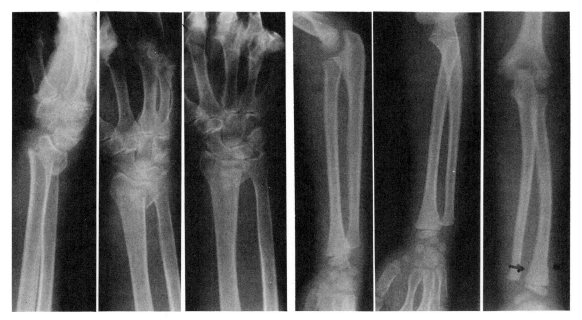

Figure 25-7 Wrist fractures. Left: Typical Colles' fracture of the right wrist, involving the distal radius and ulnar styloid. The distal fragment of the radius is displaced dorsally, producing the so-called "silverfork" deformity at the wrist. Right: Torus fracture of the left wrist of a 5-year-old girl who fell on her outstretched hand 3 days earlier. Note irregularity of the radius (arrow).

to immobilize the limb until the x-rays are initiated.

Fractures of the hand

Fractures of the hand are very commonly seen in the emergency department and probably represent the most common type of open injury to bones and joints. Such injuries usually occur as a result of a direct blow or fall and may represent a very complicated injury, particularly when due to an industrial accident. Assessment will reveal varying bone deformities as a result of muscle pull. Any angulation of metacarpals or phalanges may be quite marked, and motion of the hand or fingers may be painful or limited.

Fracture of the head of the fifth metacarpal is typically incurred by an individual striking his fist against a solid object. (See Figure 25-9.) Usually the patient will relate a history of being involved in an altercation, in which he swung at an opponent, missed and hit a wall. The distal fragment is typically dis-

placed into the palm. Careful examination will reveal the knuckle area to be swollen, and on palpation the bony projection of the involved knuckle, usually the fifth, will not be felt.

Another common injury to the fingers involves the terminal phalanx. The patient will give a history of having been struck on the end of the finger by a ball, with resultant pain and inability to extend the deformed phalangeal joint. The tip of the finger will be in a position of flexion with moderate swelling and tenderness noted on the dorsum of the joint. X-ray studies will reveal a small bone fragment torn away from the dorsal surface of the terminal phalanx. This is a typical example of an avulsion fracture, in which the extensor tendon has remained intact and the site of attachment to the bone has torn away.

After the diagnosis has been confirmed by x-ray, management can proceed in several ways. The most common and conservative method is splinting the finger. It must be

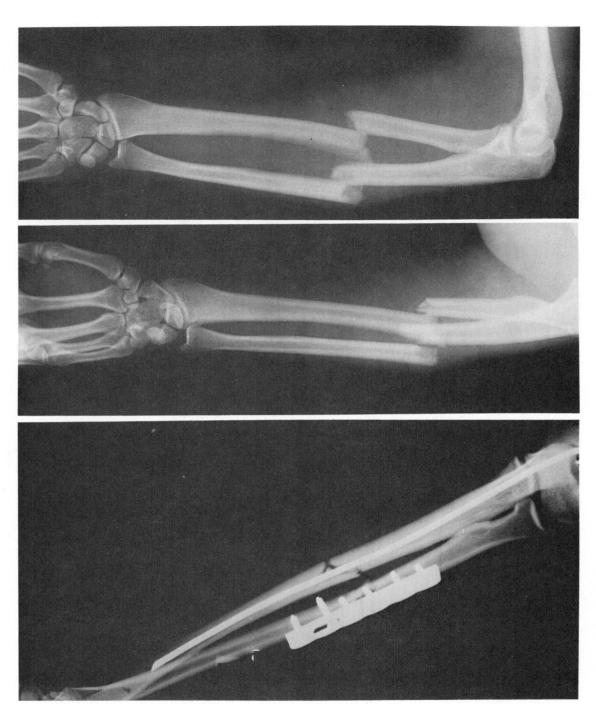

Figure 25–8 Displaced fractures of the forearm. Top: Displaced fractures of both bones of the fore-arm. Position of the fragments is the result of muscle tension in the forearm, causing displacement and overriding of the bone ends (shortening). Bottom: Treatment by open reduction and internal fixation, seen by postoperative x-ray, shows good position of the fragments. The radius was fixed with a side plate and screws, the ulna by means of an intramedullary pin.

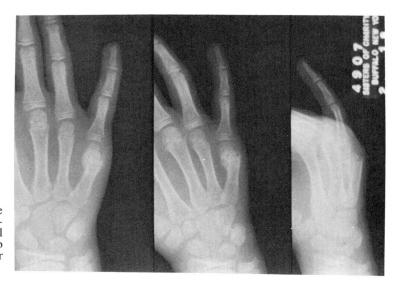

Figure 25–9 Fracture in the hand. Typical displaced fracture of the right fifth metacarpal is seen. (Note displacement into palm.) It was reduced under local anesthesia.

remembered, in treating hand fractures, that they can result in serious disability. Although they may appear minor, adherence to the general principles of fracture management is vital in such injuries.

The lower extremities

Fractures of the pelvis

Fractures of the pelvis rank very high as a cause of death after auto accidents.[21] Damage to the bladder, urethra and, in women, to the uterus are frequent. Trauma to the sigmoid colon and rectum occurs less frequently.[14] Hemorrhage is the most serious complication. One must remember that every cough, sneeze or movement can cause the unstabilized parts to shift, promoting further bleeding. Placing a draw sheet under the patient and using it as a pelvic sling can greatly reduce the hazards of moving. A Hoyer lift, using the seat part of a canvas chair, will facilitate moving the patient from the examining table to a bed. Personnel can then be freed to support the upper torso and legs.

The most common fracture of the pelvis is that of one pubic ramus. Bilateral fractures of the rami have a high incidence of related injuries. They are most dangerous because of associated abdominal injuries, and they tend to cause local and, at times, severe hemorrhage into the extraperitoneal space. The nurse should be alert for complaints of abdominal and back pain accompanied by signs of hypovolemic shock, signifying such hemorrhage. Severe ileus has been noted with fractures of the crest, or wing, of the ileum. Absent or diminished bowel sounds and vomiting should prompt the nurse to institute nasogastric suction.

Nursing care should include catheterization of the patient, to ascertain the presence or absence of urinary problems. If grossly bloody urine is viewed, a cystogram is indicated, to rule out bladder damage.

Fractures of the hip

Fracture of the hip involves the upper portion of the femur, usually in the trochanteric area, or the region of the femoral neck. It is a fairly common injury in the elderly. The usual history is that of an elderly person slipping at home or on the street, followed by severe pain in the hip area. In most instances, hip fracture victims are unable to bear weight following injury, but in the incomplete or impacted fracture, the patient may be able to bear weight, although with considerable pain. It is not unusual for the victim to remain in bed for several days after injury before presenting to the emergency department.

Pertinent physical findings are quite characteristic and reveal the injured extremity to be shortened, with the foot in external rotation. There is usually tenderness on palpation about the affected hip.

The patient is preferably examined on the ambulance stretcher prior to removal to the examining table. If the patient is in severe pain, some traction may be applied to the affected extremity by pulling on the ankle. It is rarely necessary to change the rotation of the foot at this time. With the traction being maintained on the leg, the patient may then be lifted on to the examining table by a lift team. Positioning as outlined in femur pain management is helpful.

Appropriate assessment should be carried out and x-rays ordered (Figure 25–10). It is important that both anteroposterior and lateral x-rays of the hip be taken to confirm

the diagnosis. These patients require admission, operative reduction and internal fixation. Because most are in the older age group, there is a high incidence of associated disease, particularly processes involving the cardiovascular system. The operative procedure is rarely of such an urgent nature that complete preoperative evaluation cannot be carried out. There may be a significant amount of blood loss into the area of fracture, so that blood should be drawn for type and crossmatch. Electrocardiogram and chest x-ray are also indicated.

In some instances, Buck's skin traction is used to maintain limb immobility and provide some measure of comfort for the patient. This type of traction can cause skin necrosis and complicate the postoperative care, however, and proper skin preparation is important.

Dislocation of the hip

Dislocation of the hip is a serious injury which has become more common as the incidence of automobile accidents has increased. A frequent mechanism is the sudden deceleration and the patient striking his knee on the dashboard. In the sitting position, as in a car, the hip is flexed, and if the blow is severe enough, the head of the femur can be displaced from the acetabulum. In conjunction with this injury, a contusion or fracture of the patella may also be present. The patient will complain of severe pain in the hip and inability to fully extend the hip and knee.

The findings and assessment are quite characteristic. The patient is usually apprehensive, with complaints of pain in the hip area. The characteristic position is that of the hip flexed and adducted, so that the knee is toward the mid-line. The finding is in sharp contrast to a fracture of the hip or femur, in which the hip or leg is usually in external rotation rather than adduction. The patient is unable to move from this position voluntarily, and any attempt to straighten the limb causes extreme pain.

X-ray studies will reveal the dislocation,

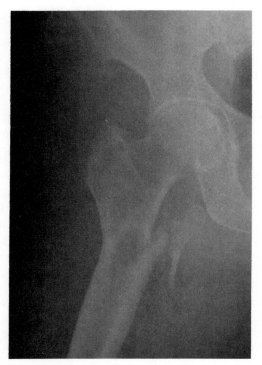

Figure 25–10 Subtochanteric fracture of the femur. This fracture required internal fixation.

which may assume a number of positions. If there is no associated fracture about the hip joint, operative reduction can be carried out. These patients are usually admitted to the hospital for reduction under general or spinal anesthesia.

Hip dislocation victims must be monitored for a considerable period of time post-injury, since there is a significant incidence of avascular necrosis of the head of the femur as a result of this injury. The blood supply to the head and neck of the femur is derived from 3 sources. Two of these sources, the ligamentum teres and the capsule, may be seriously damaged or disrupted as a result of the injury. There is no way in which the outcome can be successfully predicted.

Fracture of the femur

Of all of the extremity fractures, a fracture of the femur is by far the most important to recognize and manage properly. Although it was stated earlier that fractures of the extremities are generally not life-threatening and have a low priority of care in a multiple-injury patient, a fracture of the shaft of the femur in an adult can be serious, for it is usually associated with blood loss of between 1,000 and 1,500 ml. (see Figure 25–11). This loss occurs into the soft tissue structures about the fracture site and is accompanied by massive swelling of the thigh, although it may be quite difficult to estimate the amount of blood lost. The blood loss that occurs can be severe enough to produce severe hypovolemic shock, with no evidence of an external wound. In addition, the neurovascular structures lie in close proximity to the shaft of the femur and may be injured by a fracture.

The mechanism of injury is usually a violent incident. The patient will note severe pain, deformity and inability to bear weight

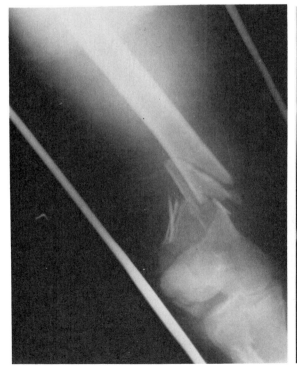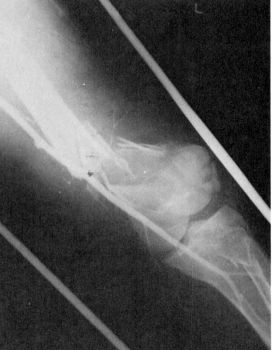

Figure 25–11 Severely comminuted fracture of the femur. Patient was struck by an auto. The injured leg was swollen, cold and pale, indicative of vascular injury. Arteriogram in emergency department x-ray revealed the intact vessel (photo at right).

on the extremity. Angulation of the fragments results from a pull of the large thigh muscles which attach along the length of the femur.

Frequently when a femur fracture victim is brought in by ambulance, a traction splint has already been applied by the trained ambulance attendant. This should be left in place while the patient is evaluated in the emergency department. Rapid but thorough physical assessment should be carried out, with recording of vital signs and complete examination of the injured extremity, including assessment for distal pulses, intact sensation and motor power of the toes.

A large-bore catheter or needle should be inserted into an appropriate vein, particularly one in the upper extremity or the opposite uninjured limb, to draw blood for complete blood count, type and crossmatch. Volume replacement should be instituted using Ringer's lactate. After the patient's vital signs have been stabilized and the limb is completely mobilized and following assessment, the patient may be transferred to the x-ray department for study.

Further management of this injury depends on the exact type of fracture. If the fracture is of the spiral or transverse type without significant comminution, some type of internal fixation, such as the use of an intramedullary rod, is the usual treatment. If, on the other hand, there is considerable fragmentation at the fracture site, the injury is perhaps better handled by the use of balanced traction, using a Steinman pin or Kirschner wire. These devices are inserted under local anesthesia through the femoral condyles or the tibial tubercle and attached to a traction device integrating the principles of a Thomas splint and a Bradford frame.

Fracture and dislocation of the knee

Dislocation of the knee typically follows a violent accident: a direct blow, a fall or torsional injury involving the knee joint.

Torsional injury to the knee, resulting in damage to both ligamentous and bony structures, is rather common. Following the episode, the patient will note severe pain,

swelling and varying degrees of deformity about the knee. Full assessment of the extremity should be done, including evaluation of both the neurological and vascular status; the popliteal artery and veins and the sciatic nerve are in close proximity to the posterior aspect of the knee joint, in the popliteal space.

Following assessment, the limb should be immobilized in a well-padded gutter splint, for transport to the x-ray department. When the limb is being moved to apply the splint, continuous traction should be applied to reduce discomfort. If there is rather marked deformity and angulation or rotation at the knee, it may be difficult, if not impossible, to straighten the joint. It is best in this instance to transport the patient without use of an external splint, using sandbags to provide immobilization.

After the diagnosis has been established, the patient will invariably require admission for surgical reduction.

Fractures of the patella are rather common and usually result from a fall with the patient landing on the knee. The patella is anatomically located within the quadriceps tendon overlying the anterior aspect of the knee joint. Injuries to the patella may thus involve varying degrees of damage to the patellar tendon, from tear to complete rupture. The fracture itself may assume a variety of shapes, from a simple transverse type to a comminuted variety with multiple fragments.

Following injury, the patient complains of pain and difficulty in walking or total inability to walk. Assessment will reveal swelling and tenderness about the patellar region. The patient should be asked to actively flex and extend the knee. This can be done in several ways. Perhaps the best is to have the patient sit on the examining table with the knee flexed and attempt to straighten out the knee. Success in this maneuver proves the integrity of the quadriceps mechanism. X-ray study will usually confirm the diagnosis.

The management of the simple transverse fracture of the patella with an intact quadriceps mechanism is usually obtained by application of a cylinder cast with the knee in full extension. This can be done in the emergency department and the patient sent home and ambulated in this manner. In severely comminuted fractures or those involving injury to the quadriceps mechanism, surgical intervention may be necessary. The usual surgical treatment is to excise the fragments of the patella and repair the damage to the quadriceps tendon.

Fractures of the tibia and fibula

Fractures of the bones of the lower leg occur quite commonly and may occur singly or together. Depending on the mechanism of injury, the fractures may occur at the same or different levels, but, because of the application of the forces involved, the fractures usually occur at the same level. The usual mechanism of injury is direct violence. In indirect violence or torsional injury, the tibia is frequently fractured at the middle and distal third and the fibula in the upper third.

Fractures involving the lower third of these bones are serious, since healing may be impaired. The incidence of non-union is higher in this area than in other portions of the bones. In addition, because of the minimal amount of subcutaneous fat, there is a higher incidence of open fractures in the lower third than in other areas of the tibia.

Physical assessment will reveal obvious deformity with tenderness at the level of the deformity. If the fracture is incomplete or undisplaced, the tenderness will be well localized at the fracture site. The nurse can determine this by carefully palpating along the anterior edge of the tibia, usually referred to as the tibial spine. Ordinarily, this should be a continuous, rather sharp edge. A history of injury combined with any disruption or lack of continuity of the tibial spine is good clinical evidence that a fracture may be present. After examination, the patient should be carefully placed in a gutter type splint and have x-rays taken (Figure 25–12).

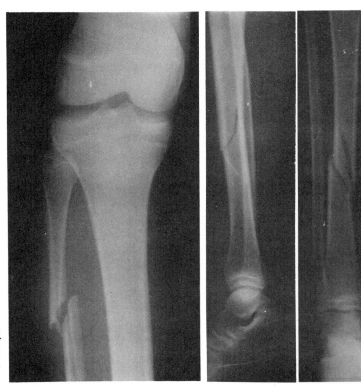

Figure 25–12 Two lower leg fractures. Left: Isolated fracture of the fibula, from a direct blow in football. Right: Isolated fracture of the tibia.

The management thereafter may vary. In incomplete or undisplaced fractures, satisfactory immobilization may be achieved by means of a long leg cast. In displaced, oblique or comminuted fracture where multiple fragments may be involved, an operative approach may be required to maintain the fragments in satisfactory position.

Fractures of the ankle

Fractures and dislocation about the ankle are rather commonly seen in adults but quite uncommon in children. The usual history is that of indirect violence; for example, the patient slips, and severe rotational forces are exerted on the ankle. A common cause of injury is stepping into a hole or walking on uneven surfaces. Following injury, the patient will complain of pain, swelling and difficulty in bearing weight on the injured limb.

Physical assessment will reveal swelling and deformity about the ankle site. Careful palpation of the medial and lateral malleoli should be carried out, and the nurse may actually be able to ascertain the exact site of fracture. In addition, vascular injuries, though rare in this type of fracture, do occur, and the patient should be thoroughly evaluated for dorsalis pedis and posterior tibial pulses. In some instances, severe swelling and pain may not be due to fracture but to a serious ligamentous injury. This should be kept in mind in these patients, particularly when the x-ray studies are negative. Further x-rays may be required, using the "stress" technique.

Management of the fracture will depend on the extent of the injury. Simple, isolated fractures of the medial or lateral malleolus may be treated by application of a short-leg walking cast. If there is significant displacement of the fragments, comminution or serious ligamentous tears, using an operative approach is necessary.

Fractures of the foot and toes

In the foot region, fractures of the heel bones and the tarsal, metatarsal and phalangeal bones are possible.

Fractures of the os calsis (the heel bone) comprise one to 2 percent of all fractures. They result from a fall in which the patient lands on the foot, with varying degrees of injury to the os calsis. Following injury, the patient complains of pain, swelling and difficulty in bearing weight on the heel or in walking at all. Assessment will reveal localized tenderness and swelling, with ecchymoses in the region of the heel and varying degrees of deformity. X-rays will confirm diagnosis (Figure 25–13).

The important point to remember in heel fractures is that the forces which result from landing on the heel are transmitted along the shafts of the long bones of the leg and up into the spine, so that it is not uncommon to have os calsis injury associated with fractures of the dorsal and lumbar vertebrae. Careful assessment must be made of the back in any patient with injury to the os calsis. The vertebral injuries usually occur in the region of the twelfth thoracic and the first or second lumbar vertebrae.

Management varies. At times, when the injury is only to the os calsis, a good supporting shoe may be effective treatment. At times, swelling, deformity and discomfort may be significant enough to warrant admission and operative reduction.

Fractures of the tarsals and metatarsals are relatively common and also result from a fall or direct violence. The patient will invariably complain of pain and inability to bear weight. Pertinent findings include tenderness, swelling and ecchymosis of the foot at the area of injury, with varying degrees of swelling of the forefoot. X-rays will confirm the diagnosis. Management will vary, depending on the degree of injury, from use of a firm shoe to application of a short-leg plaster cast.

Fractures involving the toes are rarely serious, though they may cause considerable discomfort. The usual mechanism of injury is an object dropping on the toes or striking (stubbing) the toe against a rigid object when not wearing shoes. It is not unusual to have

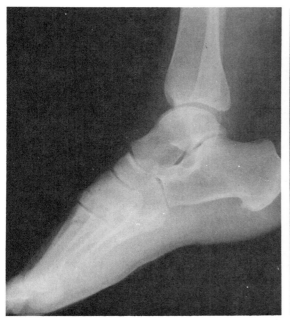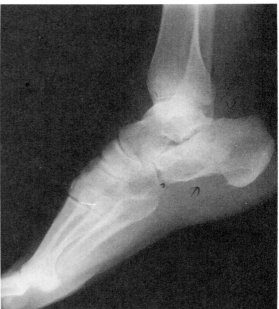

Figure 25–13 The os calcis. Left: Normal os calcis. Right: Fracture of the os calcis, received in a fall from a height.

the patient present for treatment several days after injury because of continued pain, swelling or inability to walk.

The pain is frequently described as severe and throbbing, worse when the foot is dependent and improved with elevation. Particularly after an object falls on the toe, subungual hematoma (bleeding beneath the nail) is common, which may add considerably to the discomfort.

No splinting is necessary initially. Following x-ray to confirm diagnosis (Figure 25–14), the treatment of the fracture will depend on the type of injury. In transverse fractures of the phalanges, the patient may be able to wear a shoe with comfort and bear weight as long as the normal heel and toe walking gait is altered to that of a flat-footed step. In other instances, the pain may be severe enough to require crutches. Fractures of toes other than the great toe can usually be managed by taping the injured toe to an adjacent one by means of circumferential adhesive tape wrapping. A piece of cotton or gauze

should be placed in the web space between the toes, to absorb perspiration and prevent maceration of the skin.

Evacuation of the subungual hematoma, when present, will provide considerable relief to the patient. This may be accomplished by drilling several holes in the nail using size 11 scalpel blade or a hand-operated dental drill. In instances where an entire nail bed is involved, an 11 scalpel blade can be gently inserted beneath the nail at its free edge and the hematoma evacuated. Immobilization of the toe is usually necessary for a period of 3 weeks.

NURSING CARE OF PATIENTS WITH INJURED EXTREMITIES

Nursing responsibilities assume different dimensions once the diagnosis has been established and plans for definitive treatment are outlined. Generally, patients who are to be treated in the hospital are transferred to general care areas, the casting room, operating

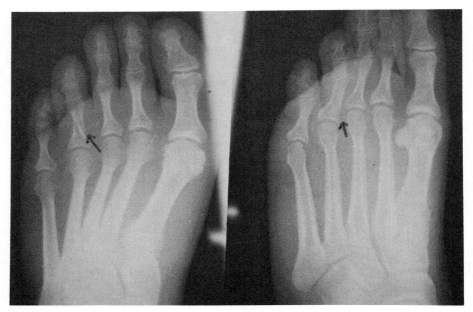

Figure 25–14 Fracture of the proximal phalanx, fourth toe. Patient was shoeless and stubbed toe on a furniture leg. Treated by taping fractured toe to adjacent toe.

rooms or an orthopedic clinic. When closed reduction and immobilization necessitating Kirschner wires or Steinman pins for extremity fractures are required, they may be accomplished under local anesthesia in the emergency department.

Complete, balanced traction, under ordinary circumstances, should not be applied in the emergency department, since transporting the patient with traction and weights in place is difficult. Beds with large traction frames rarely fit through doors. And the weights, once applied, should not be lifted.

Casts

While the principles of cast application remain standard, individual physician preferences for certain materials vary widely. The best nursing approach is to maintain a file or reference notebook recording routinely used procedures and preferences of physicians who frequently use the casting facilities.

Nurse participation in casting procedures may include preparation of the equipment and lending support and traction to the injured part while the plaster dressing is applied. While the physician's attention is directed toward applying the cast, the nurse's attention should be directed toward observing the tolerance of the patient to the procedure. Weakness, faintness and nausea may peak during closed reduction and application of the first rolls of plaster. The patient in a sitting position for cast application is especially likely to become light-headed. Sudden movement, as in the case of nausea and vomiting, could prove disastrous. Rapid consultation with the physician will determine whether casting can continue in another position or if the procedure must temporarily be halted.

Once the cast has been applied, it should be handled carefully, with the palms of the hands. While newer forms of plaster set within minutes, transmission of pressure to underlying skin is still a concern. The patient should be cautioned not to rest the wet cast on hard surfaces, such as wooden chair arms and coffee tables. A period of 24 hours is sufficient drying time for large leg casts, providing humidity is not high and the cast is not covered. The patient can be taught to test for complete seasoning of the cast by listening for a hollow sound when tapped and feeling the cast for moisture.

Cast care

The nurse can play an important role in the education of the patient concerning care of the casted extremity. Far too often, the fracture heals well, but loss of functional movement of a shoulder, hips or fingers results because adequate instruction has not been given the patient concerning range of motion exercises for unaffected joints.

The same signs and symptoms of vascular and neurological impairment previously discussed must be transmitted to the patient at a level commensurate with his understanding. A written list of instructions should be given the patient or his relatives for reference after discharge from the emergency department (see Appendix H). Reliance on verbal instructions is insufficient. Return appointments can be incorporated in the instructional format, depending upon local protocol.

Children have their own ways of destroying casts, many quite ingenious. The boy in a walking cast may discover that his casted leg kicks a soccer ball much better than before. For the smaller child, a lot of fun can be had when sand is put in one end of the cast and allowed to drain out the other. External dirt is of little consequence, however, unless it is moist, like mud. The greater danger lies with children hiding objects in the cast. Unless the child is very young, an understanding of the dangers is possible if presented well by the nurse.

The best allies in removing moisture and odors are an old toothbrush and baking soda. The baking soda can be sprinkled on the wet area, allowed to absorb the moisture and brushed away with the tooth brush. Successive applications will return the cast to a fairly odorless and dry state. A hand soap for removing grease or a nonabrasive cleanser and a toothbrush work well for removal of other stains. Use of some of the powdered, dry spray deodorants has been suggested for odor removal, but their effects are unsatisfactory in terms of removing moisture. Stockinette may be used to cover the cast and keep it clean.

Time must be taken to explain these aspects of cast care before the patient is discharged from the emergency department.

Promoting joint mobility and muscle strength

Active range of motion exercise for muscles and joints proximal and distal to cast length is important for maintaining mobility and strength of the casted extremity. At minimum, these exercises should be done at least twice a day and more frequently for optimal results.

The patient with a long arm cast extending beyond the wrist and elbow, should do active range of motion exercises for the shoulder and all noncasted joints of the hand. The patient with a fracture of the tibia or fibula will have a long leg cast, immobilizing all joints of the extremity except the toes and hip joint. "Wiggling" the toes and range of motion exercises at the hip are necessary. Hip abduction is of particular importance in enabling the patient to resume a normal gait pattern when the cast is removed.

Isometric exercises of muscles in casted extremities are effective in maintaining strength and preventing disuse atrophy. Complete instruction in and faithful adherence to an exercise program will result in a stronger and more functional extremity when the cast is removed.

Local situations will determine how emergency department personnel instruct patients in exercise procedures. If it cannot be accomplished in the emergency department, a referral mechanism for physical therapy is necessary.

Crutch-fitting

Patients with lower extremity injuries will need crutches fitted and instructions given for safe crutchwalking and transfer techniques before leaving the emergency department.

Many emergency departments utilize the hospital's physical therapists to fit crutches and instruct patients in safe crutchwalking procedures. When this is not possible, the emergency nurse should be familiar with the basics of crutch-fitting and physical therapy.

To be capable of walking on standard axillary crutches, a patient should have:

(1) Normal upper extremity muscle power (hand grasp, wrist and elbow extension).
(2) Normal, uninvolved lower extremity muscle power (hip and knee extension, ankle plantar flexion).

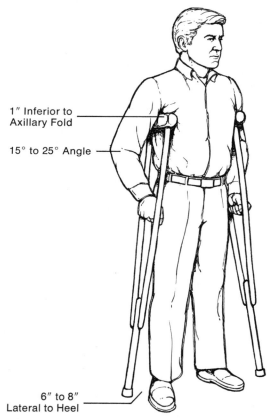

1″ Inferior to Axillary Fold

15° to 25° Angle

6″ to 8″ Lateral to Heel

Figure 25–15 Fitting axillary crutches. Note that the top of the crutch comes to within an inch of the axillary fold, the bottom of the crutch rests 6 to 8 inches to the side of the heel and the elbow is flexed 15 to 25 degrees.

(3) Unimpaired balance and coordination.

Measurement for axillary crutches can be done while the patient is supine, with the upper extremities parallel to the side of the body. Crutches can also be fitted with the patient standing erect. But, for safety, the patient must be supported by another person, a walker or a stationary object during fitting.

Measurement begins one inch inferior to the axillary fold and ends at a point 6 to 8 inches lateral to the inferior aspect of the heel. (See Figure 25–15.) The patient should be measured while wearing the shoe he will use while a crutch walker. The handpiece should be positioned so that the elbow is flexed 15 to 25 degrees, depending on patient comfort.

Crutch tips should be 2 inches in diameter to assure stable crutch positioning during walking. The patient or his family should be instructed to inspect the crutch tips periodically for excessive wear. Padding over the handpiece and axillary bar are not necessary but may be added for patient comfort. The patient must understand that weight must be borne on the hands, *not* in the axillary region.

Crutchwalking and maneuvers

The gait pattern commonly used by patients with lower extremity injury is a 3-point touch, weightbearing or non-weightbearing pattern. "Three-point" designation connotes the 2 crutches and the one uninvolved lower extremity. In this pattern, the affected extremity and both crutches advance simultaneously. Then, with the weight borne on the hands, the unaffected extremity follows through. The patient should advance the uninvolved extremity past the level of crutch placement to maintain a tripod stance for stability at each step.

Prior to practicing walking with the patient, a safety belt should be placed around the patient's waist and tightened snugly. A firm hold on the belt while the patient is practicing crutchwalking provides him with better balance control and with greater leverage should he start to fall.

Learning the gait pattern is only the beginning, for the crutch walker soon learns there are many environmental objects he has to negotiate with crutches, namely, in and out of chairs, up and down stairs and through doors. The patient needs instruction in these frequently overlooked techniques. Figures 25–16, 25–17, 25–18 and 25–19, which follow, graphically depict these techniques. Since instructions in these techniques are time-consuming and require practice, written take-home materials or follow-up physical therapy may be indicated.

From sitting to standing

Figure 25–16 illustrates how the crutch user moves from sitting in a chair to standing.

(1) The patient moves forward to the edge of the chair and places both crutches in the hand on the same side as the affected extremity. The opposite hand is placed on the arm of chair, and the unaffected leg is positioned for standing.
(2) Patient rises to standing by pushing up with unaffected leg. Both arms assist in attaining standing position.
(3) Patient shifts crutches beneath each arm, to the unaffected side first, and proceeds to ambulation.

To sit, the patient backs up to the chair, feels for the chair with the back of the uninvolved leg, and reverses the sequence outlined in the above list. For safety, all "throw rugs" should be removed from the patient's home. If possible, low chairs and soft sofas should be avoided, since these require addi-

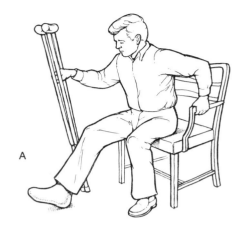

A

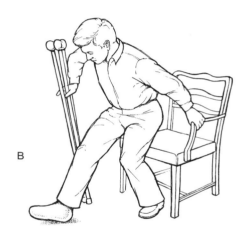

B

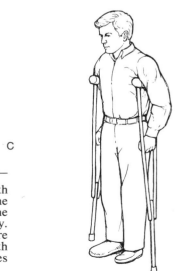

C

Figure 25–16 From sitting to standing with crutches. A: The patient moves forward to the edge of the chair, placing both crutches in the hand on the same side as the affected extremity. The arm and the leg on the unaffected side are readied for standing. B: Patient pushes up with the unaffected leg and both arms. C: The crutches are repositioned for walking.

tional effort and balance to negotiate. The above pattern can also be applied to the transfer in and out of a car.

Ascending stairs

Figure 25–17 illustrates the technique of climbing stairs with crutches.

(1) The patient uses a 3-point crutch gait to ascend stairs by bearing weight on the hands through crutches and steps up with the uninvolved leg.
(2) The patient shifts his weight to the uninvolved leg. Crutches and involved leg move up to the next step.

Descending stairs

Descending stairs is also done in 2 basic steps. Figure 25–18 illustrates.

(1) Crutches and involved leg are lowered to the step below.
(2) The uninvolved leg steps down, as the weight is borne on the hands, through the crutches.

When a railing is available, the patient may switch both crutches to one side and hold the railing on the opposite side. The patient then proceeds to descend as outlined above. (See Figure 25–18C.)

Doorways

Negotiating doorways is another difficult maneuver on crutches. When the door opens toward the patient, he should stand almost perpendicular to traffic pattern flow, grasp the door handle and open the door with the hand opposite the affected leg. (See Figure 25–19A.)

For doors opening away from patient, he stands directly in front of door, grasps the handle and opens door with hand opposite affected leg (Figure 25–19B). To proceed through the door in either case, the patient places one crutch on the floor next to door to keep it open and advances through (Figure 25–19C).

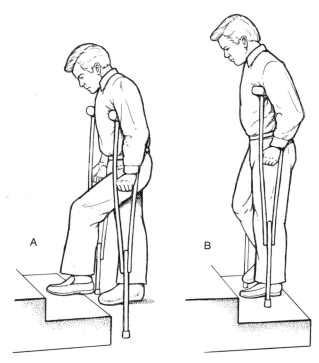

Figure 25–17 Climbing stairs with crutches. A: Using a 3-point crutch gait, the patient bears his weight on his hands through the crutches and steps up with the uninvolved leg. B: The crutches and the involved leg follow.

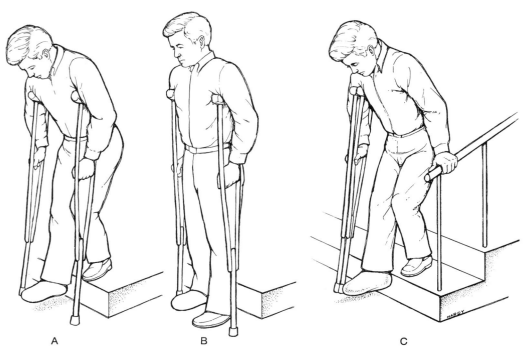

Figure 25–18 Descending stairs with crutches. A: Crutches and the involved leg are lowered to the step below. B: With weight borne on the hands through the crutches, the uninvolved leg steps down. C: When a railing is available, the patient can transfer both crutches to one side, hold the railing on the other side and proceed as outlined in A and B.

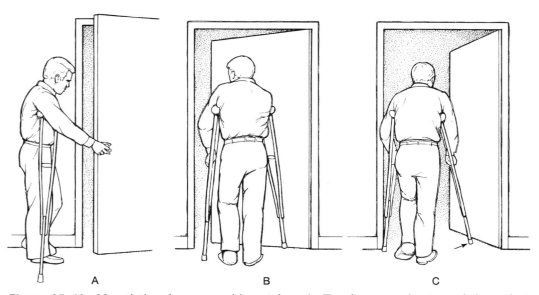

Figure 25–19 Negotiating doorways with crutches. A: For doors opening toward the patient, he should stand almost perpendicular to the traffic flow and open the door with the hand opposite the affected leg. B: For doors opening outward, the patient stands in front of the door, opens it with the hand opposite the affected leg, and proceeds as in "C." C: the patient places one crutch next to the door, thus keeping it open as he advances through the doorway.

SUMMARY

Patients with fractures and soft tissue injuries constitute a large proportion of the patients seen in an emergency department. The importance of assessment of their problems, initiation of diagnostic measures, support during treatment and education for rehabilitation cannot be underestimated, considering that the patient's very life-style depends on mobility and a functional skeletal system.

The emergency nurse plays a crucial role in each of these important steps in assessment and management, especially in insuring patient well-being in the present emergency situation and in future healing and rehabilitation.

BIBLIOGRAPHY

(1) Abraham, E. A.: McMaster, W. C.: Krijger, M., and Waugh, T. R.: "Whirlpool Therapy for the Treatment of Soft Tissue Wounds Complicating Extremity Fractures," *Journal of Trauma,* 14 (1974):222.

(2) Beck, J., and Collins, J.: "Theoretical and Clinical Aspects of Post Traumatic Fat Embolism Syndrome," *in* The American Academy of Orthopedic Surgeons, *Instructional Course Lectures,* 22 (1973):38–87.

(3) Bennett, J. E.; Hayes, J. E., and Robb, C.: "Mutilating Injuries of the Wrist," *Journal of Trauma,* 11 (1971):1008.

(4) Boucher, P. R., and Morton, K. S.: "Rupture of the Distal Biceps Brachii Tendon," *Journal of Trauma,* 7 (1967):626.

(5) Chan, D.; Kraus, J., and Riggins, R.: "Patterns of Multiple Fractures in Accidental Injury," *Journal of Trauma,* 13 (1973):1075.

(6) Connally, J., and Brooks, A.: "Vascular Problems in Orthopedics," *in* The American Academy of Orthopedic Surgeons, *Instructional Course Lectures,* 22 (1973):12–27.

(7) Eversmann, W. W.: "Injuries to the Elbow in Children," *Hospital Medicine,* 10 (1974):29.

(8) Glenn, J., *et al.:* "The Treatment of Fractures in Patients with Head Trauma," *Trauma,* 12 (1973):958.

(9) Grosz, C., *et al.:* "Volkmann's Contracture and Femoral Shaft Fractures," *Trauma,* 12 (December 1973):129–134.

(10) Harris, W. H., and Malt, R. A: "Late Results of Human Limb Replantation: Eleven-Year and Six-Year Follow-up of Two Cases with Description of a New Tendon Transfer," *Journal of Trauma,* 14 (1974):44.

(11) Heck, C. C.: "Sprained Ankle," *New York State Journal of Medicine,* 72 (1972):1620.

(12) Kerr, Avice: *Orthopedic Nursing Procedures,* ed. 2 (New York: Springer Publishing Company, 1969).

(13) Larson, C., and Gould, M.: *Calderwood's Orthopedic Nursing,* ed. 7 (Saint Louis: C. V. Mosby Company, 1970).

(14) Levine, J., and Crampton, R.: "Major Abdominal Injuries Associated with Pelvic Fractures," *Surgery, Gynecology and Obstetrics,* 116 (1963):223.

(15) McLaughlin, H. L., and Parkes, J. C., III: "Fracture of the Carpal Navicular (Scaphoid) Bone: Gradations in Therapy Based upon Pathology," *Journal of Trauma,* 9 (1969):292.

(16) Makin, G. S., and Howard, J. H.: "Arterial Injuries Complicating Fractures or Dislocations: The Necessity for a More Aggressive Approach," *Surgery,* 59 (1966):203.

(17) Markham, D. E.: "Anterior Dislocation of Hip and Diastasis of Contralateral Sacro-iliac Joint: Rear-seat Passenger's Injury," *British Journal of Surgery,* 59 (1972):296.

(18) Mital, M. A., and Patel, U. H.: "Fractures and Dislocations about the Distal Forearm, Wrist and Hand: Progress in Treatment in the Last Decade," *Amer-*

ican Journal of Surgery, 124 (1972): 660.

(19) Nixon, J. F.: "A Simple Sprained Ankle May Not Be So Simple," *Consultant* (1973):175.

(20) O'Donoghue, D. H.: *Treatment of Injuries to Athletes,* ed. 2 (Philadelphia: W. B. Saunders Company, 1970).

(21) Perry, J., and McClellan, R.: "Autopsy Findings in 127 Patients Following Fatal Traffic Accidents," *Surgery, Gynecology and Obstetrics,* 119 (1964):586.

(22) Post, M., and Haskell, S. B.: "Reconstruction of the Median Nerve Following Entrapment in Supracondylar Fracture of the Humerus: A Case Report," *Journal of Trauma,* 14 (1974):252.

(23) Reckling, F. W., and Peltier, L. F.: "Acute Knee Dislocations and Their Complications," *Journal of Trauma,* 9 (1969):181.

(24) Schweigel, J. F., and Gropper, P. T.: "A Comparison of Ambulatory Versus Nonambulatory Care of Femoral Shaft Fractures," *Journal of Trauma,* 14 (1974):474.

(25) Sims, F. H., and Detenbeck, L. C.: "Injuries of the Knee in Athletes," *Minnesota Medicine,* 55 (1972):881.

(26) Singh, I., and Gorman, J. F.: "Vascular Injuries in Closed Fractures Near Junction of Middle and Lower Thirds of the Tibia," *Journal of Trauma,* 12 (1973):592.

(27) Smith, R. F.: "Fracture of Long Bones with Arterial Injury Due to Blunt Trauma," *Archives of Surgery,* 99 (1969):315.

(28) Taylor, A. R.; Arden, G. P., and Rainey, H. A.: "Traumatic Dislocation of the Knee: Report of 43 Cases with Special Regerence to Conservative Management," *Journal of Bone and Joint Surgery,* 54-B (1972):96.

(29) Wholey, M. H., and Bucher, J.: "Angiography in Musculoskeletal Trauma," *Surgery, Gynecology and Obstetrics,* 125 (1967):730.

APPENDIX H

Cast care instructions

You have just had a cast applied as part of the treatment of your injury. Because of the nature of your injury and of the Plaster of Paris used to make your cast, there are certain precautions you should take to prevent serious problems.

(1) Keep the injured limb elevated (propped up) continuously for the next 48 hours. This is to prevent swelling of the limb, and to be effective, your arm (or leg) must be arranged so that your fingers (or toes) are at least 12 inches above your heart.

(2) Rarely, there is sufficient swelling within the cast to interfere with the circulation or nerve supply: *Signs you should look out for are excessive blueness, paleness, numbness (loss of feeling), or coldness of your fingers or toes.* This is a serious condition, and it is absolutely necessary that you return to the hospital at once.

(3) The pain of your injury should subside rapidly. You may have some mild aching, but this should respond to aspirin. If your doctor feels you need stronger medication, he will prescribe it. If the pain medication does not work within 30 to 45 minutes, you should call your doctor for advice.

Source: Orthopedic Service, Emergency Division, Santa Clara Valley Medical Center, San Jose, Ca.

(4) Do not get your cast wet. If you do, it will only fall apart and no longer perform its proper function.

(5) Never, never put anything under your cast. No matter how good it would feel to scratch that itch, you are asking for trouble from infected pressure sores or scratches if you put anything under your cast. If you have trouble with itching, call your doctor. He can prescribe medicine to deal with the problem.

(6) Your cast will be set in a few minutes, but it requires 48 hours to harden completely. If it has a walking heel, *do not walk on it* for 48 hours.

(7) For proper treatment of your injury, you should come to all your appointments on time.

(8) If for any reason you are concerned about your cast or your injury, do not hesitate to call your doctor.

26

Emergencies involving the
ears, nose and throat

JOSEPH C. SERIO

It would be difficult to cover all the acute problems that can arise in the ears, nose and throat in one chapter. Thus, this chapter includes only the problems more commonly seen by emergency department personnel. Although diseases of the ears, nose and throat frequently occur simultaneously, each sensory system will be discussed separately for purposes of clarity.

THE NOSE AND PARANASAL SINUSES

Anatomy and physiology

The nose is roughly divided into 2 parts. The upper part consists of the nasal bones and the frontal process of the maxilla. The lower, larger part consists of the cartilages and their skin and connective tissue coverings. The upper, internal part of the nose is made up of the septum and the turbinates. The bony septum divides the nose into left and right sides. The lower portion is separated into right and left chambers by the columella, which is the lowermost portion of the partition formed by the septal cartilage.

The turbinates number at least 3 on each side: superior, middle and inferior. (See Fig-

ure 26–1.) They are somewhat angulated, forming the meatuses of each of the sinuses draining into the nose. Each meatus is named for the turbinate to which it is related. The "superior meatus" contains the ostia of the posterior ethmoid and sphenoid sinuses. The *middle meatus* drains the frontal, maxillary and anterior ethmoid sinuses. The *inferior meatus* channels the drainage of the naso-lacrimal duct. (See Figure 26–2.) When the sinuses are inflamed or infected, the turbinates may be swollen, edematous and injected. Purulent material may be found in the meatuses.

The blood supply of the nose is derived from branches of the external and internal carotid arteries. The sphenopalatine branch of the external carotid supplies the turbinates, meatuses and septum. The anterior portion of the septum, called Kisselbach's triangle, contains a plexus of blood vessels and is the most frequent site of epistaxis (nosebleed).

The roof of the nose receives its blood supply from the anterior and posterior ethmoidal vessels, which are branches of the ophthalmic artery. These also supply blood

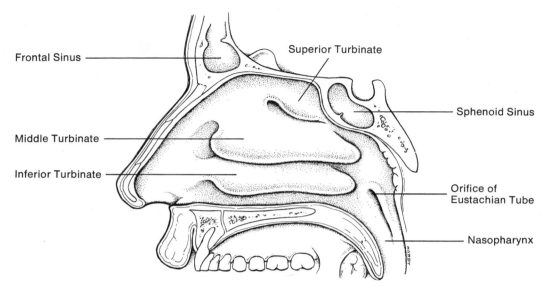

Figure 26–1 Sagittal view of right nares. This illustration shows the turbinates, which cover the meatuses of the paranasal sinuses.

to the ethmoid and frontal sinuses. The maxillary and sphenoid sinuses are served by branches of the internal maxillary artery.

The paranasal sinuses include: (1) the anterior group, consisting of frontal, maxillary and anterior ethmoids and (2) the posterior group, made up of the posterior ethmoid and sphenoid sinuses. Each sinus is named for the bone in which it is found. The bones form a part of the skull and are in contact with other structures, which may account for the symptomatology of sinus disease. For example, the floor of the frontal sinus forms a portion of the roof of the orbit. When the frontal sinus is inflamed, swelling, edema and secondary inflammation of the eye may result.

The maxillary sinus forms a portion of the floor of the orbit and also extends to the apices of the upper teeth, which accounts for symptoms of toothache associated with acute inflammation of this sinus. The ethmoid sinuses occupy the ethmoidal labyrinth. Its lateral border, the lamina papyracea, is part of the inner wall of the orbit, which is very thin. Serious inflammatory processes may perforate the wall of the orbit, causing displacement of the eye and inflammation of the

optic nerve. The roof of the sphenoid sinus is in direct contact with the base of the brain. The roof underlies the optic chiasm and the sella turcica, which contains the pituitary gland. It also lies in close relationship to the cavernous sinus and the internal carotid artery.

The nerve supply of the sinuses arises from the trigeminal (fifth) nerve and from the sphenopalatine ganglion. The latter is of clinical importance, in that it combines with autonomic nerve fibers to form the superficial and deep petrosal nerves. The superficial petrosal is also known as the facial nerve. The deep petrosal is called the vidian nerve. Some rhinologists sever this nerve in the treatment of vasomotor (allergic) rhinitis.

Only the maxillary and ethmoid sinuses are present at birth; the remainder develop during the first 7 years of life. Inflammation of the 2 original sinuses is a frequent cause of fever of undetermined origin in children.

The sinuses are lined by respiratory epithelium, a special form of mucous membrane peculiar to the respiratory tract. It is called "pseudostratified columnar, ciliated epithelium." The cilia are small, hair-like projections

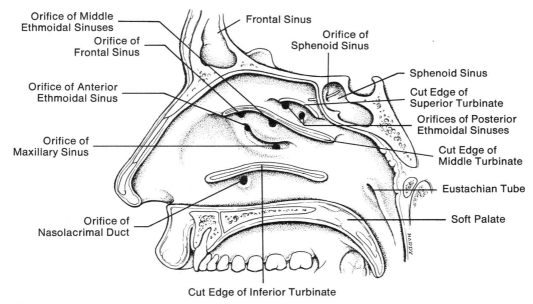

Figure 26–2 Internal anatomy of the nose. This is a sagittal view of the right nares with the turbinates removed. The sinus orifices in each meatus are identified.

in this type of epithelium, which move mucus along the epithelial surface.

The nose has many functions. It is the organ of smell through the olfactory nerve cells. It serves as an air passage and cleans, humidifies and warms the inspired air. The air conditioning process is mediated by the septum and the turbinates, and temperature control and humidification are effected through the nasal mucous membrane. Larger particles within the air are removed by the hairs within the nose, while the mucous blanket of the nose, along with its lysozyme, is bactericidal and thus serves to clean the air. The mucous blanket is moved by the cilia.

Assessment of the nose

History data collection is important. In most patients other than small children, it can be obtained directly from the patient. The most common symptom is discharge from the nose. It may be watery, bloody or purulent in nature. Knowing the duration and onset of symptoms is helpful. The nurse should note any history of nasal obstruction, difficulty in breathing through the nose, frequent colds, headaches or pain and the presence or absence of fever, chills and heavy perspiration. Whether the obstruction is chronic and persistent or only present during the acute episode should also be established. Chronic obstruction, headache or recurrent pain may indicate chronic sinus disease. In traumatic conditions, the mechanism and time of injury is important. In instances of a blow or fall, the area which was struck should be identified.

Examination begins with careful inspection of the external aspect of the nose, observing for any evidence of deformity, recent trauma, swelling, inflammation or tumors. Discharge may be noted at the external nares. In traumatic conditions, dried blood may be visible.

Palpation, particularly when swelling or bleeding is noted after injury, may reveal false motion of the nasal bones. Crepitation (grinding or crunching sound) with nasal fracture may be present.

The interior of the nose should be carefully examined, using a nasal speculum or an oto-

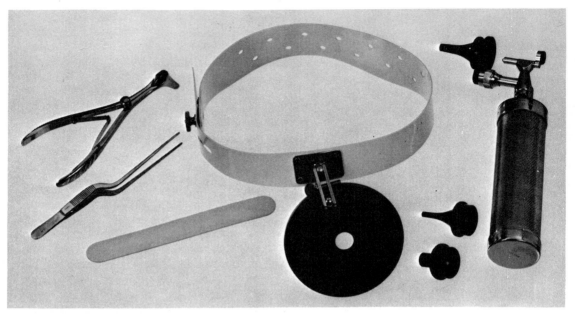

Figure 26–3 Instruments for ear, nose and throat examination. From left to right: nasal speculum, bayonet forceps, tongue blade, head mirror, aural and nasal specula with otoscope.

scope with a nasal piece attached. Figure 26–3 displays equipment used in examinations of the nose, ears and throat. Figure 26–4 illustrates the technique of speculum examination of the nose. Under normal conditions, the septum should be in the mid-line. It should be observed for any spurs or buckling (deviation) to one side, with narrowing of the nasal

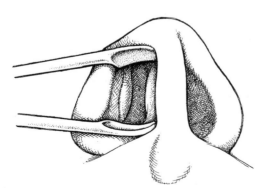

Figure 26–4 Speculum examination of the nose. Middle and inferior turbinates are visualized laterally, the septum medially.

passage as the septum contacts the turbinates. The examiner should check for any drainage in the nasal cavity and whether it is clear, bloody or purulent. The mucous membranes should be pink and moist; edema, swelling, unusual pallor, redness or excessive moisture are pathologic.

The turbinates and associated meatuses should be inspected. Involvement of a turbinate reflects a reaction in the sinus which drains into it. Except for the turbinates, the lining of the nose is smooth. Polyps are frequently found, appearing as grape-like swellings which are usually pale and moist. Irritated areas or frank ulcerations may be noted on the septum.

Transillumination of the paranasal sinuses has limited value in the diagnosis of sinus disease. X-rays are useful in the diagnosis of fractures involving the nasal bones and/or the walls of the paranasal sinuses (see Figure 26–5). Studies of the sinuses are helpful in the diagnosis of sinus disease.

Management of specific diseases of the nose

The common cold

The common cold is due to a virus. It is usually a self-limiting disease that can be associated with a secondary bacterial infection. History includes nasal congestion and stuffiness with sneezing early in the course of the disease and a burning sensation in the mucous membrane. Fever is usually absent unless a secondary infection is present. Malaise and anorexia may be noted.

Examination reveals hyperemia and injection of the mucous membrane, with purulent drainage when bacterial contamination has occurred. Management consists of isolation of the patient and supportive symptomatic care, such as encouraging fluids, rest, aspirin for fever and vitamin C.

Nasal allergy

Allergy must be considered in a patient with a history of frequent head colds associated with a profuse, watery nasal discharge. Sneezing is common. The symptoms frequently have a seasonal occurrence. Assessment will reveal a watery discharge. The mucous membranes are pale and edematous. Polyps may be visible at times.

Chronic nasal obstruction can result from inflammatory conditions of the adenoids, from tumors and, particularly in children, from foreign bodies, such as beads, buttons, erasers, marbles, beans and stones. A *unilateral* purulent discharge in a child may be indicative of an undiscovered foreign body.

Sinus disease

Involvement of the paranasal sinuses may be of the acute or chronic varieties. Acute sinusitis usually follows a cold or infection of the nose, particularly after swimming. Chronic inflammation of the sinuses is seen most frequently secondary to allergic conditions.

The victim will complain most frequently

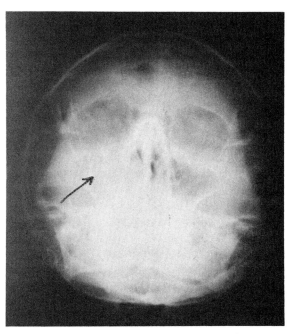

Figure 26–5 X-ray revealing obliteration of right maxillary sinus. See arrow for location of right maxillary sinus.

of a nasal discharge, which may vary from being thin and watery to thick and purulent. As the discharge enters the nasal cavity, it will drain into the pharynx, producing a postnasal drip, which is a frequent cause of sore throat. This drainage may also produce secondary inflammation of the mucosa of the pharynx and the lateral bands. Pressure may be present in sinus areas.

Headache is common in sinus inflammation and may be generalized or localized to the area of the sinus involved. Thus, the location of the headache may provide a clue to the sinus involved: frontal headache is associated with disease of the frontal sinus, while occipital headache occurs with sphenoid involvement. Neurological pain along the distribution of sensory nerves may also indicate the involved sinus. Maxillary sinusitis may cause pain or aching in the teeth, while ethmoid inflammation frequently causes pain in the area of the eye.

Assessment may reveal swelling and tenderness in the area of the involved sinus. The nasal mucosa in the area of the turbinates will appear reddened and thickened with mucopurulent or frank purulent discharge. X-ray and blood studies are rarely necessary.

Management involves supportive care. Bed rest, increased fluid intake and analgesic preparations, such as dextropropoxyphene (Darvon), oxycodone (Percodan) and acetylsalicylic acid (aspirin), for alleviation of pain and headache are advocated most frequently. Local heat by packs or steam inhalation may enhance drainage and assist in evacuation of the sinus. Vasoconstrictors and decongestants given in the form of oral preparations, (e.g., pseudoephedrine hydrochloride [Sudafed], phenylpropanolamine hydrochloride [Triaminic] and chlorpheniramine maleate [Ornade]) or, less commonly, in nasal packs provide symptomatic relief. Cultures of the drainage should be taken for predominant organisms and antibiotic sensitivity studies. In severe secondary infection, when purulent discharge is present or when systemic symptoms occur, such as fever and chills, specific antibiotic therapy is indicated. Penicillin drugs are usually effective and may be started until the sensitivity studies have been completed, usually after 48 hours.

Complications of sinusitis include orbital cellulitis or abscess, brain abscess, osteomyelitis, meningitis and cavernous sinus thrombosis. Complications relate to the blood supply and the proximity of these structures to the involved sinus.

Epistaxis

Nosebleed may be associated with trauma to or infections of the nose or may be a manifestation of systemic disease, such as hypertension or coagulation defects, especially in patients on anticoagulant therapy. Less commonly, it is due to irritation from a foreign body. Spontaneous nosebleeds associated with hypertension or anticoagulant therapy may result in massive blood loss.

The patient's general condition must be assessed and vital signs recorded. Patients with epistaxis are often apprehensive and require reassurance. Tachycardia and hypotension may indicate severe blood loss. In such patients, blood samples are drawn for complete count, type and crossmatch. If anticoagulant drugs are being used, a bleeding workup, consisting of platelet count, partial thromboplastin time and prothrombin time, is indicated.

Assessment must be careful, gentle and complete. The patient is preferably examined in a specially designed chair, with the head fixed on a headrest. The internal nares are carefully inspected with a nasal speculum. An adequate light source is necessary. Most often, the bleeding originates from Kisselbach's area, in the most anterior portion of the nasal septum. Anterior bleeding drains from the external nares. Bleeding from the posterior portion of the nose is more profuse and drains into the pharynx and mouth. If any significant amount of blood has been swallowed, nausea and emesis may occur.

Bleeding points anteriorly are easily located and may be controlled by gentle pressure. Pinching the nostrils between the thumb and index finger for 3 to 5 minutes will usually control the hemorrhage. If not, gentle pressure with a pledget of cotton containing epinephrine will arrest bleeding, and the bleeding point may then be cauterized by a silver nitrate stick. In a child, cotton moistened with hydrogen peroxide, placed in the anterior nose and combined with gentle pinching of the nostril, will be enough to control hemorrhage. Vasoconstrictor drugs (epinephrine) should be used with extreme caution in patients with hypertension.

Packing of the nose may be required when the bleeding point is located in the area of the turbinates. A petrolatum (Vaseline) gauze pack may be inserted carefully, using a bayonet forceps. If the bleeding continues after an anterior pack is in place, a posterior pack will be needed (Figure 26–6).

Placing a posterior pack is somewhat more

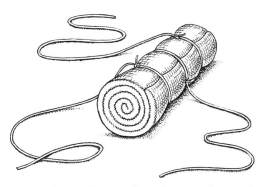

Figure 26–6 Preparation of a posterior nasal pack. A 4″ × 4″ gauze is rolled up and cut to size. Three heavy silk sutures are tied around the pack.

traumatic to the patient. (See Figure 26–7 for a visual description.) A rubber catheter is introduced into each nare until visible in the oropharynx. They are pulled out through the mouth, and an adequate size pack is tied

to the catheters protruding from the mouth, using 2 pieces of umbilical cord tape. The catheters are then gently withdrawn via the nose until the pack has been pulled upward above and behind the soft palate. It may be secured in place by a finger or a curved hemostat. The umbilical tape is tied across the columella so that the pack cannot slip down. A third string attached to the pack is brought out of the mouth and taped to the cheek. This string facilitates removal of the pack after 48 to 72 hours. An anterior pack is then inserted. Analgesics may be necessary during the time the pack is in place.

When nosebleeds occur in children, one must inspect carefully for a foreign body. If suspected, it may be confirmed by x-ray, especially if it is metallic. An alligator-type forceps may be used to remove it, and sedation may be needed.

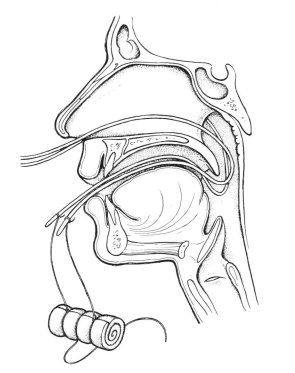
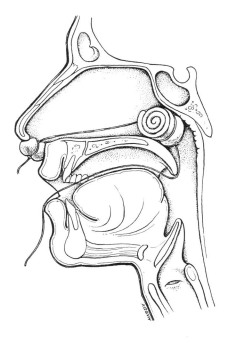

Figure 26–7 Placing of the posterior nasal pack. Left: The catheters are brought out through the mouth and tied with the lateral sutures on the pack; then the catheters are withdrawn through the nose. These sutures are then tied over a small piece of sponge at the columella. Right: The middle suture is brought out through the mouth and taped to the cheek.

Fractures of the nose

Nasal fractures occur as a result of direct trauma. The patient may complain of pain, swelling and bleeding from the nose. In those who present themselves to the emergency department hours or days after injury, difficulty in nasal breathing may be a complaint. In such instances, one should suspect a hematoma or abscess of the septum.

Examination may reveal a deformity of the nose. On careful palpation, one may feel crepitation at the fracture site when gently moving the nose. X-rays of the nose are helpful in confirming the fracture and the position of the fragments.

Management consists of reduction of the fragments to a normal position. Ice packs applied externally in the first 24 hours will reduce swelling; thereafter, heat may be used. An internal pack and a simple protective external metal splint may be needed to maintain the fragments in satisfactory position.

Nasal fractures do not take high priority in patients with multiple injuries. Reduction may be achieved successfully even several days after injury.

THE THROAT

Anatomy and physiology

The throat is made up of the nasopharynx, oropharynx and the laryngopharynx (hypopharynx).

The nasopharynx is the cavity behind the nose. Its anterior wall is the choana, the posterior part of the nose. Posteriorly, it is bounded by the coverings of the vertebral column. Inferiorly is the soft palate and superiorly, the base of the skull. The orifices of the eustachian tubes are located in the fossa of Rosenmüller, in the lateral portion of the nasopharynx. These tubes connect to the inner and middle ear, thus accounting for the high incidence of ear involvement associated with colds and sinus disease. In children, the eustachian tube is horizontal in position, while in adults it is more oblique. The fossa of Rosenmüller is an important site because of the relatively high incidence of tumors in it.

The oropharynx is behind the tongue. It is readily visualized through the mouth. Its posterior border is the vertebral column. Laterally, its boundaries are the anterior and posterior pillars which contain the tonsils in the tonsillar fossa.

The laryngopharynx lies inferior to the oropharynx and connects it with the upper end of the esophagus and with the glottis, which is the opening of the trachea. It contains the vocal cords.

The blood supply of the throat is derived from the ascending pharyngeal artery, arising from the external carotid. Innervation is through the pharyngeal plexus from the vagus and spinal accessory nerves. The vidian nerve supplies the region and when irritated may refer pain to a large portion of the head and neck.

The pharynx contains a large amount of lymphoid tissue, known as Waldeyer's ring. This ring of tissue is located in Rosenmüller's fossa and consists of the tonsils, the adenoids and faucial and lingual lymphoid tissue.

Assessment of the throat

Examination of the pharynx is preferably done with the patient in a sitting position. Necessary equipment includes a tongue blade, a dental mirror and an adequate light source. (See Figure 26–3.) Use of a head mirror will provide an excellent means of illuminating the pharynx and allowing the examiner to use both hands. When using a dental mirror, it should be heated over an exposed light bulb to prevent fogging after placing it in the patient's mouth.

Examination may be difficult if the patient is unable to open his mouth completely. The interior of the mouth should be carefully inspected. (See Figure 26–8 for a typical view.) The mucous membrane is ordinarily pink. The tonsils are located in their fossa on either side of the oropharynx, lateral to the base of the tongue. In the young, the tonsils are frequently enlarged and contain small sacs

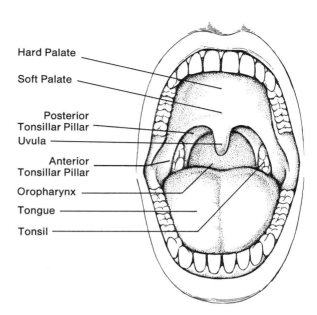

Hard Palate

Soft Palate

Posterior
Tonsillar Pillar

Uvula

Anterior
Tonsillar Pillar

Oropharynx

Tongue

Tonsil

Figure 26-8 Anatomy of the mouth, as seen by intraoral examination. When inspecting the oropharynx, the patient should be asked to say "Ah," which causes the soft palate to elevate; thus the pharynx can be better seen.

in the surface (crypts), which may be empty or contain pus. The tonsils may be covered by a purulent exudate.

The pharynx should be examined for evidence of redness or postnasal drainage. The soft palate forms the posterior portion of the roof of the mouth. Suspended from the middle of it is the uvula, which may assume many shapes. The nasopharynx cannot be visualized directly without using a dental mirror. To examine the laryngopharynx, grasp the tongue with a gauze sponge and pull it gently forward. The entire laryngopharynx, glottis and vocal cords may be seen by a dental mirror.

The presence of any exudate or membrane in the pharynx should be noted. The examiner should carefully palpate the neck for any swelling, localized masses or lymph node enlargement, as well as note any difficulty in breathing and whether the patient is breathing through the nose or mouth.

The most common diseases of the pharynx seen in the emergency department are of an inflammatory nature and involve the lymphoid tissue of Waldeyer's ring. Trauma is less commonly seen. The patient may complain of a sore throat, pain on swallowing, an associated cold, fever, chills and/or enlarged cervical lymph glands, depending on the problem.

Management of specific pharyngeal diseases

Tonsillitis

The most common problem in the pharynx for which emergency care is sought relates to the tonsils. Infection of the tonsil may be acute or of the chronic recurring variety, and the patient may present in varying degrees of severity. Infections are usually bacterial in origin and associated with symptoms of a cold or sore throat. The patient may experience a great deal of pain with swallowing, pain referred to the ear, fever, malaise and a foul odor to the breath.

Inspection of the pharynx will reveal enlargement of the tonsils with hyperemia and frequently an exudate in or overlying the crypts. The oropharynx is reddened and may have a pebble or cobblestone appearance, due to lymphoid hyperplasia. Enlarged cervical nodes may be palpated.

Management consists of supportive symptomatic care in addition to specific antibiotics. In the presence of an exudate or with recurring infections, swabs of the throat should be taken for culture of predominant organisms and sensitivity studies.

Peritonsillar abscess occurs with advanced infections of the tonsils. It usually involves the superior pole of the tonsil, trapping pus and causing difficulty in speaking clearly. The patient may speak as though he has a hot potato in his mouth and may be unable to open his jaw fully. Temporary relief may be obtained by aspiration of the pus. Definitive management is incision and drainage of the abscess, combined with antibiotic therapy and mouth irrigations.

Acute pharyngitis with membrane formation

Acute inflammatory conditions of the oropharynx may be severe and accompanied by systemic reactions of fever, malaise and anorexia. Severe infections are usually caused by specific organisms and are associated with membrane formation, a film of exudate overlying the mucosa of the pharyngeal structures.

The most common acute inflammations are: (1) septic sore throat, (2) Vincent's angina, (3) diphtheria, (4) blood dyscrasias (especially acute leukemia and agranulocytic angina) and (5) infectious mononucleosis. All are characterized by sore throat, difficulty in swallowing and talking, fever, malaise and anorexia.

Assessment will reveal a membrane, which may be wiped away, leaving a raw, bleeding surface. Regional lymphadenopathy is common in the submandibular and upper cervical areas. Management consists of supportive measures and specific antibiotic therapy. Cultures of the membrane are of the utmost importance. When diphtheria is suspected or ascertained by the organisms identified by microscopic examination of a smear of the membrane, specific diphtheria antitoxin is indicated. The patient should be in isolation. The membrane may involve a wide part of the respiratory tract. Impaired respiration is common, and the patient must be closely observed for respiratory obstruction. Tracheostomy may be necessary.

Retropharyngeal abscess is seen in infants and small children, usually under 3 years of age. Sore throat, difficulty in swallowing, stridor, fever and malaise are the most common symptoms. Examination of the pharynx will reveal reddening and edema of the mucosa. A bulging mass may be noted. Lateral x-rays of the neck will confirm the presence of the abscess by the widening of the retropharyngeal space, between the pharynx and the cervical vertebrae. Treatment consists of incision and drainage. This must be done cautiously, with the patient in the head-down position and suction ready, to minimize the possibility of aspiration. A mouth gag is used to maintain the jaws in an open position. The abscess may rupture during the placing of the gag.

Less common acute conditions arising in the pharynx include carcinoma, syphilis, gonorrhea, tuberculosis and actinomycosis. All may be associated with a chronic sore throat. Any accompanying ulcerating lesions should be biopsied for diagnosis.

Hoarseness

Diseases of the laryngopharynx (hypopharynx) are often associated with involvement of the glottic structures (vocal cords) and the upper portion of the trachea. The most common symptom is hoarseness, which may be an early sign of a serious disease. Hoarseness may occur as a result of tumors, an inflammatory or allergic condition or trauma.

The tumors may involve the larynx directly or cause pressure on the recurrent laryngeal nerve which moves the vocal cords. This nerve lies alongside the trachea and courses upward from the chest. Thus, tumors in the upper mediastinum or in the neck may cause nerve irritation and hoarseness. Tumors of the larynx are not usually cause for a patient to visit the emergency department, unless airway obstruction or respiratory difficulty is encountered.

Inflammatory conditions produce edema of the cords, with resultant hoarseness. Direct trauma to the larynx may cause damage to the cartilage about the vocal cords or to the tracheal cartilages, with hoarseness and respiratory difficulty. Inflammatory or allergic conditions in the laryngopharynx (hypopharynx) and larynx are common. The patient with acute laryngitis following a cold will complain of hoarseness or voice loss. Management consists of supportive measures, steam inhalations and rest for the larynx.

In patients with voice change or hoarseness, inspection of the vocal cords is necessary. This can be done, in a cooperative individual, with a dental mirror and an adequate light source. The vocal cords appear as 2 whitish bands which form an opening in the glottis that is roughly triangular in shape. While the cords are visualized, the patient should be asked to say the letter "E". This should cause the cords to adduct, to come together in the midline. Failure of one or both cords to adduct indicates paralysis. The cords should also be examined for tumors or thickening.

Laryngotracheobronchitis

Acute laryngotracheobronchitis is a serious condition, more commonly seen in infants and children. It is usually due to the B influenza organism. Symptoms are those of a chest cold, with nasal and chest congestion, cough, fever, chills and varying degrees of respiratory difficulty. If severe, cyanosis of the lips, earlobes and the nailbeds may be noted.

Management consists of taking smears of any drainage for culture and sensitivity studies. The child usually requires admission to the hospital. A humidified atmosphere, either cold or heated will help to thin secretions. Best results can be obtained with a properly humidified oxygen tent. Antibiotics are given in appropriate doses. When respiratory embarrassment is present, arterial blood gas determinations should be done. Tracheostomy

may be needed in instances of severe respiratory insufficiency.

Allergies

Allergic reactions in the pharynx and larynx are often due to sensitizing agents, such as drugs or pollens found in the air. As a result, edema of the larynx occurs. The patient may note difficulty in swallowing and breathing. He will often state, "My throat feels like it is closing up." Allergic reactions are particularly serious in children, because the larynx has loose areolar tissue, which responds with further swelling.

Spraying the pharynx with decongestants, such as epinephrine or ephedrine, gives rapid relief. Antihistamines given parenterally, especially diphenhydramine (Benadryl) or epinephrine may be needed. Steroids may reduce the allergic response. The patient must be observed carefully for respiratory insufficiency. In such instances, tracheostomy is indicated.

Foreign body in the air passages

Sudden respiratory distress may indicate a foreign body in the airway, particularly if the distress occurs while eating. Children commonly put toys and small objects into their mouths, and occasionally one may enter the airway. When the obstruction is at the glottic area, respiratory embarrassment is severe, cyanosis develops rapidly and death may ensue in a matter of minutes. The patient struggles to take an effective inspiration and in doing so further impacts the foreign body.

An effort should be made to dislodge the object by reaching into the mouth and sweeping the pharynx with the index finger. Curved forceps are also available for dislodgement. One must act quickly if a life is to be saved. Currently, interest has centered on the Heimlich maneuver, in which the rescuer embraces the victim from behind, with hands grasped just below the rib cage. A sudden pull of the rescuer's arms into the victim forces the diaphragm upward, which should dislodge the foreign object by the sudden gust of air from the victim's lungs. (See Chapter 13 for more details.)

Once the object has passed below the vocal cords, it will drop into the trachea and bronchi and lodge there. If it is large enough, the carina (the bifurcation of the trachea into right and left bronchi) may be obstructed. This is most unusual, however, since the carina is larger than the glottic aperture. When the foreign body has settled in the lower part of the respiratory tract, the patient will complain of persistent cough. This problem is no longer a life-threatening emergency. Partial or complete obstruction of a smaller bronchus may cause emphysema or atelectasis of the involved segment of lung.

Careful and complete evaluation is necessary, although physical findings may be minimal. Chest x-rays will usually localize the object. In cases of nonopaque foreign bodies, evidence of altered lung aeration, either atelectasis or emphysema, may be seen on x-ray and may be the first indication of an obstructed airway. Metal objects cause little reaction in the bronchi. Organic foreign bodies, such as meat or peanuts, may cause more severe reactions.

Management consists of removal of the foreign body. Extraction may be done through a bronchoscope in most instances. A variety of special instruments are available to grasp the object. Open thoracotomy is needed when the bronchoscopic approach fails.

Foreign body in the esophagus

Improper mastication or swallowing too large pieces of solid food, especially meat, may result in food in the esophagus. Non-food objects are less commonly a cause of esophageal obstruction. Symptoms result from the obstruction. The patient will complain of dysphagia and inability to swallow water, even his own saliva. The patient may frequently be able to localize the area of the block. Usually the history is of sudden onset while eating.

Chest x-ray will localize a metallic body, while use of contrast media (barium or meglumine diatrizoate [Gastrografin]) swallowed under fluoroscopic control will demonstrate where food or nonopaque bodies are caught.

Complications may result from perforation of the esophagus by a foreign object. Subcutaneous emphysema in the neck or pneumomediastinum (air in the mediastinum) on chest x-ray are diagnostic. Surgical exploration of the esophagus with drainage and repair of the perforation is then required. Antibiotics are used in large dosages.

THE EARS

Anatomy and physiology

The ears are the organs of hearing and equilibrium. Each ear consists of 3 divisions, the external, the middle and the inner ear.

The external ear consists of the auricle (pinna), a cartilaginous structure covered by skin and connective tissue which serves as a baffle to reflect sound. It connects with the middle ear by the external auditory canal, a membranocartilaginous osseus tunnel from 2.5 to 3.5 cm. in length, extending obliquely downward and anteriorly to the tympanic membrane (eardrum). The canal narrows at the junction of the external (cartilaginous) portion and the internal (osseus) segment. The size of the lumen of the cartilaginous portion will vary with movements of the mandible during chewing. A portion of the parotid gland lies in close proximity to the floor of the canal. The skin of the auricle continues into the canal. In the membranocartilaginous portion, hair follicles, sebaceous and ceruminous glands are present. The skin is densely adherent to the perichondrium and the periosteum. Inflammatory conditions resulting in edema or stretching of the skin are thus very painful.

The middle ear contains the ossicles—the malleus, incus and stapes which are attached to the tympanic membrane. The outer wall is formed by the tympanic membrane. The inner wall is the internal ear. The middle cranial fossa is above and the jugular bulb below. The tympanic membrane, or eardrum, is roughly circular in shape. The malleus attaches near the center of the drum. The upper portion is flaccid and called Shrapnell's membrane. The lower part is the pars tensa. When the ear is examined with an otoscope, a triangular area of light can be seen in the anterior portion of the pars tensa (Figure 26–9). This is referred to as the cone of light. It may vary in size depending upon the pressure in the middle ear. Similarly, Shrapnell's membrane may bulge if fluid or inflammation is present in the middle ear and retract if the eustachian tube is blocked following a cold.

The internal ear contains the organ of hearing, the cochlea, and the semicircular canals, the labyrinths, which relate to balance. The inner ear derives its blood supply from a branch of the basilar artery. The seventh and eighth nerves and the nervus intermedius are contained in the internal auditory meatus. Thus, middle ear infections extending to the inner ear may cause labyrinthitis, manifested by dizziness, loss of balance, nausea, vomiting and tinnitus.

Assessment of the ear

The only portions of the ear which can be examined are the external ear, the external auditory meatus and the tympanic membrane. The earlobes are also worth examining, since lesions such as sebaceous cysts frequently occur there.

To examine the external auditory canal, an otoscope or ear speculum with an external light source is necessary. (See Figure 26–3.) Because of the oblique direction of the canal, the pinna must be pulled upward and posteriorly. In children, the canal is more horizontal in position; thus, the ear is pulled only posteriorly. Varying amounts of cerumen (ear wax) may be found in the canal. If it obstructs the view of the eardrum, the wax may be removed by a curette or by gentle irrigation with an ear syringe and warm water. If the wax is dried, instillation of a few drops of sweet (olive) oil or peroxide will aid in

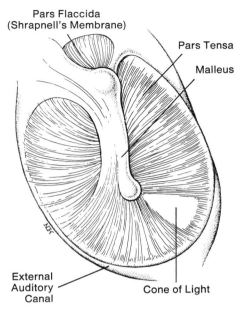

Figure 26–9 View of right ear drum through an otoscope. The important anatomical landmarks are identified.

loosening it. The wax must be removed carefully to avoid damage to the drum. In visualizing the drum, the landmarks previously described are important, especially the cone of light. Normally the drum will appear pale, gray and opaque. Any redness, bulging or retraction of the drum is pathologic.

Management of specific diseases of the ear

External ear problems

The external ear can be the site of skin eruptions, as are other parts of the body, particularly impetigo, furunculosis, herpes simplex and herpes zoster. Wounds of the pinna, such as lacerations or contusions, are managed as similar wounds elsewhere. The pinna is frequently damaged by frostbite because of the relative thinness of the skin overlying the cartilage. Frostbite reaction is similar to a burn. Initially, the skin will be blanched, and rewarming should be carried out. Later, bleb formation occurs. Blebs are managed by puncturing under aseptic conditions and by application of antibiotic ointment, such as polymixin B (Neosporin) or bacitracin. More severe cold injury will damage the cartilage which will result in deformity when healed.

Diffuse external otitis is a widespread involvement of the skin and subcutaneous tissue of the external ear. It is often referred to as "swimmer's ear." The swelling may be severe enough to completely block the auditory canal. Furuncles of the external auditory canal result from infection in the sweat or wax glands. These are usually extremely painful, especially when chewing. Management of both otitis and furunculosis is use of hot packs and instillation of antibiotic drops. Analgesics may be required for pain relief.

Foreign bodies in the external auditory canal can usually be seen by otoscopy. Insects frequently lodge in the canal. An effort should be made to wash foreign objects out with warm water irrigations. If this is not possible, the patient should be seen by a physician for object removal.

Middle ear diseases

Diseases of the middle ear affect the tympanic membrane and are usually associated with pain and hearing loss. Acute myringitis is inflammation of the drum. Otoscopy will reveal the drum to be pink and congested near the malleus and the periphery. Bullous myringitis is more severe, with pain, fever, deafness and tinnitus (ringing in the ears). On otoscopy, the drum is inflamed, with blebs present. The problem is managed by rupture of the blebs, combined with benzocaine (Auralgan) and hydroscopic ear drops. Pain is thus relieved almost immediately.

Traumatic rupture of the tympanic membrane occurs as a result of a blow over the ears, an explosion or trauma from a foreign body. Onset is accompanied by pain. Examination will reveal blood in the ear canal and a perforation in the drum. It is advisable to put no medication into the ear canal, for it will enter the middle ear. It is best to place a piece of sterile cotton in the external canal.

Acute aerotitis media results from bacterial invasion of the mucosa of the tympanum. It may vary from an acute catarrhal type to acute suppuration with perforation. The patient will complain of pain in the ear, associated with pressure, deafness and headache. In more severe forms, fever, malaise and anorexia will occur. Otoscopy will reveal the drum to be reddened and dull, with loss of normal landmarks; it may be bulging from fluid buildup behind. Tenderness over the mastoid area indicates involvement of this sinus. The regional lymph nodes may be enlarged and tender. When severe, myringotomy (incision of the drum) is necessary to evacuate the fluid. Cultures should be done on the drainage. Antibiotics and analgesics are needed. Complications must be considered if fever persists after drainage, including acute mastoiditis, meningitis, labyrinthitis, facial nerve paralysis (Bell's palsy), lateral sinus thrombosis and brain abscess.

Acute mastoiditis is the most common complication of the middle ear infection. It is marked by pain in the mastoid region and fever. Tenderness is present on palpation of the mastoid area, and swelling may be noted. Surgical drainage may be necessary.

Acute salpingitis of the eustachian tube may accompany infections of the throat or nasal allergies. It is more common in children with adenoid enlargement. The tube is occluded, preventing ventilation of the middle ear. The air in the ear is then absorbed, causing pain and impaired hearing. Treatment relates to shrinking the nasal and pharyngeal mucosa by the use of astringents (epinephrine or ephedrine). Myringotomy may be needed if fluid is present behind the drum.

Inner ear disease

Ménière's disease is an inflammatory condition of the labyrinth. The patient entering the emergency department may have an unsteady gait, nystagmus, tinnitus, nausea and vomiting. Hearing may be affected. Dizziness occurs and may be noted even when the patient is at rest. Management of the acute phase consists of sedation. Symptomatic relief may be achieved with dimenhydrinate (Dramamine), diphenhydramine (Benadryl) or meclizine hydrochloride (Antivert). Definitive management depends on total evaluation of the patient by a physician.

SUMMARY

Because the ears, nose and throat are anatomically and physiologically related, trauma or disease processes affecting one system will often also affect one or both other systems. Although this has not been stressed in this chapter on assessing and treating emergencies of the ears, nose and throat, it is an important function of emergency nursing care. The nurse should examine all 3 organ systems when a patient presents complaining of a problem with one.

BIBLIOGRAPHY

(1) Bain, J. A.: "Late Complications of Tracheostomy and Prolonged Intubation," *International Anesthesiology Clinics,* 10 (1972):225.

(2) Ballantyne, John, and Groves, John (eds.): *Scott-Brown's Diseases of the Ear, Nose and Throat,* ed. 3, vols. 1–4 (Philadelphia: J. B. Lippincott Company, 1971).

(3) Barga, J. L.: "How to Treat Nosebleed," *American Family Physician,* 8 (1973): 66.

(4) Bergner, R. K.: "Allergy, Milk and Otitis Media," *Pediatrics,* 52 (1973):144.

(5) Bowen-Davies, A.: "Methods of Examination of the Mouth and Pharynx," *in* John Ballantyne and John Groves (eds.), *Scott-Brown's Diseases of the Ear, Nose and Throat,* ed. 3, vol. 4 (Philadelphia: J. B. Lippincott Company, 1971), pp. 3–17.

(6) Brantigan, C. O.: "Delayed Major Vessel Hemorrhage Following Tracheostomy," *Journal of Trauma,* 13 (1973): 235.

(7) Bryce, D. P.: "The Surgical Management of Laryngo-Tracheal Injury," *Journal of Laryngology and Otology,* 86 (1972):547.

(8) Chadwick, D. L.: "Advances in the Treatment of Diseases of the Ear, Nose and Throat," *Practitioner,* 209 (1972): 460.

(9) Chignelli, R.: "Iatrogenic Disorders of the Nose and Throat," *Proceedings of the Royal Society of Medicine,* 65 (1972):679.

(10) Colman, B. H.: "Chronic Mucous Otitis," *Nursing Times,* 69 (1973):336.

(11) Cowen, D. E.: "Allergy of the Respiratory Tract: A Comprehensive Approach to Treatment," *Otolaryngologic Clinics of North America,* 4 (1971): 465.

(12) Empey, D. W.: "Assessment of Upper Airways Obstruction," *British Medical Journal,* 3 (1972):503.

(13) Gaskill, J. R.: "Fixation of Foley Catheter," *Archives of Otolaryngology,* 96 (1972):186.

(14) Gerwin, K. S.: "Serous Otitis," *Archives of Otolaryngology,* 97 (1973):430.

(15) Goodhill, V.: "Inner Ear Barotrauma," *Archives of Otolaryngology,* 95 (1972): 588.

(16) Harrison, D. F. N.: "Surgical Anatomy of Maxillary and Ethmoidal Sinuses, A Reappraisal," *The Laryngoscope,* 81 (1971):1658.

(17) Liebman, E. P.: "The Care of Epistaxis," *Pennsylvania Medicine,* 75 (1972):50.

(18) Norris, C. W., and Eakins, K.: "Head and Neck Pain: The T-M Joint Syndrome," *The Laryngoscope,* 84 (1974): 1466.

(19) Roydhouse, N.: "Management of Otitis Media in General Practice," *Drugs,* 3 (1972):418.

(20) Saunders, W. H.: "Nasal Packs for Epistaxis," *Journal of the American Medical Association,* 218 (1971):1830.

(21) Schofield, J.: "Conservative Treat-

ment of Subglottic Stenosis of the Larynx," *Archives of Otolaryngology,* 95 (1972):457.

(22) Sein, A. B.: "Epistaxis in the Elderly," *South African Medical Journal,* 45 (1971):1023.

(23) Shapiro, S. L.: "Some Remarks on Otitis Externa," *Eye, Ear, Nose and Throat Monthly,* 52 (1973):302.

(24) Sprinkle, R. M.; Vectri, R. W., and Kantor, L. M.: "Abcesses of the Head and Neck," *The Laryngoscope,* 84 (1974): 1142.

(25) Strome, M., and Jaffe, B.: "Epiglottitis — Individualized Management with Steroids," *The Laryngoscope,* 84 (1974): 921.

(26) Tos, M.: "Nasotracheal Intubation in Acute Epiglottitis," *Acta Otolaryngologica,* 68 (1969):363.

(27) Tucker, J. A. *et al.:* "Tracheotomy in Pediatrics," *Annals of Otology, Rhinology and Laryngology,* 81 (1972): 818.

(28) Warren, C. M., Jr.: "Treatment of Allergic Emergencies," *Otolaryngologic Clinics of North America,* 4 (1971): 599.

(29) Weiss, N. S.: "Relation of High Blood Pressure to Headache, Epistaxis and Selected Other Symptoms, The U. S. Health Examination Survey," *New England Journal of Medicine,* 287 (1972):631.

(30) Wilson, H. L.: "Otolaryngologic Problems of Skin and Scuba Diving," *Archives of Otolaryngology,* 96 (1973): 487.

(31) Wolf, C. R.: "Aerotitis in Air Travel," *California Medicine,* 117 (1972):10.

27

Care of the patient with ocular injuries

ARTHUR J. SCHAEFER

Any patient seen in the emergency department with trauma in the facial region must have a careful eye examination and x-ray studies. Too frequently, patients with other bodily injuries and in a state of shock have ocular injuries which are overlooked. One half of all monocular blindness and one fifth of all binocular blindness are due to accidents.[2] From 2 to 2.5 percent of all war casualties, according to Duke-Elder, were ocular.[3] This statistic is high, considering the eye occupies only $1/375$ of exposed body surface. Thus, the necessity of checking the eyes carefully in all victims of trauma in the facial region cannot be emphasized too strongly.

Today, automobile accidents contribute greatly to eye injuries. Orbital and ocular injuries account for almost 10 percent of all automobile injuries, according to a Cornell Medical College research project. In contrast, less than 3 percent of battle casualties in World War II involved ocular injuries, according to Keeney.[5]

ANATOMY AND PHYSIOLOGY

The eyes are paired sense organs, which move synchronously to produce binocular vision. Each eyeball, or globe, is roughly spherical.

The white portion of the eye, the sclera, surrounds the anterior portion of the globe, the cornea. The cornea is a transparent dome, which may be compared to a watch crystal. Behind the protective cornea is the iris, the colored portion of the eye. The iris is an opaque, contractile diaphragm, with a round, regular opening centrally, the pupil, behind which the lens is located.

The interior of the globe contains 2 fluids, the aqueous humor and the vitreous body. The aqueous humor, a thin fluid, lies in the anterior and posterior chambers of the eye, which are located between the cornea and the lens. These chambers communicate through the pupil.

The dense and jelly-like vitreous body fills the larger, most posterior portion of the globe, which is located between the lens and the retina. The retina forms the inner lining of the posterior portion of the globe and can only be visualized using an ophthalmoscope with special magnification. Figure 27–1 shows 2 views of the ocular structures discussed above.

Attached to the eyeball are 6 extraocular muscles, responsible for the external move-

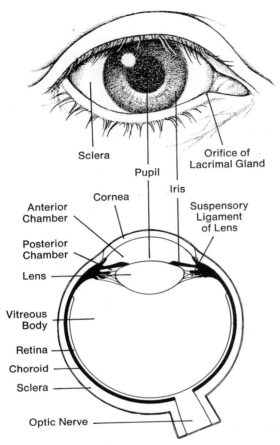

Figure 27–1   Anatomy of the left eye. Top: anterior view. Bottom: sagittal view.

ments of the eyeball. Anteriorly, the eyeball is protected by the upper and lower eyelids, which involuntarily close over the eye at frequent intervals. This reflex motion, called "blinking," serves to moisten the anterior portion of the eye, by circulating the tear fluid which flows from the lacrimal (tear) gland, located in the lateral anterior aspect of the orbit behind the superior orbital rim. The tear fluid bathes the globe, then exits via the lacrimal ducts, located at the most medial end of the upper and lower lid and draining into the nasal cavity.

The eyelids are composed of skin and muscle over a thin layer of dense connective tissue, the tarsal plate, which serves to stiffen

them. At the edge of each lid is a fringe of hair, the eyelashes, which are very sensitive to touch and, when stimulated, cause a reflex closure of the lids. Besides this protective action of the eyelids, the eyeball is further safeguarded by the orbicularis oculi muscle, a strong circular muscle surrounding the lids, which can be contracted voluntarily to produce forcible closure of the lids.

Each eyeball rests within an "orbit," surrounded by periorbital fat posteriorly and the eyelids anteriorly. The eyelids are lined by the palpebral conjunctiva, which continues onto the eyeball, covering the anterior portion (the bulbar conjunctiva). The 2 bony vaults in the cranium, the orbits, which surround and protect the eye are in direct continuity with the 4 sinuses: frontal, ethmoid, maxillary and sphenoidal.

ASSESSMENT OF OCULAR PROBLEMS

The following equipment should be on hand for ocular examination and treatment (see Figure 27–2).

(1) A small flashlight (penlight) or examining light, with a sharp beam of light to aid in critical examination of the eye and its adnexa. A flashlight with a blue beam is needed, as well, for viewing the eye after fluorescein staining.
(2) A magnifying loupe to visualize minute pathology, such as a corneal foreign body or fine corneal abrasion.
(3) A Snellen test card for visual acuity.
(4) A lid retractor or speculum to help hold the lids open if there is swelling or spasm of the lids.
(5) An ophthalmoscope.
(6) A contact lens remover (small rubber suction cup).
(7) Sterile irrigating solutions.
(8) Sterile cotton applicators.
(9) Fluorescein strips.
(10) Sterile eye pads and tape.
(11) Medications in small, sterile, dis-

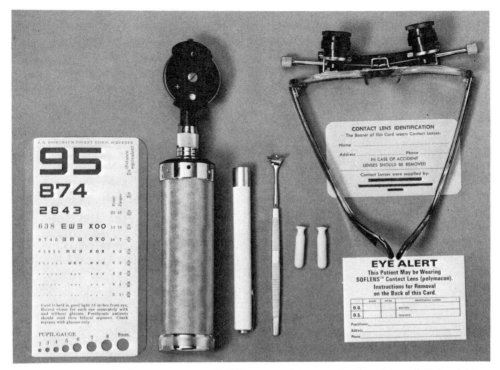

Figure 27–2 Basic instruments needed for an ocular examination. From left to right: a Snellen test card, an ophthalmoscope, a penlight, a lid retractor, contact lens removers, a magnifying loupe. The cards shown are frequently carried by patients wearing standard or soft contact lenses.

posable vials or tubes, including cycloplegics, midriatics, miotics, anesthetics and antibiotics.

Keep no atropine or steroid eye drops on the eye tray, since their misuse in some conditions can cause serious problems.

First, a good history of the injury should be obtained from the patient. If it is a child, the nurse should obtain the history from the parents or someone else familiar with the accident. It should include: (1) the time of the injury, (2) the nature of the injury (scratch, cut, foreign body, blunt instrument or flying missile), (3) the extent of pain and (4) any visual disturbance. Careful records must be maintained for the patient's benefit and medical-legal purposes.

Visual acuity should be recorded for all patients before any examination or treatment is started. If the patient cannot see or read the Snellen test card or is in critical condition, the nurse should record whether the patient can count fingers or see hand motion with each eye separately and at what distance. If even this is beyond the patient's capacity, the nurse should record whether or not he has light perception in each eye.

During an eye examination, the patient is usually frightened, upset and apprehensive. If he has pain, he will keep his eyes shut tightly as a defense mechanism. He will need reassurance and often a local topical anesthetic to permit adequate inspection of the eye. With the patient's head supported in a head rest, the eye is examined gently and carefully, being especially careful to never press against the eyeball at any time.

If the patient has moderate to severe blepharospasm (lid spasm) and cannot voluntarily open his eyelids, the examiner should use one to 2 drops of a 0.5 percent topical anesthetic, such as tetracaine hydrochloride (Pontocaine), then wait 30 to 60 seconds before raising the lid. In severe blepharospasm, the dosage of the anesthetic should be repeated in one minute, and the lids will relax. The eye can then be examined without force, alleviating the chance of further injury to the eye.

If the patient is wearing contact lenses and is conscious and able to remove them, the nurse should have the patient remove them. If the patient is unconscious or incapacitated, the nurse should remove them as follows. Hard contact lenses are removed by applying a small, hard contact suction cup to the lens and extracting the lens with it. The suction cup is pictured on the equipment tray (Figure 27–2).

Soft contact lenses are removed in a different manner. If the lens has been in the eye for some time, it may be difficult to remove if not irrigated well with normal saline. Therefore, to be sure, the nurse should irrigate the lens copiously with normal saline, directly while it is on the eye. Then she slides it gently off the cornea, onto the sclera with her index finger. When the lens is over the sclera, the nurse gently picks it off by squeezing it between her index finger and thumb. If it does not slide off the cornea easily, the lens must be irrigated again; then it will slide off. If the lens does not slide off the cornea readily, and one persists in trying to slide it off without irrigating it, the whole or part of the corneal epithelium can be denuded in removing the lens.

EXAMINATION AND TREATMENT OF COMMON INJURIES

Foreign bodies

The most common ocular injury is a simple foreign body, which may be under the upper eyelid or on the corneal or scleral conjunctiva. If a patient has the sensation of a foreign body and if it is difficult for him to open

his eye, the nurse should instill one to 2 drops of 0.5 percent topical anesthetic, such as tetracaine hydrochloride (Pontocaine), and wait about a minute. Then the cornea is inspected carefully with magnification. If no foreign body is seen, the nurse should evert the upper eyelid and inspect the tarsal conjunctiva (inner lid). This is where the foreign body is usually lodged.

To evert the upper eyelid: (1) The patient looks down toward his feet with both eyes, and the nurse gently grasps the eyelashes of the upper lid and gently pulls the lid down and slightly outward, away from the eye. This step is illustrated by Figure 27–3.* (2) While grasping the eyelashes in this downward and outward position, the nurse applies gentle pressure directly on the lid (on the upper edge of the tarsus on the skin side, about 10 mm. above the upper lid margin), using a small cotton-tip applicator, and simultaneously pulls the lashes upward. (See Figure 27–4.) The lid will evert easily (Figure 27–5).

Use a sterile cotton-tip applicator, moistened with normal saline or ocular irrigating solution to wipe the foreign body off the upper tarsal conjunctiva (Figure 27–6). When the nurse has finished, she releases the upper lid and asks the patient to look up. The lid will readily flip back to its normal position. The patient is then prescribed local ophthalmic antibiotic drops, to be used 4 times a day for 5 days, to prevent infection.

If a foreign body is not found under the upper lid, the next approach is to stain the cornea with a sterile fluorescein strip. (Never use fluorescein drops, since the solution is easily contaminated with pyocyaneous organisms.) The end of a sterile strip is moistened with ocular irrigating solution or sterile normal saline. The nurse then touches the tip of the strip to the inner side of the lower eyelid, removes it and asks the patient to blink a few times. The fluorescein will mix with the tears and flow over the cornea. A minute corneal foreign body can then be seen by the

* Figures 27–3, 27–4, 27–5, 27–6, 27–8, 27–9, 27–10, 27–11, 27–12 and 27–13 appear on the color plate included in this text.

concentration of fluorescein in the area surrounding it.

If a corneal foreign body is present, the patient is given one to 2 drops of 0.5 percent topical anesthetic before it is swabbed away lightly with a moist cotton-tip applicator. If the particle does not dislodge with this gentle brushing maneuver, stop. The corneal epithelium could be damaged by continued swabbing. The nurse should then refer the patient to an ophthalmologist for removal.

If the nurse is alone, with no immediate help available, she should carefully lift the foreign body off the cornea with the point of a sterile number 25 hypodermic needle, ocular foreign body spud or sharp-pointed number 11 Bard-Parker knife blade. An antibiotic ointment and sterile eye pad are applied to protect the eye and lessen discomfort to the patient. She should advise the patient to be checked by an ophthalmologist in one day.

If the foreign body was iron in content and a rust ring is present on the eye and does not dislodge easily with the foreign body, the patient should see an ophthalmologist for removal of the rust ring under slit lamp observation. An antibiotic drop is instilled and a sterile eye pad applied before sending the patient to the ophthalmologist. Eye pads should be taped to the side of the eye, rather than above it, near the eyebrow.

If there is no foreign body present on the cornea, the nurse must check the cornea with a good focal light for a stain on the cornea, indicating an abrasion, erosion or scratch. These conditions will give rise to the same symptoms as a foreign body. The treatment for corneal abrasions is installation of an antibiotic ophthalmic ointment and application of a sterile eye pad, instructing the patient to keep both eyes closed. Healing of scratches, abrasions and erosions usually occurs in 24 hours, barring infection. The patient should see an ophthalmologist for follow-up examination in 24 to 48 hours.

Although these are very painful conditions, the nurse must *never* give a topical anesthetic to the patient to take home. Continued use of topical anesthetics promotes further corneal epithelial breakdown and slows the healing process. The patient can take analgesics by mouth to relieve the pain.

Burns

Ultraviolet and flash burns

Ultraviolet and welder's flash burns (actinic keratitis) are also very painful conditions, producing a diffuse punctate keratitis in the exposed cornea, severe blepharospasm and sensitivity to light. The patient usually states he was using a sun lamp, was welding or was near a welder without proper ocular protection about 6 to 8 hours prior to the onset of symptoms.

To relieve the blepharospasm and facilitate examination, one to 2 drops of a 0.5 percent topical ophthalmic anesthetic should be instilled. The lids will relax in 30 to 60 seconds, and the eye can then be examined. Then, the eye is stained with a fluorescein strip, as described above. A diffuse punctate staining of the cornea can be seen on examination with magnification. To treat, instill a cycloplegic, cyclopentolate hydrochloride (Cyclogel) or homatropine drops, an antibiotic ointment and binocular eye pads. Again, give an analgesic and sedation by mouth, and send the patient home for 24 hours of complete rest. These injuries usually heal quickly if treated promptly.

The following is a history of a patient with the typical symptoms of an ultraviolet burn and the typical corneal changes.

> On questioning of her activities of the last 12 hours, the patient stated she had been ironing white bed linens. Because of the heat, she moved her work into the yard and ironed in direct sunlight. She received enough ultraviolet light from the sun rays reflecting off the linen into her eyes to produce an ultraviolet burn. She responded rapidly and healed with the usual therapy for flash burns.

Chemical burns

Any chemical splashed into the eye should be treated by immediate and copious irrigation with tap water if normal saline or other commercial irrigating solutions are not immediately at hand. Irrigation should be continued for at least 10 minutes.

Chemical burns can be due to acids, alkalis or organic irritants. Acid burns coagulate their own protein barrier on contact and, as a rule, show an immediate and sharp demarcation of extent. If irrigated immediately and properly, they do not penetrate deeply. Their clinical course is usually predictable within a few hours after injury. Another history:

> This resourceful patient, who splashed acid in his eye, was some distance from tap water. He had a full bottle of beer with him, which he poured into his eye to irrigate it when he experienced the sudden pain and irritation from the acid. He then went to a tap and irrigated the eye further with water. His fast action, even with beer, probably saved him from more serious corneal damage.

Alkali burns are much more serious than acid burns, because they are proteolytic and break down the protein barrier of the eye. The end products of alkali burns are alkaline, and they are further augmented by the alkaline tears. Alkali particles will continue to lyse the corneal protein and burn deeper if not removed. The severity of the burn is determined by the alkali concentration and by the duration of contact. Therefore, it is imperative to irrigate immediately and copiously at the scene of the accident with plain tap water. A shower can be used if available. The eyelids must be held open to let the stream wash the eye and fornices directly. Then someone must transport the patient to the nearest emergency facility for further care and evaluation.

At the emergency department, a topical anesthetic is instilled; all foreign particles are removed with a moist cotton applicator or foreign body spud; and the eye is irrigated at frequent intervals. In severe burns, a topical anesthetic should be repeatedly instilled between long courses of irrigation. An ophthalmologist should see the patient as soon as possible if the burn is severe. Frequently, with many particles of alkali penetrating the

corneal epithelium, he will have to debride the entire corneal epithelium to remove all alkali particles and prevent further penetration into the cornea and permanent scarring.

Organic burns, such as those produced by brake fluid, cause mild reaction, with edema of the conjunctiva and cornea. They are painful but usually do not result in permanent damage.

To summarize, treatment of chemical burns begins with immediate copious irrigations with tap water, saline or any available ocular irrigating solution. In severe cases, irrigation should be done every few minutes for several hours. A local anesthetic, such as 0.5 percent Pontocaine should be repeatedly instilled between irrigations to relieve the patient and enable him to relax the lids for thorough irrigation.

After irrigation is completed, antibiotic drops are started, and the eyes are patched in patients with corneal involvement. In serious burns, a cycloplegic, such as homatropine or Cyclogel, can also be instilled to relieve ciliary spasm. At night, antibiotic ointments and binocular patching is continued, even if only one eye is involved, until the cornea has healed. Binocular patching is necessary to keep both eyes immobile and at rest. Oral medication for pain and sedation for sleep are needed for patients with these painful injuries. Patients with chemical burns should be referred to an ophthalmologist for further therapy and follow-up, as soon as possible.

Success in treating patients with acute chemical burns of the eye using the "Water Pic" device and distilled water has been reported.[4] It directs a pulsating stream of water to the eye and fornices to thoroughly remove all chemicals. Sterile disposable devices specifically designed for continuous eye lavage and medication are also available (see Figure 27–7). These are plastic disposable units similar to those used in intravenous therapy. On the distal end, are plastic scleral-type shells, like scleral contact lenses, which fit under the lids to cover the cornea and

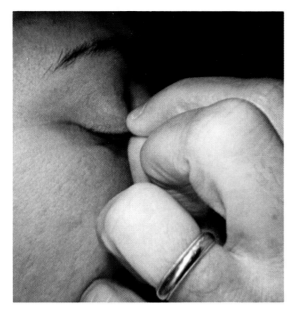
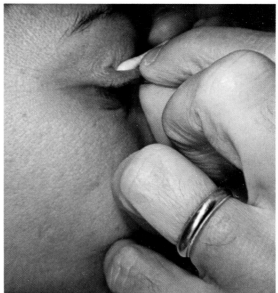

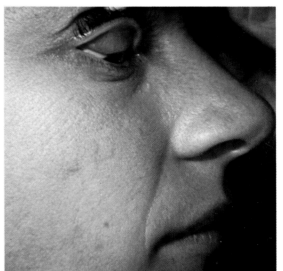

Figure 27–3 (top left) Everting the upper eyelid, step one.

Figure 27–4 (top right) Everting the upper eyelid, step two.

Figure 27–5 (center) Eversion of the upper eyelid.

Figure 27–6 (bottom left) Foreign body on the upper eyelid.

Figure 27–8 (bottom right) Hyphemia (note the blood fluid level at the lower part of the cornea).

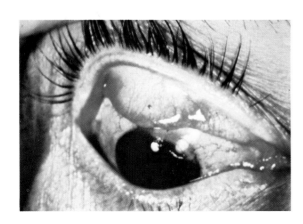
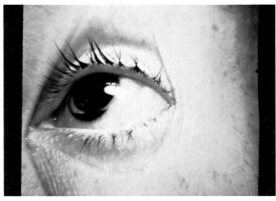

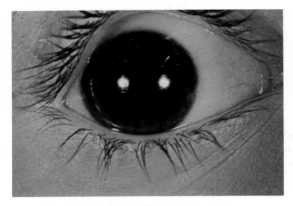

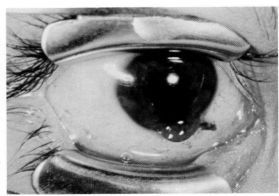

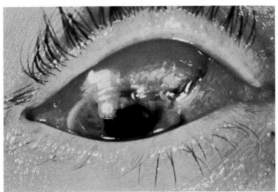

Figure 27–9 (top left) Tear of the iris (iriodyalisis).

Figure 27–10 (top right) Perforation of the cornea, with prolapse of the iris.

Figure 27–11 (center) Lacerating wound of the cornea and sclera, with prolapse of the iris and ciliary body.

Figure 27–12 (bottom left) Subconjunctival hemorrhage.

Figure 27–13 (bottom right) Multiple lacerations involving the edge of the eyelid and the tear duct.

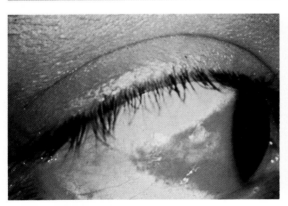

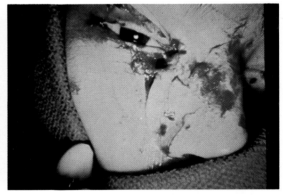

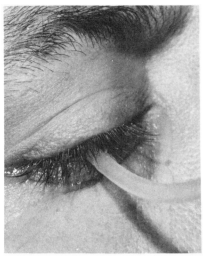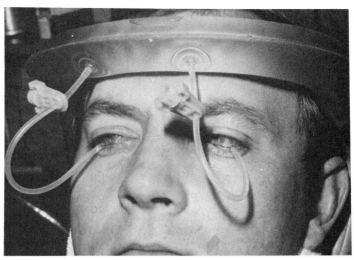

Figure 27–7 Continuous eye lavage. "MedCap" combines a headband with a capacity of 400 ml. of irrigating fluid and 2 MorTan therapeutic lenses, which fit under the eyelids. This allows for continuous irrigation of the surface of the eyeball.
Source: Photos courtesy of MorTan, Inc., Torrington, Wyo.

through which a constant drip of irrigating fluid or medication can be delivered to the eye. They are used for continuous ocular irrigation in severe chemical burns following emergency treatment and in other conditions of the eye requiring continuous irrigation with local medication and/or fluids.[6]

Tear gas and mace

Tear gas and mace injuries to the eye are becoming more common as these products are put to wider use. The treatment is as outlined for chemical burns. In patients with severe injuries requiring admission, 200 mg. of hydrocortisone sodium succinate (Solu-Cortef) in 1,000 cc. of dextrose given daily through a continuous eye lavage unit has been beneficial, in conjunction with the usual medication given in severe chemical burns of the eye.[4]

Thermal burns

Thermal burns may be due to either flame or external contact and are similar, pathologically, although the flame usually just singes the lashes and lids unless the heat is intense and prolonged. The contact burn involves the eyes directly by the splashing of

drops or particles of hot substances into the eye, such as hot lead, tar, water, ashes.

Treatment depends on the degree of injury. Superficial burns will require only protection from contamination and local antibiotics. Whole thickness burns of the lids require a new covering with grafted skin and tarsorrhaphies between the upper and lower lids to counteract the vertical contractures that can occur in the healing processes of deep burns of the eyelids. The burned areas must also be cleansed of all foreign material. In severe burns of the eyeball and cornea, a cycloplegic eye drop is used to relieve ciliary spasm and 0.5 percent Pontocaine is administered to relieve local pain so that examination and treatment can be carried out. Local antibiotic ophthalmic drops and ointments are used, as well. The earlier treatment is carried out, the better the prognosis.

Contusions

Superficial contusions may only involve the eyelids, resulting in the common "black eye" appearance due to hemorrhage into the tissues of the lid. Application of cold packs for 20 minutes, 4 times a day for 2 days usually is adequate therapy, followed by warm packs, 4 times a day thereafter. If marked ecchymosis of the lids occurs, oral administration of a proteolytic enzyme, such as Ananase, may be helpful.

In moderately severe contusions, the anterior segment of the eye may show: (1) traumatic mydriasis (dilatation of the pupil), (2) hyphemia (blood in the anterior chamber, note the blood fluid level at the lower part of the cornea in Figure 27–8), (3) small peripheral iris tears or larger tears with separation of the iris from its root (iridodialysis, as illustrated in Figure 27–9) and (4) punctate lens opacities and iridodenesis (a tremulous iris due to posterior dislocation of the lens, thus removing the support of the lens to the posterior iris surface). The posterior segment in moderate contusions may show retinal edema without hemorrhage, choroidal tears or ruptures and macular changes including edema and holes.

Severe contusions involve the eyeball and the orbital bones. Any impact against the eyelids and the eye by blunt force, whether it be a door knob or a flying object, can cause a contusion of the eye. Patients with severe contusions should be x-rayed to rule out fractures of the orbital bones and intraocular foreign bodies. In very severe contusions, clinical manifestations of intraocular hemorrhage may occur, including: (1) anterior chamber hyphemia, (2) hemorrhage in the retina and the vitreous body or both, (3) cataract (opacification of the lens), (4) iris tears and (5) gross detachments of the choroid and retina.

Contusions of the eyeball, by their serious nature, demand immediate and proper treatment, which includes admission to the hospital, sedation, binocular eye pads, absolute bedrest (with elevation of the head if hyphemia or vitreal hemorrhage is present) and care by an ophthalmologist.

Whenever a patient arrives in the emergency department with a history of blunt trauma to the ocular region, he should be considered to have a serious injury until all the previously listed serious ocular lesions have been ruled out. For example, a patient with hyphemia, even without signs of severe ocular trauma, is considered to be in serious condition, since recurrent hemorrhages, absolute glaucoma and eventual blindness are real possibilities. The nurse must always be on the lookout for these potentially blinding injuries.

Perforating ocular wounds

Perforating ocular wounds are more common in children and in victims of automobile accidents. Industrial wounds have been greatly reduced through safety programs. Perforations or ruptures of the globe can be seen grossly on examination by lacerations or cuts on the eyeball, with pigment protruding or showing in the lips of the wound (see Figure 27–10). If the cornea is perforated, the iris is nearly always prolapsed (Figure 27–11). It may even appear to be a foreign body, since it is black. The nurse must never try to remove it or wipe it away. She must also be sure not to press on the globe, since this may cause further injury.

If a perforation is suspected, both eyes are bandaged and no medications are instilled. The patient must be admitted to the hospital for complete examination, evaluation and repair under general anesthesia by an ophthalmologist. More damage, such as severe hemorrhage and increase in tissue prolapse, can be produced in an excited child or adult with marked blepharospasm by trying to examine the eye further after a perforation is seen or is reasonably suspected from the ocular signs.

Blow-out fractures of the orbit

A blow-out fracture of the orbit is caused by a sudden increase in intra-orbital hydraulic pressure, resulting from the application of a traumatic force over the orbital area, such as a fist or baseball. The eye and orbital contents are compressed into the orbit, an essentially closed area. If the force is great enough, either the eye will rupture or the very thin orbital floor (one mm. or less thick) will break and blow out into the maxillary sinus. The compressed orbital contents then herniate into the maxillary sinus. If a patient presents with a history and signs of such an injury and with symptoms of double vision, a blow-out fracture must be considered first. Special radiological studies must be made and consultation with an ophthalmologist obtained. Repair can be done as late as 5 to 7 days after injury, allowing time for an adequate and thorough workup and diagnosis.

Subconjunctival ocular hemorrhage

A common ocular problem, which is also very alarming to the patient, is a subconjunctival hemorrhage on the eyeball (see Figure 27–12). The conjunctiva, which lines the eyelids and covers the eyeball, is transparent and not firmly attached to the eyeball. A small hemorrhage appears bright red below the conjunctiva. Usually it is a benign, innocuous entity. Rarely, it can be serious when the hemorrhage occurs after a head injury.

Treatment for the common benign subconjunctival hemorrhage is reassurance for the patient that the condition is not serious and that his vision will not be affected.

Conjunctivitis

Conjunctivitis is commonly seen in the emergency department. The conjunctival lining of the lids is usually inflamed, and a purulent or mucopurulent discharge is present in bacterial conjunctivitis. It can also be of a viral, fungal, chemical or allergic etiology, with different signs and symptoms in each type. Treatment consists of local antibiotic drops during the day and ointment at night.

Dendritic keratitis

Dendritic keratitis is a specific viral infection of the cornea. The eye is injected; photophobia is present; and a foreign body–like irritation is present. When the cornea is stained with a sterile fluorescein strip, a fine lesion can be seen, like the branching of a tree.

Steroids must never be given, as they lead to rapid progression and extension into the depth of the cornea, with permanent scarring and loss of vision. Patients with this condition should be referred to an ophthalmologist.

Lacerations of the eyelids

Lacerations through the skin of the eyelids, eyebrows and surrounding tissues should be first checked for associated ocular injury. When serious ocular injury is ruled out (as in Figure 27–13), the lid lacerations can be closed. Repair of lid lacerations not involving the lid margins, tear ducts (canaliculus) or levator (elevator) muscles of the upper lids is well within the province of the well-trained general surgeon.

An ophthalmologist should always be called for repair of lid lacerations involving the lid margins, tear ducts or levator muscles. Primary repair of these lacerations should be done as soon as an ophthalmologist and an operating suite are available. Emergency management consists of protecting the fresh wound with a sterile dressing and giving appropriate systemic supportive treatment.

Chalazion

A chalazion is an infection of one or more of the Meibomian glands in the eyelid. The patient usually complains of a swollen, erythematous and tender lid. Many times, in subacute cases, there will be a localized swelling, with point tenderness in the area of the lid involved.

To treat, very warm soaks are applied for one to 2 hours daily, and local antibiotic drops are instilled. If the chalazion does not improve and a chronic, small, localized swelling in the lid forms, the patient is referred to an ophthalmologist for surgical treatment.

Acute glaucoma and iritis

Acute glaucoma or iritis (iridocyclitis) must be ruled out in a patient with acute severe pain in the eye and around the brow region. The eyeball is usually red and appears very inflamed in both conditions. The following observations are useful in distinguishing the 2 conditions.

In glaucoma, the cornea is steamy and with tactile tension (finger tension on the eyeball) feels hard; the pupil is mid-dilated, the vision is poor; and the onset is usually sudden. In iritis, the cornea may be slightly hazy, with a loss of luster, but is not steamy; the tactile tension is normal or lower than normal; the pupil is small (miotic, constricted); the vision is fair; extreme photophobia (sensitivity to light) is present; and the onset is usually gradual. In both glaucoma and iritis, the patient must be referred to an ophthalmologist for care. In both conditions, the affliction is bilateral.

Medical management of acute glaucoma consists of constricting the pupil with a miotic, such as pilocarpine, giving acetazolamide (Diamox) or other carbonic-anhydrase inhibitors (which act directly on the ciliary body) and intravenous mannitol if necessary. Oral or injectable medication may be needed for pain. Surgery may be indicated in some patients, to provide a new outflow channel for intraocular fluid.

In iritis, the pupil must be dilated to prevent scarring and adhesions. A mydriatic, such as phenylephrine hydrochloride (Neo-Synephrine) ophthalmic drops is useful for this purpose. Cycloplegic drops are given concurrently, and oral pain medication may be prescribed. Photophobia can be relieved in part by dark glasses, a good idea whenever mydriatic drops are instilled. A complete medical workup is needed to determine and treat the underlying cause.

SUMMARY

The following list summarizes the important considerations involved in nursing care of the patient with ocular injuries.

(1) Local ocular steroids should not be used in an emergency department, unless prescribed by an ophthalmologist. They should never be included on an eye tray. They can promote bacterial, viral and yeast infections, as well as induce glaucoma in susceptible patients.

(2) For all chemical burns, the eye must be irrigated immediately, copiously and sufficiently long (10 to 15 minutes) with ordinary tap water, unless normal saline or sterile ocular irrigating solutions are immediately available.

(3) Ophthalmic antibiotic drops and ointments that should be available in an emergency department are listed in Table 27–1. It must be remembered that ophthalmic ointments are *never* interchangeable with topical ointments. The mydriatics and cyclopegics are topically applied autonomic drugs which produce mydriasis (pupillary dilatation) and cycloplegia (paralysis of accommodation), respectively. The miotics serve to constrict the pupil.

(4) To prevent cross-contamination, it is important that a new sterile bottle of drops or a new tube of ointment be used for each patient. If the drops or ointment are not given to the treated patient to take home, they should be discarded.

(5) Sterile fluorescein strips, such as Fluor-I-Strips, are preferable to fluorescein liquid drops for staining the eyes because of the danger of pyocyaneous contamination of fluorescein eyedrop bottles on treatment trays in the emergency department. Pyocyaneous infection can cause a rapid fulminating infection, enophthalmitis and loss of the eye. If fluorescein drops are used, the bottle must be discarded after each use and a new sterile vial of fluorescein opened for each patient.

(6) In all eye injuries, the patient is usually frightened, apprehensive, in pain and keeping his eyes closed tightly as a defense mechanism. He needs and must have reassurance, very gentle care and manipulation and often local anesthetic drops to permit nontraumatic inspection of the injured eye. The nurse must never press against the eyeball at any time during the examination. It is important to be gentle and reassuring.

TABLE 27–1   OCULAR MEDICATIONS IN THE EMERGENCY DEPARTMENT

Drug type	Drug generic name	Drug trade name and dose
Common mydriatics		
(1) Sympathomimetic ophthalmic solutions	Phenylephrine	Neo-Synephrine, 10%
	Epinephrine	Adrenalin, 1:1,000
	Hydroxyamphetamine	Paredrine Hydrobromide, 1%
	Ephedrine	Ephedrine, 5%
(2) Parasympatholytic ophthalmic solutions (cycloplegics)	Atropine	Isopto Atropine, 0.25% to 0.5%, 1%, 2%
	Homatropine	Homatropine Hydrobromide, 1% to 5%, Isopto Homatropine, 2%, 5%
	Hyoscine (Scopolamine)	Hyoscine (Scopolamine), 0.25% to 0.5%
	Cyclopentolate	Cyclogyl, 1%, 2%
	Tropicamide	Mydriacyl, 1%, 2%
Miotics		
(1) Parasympathomimetic ophthalmic solutions	Pilocarpine	Isopto Carpine, Pilocar, P. V. Carpine Liquifilm, 0.25% to 10%
	Carbachol	Isopto Carbachol, P.S. Carbachol Liquifilm, 0.25% to 3%
	Eserine (Physostigmine)	Eserine, 0.25% to 1%
	Neostigmine	Neostigmine, 3% to 5%

(7) *Every patient seen in the emergency department with trauma around the facial region requires a careful eye examination.* When all life-sustaining measures have been carried out, a careful inspection of the eye by the emergency nurse and physician, if present, will uncover any serious ocular injuries. Institution of prompt and proper treatment will result in saving the sight of many an injured eye.

(8) A patient who has had an anesthetic instilled should have that eye patched until the effects of the anesthetic wear off. This precaution will protect the eye from foreign body invasion or further trauma. A patient should never be given an anesthetic for outpatient use. Examples of anesthetics are tetracaine, proparacaine hydrochloride (Ophthaine), ophthetic and butacaine (Butyn).

(9) Drops are properly instilled by having the patient assume a supine or a head-back position while sitting. The patient is instructed to look up while the nurse, using a small piece of gauze, everts the lower eyelid, exposing the conjunctival sac. The medication is dropped in the conjunctival sac. Any excess splashed onto the face by reflex blinking is removed by the gauze. An ointment is applied similarly, spreading it from the inner to outer canthus of the conjunctival sac.

(10) The eyes, being man's windows to the world, are important, indeed. Even though an injury to the eye may appear innocuous and nonacute, the very importance of the eyes mandates careful assessment and accurate, complete treatment. Teamwork among alert, well-trained emergency nurses and physicians and the ophthalmologist is imperative for the preservation of sight in patients with ocular injuries.

BIBLIOGRAPHY

(1) Alexander, M., and Brown, M.: "Physical Examination . . . the Eye," *Nursing '73,* 3 (December 1973):41–46.

(2) Dockery, R. W.: "Role of the Ophthalmologist in Acute Trauma," *Journal of the Kentucky Medical Association,* 56 (May 1958):449–452.

(3) Duke-Elder, S.: *Textbook of Ophthalmology,* ed. 6 (Saint Louis: C. V. Mosby Company, 1954).

(4) Forberg, P. K., and Byers, L. W.: "Chemical Mace: A Non-Lethal Weapon," *Journal of Trauma,* 9 (April 1969): 339–342.

(5) Keeney, A. H.: "Ocular Injuries in Automobile Accidents," *Symposium on Industrial and Traumatic Ocular Injuries* (New Orleans: New Orleans Academy of Ophthalmology, 1963).

(6) Morgan, L. B.: "A New Therapeutic Scleral Lens," *Rocky Mountain Medical Journal,* 68 (1971):26.

(7) _____: "Plastic Scleral Lens Helps to End Pain in Injured Eyes and Promotes Healing," *Journal of the American Medical Association,* 214 (1970):835.

(8) Weinstock, Frank: "Emergency Treatment of Eye Injuries," *American Journal of Nursing,* 71 (October 1971):1928–1931.

28

Dental emergencies

WILLIAM D. ZITER

In the past decade the distribution of health services in America has clearly been altered. The community hospital, once a storehouse for the hopelessly ill and a treatment center for patients with acute medical or surgical problems, has gradually become a truly comprehensive community health facility.[4] As the center of the community's health resources and services, the hospital seeks to advance the care of the individual as a complete being living in a complex society, taking into account all influences on general health; that is, *total health care*.

The obvious relationship between oral/dental health and health in general indicates without question that dentistry plays an important part in a total health plan and should become an integral part of the operation of all community and general hospitals. Naturally, as dental services become available, the emergency department will be faced with an increasing number of patients whose complaints will be primarily dental in origin. It is hoped that the following information will serve to orient emergency department nurses in behalf of these patients.

The dental patient rarely presents to the emergency department with an acute, life-threatening emergency. Occasionally, a patient with serious post-operative hemorrhage is encountered, and uncommonly a patient with a compromised airway as the result of extension of dental infection is seen, but these situations represent rare exceptions. More commonly, dental patients present with a variety of more routine complaints, such as pain and/or swelling, related to trauma, oral infection or previous dental therapy; and although these conditions are not immediately dangerous, they may be of considerable distress to the patient and thus deserve prompt, considerate attention.

It should be noted that the indicated emergency therapy is generally *not* the definitive treatment. Rather, it usually consists of simple procedures that can be carried out quickly to alleviate the patient's immediate problem until a definite diagnosis can be made and a specific treatment plan instituted. With a small amount of indoctrination and experience, emergency nurses can manage many of these emergency measures.

GENERAL CONSIDERATIONS

When a patient presents with a dental complaint, it is important to obtain as much information as possible about the patient's previous dental experience, in addition to the standard medical history. It should be obvious that there is a great variety of dental problems an emergency department could be faced with. It is reasonable to assume, therefore, that information regarding the type and extent of treatment, if any, the patient has previously undergone could be extremely helpful in arriving at a working diagnosis of the problem at hand. This is particularly true when dental procedures have been recently performed. Most patients are well aware of the type of treatment that has been carried out and in many instances can provide valuable insights to the examining emergency personnel.

If sophisticated dental treatment, such as extensive bridgework or multiple root canal procedures, has been undertaken, it is doubtful whether untrained personnel will be able to provide other than symptomatic treatment without potentially doing more harm than good. In such instances, immediate dental consultation is advisable. Conversely, patients with a toothache who have never been to a dentist and have obvious uncomplicated dental caries probably require only systemic analgesics as emergency therapy. Subsequent referral to the proper clinic or office for definitive treatment would then be in order.

To properly evaluate dental patients, however, in addition to the dental history, a thorough, carefully performed oral examination is mandatory. In order to accurately perform this exam, it is necessary to have only a very small amount of special equipment, including a dental chair, or a substitute, with a headrest; a source of light that can be focused directly into the mouth, such as a dental light or headlight; an adequate source of suction; and a mouth mirror. The remaining prerequisites include 20/20 vision, probing fingers and a high degree of suspicion.

The examination of the mouth itself must be detailed and systematic. Each examiner should develop his or her own approach, to be followed each time as a routine, so that no portion of the exam will be omitted. All removable dental appliances, such as complete dentures or removable partial dentures, should be taken out of the mouth before the examination. Inspection and/or palpation of the lips, the labial and buccal mucosa, the hard and soft palates, the tonsillar regions, the floor of the mouth, the tongue, the gingivae and the teeth must be standard procedure. The examiner should note changes in color, texture, size, position and function of these organs, as well as any indication of overt pathology or trauma. Any abnormal findings should be recorded, and the information revealed to the dentist who will ultimately manage the case.

It is particularly important to be thorough when examining a patient who has received oral trauma or has sustained multiple trauma, including trauma to the oral region. Hidden contusions or lacerations, especially of the tongue, floor of the mouth or oropharyngeal region, could lead to difficulty in breathing or swallowing or to unwarranted blood loss. In addition, foreign particles, such as detached teeth or pieces of teeth, parts of dentures or dental restorations, blood clots and other debris, represent a potential hazard to the airway, particularly in a comatose or semicomatose patient. They should be actively sought and, when found, carefully removed. A good source of light and appropriate suction will aid immeasurably in this task.

The only study adjunct to history and physical examination commonly used in oral diagnosis is the radiograph. Analysis of the blood or urine and the use of sophisticated electronic equipment is of lesser value in the management of patients with dental emergencies. Therefore, in most cases, when the patient's complaints are related to the teeth or other hard structures of the head and neck, radiographs will be desirable and perhaps should be ordered prior to consultation. Although dental x-rays, such as the periapical and occlusal views, are not routinely taken by medical radiologists, the standard facial series will probably be of value. In the future, it is hoped that dental radiographs will also be available in emergency departments, so that more accurate assessment of the teeth and jaws can be made.

The remainder of the material in this chapter applies to specific problems that may be seen by emergency department personnel. In order to simplify matters, they will be considered under 7 main headings:

(1) Pain.
(2) Hemorrhage.
(3) Swelling.
(4) Reactions to local anesthesia.
(5) Trauma to the face, mouth and jaws.
(6) Dislocation of the temporomandibular joint.
(7) Acute oral lesions.

Invariably, material will overlap from one category to another. It is hoped, however, that this classification will serve to reduce confusion.

PAIN

Pain is, of course, the most common complaint of dental patients who present to the emergency department of a hospital. The pain is usually related to decayed teeth but may also reflect trauma or pathology in adjacent structures. Because of the wide variety of conditions that are manifest in the oral cavity as pain and because of the frequency of referred pain, the differential diagnosis in these circumstances is often quite confusing and occasionally very difficult. General descriptions of the more common presenting problems follow.

Odontalgia

Almost everyone has experienced the distress and discomfort of a toothache and can appreciate why patients sometimes appear in misery at the hospital emergency department in the middle of the night. The usual etiology is dental caries, a disease of the calcified tissues of the teeth, which is unique in respect to all other diseases in that it is *unhealing* and irreversible.[15]

Clinically, in its early stages, dental caries

cause the enamel of the crown of the tooth to appear opaque and chalky white. As the process progresses, the lesion discolors to brown or black, and the enamel is soft. As the enamel is completely destroyed, a visible cavity occurs, which has an opaque or whitish periphery. The base of the cavity is composed of brownish, soft, leathery material.

When the etiology is dental caries, the toothache, in its early stages, is best described as a sharp, shooting pain that persists for a short time after removal of the precipitating stimulus. Later, when damage to the pulp of the tooth is irreversible, the pain becomes more intense and is persistent and more throbbing in character. Heat generally aggravates the pain, whereas cold may relieve it.

The pain can often be accurately localized by the patient to a single offender, but in many instances localization is not possible. Referred pain is very common when dealing with pulpal disease, and the patient may even have difficulty differentiating which jaw the pain is emanating from. At this time, however, the tooth is usually quite sensitive when percussed with a metal instrument, such as the handle of a mouth mirror. When this simple test is positive, it is evidence of probable irreversible pulp damage, and it is likely that endodontic therapy or extraction of the tooth will be indicated.

Toothaches can also be the direct result of inflammation of the gingivae, or gums, a condition which is referred to as periodontal disease. In this chronic disease, the supporting structures of the teeth, both hard and soft tissues, are progressively destroyed. This is a consequence of the irritation of the periodontal tissues by local factors, such as calculus or tartar, and by the action of certain bacteria which accumulate on the teeth in a soft, filmy substance, referred to as dental plaque.

Clinically, periodontal disease is characterized by sore, reddened, edematous gingival tissues, which bleed freely and easily on provocation. The examiner may also note a purulent exudate around affected teeth, which often become quite loose in the later stages of the disease. "Bleeding gums" and "loose teeth" are almost as common presenting complaints as dental pain.

Although periodontal disease is not always painful, certain periodontal conditions can cause distress. This type of pain can be differentiated from pulpal pain by its character, which is usually dull and gnawing, as compared to the sharp, pulsating pain seen in pulpitis. This is because the inflammation is not confined in any unyielding pulp chamber.[10] The discomfort of periodontal disease is often intensified during function, due to irritation of the tissues by the forceful wedging of food, which results in shifting of mobile teeth.[5] Localization of pain here is much more accurate; the patient can usually point to the etiology of the distress immediately, and no other diagnostic effort is required.[2]

Patients who are in discomfort as the result of recent dental therapy will be also seen periodically. Any one of a number of procedures performed in the dental office can produce lingering oral pain. This list includes dental restorations (fillings), bridges, dentures, root canal or periodontic therapy, surgery, even orthodontic treatment. In such cases, conservative measures should be adopted until the patient's dentist can be contacted.

The management of patients with uncomplicated dental pain in the hospital emergency department is usually quite elementary. In almost all such cases, the definitive treatment that is indicated will require specialized, often sophisticated equipment that is available only in the dental office. Even an experienced dentist will be able to do very little in an emergency department setting. A simple, conservative approach is therefore advocated, consisting primarily of the administration or prescription of systemic analgesics to control the pain until the patient can be seen and evaluated in the proper clinic or office environment.

The drugs that are usually used for pain relief are mild- or moderate-strength narcotics, such as codeine or meperidine, in appropriate doses. The topical administration of commercially prepared gels or drops is usually ineffective, and the topical administration of mild over-the-counter analgesics, such as aspirin, is definitely contraindicated.

If the etiology of the pain is dental caries, and an obvious cavity is present, a sedative dressing, such as zinc oxide and eugenol, can be carefully placed into the cavity and may be successful in controlling the discomfort until definitive treatment can be undertaken. Naturally, common sense instructions regarding oral hygiene, limited activity, and abstention from hot, cold or sweet foodstuffs or beverages should be stressed.

Postsurgical pain

Almost every surgical procedure is associated with some postoperative distress. Oral surgery is no exception; in fact, due to the extremely sensitive nature of the oral area, even minor procedures, such as simple extractions, may produce marked discomfort. The problem is treated with intermittent cold applications to the surgical site during the first 24 hours postoperatively and by the administration of one of the analgesic drugs mentioned above. This simple regimen is followed even when extensive oral surgical procedures, such as the removal of impacted teeth, have been performed.

There is one postsurgical problem that warrants special management. This syndrome is correctly termed alveolar osteitis but is commonly referred to as a "dry socket." The etiology of this condition is unknown, and although it can be seen following the removal of any tooth, the vast majority of cases follow surgical removal of mandibular third molars (wisdom teeth). Signs and symptoms include severe throbbing pain, often radiating to the ear, which classically begins 2 to 4 days after surgery. The mucosa adjacent to the socket usually appears normal, but the blood clot within the socket is necrotic or absent. The patient complains of a foul taste in his or her mouth, and a fetid odor to the breath is apparent. Vital signs, including temperature, are generally normal.

Treatment of an alveolar osteitis includes inspection of the wound for the presence of a foreign body, irrigation of the socket with a warm isotonic saline solution and careful placement of a medicated dressing into the unprotected alveolus. The dressing usually consists of a length of sterile iodoform gauze, with the medication applied in the form of a paste. The medications recommended include anodynes (eugenol or guaiacol), topical anesthetics (butacaine or benzocaine) and antiseptics (iodine). The socket should not be curetted. Antibiotics are not indicated, unless concomitant systemic infection exists. Systemic analgesics may be considered, depending on the severity of the pain, but generally the local dressing is more effective than analgesics in controlling the pain of alveolar osteitis.

Tooth eruption

Pain related to tooth eruption, with one exception, is a problem of very young children. The pain is frequently accompanied by agitation, a slight elevation of the temperature and, occasionally, rhinitis or nasal discharge. Intraorally, the tissues over the erupting tooth are tender and appear reddened and edematous.

Immediate management of this situation includes application of a topical anesthetic and gentle massage to the overlying tissues. Mild systemic analgesics may be prescribed. The parent should then be instructed to have the child bite on a teething ring to encourage eruption through the mucous membrane, but the tissues should never be incised, unless an eruption cyst is present, as surgery may predispose to secondary infection.[11]

The only eruption problem seen in adults involves the eruption of the third molar teeth (wisdom teeth), around the ages of 18 to 20. The clinical situation is termed "pericoronitis" and is predominately related to the mandibular third molars. The soft tissues around the crown of the partially erupted tooth are red and inflamed, and suppuration may be seen under the gingival flap. The infection may spread anteriorly and localize as a fluctuant area opposite the first or second molar or it can spread posteriorly into the masticator space and cause moderate muscle trismus. Tender submandibular lymphadenopathy may also be seen.

The immediate management of this clinical problem includes irrigation under the pericoronal flap with a warm isotonic saline solution to remove accumulated debris and giving instructions to the patient to continue warm saline mouth rinses 4 to 6 times each day. Analgesics should be considered, and if a vestibular abscess is present, it should be drained. Antibiotic therapy is indicated only when there is evidence that the infection is spreading (lymphadenopathy or trismus), or when significant suppuration is present. Ultimately, when the acute symptoms subside and when infection has been controlled, definitive treatment, usually extraction, can be considered.

Pain of maxillary sinus origin

A brief discussion of maxillary sinusitis is included here, because pain associated with infection in the sinus is very often referred to the maxillary teeth in the vicinity and may confuse the clinical picture. Anatomically, the maxillary bicuspids and molars are intimately related to the antrum. Indeed, in many instances, the roots of these teeth project into the sinus, and the 2 are then separated by only a thin lamina of bone. It is common sense to assume that pathology in one area might well be confused with disease in the other.

Maxillary sinusitis is characterized by a continuous throbbing ache, which is mainly in the infraorbital region, is often bilateral and may intensify on postural change. The pain can radiate to the maxillary posterior teeth, the cheek and the frontal region. The infraorbital area is often quite tender when palpated.

The significance of this entity is that it tends to confuse the differential diagnosis of facial pain. The patient is certain that his teeth are the source of his problems, so much so that a great many perfectly good teeth have been sacrificed unnecessarily and unwillingly in a fruitless attempt to alleviate the patient's distress. It is thus important to consider maxillary sinusitis as a potential etiology whenever the presenting complaint is pain in the maxillary posterior teeth. This is particularly important when there is no obvious dental pathology. Once the diagnosis of maxillary sinusitis has been established, the patient should be given systemic antibiotics and analgesics and referred to an otolaryngologist for definitive care.

Pain in the temporomandibular joint area

Patients occasionally present to the emergency department complaining of diffuse pain in the ear and in the preauricular area. Once the presence of pathology in the ear has been ruled out, the examiner should consider the temporomandibular joint and the associated masticatory muscles as potential sources of difficulty. The classical presenting symptoms of this pain dysfunction syndrome include a continuous, dull, diffuse ache in the preauricular region. The pain is usually unilateral, may intensify upon mandibular movement, such as during mastication, and may be referred to the ear, the temporal region or the angle of the mandible.

The etiology of this clinical problem may be related to definitive pathology within the temporomandibular joint. Traumatic, degenerative and rheumatoid changes have been reported.[11] A careful history and precise radiographs will aid in establishing the diagnosis of disease within the joint proper. In such cases, initial management would consist of the administration of systemic analgesics, the application of moist heat to the affected area and restriction to a soft diet.

More commonly, the underlying cause of this clinical syndrome is spasm in one or more of the muscles of mastication. This problem is seen predominantly in women, is related to psychological stress and is usually associated with some hyperactivity of the masticatory muscles, such as clenching or bruxing. The term presently used to describe this symptom complex is the myofascial pain dysfunction (M.P.D.) syndrome. Symptoms, in addition to those discussed above, include tenderness on palpation of one or more of the muscles of mastication and pain that is either worse on arising in the morning or mild in the morning and gradually worsening as the day progresses. The patient is often unable to open his mouth widely, and the mandible may deviate on opening. Radiographs of the joint are consistently normal.

Emergency department management of the M.P.D. syndrome, in addition to moist heat, soft diet and analgesics, includes the administration of drugs, such as diazepam, to relieve tension and anxiety and provide muscle relaxation.

Trigeminal neuralgia

Neuralgias are disturbances of nerves, characterized by paroxysmal pain which extends along the course of the impaired nerve trunk. The pain is usually felt in the terminal peripheral branches of the nerve trunk affected and follows precise anatomical somatic pain pathways. Many varieties of neuralgia have been distinguished, primarily according to the part of the body that is affected. The facial area is no exception, and several facial neuralgias have been described. All are rare, but when they do occur, they are the cause of great distress to the patient and a source of much consternation to the diagnostician. Of the facial neuralgias, the most common and most important is trigeminal neuralgia.

Trigeminal neuralgia, or tic douloureux, is an idiopathic disease most commonly seen in middle-aged and older people. It involves the trigeminal nerve, which supplies the teeth, jaws, face and associated structures, and is characterized by excruciating, paroxysmal, lancinating pain, lasting seconds or minutes. The initiation of the distress is classically related to stimulation of a particular area of the face, that is, a trigger zone. The pain is unilateral in any one paroxysm, is confined to one or more of the branches of the trigeminal nerve and is associated with no objective sensory loss.[17] The intermissions between paroxysms are generally pain-free.[2]

The treatment of trigeminal neuralgia has

been extremely varied over the years, and success has not been outstanding. Peripheral and central injections of absolute alcohol have been performed with modest success, as has peripheral surgery. Neurosurgical sectioning of the trigeminal sensory root by any of a number of techniques is recognized by many surgeons as the treatment of choice when attempting a permanent cure.[15] Recently the use of anticonvulsant medications, such as carbamazepine, has been advocated to control the paroxysms rather than destroy the nerve. Success with this approach has been promising, but serious side effects have been reported following prolonged use of these drugs.

Unfortunately, there seems to be no effective emergency treatment for this condition. Patients who report to the emergency department during or just after a bout of pain can only be comforted verbally and directed to where a definitive workup can begin. Systemic analgesics, sedatives and tranquilizers seem to be of little value.[11]

Idiopathic pain

Many patients present for treatment complaining of pain for which no immediate cause is apparent. In most instances, the complaint is of long duration, although from the patient's standpoint it has now become so severe or so intolerable it is considered an emergency. Despite careful search no pathology can be discovered; often the pain does not even follow basic anatomic pathways.

For such persons, an analgesic drug plus a sedative or tranquilizer may provide some comfort during the time necessary for establishing a diagnosis and starting definitive treatment.

HEMORRHAGE

Intraoral hemorrhage is a relatively common occurrence, which may follow a surgical procedure or a traumatic accident. When it is encountered, it represents an "honest" emergency, which should be managed quickly and efficiently. The majority of patients who present in pain can be delayed a reasonable period of time prior to definitive treatment, provided adequate systemic analgesics are administered, but the patient with bleeding cannot wait. If simple emergency measures are not effective in controlling the hemorrhage, a dental consultant should be called immediately.

Active hemorrhage in any region of the body is extremely disconcerting to essentially all patients. Bleeding in the mouth, however, is even more likely to produce marked anxiety, for several reasons. The patient cannot see where the blood is coming from and, therefore, tends to exaggerate the extent of the blood loss. Also, the hemorrhage is usually mixed with large volumes of saliva, again distorting the true clinical picture.

Swallowing of some blood is unavoidable, and unfortunately even a modest amount creates distressing nausea and sometimes vomiting. Patients often attempt to clear the mouth through constant expectoration, which not only aggravates the hemorrhage but adds to the thought that blood loss may be reaching serious proportions. The end result is a patient who may be exceedingly apprehensive, a situation which leads to an increase in blood pressure and heart rate, which in turn tends to promote further hemorrhage.

The emergency management of patients with oral bleeding is not complicated. Once the patient has been reassured, the initial effort should be directed toward application of pressure. Intraoral bleeders can rarely be clamped and tied, and electrocoagulation is of little value. Therefore, time and effort should not be wasted in behalf of these techniques. Rather, all efforts should be extended toward the careful application of pressure directly onto the bleeding site. This is best accomplished by having the patient bite firmly on a large gauze pad. To be effective, however, the gauze must be precisely placed.

First, using adequate light and suction, the mouth should be carefully cleaned of blood, saliva, blood clots and other debris. Then, the exact source of the bleeding can be determined and the gauze pad accurately placed. Firm pressure should be maintained for 20 to 30 minutes while the patient rests comfortably. If, at the end of the prescribed period of time, the bleeding has been controlled, the patient should sit quietly for an additional 10 minutes before being dismissed, in order to determine if the bleeding will reoccur. If the above regimen is not effective in controlling the hemorrhage, a dentist should be called immediately, who would then under local anesthesia undertake specific measures to control the bleeding. These include the use of hemostatic agents, such as oxidized cellulose, and the placement of sutures.

In addition to directing efforts toward the application of pressure, emergency department personnel should consider the patient's general condition, as well. Vital signs should be taken and recorded, and if the patient shows signs of shock, immediate medical assistance should be obtained. It is extremely uncommon for hypovolemic shock to result from intraoral bleeding, but it has happened.

If possible, a brief medical history should be taken to determine whether a systemic factor is contributing to the bleeding problem. Previous difficulty with excessive bleeding, a history of a blood dyscrasia, liver disease, anticoagulant therapy and salicylate therapy are all factors that could seriously complicate oral surgery or facial trauma. If medical problems such as these do exist, medical consultation should be obtained.

SWELLING

The diagnosis of tumors or swellings which affect the soft tissues of the face and mouth is often difficult because of the variety of lesions that manifest themselves in that area. Certainly the swellings most commonly seen in emergency departments are related to bacterial infections, but in order to arrive at an accurate diagnosis, differential diagnosis must include trauma and previous surgery, tumors, systemic diseases, allergies, salivary gland obstructions and subcutaneous emphysema, in addition to infections.

The principal swellings which affect the face and neck are considered below. Characteristic features and initial management are emphasized.

Infections

Infections that manifest in and about the face and mouth can be produced by a wide variety of bacterial, viral and mycotic organisms. Diseases such as tuberculosis, syphilis, cat scratch fever, actinomycosis and many more can produce infectious swellings and are occasionally encountered in the emergency department. However, the vast majority of swellings related to infections are the direct result of dental pathology, that is, dental caries or periodontal disease.

Acute alveolar abscess

The acutely infected tooth, or acute alveolar abscess, is one of the most common dental emergencies encountered. These abscesses are related to a nonvital or degenerative pulp, usually the result of advanced dental caries, and are characterized clinically by a swollen face, an elevated temperature and varying amounts of pain. The swelling has a relatively distinct outline, and fluctuation can often be elicited. The patient usually has spent one or more sleepless nights, is dehydrated and may have eaten little since the onset of the condition. Local examination reveals an extremely tender tooth, which the patient can identify with precision.

Initial management of the acute alveolar abscess will vary widely, depending on the individual case. Consideration should be given to antibiotic therapy, incision and drainage and supportive care.

Systemic antibiotics should be administered if the patient exhibits signs of toxicity, such as malaise, elevated temperature or leukocytosis. The overwhelming drug of choice for odontogenic infections is penicillin.

The drug is exceedingly effective when administered orally in appropriate doses and is associated with very few side effects. For patients who are allergic to penicillin, erythromycin may be substituted. If the patient is nontoxic and the infection is localized, antibiotics may be omitted.

Incision and drainage, with placement of an appropriate sterile drain, should be considered in every case of alveolar abscess where fluctuance is present, denoting an underlying collection of pus. The incision and drainage is indicated whether the patient is toxic or not and may be carried out intraorally or extraorally, as indicated. It may or may not be accompanied by extraction of the offending tooth. The procedure should be performed as quickly as is reasonable, because the problem will not resolve on antibiotics alone, regardless of the dose. Cultures of the exudate should, of course, be taken and sent to the laboratory for examination.

Supportive therapy is critical in managing patients with dental infections. Good nursing care is as important as the pharmacological or surgical phases of treatment. However, since most patients with dental infections are treated on an outpatient basis, verbal instructions regarding home care must be relied on and, therefore, should be thorough, clearly presented and include the following considerations.

(1) Complete rest is necessary.
(2) Analgesics and sedatives will relieve pain and anxiety and promote sleep.
(3) Fluids in several forms should be administered to reverse dehydration.

In severe cases, input-output records should be kept. Adequate nourishment is essential and may be given in liquid or soft form if required. Liquid high protein dietary supplements may be beneficial.

Cellulitis

The above description of an acute alveolar abscess is obviously based on the classical definition of an abscess, which states that it is a localized collection of pus. The process remains localized because the defensive factors in the region are capable of walling off the infection and preventing it from spreading.[14] Occasionally, the bacterial infection is overwhelming, either because the bacteria are extremely virulent or because the resistance of the host is impaired. The bacterial invasion under these circumstances is unimpeded as it progresses through surrounding tissues to areas remote from the original site of infection. The process is then termed a "cellulitis."

An acute cellulitis of dental origin is usually confined to the general area of the jaws. The tissues become grossly edematous and firm to palpation. The swelling is diffuse and not sharply demarcated, and no fluctuation is noted. At this stage, suppuration has not occurred.

The patient may show a severe systemic reaction to the infection. The temperature is usually elevated, the white count is increased and the differential count may "shift to the left." The sedimentation rate is also increased, and the pulse rate is accelerated. The fluid and electrolyte balance may be changed, and the patient frequently experiences weakness and malaise. In short, this is an acutely ill patient.

The treatment of an acute facial cellulitis involves the same basic principles as previously enumerated but emphasizes some special considerations. Hospitalization may be indicated. Antibiotic therapy should be aggressive, utilizing parenterally administered drugs. Supportive care must be meticulous. Incision and drainage should be considered in each case but may not be indicated in every case, as suppuration may never occur. Definitive surgery is generally postponed until the patient is nontoxic.

A special cellulitis is classically referred to as Ludwig's angina. This is best described as an overwhelming generalized septic cellulitis of the submandibular region.[14] This infection differs from other types of facial cellulitis in several ways.

Ludwig's angina

Ludwig's angina is a descending infection, spreading downward from the jaws toward the mediastinum, and is characterized by a board-like, brawny induration of the involved tissues. Three fascial spaces are involved bilaterally: submandibular, submental and sublingual. If the involvement is not bilateral, the infection is not considered a true Ludwig's angina.

Because of the massive involvement of the sublingual spaces, the floor of the mouth and tongue are markedly elevated toward the palate. This represents a significant threat to the patient's airway, and, therefore, all cases of suspected Ludwig's angina should be treated as distinct emergencies. The patient should be hospitalized and observed closely. Tracheostomy must be considered if there is the slightest hint of respiratory embarrassment. Massive antibiotic therapy, usually administered intravenously, is indicated. Despite the fact that the involved tissues are board-like, incision and drainage, performed intra-orally, may be productive. Nursing care should be as intense as with any other life-threatening emergency.

Postsurgical swelling

Postoperative edema following oral surgery is quite common. This is particularly true following the surgical removal of impacted teeth, where moderate facial swelling is the rule rather than the exception. Patients are generally warned of this occurrence, but occasionally one will become alarmed and present as an emergency.

Substantial facial edema, either unilateral or bilateral depending on the surgery, will be immediately apparent, and a history of recent surgery will be obtained. Although this situation is generally not serious, it is important to differentiate between postsurgical edema and a postoperative infection. Both entities will cause pain, swelling and limitation of func-

tion, but the infectious process will, in addition, be characterized by the classic signs of abscess or cellulitis previously discussed, including malaise, increased temperature, leukocytosis, fluctuation.

Management of this patient includes reassurance that the swelling is to be expected, that it may not reach its maximum until 48 to 72 hours following surgery and that it will resolve in 5 to 7 days. Intermittent cold applications to the operative site (30 minutes per hour) should be used during the first 24 hours after surgery to limit the degree of edema. After the first day, intermittent moist heat (30 minutes per hour) is used to increase circulation and aid in dissipation of the edema. Intraorally, heat is achieved by the use of hot isotonic saline rinses.

The various enzyme preparations and antihistamines suggested for the treatment of postoperative swelling should not be used routinely. Enzymatic agents do not prevent edema but rather redistribute the fluid over a wider area by breaking down connective tissue and fibrin barriers. Some degree of localized swelling may be a desirable physiological response to tissue injury; in addition, disturbance of the tissue barriers can predispose to the spread of infection.[11]

Salivary gland obstruction

Diseases of the salivary glands may affect an individual gland or may involve several at one time. Enlargement may be due to an inflammatory process, a degenerative process, a cyst, a neoplasm or the obstruction of a duct.[8] A brief discussion of salivary gland enlargement resulting from obstruction is included here, because it may appear quite similar to many dentally related conditions and, therefore, must be considered in the differential diagnosis of facial and oral swellings.

The location of the swelling is often helpful in making the diagnosis of major salivary gland enlargement. The parotid, submandibular and sublingual glands have distinct anatomic locations that are not easily confused.

Occasionally, however, an enlarged lymph node can be mistaken for a swollen submandibular gland.

When duct obstruction is present, it is related to a stone (sialolith), a mucous plug, cell debris or a foreign body. Obstruction is generally followed by a varying degree of infection, resulting in signs and symptoms including pain and swelling, which usually increase at mealtime, and the absence of salivary flow from the affected duct. Pus may be excreted if the gland and duct are milked, and signs of systemic involvement, such as an increased temperature, may also be noted.

Minor salivary gland obstructions can occasionally occur on the palate, cheek, lip or floor of the mouth. They are usually asymptomatic unless traumatized and should not be confused with intraoral swellings related to infected teeth.

If obstruction of a major salivary gland is suspected, the gland should be examined roentgenographically for the presence of a sialolith. Anteroposterior and lateral views are used for visualization of the parotid gland; an occlusal view is used for the sublingual gland and anterior extension and duct of the submandibular gland; and a lateral oblique view is used for the main portion of the submandibular gland.[13]

If a stone is present within the duct and is readily accessible and if the patient is having considerable discomfort, the surgical removal of the stone can be considered an emergency measure; consultation is urged. When the stone is within the gland or if the obstruction is due to other causes, the immediate treatment consists of analgesics for pain, belladonna drugs to diminish salivation and relieve the distension and a broad spectrum antibiotic to combat infection. The patient may then be referred for definitive workup.

Neoplasms

Neoplasia is a poorly understood biological phenomenon, which, in some instances, cannot be clearly differentiated from other processes or tissue reactions. While no precise definition of neoplasia exists, a neoplasm is often considered to be an independent, uncoordinated new growth of tissue which is potentially capable of unlimited proliferation and which does not regress following removal of the stimulus which produced the lesion.[15]

Neoplasms of the oral cavity and adjacent structures are important in the dental profession because of the role the dentist plays in the diagnosis and treatment of these lesions. While tumors do not make up a majority of the pathologic conditions seen in the dental office, they are of great significance, since they have the potential to jeopardize the life, health and well-being of the patient. For this reason, a brief description of serious neoplasms that may be discovered during oral examination follows.

Squamous cell carcinoma of the oral mucosa is a relatively common lesion, which comprises over 95 percent of oral malignancies and approximately 10 percent of all malignant tumors affecting the body. Because of its frequency of occurrence, clinical variability and potential danger, carcinoma must always be considered in the differential diagnosis of swellings and lesions of the oral cavity.

Clinically, in its early stages, epidermoid carcinoma presents as one of 3 general patterns: (1) a papillary or verrucous lesion, which is an exophytic growth; (2) an ulcerative type, which has a raised, indurated margin; or (3) a white, raised plaque, which represents a degeneration of the premalignant lesion leukoplakia.

As an oral cancer progresses, the pattern becomes more irregular, and surface trauma and infection invariably complicate the lesion. Oral carcinoma is easily traumatized, and hemorrhage of varying degrees is a relatively common sign. In larger lesions, tissue necrosis may be an obvious feature.

Symptoms of oral carcinoma are of little clinical significance. The lesions are not painful, unless ulcerated and infected and, in this condition, are not more painful than other oral ulcerations. Lesions of the tongue tend to cause some abnormality of function in this highly active and motile organ. The patient may complain of difficulty in normal speech, and the infiltration of the lingual musculature by carcinoma may also result in symptoms of burning as well as abnormalities of taste sensation.[12]

Oral cancer is seen predominantly in males and is generally a disease of the sixth and seventh decades. Poor oral hygiene and abuse of tobacco and alcohol are common associated findings. Although lesions of carcinoma can be seen affecting all areas of the oral mucosa, certain sites, such as the lip and tongue, are more common than others.[15]

The treatment of oral carcinoma at present involves surgery, radiation, chemotherapy or combination therapy. The success of the treatment depends upon the differentiation of the tissue and the extent of the tumor. As with malignant disease in other parts of the body, the survival rate following therapy for oral cancer is highest for small lesions detected early in development.

It is crucial, therefore, that all personnel, professional and paraprofessional, who are engaged in oral examination for any reason be aware of the presenting signs and symptoms of this disease and be highly suspicious of *any* intraoral abnormality. Since lesions in the mouth are generally superficial and accessible to examination, it should be possible to discover a great many early lesions. Referral for consultation and perhaps biopsy of such lesions might well be a life-saving procedure. Indeed, biopsy should be seriously considered in every case when an abnormal lesion, especially an ulcer, has been present for 2 weeks and does not show signs of improvement.

There are, of course, a great many benign tumors and tumor-like conditions that present as swellings of the face or mouth. They may be seen in all parts of the oral cavity and generally produce no interruption in function. Nevertheless all such pathology should be properly evaluated by professional personnel, and referral in *all* cases is indicated.

Subcutaneous emphysema

Submucosal or subcutaneous emphysema is an uncommon condition, where air is present in the subcutaneous tissues. It most frequently accompanies fractures of the zygoma or maxilla when the maxillary sinus is involved. Air may also be forced through a surgical incision or intraoral laceration by sneezing with the mouth closed or by forceful blowing, such as is seen when certain musical instruments are played. In addition, the condition may be iatrogenically produced if the air syringes commonly utilized in dentistry are not used with caution.

Clinically, a swelling of the face and/or neck of rather sudden onset will be seen. The tissues affected will have a spongy, crepitant feeling on palpation. The process is nontender, and systemic signs and symptoms are absent.

No treatment is necessary for this condition, as the air in the tissues will be absorbed spontaneously within a few days. A few words of reassurance to the patient would, of course, be in order.

REACTIONS TO LOCAL ANESTHESIA

Local anesthetics are the most commonly used drugs in dentistry. Literally hundreds of injections are given weekly by the average practitioner, with unbelievably few complications. In fact, the use of local anesthetics has become such a routine procedure in office practice that one is apt to ignore the possible hazards in their employment. However, complications do occasionally occur and may present as emergencies to the hospital. Some of the more common problems are discussed below. Discussions of systemic reactions, such as allergy and toxicity, will be omitted so that complications unique to local anesthetic injections in dentistry can be emphasized.

Facial paralysis

Penetration of the anesthetic solution into the parotid gland after a misdirected mandibular block can produce facial nerve paralysis, similar in appearance to Bell's palsy. This condition is characterized by inability to close the eyelid, obliteration of the nasolabial fold, dropping of the corner of the mouth and deviation of the mouth to the unaffected side.

This is a temporary condition, requiring no treatment except covering the eye to prevent corneal abrasion when the lid cannot be closed. The patch should remain in place for the duration of the paralysis.

Visual disorders

Temporary loss or blurring of vision (amaurosis) can follow any one of several different injections and results when anesthetic solution diffuses into the orbit and affects the optic nerve. The patient can be assured that the condition is transient, not serious and will subside when the effects of the anesthetic have worn off.

Transient paralysis of one or more of the extraocular muscles can follow some maxillary injections if the anesthetic solution diffuses into the orbit to affect the oculomotor nerve. This results in asynchronous ocular movements and temporary diplopia. No treatment other than reassurance is indicated.

Hematoma

Extravasation of blood into the tissues can result when a blood vessel is damaged during injection. This problem usually follows a posterior superior alveolar block, which is used to anesthetize maxillary molar teeth and results from damage to the posterior superior alveolar artery or the pterygoid venous plexus. Clinically, this hematoma presents as a rapidly enlarging swelling in the cheek.

If recognized quickly, excessive bleeding can be prevented by firm pressure over the region, along with use of ice packs. Otherwise, the condition is self-limiting, and the hematoma requires no immediate treatment. After 24 hours, hot, moist applications may aid in resolution of the swelling, which usually takes 3 to 5 days. Antibiotics are used only if signs of secondary infection appear. The patient should

be advised that the tissues in the area of the hematoma will change color as resolution occurs and that, despite a rather ominous appearance, the condition is not serious.

Tissue sloughing and ulceration

Sloughing and ulceration of the tissues are rare complications which may result from injecting excessive amounts of an anesthetic agent under a firmly attached mucosa or from the use of too high a concentration of vasoconstrictor in the anesthetic solution. Occasionally, especially in children, the lip or cheek may be chewed while anesthetized.

If painful, the lesions can be coated with tincture of benzoin, or a topical anesthetic can be applied. The healing area should be kept meticulously clean, but the use of irritating mouthwashes or antiseptics should be avoided. Antibiotic therapy is generally not indicated.

Trismus

Muscle soreness and difficulty in opening the mouth are commonly seen after an inferior alveolar nerve block, which is used to anesthetize mandibular teeth. This is usually caused by trauma to the medial pterygoid muscle, resulting in spasm of the muscle, or by the accidental injection of an irritating solution. Delayed trismus generally is the result of a needle tract infection.

These conditions are treated by hot saline mouth rinses and external hot, moist compresses. Antibiotics are used only if there are overt signs of infection. Gentle jaw exercise is helpful in limiting fibrosis and in reestablishing normal opening. In instances of infection, however, motion should be limited until the inflammatory process has been controlled.

Prolonged anesthesia or paresthesia

Persistent loss or alteration of sensation after a nerve block may be caused by trauma from the needle, hemorrhage into the neural sheath or, rarely, from a contaminant in the anesthetic solution.

There is no treatment for this condition. The patient should be advised that in most instances nerve regeneration will occur, although this may take 6 months or more.

TRAUMA TO THE FACE, MOUTH AND JAWS

Emergency treatment of patients with maxillofacial trauma is an important aspect of hospital practice. Professional personnel, including physicians, dentists and nurses, who are called on to evaluate and treat such patients must cooperate and work together so that a broad range of knowledge and experience will be available and correct therapy will be administered.

The treatment of traumatic injuries of the face, teeth and facial bones should be directed toward restoration of occlusion of the teeth, normal function of the jaws and normal appearance of the face. Careful attention must be given to every injury in this region, to minimize subsequent deformity. In few other injuries is the result so dependent on proper early care and meticulous attention to detail.[16]

General patient care

Unless associated with fractures of the skull, intracranial injuries or serious injuries to other parts of the body, even severe facial injuries are usually not life-threatening. Although definitive care of facial trauma should be instituted as soon as possible, management of this trauma should never take precedence over the general care of the patient. Therefore, initial attention should be directed to any concomitant condition, which if uncorrected might have serious or fatal consequences.

First priority must be given to establishment and maintenance of a patent airway, control of hemorrhage, management of shock and recognition and treatment of severe head injuries and trauma to the thorax or abdomen. Airway maintenance and control of hemorrhage are considered below. All other associated injuries are covered in other chapters in this text. The reader is particularly advised to consult Chapter 6 on triage, Chapter 9 on shock, Chapter 10 on tetanus prophylaxis, Chapter 16 on the comatose patient and the chapters covering the specific injuries encountered.

Airway maintenance

Since injuries about the face and jaws are likely to produce an obstruction of the upper airway, conditions that interfere with patency of the airway should be sought out and corrected without delay. Blood, in the form of active bleeding or blood clots in the oropharynx, must be controlled. The tongue may also be a threat to the airway, because in an unconscious patient, it may fall against the posterior pharyngeal wall. Foreign bodies, such as dentures, broken teeth, mucus, vomitus, are common causes of obstruction. Lastly, fractures of the maxilla can be displaced posteriorly and interfere with the airway, and mandibular fractures may result in loss of support for the tongue, permitting it to fall back into the oropharynx.

The most important sign of a compromised airway is labored, noisy respirations. For all intents and purposes, noisy breathing is obstructed breathing. Other signs of airway obstruction include gasping for breath, laryngeal stridor, restlessness and apprehension, cyanosis and circumoral pallor.

When signs of airway problems are encountered, immediate measures must be taken to relieve the obstruction. The tongue should be grasped and pulled forward, and the pharynx should be cleared of all foreign material. This may be done manually or with the use of forceps and suction. Once the airway has been cleared, it can be maintained by positioning the patient on his side, with the face up and the chin extended. The tongue can be held forward with an oral or nasal airway; then oxygen can be administered. If the above measures do not relieve the obstruction, consideration must be given to a tracheostomy or the insertion of an endotracheal tube.

Control of hemorrhage

Hemorrhage associated with facial injuries is seldom a serious problem. Although the blood vessels of the facial areas are numerous, they are small and well supplied with elastic fibers. When severed, they normally retract within bony canals and are occluded by thrombosis.[16] Thus, bleeding related to facial injuries usually stops spontaneously.

When bleeding does persist, it may be extraoral or intraoral. Since most extraoral hemorrhage is of the "seeping" or "oozing" type, the application of a firm pressure dressing over the involved region is usually all that is necessary to control the bleeding. If pressure dressings are ineffective, the margins of the wound must be retracted and the bleeding points identified, clamped and tied.

Intraoral bleeding is generally controlled by applying pressure with gauze to the bleeding area. When hemorrhage from fracture sites is extensive, it is managed by reducing the bony fragments which are then maintained in position with circumdental wires.

Care of soft tissue injuries

Although the management of facial fractures may be delayed, wounds to the soft tissues of the face should be treated, whenever possible, within a few hours after the injury. The patient is seldom injured so severely that early closure of facial lacerations cannot be accomplished. Early primary closure stimulates prompt healing, limits the degree of inflammatory reaction and minimizes subsequent development of scar tissue. In addition, such closure seals off avenues of contamination and, therefore, assists in the prevention and control of infection.[3]

When the general condition of the patient permits, reduction of facial fractures should be carried out prior to closure of the soft tissue wounds. If the soft tissues are closed first, the subsequent manipulative procedures necessary for reduction of the fractures frequently cause disruption of the wounds.[9] It is, therefore, imperative that oral surgical consultation be obtained at the outset of treatment.

Management of soft tissue injuries involves, first, proper cleansing and debridement of the wound. The area around the wound is scrubbed with surgical detergent soap and a brush. Then the area should be thoroughly lavaged with copious amounts of sterile saline. All hematomas should be removed. Radical debridement is not indicated; however, all necrotic and devitalized tissue should be meticulously removed, along with all foreign material. Rough, irregular, ragged or lacerated margins are then removed, and following complete hemostasis, the wound is closed in layers. Larger wounds are then completely covered by a firm pressure dressing.

Since all major maxillofacial wounds are contaminated, every effort must be made to prevent infection. Prevention is accomplished for the most part by strict adherence to sterile technique, thorough cleansing of the tissue, complete hemostasis, conservative but adequate debridement and wound closure that eliminates all dead spaces.[16] In addition, antibiotics are generally indicated in major trauma, especially if there is a communication with the oral cavity, which is, of course, contaminated. Penicillin in appropriate doses is generally the drug of choice. Naturally, a negative history of sensitivity must be obtained prior to administration.

Fractured or avulsed teeth

Patients with fractured or avulsed teeth should generally be seen immediately by a member of the dental service. The sooner the injured teeth are treated, the better the prognosis.[1] If only the enamel of the tooth is fractured, the patient is usually asymptomatic. The treatment is to smooth off the sharp edges, to prevent laceration of the tongue or lips. This is not necessarily an emergency.

If, however, the fracture of the crown of the tooth involves the dentin or the pulp, the tooth will be sensitive to touch and thermal changes, such as air passing over the tooth. In such cases, desensitization and restorative procedures must be carried out as soon as is reasonable.

Displaced or avulsed teeth will need substantially more treatment, including realignment or replacement with adequate splinting to stabilize the tooth for 6 weeks. This will require local anesthesia, professional attention and prolonged follow-up. Avulsed teeth should be kept moist in a clean handkerchief until the patient arrives at the hospital. Then the tooth should be placed in sterile saline.

No attempt should be made by nondental personnel to remove dirt or debris, as critical periodontal fibers still attached to the cementum of the tooth may be destroyed. Attention should be given to controlling hemorrhage in the mouth and to calming and reassuring both the patient and the family until professional help arrives.

Fractures of the facial bones

After the patient's general condition has been deemed satisfactory, a detailed examination is indicated to determine the extent of the facial injuries. Diagnosis of fractures is made from the information obtained from the history, clinical examination and roentgenographic studies. (See also Chapter 25, "Injuries of Bones, Joints and Related Soft-Tissue Structures.")

The history should include information regarding the time of injury, the type of accident, any loss of consciousness, prior treatment and associated medical problems. This information can be valuable in assessing the patient's general condition and in planning therapy.

Visual examination will often reveal conditions suggestive of a fracture. Edema, ecchymosis, obvious deformity, limited opening or deviation of the mandible on opening, obvious malocclusion and pain on movement of the jaws are suggestive signs and symptoms.

Intraoral examination will also reveal telltale signs of fracture, including lacerations of the oral mucosa, abnormal alignment of teeth, inability to bring the teeth into occlusion and independent movement of fragments when the patient attempts to bring the teeth into occlusion.

Digital examination will yield additional information. Extreme tenderness, inability to manually move the mandible through its normal excursions, palpable fracture lines, abnormal mobility of fragments and crepitus are indications of possible fracture.

Radiographs are reliable aids in the diagnosis of fractures. They must be adequate in quality and quantity to clearly demonstrate all fracture lines. To describe mandibular fractures, in addition to the standard facial series, the exaggerated Townes' position and temporomandibular joint films are often needed. Intraoral and occlusal views are also of value in certain cases. In maxillary and zygoma fractures, the Waters and vertex-submental views are most frequently utilized.

It should be noted that radiographs in general are not as helpful in diagnosing maxillary and zygomatic fractures as they are in evaluating mandibular trauma. This is related to the amount of superimposition in this area. To compensate, clinical evaluation must be that much more astute.

Clinical signs of fractures

The following list summarizes the signs which indicate facial fractures.

(1) *Pain.* After trauma, a fracture should be suspected when pain is elicited as the jaw is moved. However, pain is not always a reliable sign, since fractures of the maxilla and zygoma are accompanied by little or no pain.

(2) *Swelling.* Swelling is not a completely reliable sign of fracture, even though most traumatic injuries producing fractures are accompanied by swelling. Many traumatic injuries, however, produce swelling without concomitant fractures.

(3) *Hemorrhage.* When bleeding from the nose is encountered following an injury, suspicion of a fracture of the maxilla, zygoma or nasal bones is warranted.

(4) *Ecchymosis.* Ecchymosis is not constantly associated with fracture. However, when ecchymosis follows a traumatic injury, a thorough examination to determine whether a fracture has occurred is justified. Ecchymosis behind the ear over the mastoid process is known as Battle's sign and is usually associated with a basal skull fracture.

(5) *Crepitus.* The grating sound or sensation that is heard or felt when the ends of a fractured bone are brought into contact with each other is a reliable sign of fracture. However, manipulation of the fractured bone is usually accompanied by considerable pain, and since other less traumatic tests for fractures are available, the manual movement of fractured bones as a diagnostic procedure is seldom necessary.

(6) *Loss of function.* Inability to move the mandible through its normal excursions, as well as trismus and altered occlusal relationships are reliable signs of fracture.

(7) *Abnormal movement.* Mobility in any part of the facial bones other than at the temporomandibular joint is a reliable indication of fracture.

(8) *Displacements.* Grossly displaced fragments often produce facial deformities that are pathognomonic of fractures.

(9) *Malpositions.* Disruption of normal occlusion or malposition of various segments in the same arch are reliable signs of fracture.

(10) *Paresthesias.* After trauma, altered sensation is a suspicious sign. Paresthesia of the lower lip suggests a fracture of the body of the mandible, and infraorbital numbness is suggestive of a maxillary or zygomatic fracture.

(11) *Fluid seepage.* Loss of cerebrospinal fluid from the nose or ear is pathognomonic of fracture of the facial bones.

(12) *Other signs.* Periorbital edema, periorbital ecchymosis, subconjunctival hemorrhage and impaired ocular movements should arouse suspicion of zygomaticomaxillary complex fractures.[16]

When a facial fracture has been diagnosed, the nurse should attempt to make the patient comfortable, and immediate oral surgical consultation should be requested. Generally, the swelling and muscular trismus that frequently accompany fractures of the facial bones are very effective in limiting movement and, hence, tend to minimize pain. Manipulation of the fractures or attempts at mastication generally stimulate considerable pain and should be avoided.

Sedation is to be avoided until the condition of the patient is determined and an accurate diagnosis has been made. Heavy sedation will often mask signs of increased intracranial pressure. In the presence of associated head injuries, strong narcotics are to be avoided. Chloral hydrate may be used if sedation is necessary, and codeine sulfate is usually sufficient to control pain.[16]

Antibiotics should be considered in all cases, since most facial fractures are compounded into the mouth or the paranasal sinuses. Penicillin is generally the choice.

DISLOCATION OF THE TEMPOROMANDIBULAR JOINT

Dislocation of the temporomandibular joint occurs with relative frequency when the capsule and the temporomandibular ligament are sufficiently relaxed to allow the condyle to move anterior to the articular eminence during opening. Muscle contraction and spasm then lock the condyle into this position, so it is impossible for the patient to close his jaws to their normal occluding position. Dislocation may be unilateral or bilateral and may occur spontaneously following stretching of the mouth to its extreme open position, such as during a yawn or a routine dental operation.

Dislocations can usually be reduced by inducing downward pressure on the posterior teeth and upward pressure on the chin, accompanied by posterior displacement of the entire mandible. It is preferable for the operator to stand in front of the patient. Generally, reduction is not difficult. However, muscle spasm may occasionally be sufficient to prevent simple manipulation of the condyle back to its normal position, and it becomes necessary to obtain muscle relaxation to allow proper reduction of the condyle. This can be accomplished by the administration of a general anesthetic, supplemented, if necessary, by a muscle relaxant.[6]

ACUTE ORAL LESIONS

Acute lesions of the oral mucosa are not seen routinely, either in dental practice or in the hospital emergency department. When they do present, they must initially be recognized as such, so that they can be evaluated intelligently. The patient, at such time, may be in acute distress, and efforts must be extended to first relieve discomfort and then to begin the process of diagnosis.

There are, indeed, a great variety of conditions that present as an acute stomatitis. Burns, drug idiosyncrasies, infectious processes, dermatological disorders and oral manifestations of systemic diseases can all present with a chief complaint of a "sore mouth." Common initial symptoms, in addition to pain, include a tender mucosa which is generally reddened but may also exhibit whitish areas, due to necrosis of tissue, swollen and perhaps ulcerated gums and, in many cases, the presence of vesicles or ulcers on the mucosa.

Burns may be thermal, that is, related to hot foods (the hot pizza syndrome), or they may have a chemical etiology. One of the most common chemical burns seen by dentists is caused when aspirin has been topically applied by a patient to the mucosa next to an aching tooth. A whitish area of tissue necrosis is produced, which will slough off, leaving a reddened, ulcerated base. Chemical burns may also be produced by phenol, commercial toothache drops and other caustic agents.

Local reactions to drugs or materials used in contact with the oral mucosa are termed "stomatitis venenata." These reactions are occasionally related to mouth washes, dentifrices, lozenges and acrylic, the plastic material used to construct dentures. "Stomatitis medicamentosa" refers to the oral mucosal reaction related to drugs administered systemically. Antibiotics, sulfonamides, salicylates and halogens have all been causative in this type of reaction.[7] The oral mucosa and gingivae may become ulcerated, swollen and very painful.

Viral, bacterial and fungal diseases can all produce disabling oral infections. Such systemic diseases as herpes simplex, tuberculosis, syphilis, histoplasmosis, moniliasis and others can be associated with serious oral lesions, in addition to systemic manifestations. Vesicles and ulcers are the most common oral signs.

Acute necrotizing gingivitis, also known as Vincent's infection or trench mouth, is a common local bacterial infection of the oral cavity. It is a nontransmissible inflammatory disease of the gingivae, caused by a combination of lowered resistance of the patient and local irritation, with superimposition of Vincent's organisms (fusiform bacilli and spirochetes) normally found in the oral cavity. In the acute phase, there is swelling, ulceration, bleeding and pain primarily in gingival tissues. Systemic signs of infection may be noted.

"Aphthous stomatitis" (canker sores) may occur in any area of the mouth. The lesions are the most painful ulcerations of the oral cavity and are characterized as being of varying sizes and yellow-white in color and as possessing margins which are erythematous and indurated. The ulcers are present for about a week and heal completely in 10 to

14 days without scarring. The etiology of the condition is speculative.

Dermatological disorders, such as Erythema multiforme, Pemphigus vulgaris, lupus erythematosus and others, may affect the oral mucosa in addition to the skin. Clinically, in the oral cavity, they present as vesicles, bullae or ulcers that are prolonged and associated with systemic signs of infection and generalized disease.

Oral manifestations can be noted with a number of systemic diseases, such as diabetes mellitus, vitamin deficiencies, blood dyscrasias and renal failure. The lesions are nonspecific, unhealing unless the primary disease is controlled and frequently accompanied by spontaneous bleeding from the gums and other parts of the oral mucosa.

It should, indeed, be obvious that a great variety of conditions can present as a "sore mouth," and making a definitive diagnosis in many instances is a significant task. Emergency management, however, is less complicated. The patient should be treated with sympathy and reassurance. Mild analgesics and topical anesthetics may be utilized to reduce pain. A soft, bland diet should be suggested and fluids encouraged. Bed rest is indicated, along with warm saline mouth rinses, which of necessity must be substituted for normal oral hygiene. Consultation or referral should then be undertaken.

Acute lesions of the oral mucosa usually heal completely in 2 weeks time. If this does not happen, further investigation, including biopsy, will probably be in order.

SUMMARY

The modern general hospital is faced with an amazing variety of urgent situations. Dental emergencies are not the most glamorous or dramatic, but they do occur with monotonous regularity. Unfortunately, hospital physicians and nurses generally have little orientation toward dentistry and are able to do little in behalf of these patients.

In this chapter, information regarding many phases of dentally related problems has been presented. It is hoped that it will aid in the management of emergency patients and that it will promote consultation and a sincere spirit of cooperation between physicians, dentists and nursing personnel.

BIBLIOGRAPHY

(1) Andrews, R.: "Injured Anterior Teeth," *in* F. McCarthy (ed.), *Emergencies in Dental Practice,* ed. 2 (Philadelphia: W. B. Saunders Company, 1972), Chapter 18.

(2) Bell, W.: *Synopsis of Oral and Facial Pain and the Temporomandibular Joint* (Dallas: published by the author, 1967).

(3) Chipps, J.; Canham, R., and Makel, H.: "Intermediate Treatment of Maxillofacial Injuries," *U.S. Armed Forces Medical Journal,* 4 (1953):951.

(4) Friedrich, R.; Gambuti, G., and Linz, A.: "Role of the Hospital in the Future of Dental Education," *Journal of Oral Surgery,* 25 (1967):47.

(5) Glickman, I.: *Clinical Periodontology,* ed. 4 (Philadelphia: W. B. Saunders Company, 1972).

(6) Henny, F.: "The Temporomandibular Joint," *in* G. Kruger (ed.), *Textbook of Oral Surgery,* ed. 4 (Saint Louis: C. V. Mosby Company, 1974), Chapter 20.

(7) Huebsch, R.: "Acute Oral Lesions," *in* F. McCarthy (ed.), *Emergencies in Dental Practice,* ed. 2 (Philadelphia: W. B. Saunders Company, 1972), Chapter 21.

(8) Irby, W., and Baldwin, K.: *Emergencies and Urgent Complications in Dentistry* (Saint Louis: C. V. Mosby Company, 1965).

(9) Kruger, G.: "Fractures of the Jaws," *in* G. Kruger (ed.), *Textbook of Oral Surgery,* ed. 4 (Saint Louis: C. V. Mosby Company, 1974), Chapter 19.

(10) Kruger, G., and Reynolds, D.: "Maxillofacial Pain," *in* F. McCarthy (ed.), *Emergencies in Dental Practice,* ed. 2 (Philadelphia: W. B. Saunders Company, 1972), Chapter 20.

(11) Laskin, D.: "Treatment of Common Emergencies of the Hospital Dental Patient," *in* B. Douglas (ed.), *Introduction to Hospital Dentistry,* ed. 2 (Saint Louis: C. V. Mosby Company, 1970), Chapter 12.

(12) McCarthy, P., and Shklar, G.: *Diseases of the Oral Mucosa* (New York: McGraw-Hill Book Company, 1964).

(13) Mandel, L.: "Salivary Gland Disease," paper read at St. John's Hospital, Queens, N.Y., April 19, 1974.

(14) Moose, S.: "Acute Infections of the Oral Cavity," *in* G. Kruger (ed.), *Textbook of Oral Surgery,* ed. 4 (Saint Louis: C. V. Mosby Company, 1974), Chapter 11.

(15) Shafer, W.; Hine, M., and Levy, B.: *A Textbook of Oral Pathology,* ed. 2 (Philadelphia: W. B. Saunders Company, 1963).

(16) Shira, R.: "Emergency Treatment of Patients with Facial Trauma," *in* B. Douglas (ed.), *Introduction to Hospital Dentistry,* ed. 2 (Saint Louis: C. V. Mosby Company), Chapter 13.

(17) Sweet, W.: "Trigeminal Neuralgias," *in* C. Alling (ed.), *Facial Pain* (Philadelphia: Lea & Febiger, 1968).

29

Acquiring donor organs for transplantation

ALBERT D. MENNO
DIANN ANDERSON

HISTORICAL CONSIDERATIONS

The use of human tissues in one human being from the body of another is largely a twentieth century development. Many slow, progressive steps were taken in the latter half of the nineteenth century, mostly with various methods of transplanting skin. Among several skin transplant surgeons, Thiersch, in 1874, described the microscopic details of how a graft "took," that is, how the graft adhered in its new bed. A similar period of development occurred with corneal transplantation, beginning in 1884.

It was not until 1943, however, that Gibson and Medawar first appreciated the significance of the *source* of tissue for transplantation and initiated research on the immunological reactions that occurred in allografting and xenografting.* Organ transplantation, because of technical difficulties, was not attempted until the first decade of the twentieth century, at a time when vascular surgery was just coming of age. Success was only short-term, however, until the classical work of

* Definitions of terms will follow.

Medawar, which described the standard rejection reaction occurring in transplantation of tissues and its variations.

The first successful transplantation with prolonged survival occurred in 1955, when a human kidney was taken from one person and transplanted in an identical twin. Since then, approximately 2,500 kidneys have been transplanted in the United States, and at least 5 times that number have been transplanted worldwide. Other tissues which have been transplanted, with varying degrees of success, include blood vessels, bone, blood, skin, cornea, lung, heart, intestine, endocrine glands, marrow and liver.

IMPLICATIONS FOR EMERGENCY NURSES

Although its history has been brief, transplantation of organs is now common in the practice of many medical specialties. Nurses in a wide variety of settings are caring for patients who have undergone transplant procedures, such as skin grafts, corneal transplants, kidney transplants and, in some locales, heart and liver transplants.

The nurse in an emergency setting is not frequently involved in care of patients during or following transplantation procedures. Skin grafting for a wound is probably the most notable exception. More often, emergency nursing centers around the care of a possible donor, the emotional support of his family or the mechanisms for acquiring permission to obtain donor organs from the family of a dying patient. In addition, the nurse may serve as a facilitator and liaison person among those concerned with the acquisition, transport and maintenance or storage of donor organs.

Thus, part of the nurses's responsibility may include the initial handling and storage of donor organs until they can be transported to the appropriate location. In other instances, where the donor organ must be supported in vivo, the nurse may become involved in life-support measures of the dying patient to provide adequate perfusion of the donor organ(s) until the necessary arrangements can be made. The specific nursing responsibilities will depend a great deal on where the nurse practices and the types of transplants done in that area. Since this varies widely, it is advisable for each emergency nurse to become acquainted with the community and regional resources available for procuring, storing and transplanting various donor organs.

TERMINOLOGY

Terms have evolved over the years to express the relationship of the donor source to the recipient. An understanding of the following terminology is necessary to comprehend the variety of transplants that can be done.

The transplantation of any tissue or organ from one place in a given individual to another place in the *same individual* has been called an "isograft" in older literature and an "autograft" in more modern literature. The trans-plantation of any tissue or organ from one individual to another individual of the *same species* has been called a "homograft" in older literature and an "allograft" more recently. The transplantation of any tissue or organ from an individual of one species to an individual of *another species* has been called a "heterograft" in the past and a "xenograft" in more recent literature.

Under normal circumstances, autografts do not involve immunological reactions. Success is more dependent on mechanical factors, such as the size of vessels, characteristics of the donor organ and the recipient space for the organ. Xenografts and allografts, on the other hand, involve very clear-cut immunological reactions, and success is dependent on both mechanical factors and the degree of similarity or difference between the donor and the recipient (see "Tissue-Typing").

KIDNEY TRANSPLANTS

Kidney transplantation is a common type of transplant, and the matching of donor kidneys to potential recipients has been well organized. For these reasons, this chapter will provide a framework for understanding this one type of transplantation and how it is facilitated through a network of mutual cooperation. Similarities and differences which exist among the various types of organ transplants are outlined later in the chapter.

Selection of the donor

Whenever siblings, parents or children of patients are available, an attempt is usually made to use one as the source of the kidney for transplantation. These donations are usually completely elective and dependent on a detailed study of the function of the donor organ, in addition to its tissue match to the recipient.

A problem arises when a relative is not available, not willing or not physically healthy enough to donate an organ; a cadaver becomes the only possible source for a kidney. Cadaver kidneys, however, are rarely used in children.

Size and age factors

The practical limit on youth of a donor of a kidney for use in adults is dependent primarily on the size of the organ rather than on the age. In the average-size child, the limit falls at 7 to 8 years. The kidney at this age is almost always large enough to sustain a small- to average-size adult; evidence shows the organ rapidly enlarges within the first few weeks after transplantation.

Although transplantation has occurred from donors as old as 75 years of age, the common practical age limit for adult donors is approximately 50 to 55 years. Individuals older than this commonly have sufficient sclerosis of the aorta or renal arteries to make the anastomosis of the artery technically very difficult. In addition, organs beyond this age are more likely to have undesirable vascular changes, glomerular changes or pyelonephritic fibrosis. A rapid, complete evaluation of function on such donors would be necessary if they are to be considered seriously at all.

Cadaver donors

The usual donor of cadaver kidneys is most likely to fall between the ages of 15 and 45, due to the prevalence of automobile accidents, the producer of most cadavers at those ages. The most appropriate cadaver donor for organs is one with an almost pure, severe cerebral injury; however, most severely injured patients have multiple injuries.

Dying patients with injuries of the extremities can be considered, but those with a potentially contaminated abdomen, as from recent surgery, leakage of intestinal content or obvious peritonitis, should be avoided. Whenever there is suspicion of renal injury, such as mild gross hematuria or microscopic hematuria, an I.V.P. should be done to prove the integrity of the kidneys. Many contused but not otherwise damaged kidneys can be salvaged by this maneuver.

Most transplant surgeons presently avoid cadaver donors with injuries resulting from criminal assault or when a criminal charge is pending against a party of the associated accident. A suicide victim may be used, depending on the attitude of the medical examiner in the locality and if the suicide is clear-cut and unquestioned.

A good working relationship with the coroner or medical examiner is absolutely essential. Whenever a potential donor becomes available, it should be the custom to call the coroner or medical examiner to be sure he sees no medicolegal impediment to salvaging the kidneys.

It is necessary to transplant only one healthy kidney to maintain a person who is otherwise without kidney function. Therefore, when a cadaver donor becomes available and both kidneys can be salvaged, 2 different recipients may receive a kidney simultaneously, often in 2 separate hospitals, each with their own transplant teams. Obviously, a closely knit communications network is necessary to coordinate all these activities. Since 4 to 6 hours are necessary for tissue typing (discussed below), the person who arrives dead (DOA) or dies shortly after arrival at the hospital is usually not considered a donor candidate unless an organ perfusion apparatus is available. Local practice governs what can be done. A few transplant centers are willing to salvage kidneys from a recent DOA donor, place them in supportive perfusion and assess their function for possible use. More often, kidneys are used from patients who die a short time after arrival. Such kidneys are placed on a perfuser before transplantation.

Belzer initially developed a perfusion apparatus that circulates serum made from AB negative blood through the refrigerated kidney. Although clinically capable of sustaining the kidney for 72 hours, it is more commonly used for periods of 10 to 18 hours.

Several similar machines are now on the market. The use of an organ perfuser is desirable for a number of reasons:

(1) Sustaining the organ while tissue-typing is being completed.
(2) Obtaining more time for recipient preparation.

(3) Providing a means of testing the functional viability of the organ after salvage and before recipient implantation.
(4) Transporting the organ over long distances.

Salvaging the organs

In the past few years, salvaging kidneys from cadavers has become a very highly organized procedure. This is necessary, because with death and cessation of cardiac action, circulation through the kidney ceases. The absence of renal blood flow from the time of death until vascular anastomosis is completed in the recipient is called the "ischemia time." The total ischemia time is the sum of the "warm" and "cold" ischemia times.

It is generally accepted that no more than 45 minutes should elapse from the time of death to the time when the kidney is cooled to near-freezing temperatures. This is the warm ischemia time. Three and a half to 4 hours are allowed to place the donor kidney in the recipient, anastomose the renal artery and vein to the recipient vessels and reestablish blood flow. This is the cold ischemia time. Generally, the shorter the warm ischemia time, the longer the donor kidney can tolerate the total time of ischemia. When the warm ischemia time is as little as 10 minutes, the surgeon can work with approximately 10 *hours* of tolerance to total ischemia.

The donor kidneys are removed by surgeons in an operating suite, under sterile conditions. Once the blood vessels are divided, arterial perfusion is initiated, using a solution which has been cooled to 4° C. (see Figure 29–1). This perfusion is effected by gravity only; it flushes out the renal arteries and veins, rinsing out all the blood and cooling the kidney from within. The fluid most commonly used is a 5 percent glucose/Ringer's lactate solution with 50 mg. of heparin and 1.0 gm. of procaine added. A special solution, somewhat similar but with additional magnesium and dibenzyline, is preferred. It can be prepared by the hospital pharmacy.

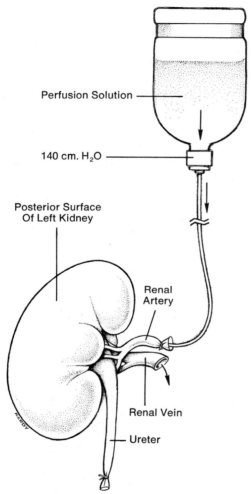

Perfusion Solution

140 cm. H$_2$O

Posterior Surface Of Left Kidney

Renal Artery

Renal Vein

Ureter

Figure 29–1 Technique of kidney perfusion. Sterile intravenous tubing is inserted into the main renal artery and held in place by a suture tied around the exterior of the artery. The perfusion solution (4° C. lactated Ringer's, with 50 mg. heparin and 1 gm. procaine per liter) is raised to a height of 140 cm. of water above the donor kidney and allowed to run through the kidney by force of gravity. The cut end of the renal vein is open, to allow the fluid to flow from the kidney.

After 500 to 1,000 cc. are flushed through each kidney, they are placed in sterile plastic bags, then in a one to 2 liter nalgene jar and transferred in styrofoam-insulated cartons (Polyfoam Packers) to the recipient hospital. Each kidney should be labeled "left" or "right," since, for technical reasons, it is desirable to place a right kidney in a left iliac fossa and vice versa.

Tissue-typing

The success of autotransplantation is dependent, in part, on matching compatible donors and recipients by tissue-typing. This is a most delicate procedure, requiring 4 to 6 hours to complete. It involves the collection of 20 to 25 cc. of blood, which is defibrinated and passed through a column of resin material to separate out the lymphocytes. The lymphocytes are then tested with antisera, and the positive reactions are noted. In this manner, the HL-A (human lymphocytic antigen) type of the donor is identified and compared with that of all possible recipients until a match is found.

Terasaki, among others, classified the antisera used in typing.[9] Formerly, as many as 200 might be used in a single typing. With the work of Teresaki and others, it was possible to define human lymphocyte antigens reacting against groups of antisera. Presently, there are 13 groups of transplantation antigens accepted and used internationally in tissue-typing. Many more are being used by various immunologists throughout the world, who are engaged in various stages of analysis of these antigens. Undoubtedly, some of these may later become accepted. Those fully accepted bear the designation "HL-A" (human lymphocyte antigen) plus a number.

Only those antigens within the "HL-A" system are significant for the purposes of transplantation. They are present on all somatic body cells, but the lymphocyte, being a readily available "circulating cell," is used as typical for testing purposes. The lymphocyte is also a mediator in the immunological response of rejection, making its choice as the model cell all the more significant. From the technical standpoint, difficulties sometimes arise because of inability to separate the lymphocytes from other white blood cells, particularly after trauma, when excessive numbers of polymorphonuclear leukocytes may be present.

The red cell ABO antigens, so well known in blood crossmatching for compatibility, are also most important to match in transplants. These are very strong antigens which can evoke massive, rapid and acute responses in the recipient within minutes of exposure to them. This phenomenon is called "hyperacute rejection." Mismatching in the ABO system dooms the transplant to failure.

On the other hand, the red cell Rh antigen is very weak and of little significance. It is usually completely ignored when matching donors to recipients, and no transplant rejections are known to have resulted from ignoring this antigen.

Medicolegal considerations

Almost all states have now adopted a *Uniform Anatomical Gift Act,* stating: (1) an individual of age 18 or older can, prior to his death, consent to the removal of any or all organs from his own body after death and can carry a signed, witnessed card to that effect; (2) only the most available ranking next of kin need sign a consent for removal of organs from a dead relative for transplantation (whereas *all* of the ranking next of kin must sign for postmortem examinations); and (3) a state of "cerebral death" acceptable to both medical and legal communities can be determined when 5 criteria are met.

The 5 criteria for cerebral death, all of which must be present, are: (1) the absence of spontaneous respirations, (2) the absence of all reflexes, (3) dilated fixed pupils, (4) a completely flat electroencephalogram, taken on 2 occasions 24 hours apart and (5) an unstable blood pressure. *All 5 criteria must be present* for "cerebral death" to be declared (obviously with the consent of the family) in hopeless situations so that salvage of the kidneys can be accomplished and the respirator turned off in an acceptable legal manner.

For consent to be signed by relatives, a standard consent form, specifying the operative procedure as "removal of (specified organ) after death for transplantation purposes" is all that is required. For the individual over 18 who wishes to sign his own consent, a card is presently available from headquarter offices, National Kidney Foundation, which can be carried in the wallet (see Figure 29–2). It must be signed by 2 witnesses. This card then represents the complete legal consent form in itself and can be used even when relatives cannot be contacted. Such cards are now acceptable in all 50 states. It specifies whether certain organs, all available and desired organs or the entire body may be used for scientific purposes.

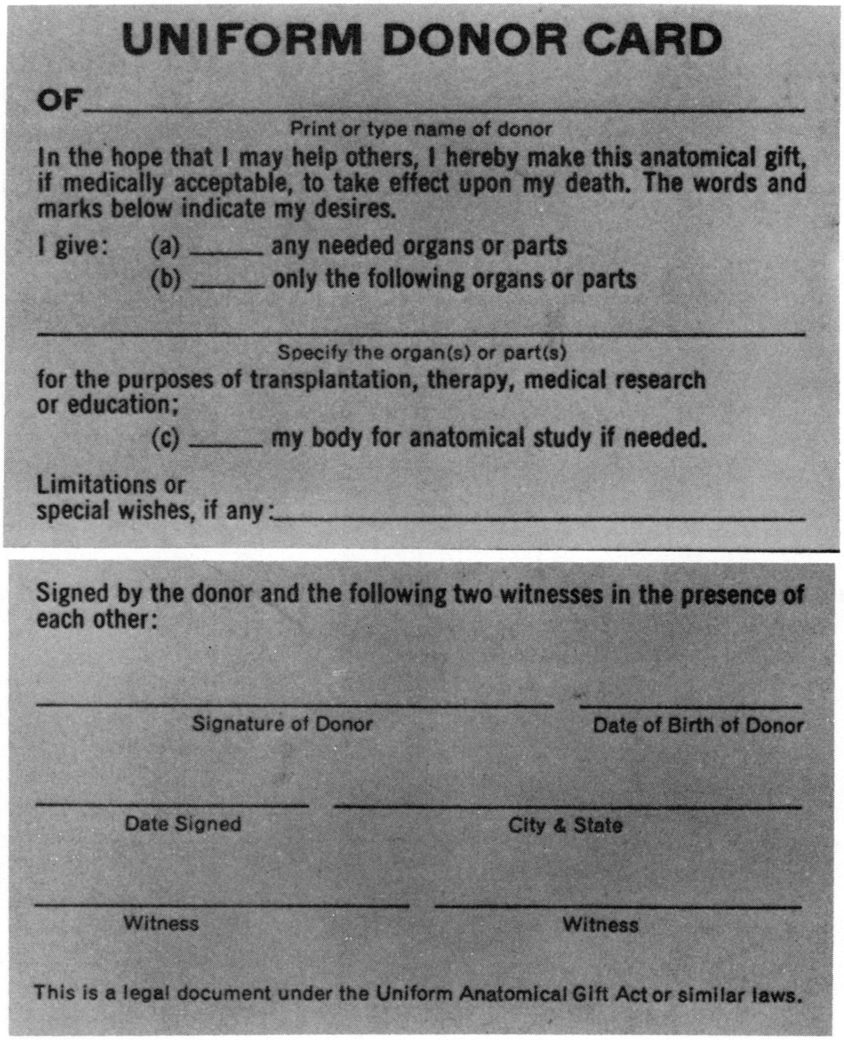

UNIFORM DONOR CARD

OF ______________________

Print or type name of donor

In the hope that I may help others, I hereby make this anatomical gift, if medically acceptable, to take effect upon my death. The words and marks below indicate my desires.

I give: (a) ____ any needed organs or parts

(b) ____ only the following organs or parts

____

Specify the organ(s) or part(s)

for the purposes of transplantation, therapy, medical research or education;

(c) ____ my body for anatomical study if needed.

Limitations or special wishes, if any: ______________________

Signed by the donor and the following two witnesses in the presence of each other:

______________________ Signature of Donor

______________________ Date of Birth of Donor

______________________ Date Signed

______________________ City & State

______________________ Witness

______________________ Witness

This is a legal document under the Uniform Anatomical Gift Act or similar laws.

Figure 29–2 Legal consent for donation of an organ or body part. This form is a legal document, when properly completed, under the Uniform Anatomical Gift Act and similar laws.

Establishing a system to facilitate transplants

A community-wide communication system is essential for matching donor kidneys to needed recipients. This system must possess at least 2 capabilities: (1) rapidly informing appropriate sources that donor kidneys have been obtained and (2) providing a continuously updated list of needed recipients and related information. While system differences exist, depending on locale, the model discussed below is common to many areas. The reader is best advised to become familiar with the procedure in her own locale by contacting the nearest hospital known to be transplanting organs of any type, contacting the regional chapter of the National Kidney Foundation or contacting the chairman of the department of surgery of the nearest medical school.

The operation of one system

In upstate New York and southern Ontario, lines of communication have been developed, as shown in the accompanying diagram (Figure 29-3). The hospitals involved supply representatives on rotation to receive calls from hospitals with potential donors, arrange for tissue-typing, select appropriate recipients and salvage kidneys in hospitals anywhere in the region. In addition, a continuously updated list is circulated to participating hospitals, containing names of potential recipients who have previously been tissue-typed, their ABO types and the names of their attending physicians. The salvaged kidneys are sent to the best-matched recipients, preferably in 2 different hospitals. When many equally matched recipients are found, the patients who have been waiting the longest are given preference.

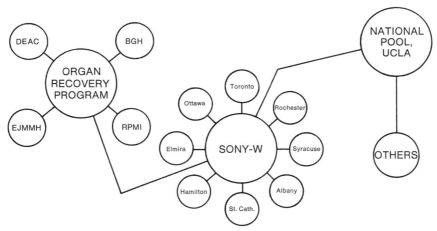

Figure 29-3 Interlinkage of transplant centers. When a donor kidney becomes available, physicians on call to the Buffalo organ recovery program proceed to the hospital where the patient is and salvage the kidneys. Tissue-typing is completed, and the kidneys are made available to compatible recipients. If a good match is not obtained locally, contact is made with the SONY-W listing in Rochester, which includes the cities shown in the illustration above. If a satisfactory match is still not obtained, the national pool at UCLA (University of California at Los Angeles) is contacted.
Key: DEAC-Deaconess Hospital; EJMMH-E. J. Meyer Memorial Hospital; RPMI-Roswell Park Memorial Institute; BGH-Buffalo General Hospital; SONY-W-Southern Ontario–Western New York. Each circle around SONY-W represents a city: Buffalo, Rochester, Syracuse, Albany, Elmira in New York State and St. Catherines, Hamilton, Ottawa and Toronto in Canada.

When one kidney or both kidneys cannot be used locally because of poor match, contact is made with the SONY-West listing in Rochester, New York. This is an organization formed by representatives from hospitals in Buffalo, Rochester, Albany and Syracuse, New York, in addition to Hamilton, Toronto, St. Catherines and Burlington, Ontario. SONY-West supplies a listing of the recipients in this larger area. Problems with custom officials are averted through proper notification by telephone and transportation provided by state and provincial police.

If no suitable recipient match is found within this larger area, similar contact may be made with a more distant regional listing such as that located in Los Angeles, California. This listing contains a large number of patients in California and other western states, in addition to some in foreign countries.

OTHER TRANSPLANTABLE ORGANS

Cornea

The next most publicized transplantable tissue is the cornea, though this was actually transplanted long before the kidney. Indeed, the patterning of the renal "organ recovery" programs follows the patterns set forth by the eye banks in many areas of the country.

Corneal transplant has several unique advantages. The first is that of time, since several hours are available from the time of death to the time when the cornea must be salvaged, treated with antibiotic and saline solutions and cooled. This allows for obtaining consent from relatives and preparing the recipient. Secondly, there are no agonal physiological changes in the cornea that limit its capabilities after transplantation. Thus, the corneas from a person who is DOA may be salvaged. Thirdly, no tissue-typing is necessary, since the cornea acquires no vascularization after transplantation. Indeed, its function requires that it *not* become vascularized; thus, there is no way for tissue-antibodies to reach it.

The most important activity to be taken by the nurse when cornea salvage is a possibility is taping the lids of the donor closed, to prevent drying. All remaining steps should be taken by a representative of the local eye bank, who should be called immediately. He has about 3 hours to complete the salvage.

Skin and bone

Skin and bone are the tissues which presently can be "banked" in the strict sense of the word. Both are stored by cleansing and rinsing in saline solutions, treated with antibiotics, and freezing. Both skin and bone are removed as soon after death as convenient. No time limit is presently stated, although 12 to 24 hours is a practical limit. Only diseased tissues or tissues with tumors in them need be excluded from salvage.

Of all organs used, bone creates the least problem in transplantation, because eventually it is completely replaced by the recipient's own tissues and merely acts as a strut and a source for calcium. No attempt is ever made to tissue-type the donor or the recipient for this type of transfer.

Skin is handled very similarly and is presently most useful for transplantation in burned patients. For this purpose, it mainly acts as an organic dressing to prevent the problems that occur with infiltration of bacteria into the burn wound. When it is used solely in this fashion, there is usually no attempt at tissue-typing, as it is expected that it eventually will slough and disappear. Organic dressings allow the burned patient to recover more completely and to regenerate sites on his own body where skin may be obtained for an autograft. (See Chapter 17, "Care of the Burned Patient.")

When the allografted skin is intended to become permanently attached, tissue-typing is necessary. A relative is usually a good donor for skin transfer. Well-organized skin and bone banks exist in many metropolitan areas, as well.

Blood vessels

Salvage of blood vessels has become very unimportant in recent years because of the availability of prosthetic vessels. But, whenever natural vessels are desirable, the saphenous vein is usually chosen, and an autograft is done.

Aortic valves or aortic valve cusps are presently being used as allografts in open heart surgery. These are salvaged and stored by the individual surgeons who use them, usually from cadavers within their own institutions. They are rinsed in saline solutions, treated with antibiotics and frozen, much as bone and skin are handled. No tissue-typing is necessary, since they merely act as struts in the formation of new cusps within the aorta.

Other organs

At the present time, transplants of endocrine glands, marrow and spleen are being done only in isolated institutions. No detailed information is presently available regarding widespread usage of these donor organs.

Transplantation of lung, heart and liver is presently widely publicized but always extremely difficult to perform. Each of these organs can be sustained outside the body for only short periods of time and always only with the use of pump oxygenators during the transfer between the cadaver and the recipient. Therefore, salvage from patients dying within the institution where the transplantation will occur is most practical. Portable perfusion techniques are being perfected, however, to thwart this limitation.

Lung, heart and liver transplants are being performed presently in very few centers in any one country, and tissue-typing is always necessary. The success rate with these organs is presently only mediocre, due to inability to control immunological reactions.

SUMMARY

The transplantation of human tissues occurs every day in the United States. The tissues most commonly used are skin, corneas and kidneys. While some tissues may be preserved and stored for long periods of time, others such as the kidneys must be implanted in the recipient within a matter of hours.

In many areas of the United States, transplant centers are established. Many of these centers are linked across the country to allow for complete utilization of donor organs as they become available. The emergency nurse should familiarize herself with the transplantation services available in or near her region, help establish procedures to obtain suitable organs for human transplantation and facilitate their use.

The Uniform Anatomical Gift Act has been enacted in most states. Many persons carry uniform donor cards. When properly completed and witnessed, such a card constitutes a legal document. Consideration must be given, however, to which persons are and are not suitable as organ donors.

The primary limiting factor in transplantation is the availability of donor organs. The emergency nurse can play an important role by being aware of a seriously injured patient as a potential organ donor after death. When such a patient is seen in the emergency department, she should initiate measures aimed at facilitating the acquisition of usable organs.

BIBLIOGRAPHY

(1) Alexander, J. W., and Good, R. A.: *Immunobiology for Surgeons* (Philadelphia: W. B. Saunders Company, 1970).

(2) Brooks, J. R.: *Endocrine Tissue Transplantation* (Springfield, Ill.: Charles C Thomas, 1962).

(3) Juul-Jensen, Palle: *Criteria of Brain Death* (Copenhagen, Denmark: Munksgaard Company, 1970).

(4) Menno, A. D., and Giordano, M. L.: "The Operation of the Kidney Bank of Buffalo," *Cryobiology,* 7 (September–October 1970):179.

(5) Moore, F. D.: *Give and Take* (Philadelphia: W. B. Saunders Company, 1964).

(6) Rappaport, F. T., and Dausset, J.: *Human Transplantation* (New York: Grune & Stratton Company, 1968).

(7) Starzl, T.: *Experience in Renal Transplantation* (Philadelphia: W. B. Saunders Company, 1964).

(8) Starzl, T. E.; Porter, K. A.; Husberg, B. S.; Ishikawa, M., and Putnam, C. W.: *Renal Homotransplantation in Current Problems in Surgery* (Chicago: Yearbook Medical Publishers, 1974).

(9) Terasaki, P.: *Histocompatibility Testing* (Baltimore: Williams & Wilkins Company, 1970).

index